Transforming essential principles into practical nursing skills

Clinical nursing skills from Oxford will take you, step-by-step, from student to nurse, giving you the knowledge to perform clinical skills with accuracy and confidence.

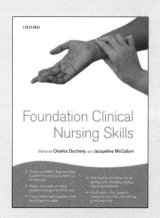

Starting with *Foundation Clinical Nursing Skills* for first years and working your way up through the series you'll find essential background theory explained and supported with evidence-based rationale. Each clinical skill is set out in a step-by-step process, richly illustrated with diagrams and photographs, whilst a range of scenarios help you apply theory to practice.

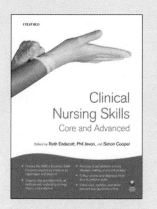
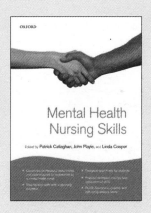
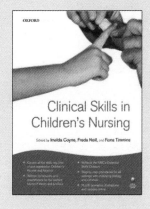

Visit the website to reinforce your learning, with tips, exercises, video examples, to prepare you for placement and exams

www.oxfordtextbooks.co.uk/orc/clinicalnursingskills

Smart nursing from Oxford

Clinical Skills in Children's Nursing

EDITED BY

Imelda Coyne
Freda Neill
Fiona Timmins

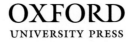

OXFORD
UNIVERSITY PRESS

OXFORD

UNIVERSITY PRESS

Great Clarendon Street, Oxford OX2 6DP

Oxford University Press is a department of the University of Oxford.
It furthers the University's objective of excellence in research, scholarship,
and education by publishing worldwide in

Oxford New York

Auckland Cape Town Dar es Salaam Hong Kong Karachi
Kuala Lumpur Madrid Melbourne Mexico City Nairobi
New Delhi Shanghai Taipei Toronto

With offices in

Argentina Austria Brazil Chile Czech Republic France Greece
Guatemala Hungary Italy Japan Poland Portugal Singapore
South Korea Switzerland Thailand Turkey Ukraine Vietnam

Oxford is a registered trade mark of Oxford University Press
in the UK and in certain other countries

Published in the United States
by Oxford University Press Inc., New York

© Oxford University Press 2010

The moral rights of the authors have been asserted
Database right Oxford University Press (makers)

First published 2010

British Library Cataloguing in Publication Data
Data available

Library of Congress Cataloging in Publication Data
Data available

Typeset by MPS Limited, A Macmillan Company
Printed in Italy
on acid-free paper by L.E.G.O. S.p.A

ISBN 978-0-19-955903-9

10 9 8 7 6 5 4 3 2 1

Preface

This book addresses the clinical skills component of pre-registration children's nurse education. Clinical skills are a fundamental component of nursing curricula that prepare practitioners for practice. Clinical skill competency requirements are usually outlined in regulatory guidelines such as the Nursing and Midwifery Council UK (Essential skills clusters).

The primary readership for this text is undergraduate pre-registration nursing students studying on a children's branch of the programme, or adult branch nursing students undertaking their children's module.

Our impetus for writing this is the perceived need for a comprehensive integrated textbook that will provide up-to-date, detailed information on clinical skills for children's nurses. Children's nurses now undertake more advanced clinical and technological skills and therefore need a textbook that clearly illustrates the essential skills and the rationale for each skill.

However, the aim of this book is to provide a resource that will truly meet the needs of children's nursing students in content and style. The book is written in such a way as to aid learning and recall in the clinical environment, helping the student to attain competency. It has been written to meet the unique needs of children's nurses by taking a family centred approach.

This book has been edited by Prof. Imelda Coyne, who is Head of Children's Nursing Discipline and Associate Professor in Nursing at Trinity College Dublin. She has over twenty years' experience in children's nursing and has published widely in the field. Freda Neill, co-editor, is Clinical Skills Manager at Trinity College Dublin and has extensive experience in Health Visiting and Public Health. She currently manages the Clinical Skills Centre for Nursing and Midwifery at Trinity College Dublin, and has published and presented in the area of clinical skills. Dr Fiona Timmins, a Senior Lecturer at Trinity College Dublin and a general nurse specializing in Intensive and Coronary, has extensive experience in writing for publication.

It has been a great pleasure for us to draw this book together and we hope that you enjoy reading this book and find it useful. All information is correct at time of publication; however, we are cognisant of continual changes to practices in the field and policy changes at both local and national level. In light of this we will be offering you updates and further information at ⓦ **http://www.oxfordtextbooks.co.uk**.

Professor Imelda Coyne
Ms Freda Neill
Doctor Fiona Timmins

Acknowledgements

We are indebted to our commissioning editor, Geraldine Jeffers, and her team for their guidance and helpful support throughout the production of this textbook. We are also grateful to all those authors who have contributed to the book and would like to thank them for their hard work and commitment. We would also like to remember the children and families we have had the pleasure to meet in our clinical practice, as their experiences informed the content. Finally we would like to acknowledge and thank our own children and families for their support and love.

Artwork acknowledgements

OUP would like to acknowledge the following sources of artwork: Figures 3.8, 14.1, and 16.1 to 16.5 inclusive reproduced with kind permission of Patient.co.uk; Figures 4.1 and 4.2 the Department of Health, Crown copyright; Figure 13.1 reproduced with kind permission of Churchill Livingston, Edinburgh, from their book by Chamley, CA, Carson, P, Randall, D, Sandwell, M (2005) *Developmental Anatomy and Physiology of Children*, 1st ed.; Figure 3.1a © Corbis/Digital Stock; Figure 3.1b © Valueline; Figure 3.6 © Photodisc; Figure 3.7 © Image Source; Figure 10.6 © Fotolia.com; Figure 14.2 © istock.com.

Figures 10.1 and 10.2 were previously published in *The Human Body: An introduction for the biomedical and health sciences*, by Gillian Pocock and Chris Richards (2009), Oxford University Press. Figures 7.1, 9.2, 11.4, 12.1, 14.2, 15.1, and 15.3 were originally published in *Clinical Nursing Skills: Core and Advanced* by Ruth Endacott, Phil Jevon and Simon Cooper (2009), Oxford University Press. Figures 8.1, 11.1, and 11.3 were originally published in *Foundation Clinical Nursing Skills* by Charles Docherty and Jacqueline McCallum (2009), Oxford University Press. Figure 15.4 was published in Total Burn Care, 3rd Edition, by David N. Herndon, MD, FACS, 880 pages. Copyright Elsevier (2007).

Brief contents

Detailed contents

About the authors

The editors

Imelda Coyne   PhD, BSc (Hons), Dip N, RNT, RSCN, RGN FEANS is an Associate Professor and Head of Children's Nursing at the School of Nursing and Midwifery, University of Dublin, Trinity College.

Freda Neill   MSc, BSc (Hons), Cert Ed, Dip Health Visiting, RGN, RM currently works as the Clinical Skills Manager in the School of Nursing and Midwifery, University of Dublin, Trinity College.

Fiona Timmins   PhD, MSc, MA, FFNRCSI, BSc (open), NFESC, BNS, RNT, RGN currently works as a Senior Lecturer in the School of Nursing and Midwifery, University of Dublin, Trinity College.

The contributors

Carol Barron   MSc, BA (Hons), Dip Pharm, RNT, RSCN, RGN works as a Lecturer at the School of Nursing, Dublin City University (DCU), Dublin.

Isabel Byrne   RPN, RGN, RNT, PGDip Clinical Practice, MSc (CHSE) works as a Clinical Tutor teaching clinical skills to both general and children's undergraduate nurses in the Clinical Skills Centre, School of Nursing and Midwifery, University of Dublin, Trinity College.

Margaret Chambers   MSc, BSc (Hons), DPSN, PGDip Ed, RN, RSCN, RNT works as a Lecturer in Children's Nursing at the University of Plymouth, Devon, England.

Hazel Chamberlain   PhD, MA, BSc (Hons), RGN, RSCN, DPSN currently works as the Named Lead Nurse for Child Protection/Safeguarding for the Central Manchester area and Manchester Children's University Hospital Foundation Trust.

Sam Chenery-Morris   RGN, RSCN, RM, Dip HE, BSc Midwifery Practice, PGDip in Interprofessional Education works as a Lecturer in midwifery at University Campus Suffolk, Ipswich.

Mary Clynes   MSC, BA (Hons), RNT, RCN, RGN works as a Lecturer at the School of Nursing, Dublin City University (DCU), Dublin.

Yvonne Corcoran   MSc, RGN, TCN, RM works as a Lecturer at the School of Nursing, Dublin City University (DCU), Dublin.

Dr Paul Costello   works as a Lecturer in biological sciences in the School of Nursing and Midwifery, University of Dublin, Trinity College. He has worked in clinical medicine and lectured at undergraduate and postgraduate level.

Amanda Driffield   RGN, RSCN, BHSc, PGDip works as a Lecturer in Children's Nursing, School of Nursing, University of Leeds, Leeds.

Michelle Green   MSc, BSc (Hons), RGN, RSCN works as a Child Health Lecturer in the School of Healthcare, University of Leeds, Leeds.

Eleanor Hollywood   MSc, HDip Children's Nursing, BSc (Hons), RNT, RCN, RGN is a Lecturer in Children's Nursing to both postgraduate and undergraduate nursing students in the School of Nursing and Midwifery, Trinity College, Dublin.

Kirsten Huby   MA, BN (Hons), RN (Child) works as a Child Health Lecturer in the School of Healthcare, University of Leeds, Leeds.

Denise Jonas   RSCN, RGN, MSc, BSc, PGCert HEPR works as a Lecturer/Practitioner in child health and children's pain management at the School of Nursing, University of Salford and Central Manchester & Manchester Children's University Hospitals NHS Trust.

Jacinta Kelly   MSc, RGN, HDip Critical Care, FFNMRCSI is currently a Lecturer at the School of Nursing and Midwifery, University of Dublin, Trinity College.

Carole King   MSc, RCN, RGN, RCT, RNT works as a Children's Lecturer at the School of Nursing and Midwifery, University of Dublin, Trinity College.

Joan Livesley   works as a Senior Lecturer at the School of Nursing and also works for the Institute for Health and Social Care Research at the University of Salford, Manchester.

Dr Aileen Lynch   BSc (Hons), MSc, PhD works as a Lecturer in the School of Nursing and Midwifery, University of Dublin, Trinity College, Dublin and teaches Anatomy and Physiology on the Undergraduate Nursing/ Children's and Midwifery programmes.

Siobhan McDermott   MSc, RGN, RSCN currently works as a Lecturer at the School of Nursing, Dublin City University (DCU), Dublin.

Moira McLoughlin   MSc, PGDip ED, BSc (Hons), OND Dip Nursing, RSCN, RGN is a Senior Lecturer at the School of Nursing, Faculty of Health & Social Care, University of Salford, Manchester.

Aoife Moran   RGN, Dip HE (Nursing), BNS (Hons), PhD works as a Lecturer in the School of Nursing, Dublin City University, Dublin.

Yvonne Muldowney   RGN, BSc, MSc (Ed) works as a Clinical Nurse Tutor in the School of Nursing and Midwifery, University of Dublin, Trinity College. Specialties include Critical Care Nursing and General Nursing with a special interest in skin care.

James Mulkerrins   MSc, RNT, RN works as a Clinical Tutor teaching clinical skills to both general and children's undergraduate nurses in the Clinical Skills Centre, School of Nursing and Midwifery, University of Dublin, Trinity College.

Therese Nestor   is a Clinical Nurse Specialist in Neurology at the Children's University Hospital, Temple Street, Dublin. She has years of experience working with children and families suffering from neurological disorders.

Mary Nevin   MSc, RNT, RN works as a Clinical Tutor teaching clinical skills to both general and children's undergraduate nurses in the Clinical Skills Centre, School of Nursing and Midwifery, University of Dublin, Trinity College.

Liz Nolan   GN, RCN, HDip in Sick Children's Nursing, BSc in Practice Development, Dip Management works as a Clinical Placement Coordinator in the Children's University Hospital, Temple Street, Dublin.

Caroline O'Connor   MSc, BNS (Hons), Higher Dip in Children's, NCEA Applied Chemistry, RCN, RGN works as a Nurse Development Coordinator in the Children's University Hospital, Temple Street, Dublin.

Colleen O'Neill   RGN, RCN, MSc in Nursing, BSc (Hons), works as a lecturer at the School of Nursing, Dublin City University, Dublin.

Jan Orr   PGDip, RNT, BSc (Hons), RSCH, works as a lecturer/practitioner and works as Deputy Sister, St Michaels Hospital, Cornwall and is a Children's Clinical Skills Lecturer at the Faculty of Health and Social Work, University of Plymouth.

Joan Simons   RGN, RSCN, RHV, BA (Hons), PGDE, PGDAHP, DMS, MA, PhD works as the Professional Lead Child Health, Faculty of Health and Human Sciences, Thames Valley University, London.

Hilary Southern   RGN, BNS, RNT, MSc (Ed) works as a Clinical Tutor teaching clinical skills to both general and children's undergraduate nurses in the Clinical Skills Centre, School of Nursing and Midwifery, University of Dublin, Trinity College.

The Online Resource Centre

This textbook is accompanied by an Online Resource Centre that provides students, lecturers and mentors with interactive resources to develop clinical nursing skills. You can access the website from any computer with internet access and so you will find it helpful to save the web address in to your 'favourites' at the earliest opportunity: **www.oxfordtextbooks.co.uk/orc/coyne**

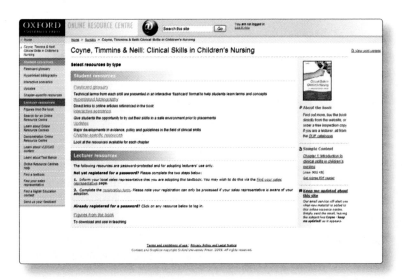

Updates

Major developments in evidence, policy and guidelines in the field of clinical skills will be posted to the Online Resource Centre every six months. Sign up to be alerted to the updates by clicking on the link 'Keep me updated about this site' on the home page.

Chapter specific resources

Each chapter is supported by the following resources to help you apply and develop your skills:

- **Videos** Selected chapters have accompanying videos to demonstrate skills.

  You will see this icon in the book to indicate a video is available.

- **Interactive scenarios** Give you the opportunity to try out your skills in a safe environment prior to placements.

- **Hyperlinked bibliography** Direct links to online articles referenced in the chapter (institutional subscriptions are required for access to full papers).

- **Interactive glossary** Technical terms from each skill are presented in an interactive 'flashcard' format to help you learn terms and concepts.

For lecturers

(In addition to the resources listed above): Figures from the book to download and use in teaching.

How to use this book

Clinical Skills in Children's Nursing explains and demonstrates the clinical skills required of all children's and general nursing students through the use of specific features and learning tools. This brief tour shows you how to get the most out of this textbook package.

Background knowledge

The essential principles, evidence and important considerations for each skill are introduced and discussed before the procedure is presented so you understand why, when, and if to undertake a clinical skill.

Table 9.1 Normal heart rates in children

Age	Heart rate
Premature	100–180
0–1 month	100–180
1–3 months	100–160
6–12 months	80–140
1–5 years	75–120
6–10 years	70–110
11–16 years	60–100

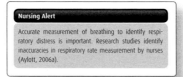

Nursing Alert

Accurate measurement of breathing to identify respiratory distress is important. Research studies identify inaccuracies in respiratory rate measurement by nurses (Aylott, 2006a).

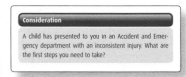

Consideration

A child has presented to you in an Accident and Emergency department with an inconsistent injury. What are the first steps you need to take?

Physiology across children's age ranges

Physiological variables in babies, infants, children and adolescents are summarised in tables to help you remember key biology.

Nursing alerts box

Important implications for practice, including precautions and potential 'warning signs' are highlighted to aid decision making and problem solving.

Considerations box

Readers are asked to consider underlying core principles and issues in children's nursing and how they may influence clinical skills.

Visual demonstration

Drawings help to relate the underlying anatomy to the clinical skill whilst photographs demonstrate how to undertake a skill.

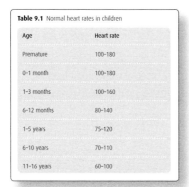

Figure 8.1 The respiratory system

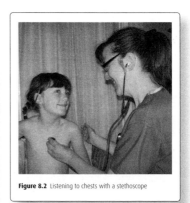

Figure 8.2 Listening to chests with a stethoscope

Step-by-step guide to IV fluid administration

Step	Rationale
1 Ensure you have undertaken the preparation as outlined above.	To ensure the prescription has been correctly drawn up and the nurse and patient have been prepared.
2 Check the patient's name and date of birth verbally and against their ID band.	Ensures that the correct fluid is administered to the correct patient.
3 Open administration sets and if more than one is needed connect together using an aseptic or non-touch technique in line with local policy. Ensure all lines are clamped. The number of lines and additional connections should be kept to a minimum. If more than one type of fluid is to be administered through one vascular access device at the same time then both fluids must be compatible.	Aseptic or non-touch technique should be used to prevent contamination of the fluid. Lines and connection should be kept to a minimum to reduce the risk of infection (DH, 2003).
4 Expose port on fluid bag by removing the protective covering. Remove the protective cap from the spike of the administration set.	Administration sets need to be primed to remove air from the system.
Spike the bag of fluid with the bag held below eye level. Hang the bag on the IV stand.	Holding the bag below eye level prevents splashes into eyes.

Step-by-step guidance

Each procedure is broken down into clear steps with accompanying rationale so you can see what to do and why. These have been carefully laid out to help learning.

Step-by-Step guide to ECG monitoring

This is an advanced skill. You *must* check whether you can assist with or undertake any aspect of this skill, in line with local policy.

Step	Rationale
1 The leads for the ECG monitor are connected to the child through use of electrodes. There are a range of sizes and types on the market and the nurse must be familiar with the type used locally.	To ensure they can carry out the procedure correctly.
The electrodes have a metal stud on one side (or an integrated lead) and conductive adhesive on the other.	This adhesive allows the electrode to stick to the chest and conduct the electrical impulses from the heart.
2 Ensure the skin is clean and dry.	If the skin is wet or oily the electrodes will not adhere and may give a poor or inaccurate trace on the monitor.
3 Peel the backing off and place the electrodes at the left and right shoulders of the patient with the third electrode on the left side of the abdomen or on the leg (see Figure 9.3).	Correct placement of the electrodes and leads is important; if misplaced the ECG recording will be affected.

Advanced skills

These are identified by these icons and **colour coded in black** to remind students and newly qualified nurses that you must check if you are allowed to undertake these skills in line with local policy.

Support for further learning and assignments

At the end of each skill there are specific sections to aid reflection and further learning as well as reminders of key points. Each skill ends with references and a list of key further reading material.

Part One

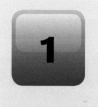

1 Introduction to clinical skills in children's nursing

IMELDA COYNE, FREDA NEILL, AND FIONA TIMMINS

This book aims to provide nursing students with information about a broad range of clinical skills that they may use while nursing children. In recognition of the challenges in the healthcare setting, there is now greater emphasis on ensuring that nurses are prepared adequately to deliver safe and competent care, and that nurses are equipped with both the knowledge and practical skills to enable them to perform procedures safely and sensitively for children. This text aims to take account of these issues and serve as an essential resource for nurses and nursing students.

The context of clinical skills in children's nursing

Changing trends such as the move away from hospital care, shorter hospital stays, increased use of day surgery and outpatient care, parents undertaking procedures in the home supported by community care teams, and development of primary care services, present challenges to contemporary children's nursing practice. Technological advances also mean that children now undergo more intensive technical procedures and complex treatment protocols, and the nurse has to be equipped with a diverse range of clinical skills. In this book we try to provide a comprehensive guide by addressing the following themes and challenges:

Family and child centred care

In addition to the fundamental physical clinical skills that are required of a nurse, attention is also drawn to the important psychosocial aspects of skill delivery throughout this book. In particular skills of communication and family centred care are presented as overarching themes. This emphasis is consistent with changing trends in children's nursing, whereby shorter hospital stays, and increased acuity of children, means that there is now less time to develop a relationship with the **child** and family, less time to build rapport and trust, which could ultimately impact negatively on the hospital experience for that family. Building relationships, developing trust, and family centred care are pivotal to the success of modern children's nursing.

In an attempt to negate the potential for adverse aspects of hospitalization, increasingly families are encouraged to remain with their child during their hospital stay. This presents a unique challenge for nursing students, who may find themselves daunted by the fact that they are caring for not one child, but both the child and family. Furthermore, a unique challenge of children's nursing is the performance of vital nursing procedures on children who are reluctant to cooperate due to fear of pain, anxiety, or distress, whilst being observed by concerned parents.

Technical and integrated knowledge

Children's nurses now undertake more advanced clinical and technological skills in both hospital and the community. Nursing students need to feel confident about performing clinical skills as they have a responsibility for patient safety and for the emotional support of the child and family. Therefore they need a textbook that clearly illustrates the essential skills and the rationale for each skill. We welcomed the opportunity to produce such a new text and the impetus for writing this children's skills textbook is the need for a comprehensive textbook that will integrate knowledge on a variety of topics, from anatomy and physiology content to child and family centred care, with up-to-date and detailed information on clinical skills for students of children's nursing. We wanted to incorporate not only skills teaching, but also learning underlying evidence and practice of holistic nursing, including issues of safety, legality, and patient centred care.

There are many excellent anatomy and physiology texts available for students but such texts rarely discuss clinical skills in tandem. Students can experience difficulty understanding the rationale for nursing procedures when the skills are not supported by the relevant anatomy and physiology of the body systems. This is illustrated by one nursing student who recalled:

> *I was recently on ward placement where one of the nurses had to catheterize a female patient and was unsuccessful as she was not sure where the urethra was. She had to look up a picture on the internet before she did it again but this time successfully.*

As more nursing programmes at university level become modularized, students are frequently expected to be able to integrate knowledge on a variety of topics in their performance of clinical procedures. This can prove challenging for many students as they find it difficult to integrate disparate bits of information to produce a coherent performance of skills delivery. This book will be very useful in this regard as it contains detailed information on the essential clinical skills prescribed in pre-registration children's nurse education, and the early chapters bring together the essential, underlying knowledge to provide the wider context in which clinical skills are carried out.

Developing competencies from student to registered nurse

This textbook is written specifically for the new generation of children's nurses. In particular, it is written for pre-registration student nurses and so it reflects the content of the pre-registration curricula and the level of knowledge needed at this stage of training. Pre-registration students may be studying on a children's branch of the programme in the UK, undertaking an integrated general and children's nursing programme, or be qualified nurses undertaking children's nursing courses. The text is also relevant to newly qualified staff working with children (particularly the advanced skills sections).

Clinical skills are a fundamental component of nursing curricula that prepare practitioners for practice and so clinical skills acquisition has become a central topic for discussion and debate within pre-registration nursing education. Clinical skills competency forms a component of the nursing skills required by nursing students before being permitted entry to the professional nursing register. These competencies are usually outlined by regulatory guidelines such as the Nursing and Midwifery Council UK (Essential skills clusters) and An Bord Altranais (Republic of Ireland), and thus mirrored within nursing curricula.

Reading a text such as this is essential to develop these competencies; however, it is important to remember that performing skills in practice requires the support and guidance of your mentor or preceptor, compliance with local policies and guidelines, and appropriate education and/or preparation. This textbook is simply a guide towards developing an understanding of a number of skills required to nurse children—it must be supplemented by clinical experience that complies with local policies and guidelines.

Important note: You will need to remember that since practice can vary between some countries, it is important to adhere to local guidelines and policies when in practice.

Advanced skills

The competencies expected of student nurses, newly qualified nurses, and registered nurses can vary from country to country as well as from one local healthcare service to another. We appreciate that in some universities, students may need to develop competency in a skill that is not required of a student 50 miles away. Likewise some employers can expect newly qualified nurses to develop competencies in some advanced skills within the first year post-qualification. To ensure that we have provided the right breadth of content we have covered extra skills that are often considered 'advanced'.

The advanced skills have been clearly marked with an icon in the table of contents and in the chapters themselves and are presented in special black boxes. Before each advanced skill, readers are asked to check if they are allowed to undertake or assist with these skills in line with local policy. It is imperative that readers act within the limitations of their knowledge, experience, qualification, and local policies.

How to use this book

The purpose of the book is to provide a resource that will truly meet the needs of children's nursing students in content and style. It is written to meet the needs of children's nurses by providing research-based evidence on how to perform skills and nursing procedures in the clinical environment and community setting. It provides an optimal balance of theory and practice, so that students will understand the rationale and evidence for a skill as well as when and how to undertake it.

The principle of family centred care is threaded throughout all of the chapters, as the involvement of children and their families is essential for high quality care. It is important that parents are involved in the care of their hospitalized child since parents are increasingly expected to learn and perform nursing procedures for their children at home and in the community.

The content is written in such a way as to aid learning and recall in the clinical environment, helping the student to attain competency. Students can find it difficult to wade through large pieces of dense text when time is short and they need the information quickly. To guard against this problem and ensure a student-friendly layout, the content is enlivened with many pedagogical features such as easy-to-find procedure tables, drawings, photos, tables, and nursing alerts highlighting key points. This 'how to use this book' section illustrates these features but we also want to draw your attention to other features, such as:

- A clear, accessible, and memorable writing style, presented in short sections with clear headings for easy reading and recall.

- The content is related to family centred care at the different life stages, incorporating areas of community care and cultural awareness throughout.
- It takes a family centred approach and includes suggestions on how to respect the child and family and how to involve them safely in the performance of procedures.
- The material is linked to life sciences and **child development** so that students understand the rationale behind procedures.
- Normal physiological/developmental ranges are set out in the early chapters.
- Physiological/developmental ranges specific to each skill are outlined clearly and helpfully in each skill chapter.
- The anatomy and physiology content in each chapter is illustrated with diagrams and photos.
- The skills are mapped against competencies for practice, giving the student a clear 'road map' to work to.
- Key points are summarized in helpful tables.
- It is highly illustrated with lots of photos and line drawings, including pictures demonstrating practical information such as how to position the baby/child etc.
- Each chapter is supported by online resources including case scenarios that test recall and application of knowledge, which is a good way of reinforcing knowledge and enhancing understanding.

Outline of content

This book assumes that students have finished the first year of the nurse education programme; however, an introduction section addresses the core principles of children's nursing and the unique aspects of skills required in children's nursing, and summarizes key foundation material such as child development, major milestones, and key ranges in physiology, so the reader has the necessary material before they read the more clinical content in the rest of the book. While this book does not aim to provide detailed information that may be found in anatomy and physiology texts, it will provide essential practical anatomy and physiology information required by students to perform specific clinical skills. The content is structured into three sections with sixteen chapters in total.

Section One includes the opening four chapters that cover the unique aspects of skills required in children's nursing and can be referred back to as the reader works their way through the skills. Chapter Two provides an essential pillar for the book. It introduces the reader to the core principles in children's nursing: communication and family centred care. It discusses the potential effects of hospitalization on the child and family, attachment and loss theory, play and safety, and the important role that the nurse has in facilitating family centred care to address these aforementioned issues. Chapter Three provides a summary of normal child growth and development, and outlines ranges of anatomical and physiological differences from neonates to teenagers. This provides fundamental knowledge that acts as a basis for reading further through the book. Chapter Four details important information on child consent and legal and ethical matters, a fundamental knowledge of which is essential to the nursing care of children.

Section Two consists of three chapters that outline core clinical skills of interest to pre-registration students. These essential skills include admission procedures and discharge planning, models of care, and principles of good record keeping (Chapter Five). Chapter Six follows on from this with a discussion and outline of mobilization, pain assessment and management, wound assessment and management, and other relevant procedures. Principles of drug administration are outlined in Chapter Seven.

In **Section Three,** skills are discussed and outlined according to body systems in order to provide a logical structure. There are nine chapters, which link each system with the clinical skills suitable for pre-registration students. The *Essential Skills Clusters* (ESCs) identified by the NMC (2007) for pre-registration nursing programmes are addressed comprehensively within all of the systems chapters. The nursing procedures relate to respective outcomes and proficiencies within the *Standards of proficiency for pre-registration nursing education* (NMC 2004).

A note from the editors

This book is meant as a useful and essential resource for nurse students and qualified nurses working with children and families. We hope that the evidence base related to clinical skills that has been assembled for this edition, together with the unique range of contributors and their approaches, provides a rich source of information for your future nursing practice.

2 Introduction to core principles in children's nursing

IMELDA COYNE AND JOAN LIVESLEY

Introduction

The aim of this chapter is to discuss the core principles in children's nursing and the application of these principles in everyday practice for nurses working with children and families. These essential principles are fundamental in the delivery of high quality care and as such will be evident throughout this textbook. This chapter will explain these principles in the context of community and hospital care and illustrate how nurses can use this knowledge in their clinical practice.

Learning outcomes

There is no doubt that clinical skills are an essential component of high quality healthcare, but they are on their own insufficient to ensure that the needs of children and their families are met. Clinical skills need to be embedded in children's services that are child centred and clearly focused around the needs of children and their families; but how is this possible? To ensure high quality care for children in hospital and the community you need to incorporate the core principles of family centred care into your everyday nursing practice and interventions. It is essential to understand the principles of family centred care and the importance of partnership and negotiation in the delivery of clinical skills.

Knowing where to begin can be difficult, but we think that you can start with the concept of **attachment** and loss. Understanding this in relation to children's separation from their family and home will help you to understand

the impact of hospitalization on children, particularly those younger than five years old. The adverse aspects of hospitalization have been a substantial driving force in delivering more nursing services to children at home. However, it is also important to remain aware of the ongoing impact of lifelong illness on children and their families and why it is essential to use effective communication skills, maintain safe environments, and incorporate play into your practice. Together with evidence-based clinical skills, these facets of practice will enable you to maintain and promote children's and families' health and well-being. Specific learning outcomes are as follows.

At the end of this chapter you will:

- Understand the basic elements of attachment and loss theory.
- Have an understanding of the effects of hospitalization on child and family.
- Develop an awareness of the standards required for children in hospital.
- Begin to understand strategies for reducing the adverse aspects of hospitalization.
- Have a knowledge of the philosophy of family centred care.
- Understand the principles of communicating with children, safety and safeguarding children, and the importance of play.

Prior knowledge

The principles discussed in this chapter may be viewed as the core concepts underpinning children's nursing and all clinical skills that follow in later chapters. The principles are closely linked to other concepts such as accountability, advocacy, consent, and safeguarding children, which are discussed in detail in Chapter Four. For example in family centred care, various caring procedures are often shared between nurses and parents and this raises issues around education, support, accountability, and role boundaries. Understanding families is an important aspect of working with children. It is important to remember that it is the family, not healthcare professionals, who raise children. Children most often live in the context of a family and are usually reliant on adults for physical and emotional care and support (Mayall, 2002).

The concept of the family is a complex phenomenon and a complete overview is beyond the scope of this chapter. However, it is necessary for you to explore the key features of families and family structures in order to understand the importance of delivering care that is family centred. Families can differ considerably in their makeup and it has been postulated that the family environment impacts upon children and their achievements. For further information on this topic it would be helpful for you to read **http://www.statistics.gov.uk/focuson/families/**. It would also be helpful for you to have some prior knowledge of major concepts associated with childhood that are discussed within sociological and child development texts. Hence taking time to read some general sociological texts on childhood and families such as James and James (2004) or Mayall (2002) will enhance your understanding of the key issues discussed in this chapter.

Children and families

Anne Casey's seminal work (Casey & Mobbs, 1988) is fundamental to the introduction of the concepts of parent participation and partnership nursing as core principles for nursing children in hospital or the community. These concepts have evolved to a more inclusive term of family centred care, which recognizes the importance of including both children's and families' needs in planning care delivery. Underpinned by partnership working and negotiation with parents and children, family centred care has become an important philosophy for work with children and their families.

However, before we examine the concept of family centred care it is important to consider other theoretical perspectives that underline the importance of child-adult relationships to children's growth, development, and well-being. It is also important to consider the potential detrimental impact of hospitalization and lifelong illness on children and families.

Attachment and loss

To understand the effects of hospitalization on children and families, you need to understand the body of knowledge on attachment theory and attachment behaviour. The work of John Bowlby (1952; 1956; 1980) and James Robertson (1958a; 1958b; 1989) made a significant contribution towards understanding the impact of hospitalization on infants and children. John Bowlby was an eminent psychiatrist who developed a theory to explain the process of attachment and separation.

Attachment behaviour was developed from an understanding of **ethology** (the study of animal behaviour), psychoanalysis (the study of human psychological functioning), human evolutionary biology (the origin of human species), and cognitive psychology (the study of internal mental processes). It was also developed using observations of children in many different situations and environments. Bowlby defined attachment as need for the infant/child to stay in close proximity to the primary caregiver, usually the mother, and to be comforted by her presence, sound, and touch. Attachment theory was developed through testing the following three propositions: (1) children who are able to predict the availability of their caregiver will suffer less fear and alarm in frightening situations than children who cannot predict the behaviour of their caregiver; (2) attachment behaviour and the internalization of how the caregiver will respond is most acutely developed between six months and five years of age; and (3) the child's experience of seeking care and receiving protection is pivotal to continued healthy development.

Attachment theory is considered to be universal in that it is applicable to child-adult relations across different cultural groups. This means it is an important theory for children's nurses and the following explanation of the key concepts of attachment theory will help you to understand the importance of children's relationships with adults. There are four concepts central to attachment theory.

These are: **attachment figures**; attachment behaviour; **separation anxiety**; and **internal working models** (or mental representations of self in relation to others).

Attachment figures

Attachment figures can be defined as any person with whom the child has an emotional bond, and these are most often the child's parents or main caregivers. An important facet of the relationship between a child and their attachment figures is how the child will seek out or search for their attachment figures when they are feeling fearful, frightened, or anxious (Ainsworth, 1989). This means that the child will seek out physical and emotional closeness to their attachment figures when strangers, strange places, or strange situations face them. Being admitted to hospital means the child is confronted by all three so it is important that you identify those adults to whom the child is psychologically attached in order to provide emotional security during hospitalization and episodes of illness at home.

> **Nursing Alert**
>
> Since all families are different, it is important that you identify early on in the admission process the family members that are closest to the child. This will help the child's emotional welfare and avoid the possibility of key members being excluded unintentionally.

Attachment behaviour and separation anxiety

Understanding the relationship between an attachment figure and a child is a very important part of attachment theory; however, it is also necessary to understand attachment behaviour. Attachment behaviour is activated when a stranger, strange place, fear, darkness, or separation from their attachment figure confronts a child. As Bowlby (1980) stated: 'Attachment behaviour is commonly shown by a parent, or other adult, towards a child or adolescent, but is also shown by one adult towards another especially in times of ill health …' (p 39). Active attachment behaviour focuses the child's attention on seeking and maintaining proximity to their caregivers.

In other words, attachment behaviour is the term used to describe how the child signals a need for care. Should the child's attachment behaviour remain ungratified (or unfulfilled) by the close proximity of their attachment figure, the child may 'collapse into distress' (p 209).

Internal working models

It is necessary to consider how the child experiences the attachment figure's response to the care-signalling, as this leads to different 'adapted' styles of attachment behaviour. This is explained through the construct of internal working models, which are mental representations of self. Mary Ainsworth's work (1989) confirmed Bowlby's hypothesis that the presence of a sensitive and available attachment figure enables a child to feel safe and secure.

Infants and children who are unable to break through their attachment figure's insensitivity, or those children who experience a negative or harmful response, learn to adapt their attachment behaviour. In other words, they may become clingy or 'whinge' in order to break through insensitivity, or learn to hide their need for care in order to avoid harm. The terms used for adaptive styles of attachment behaviour are: secure, ambivalent, and avoidant. More recently, a fourth category, disorganized, has been added to describe the attachment behaviour of children who have been unable to do anything to provoke the required response from their attachment figure. This also explains why children may behave differently with different caregivers. Hence a child's experience of their relationships with their attachment figures or caregivers can exert a powerful influence on the child's concept of 'self' and 'self value' in relation to others.

These internal working models enable the child to construct models of how they are valued by others. In turn, this translates into how they value themselves and sets the course for how they grow and develop a sense of self. A lack of felt security is considered a risk factor for psychopathology in adulthood and intergenerational and maladaptive parenting (Howe, 2005). For a more detailed explanation of this please read Howe (2005).

Maternal deprivation

The relationship between attachment figures, attachment behaviour, and emotional well-being was further developed by James Robertson in collaboration with Bowlby. Robertson filmed observations of young hospitalized children who had been separated from their mothers. His initial work was undertaken in the 1950s in hospital wards that prohibited or severely restricted parents from visiting sick children.

Robertson's film of a two-year-old child admitted to hospital captured the adverse effect of maternal separation as the child cries and protests in an attempt to prevent her mother leaving. But her mother was not allowed to stay. Robertson's observations enabled Bowlby (1975) to delineate a child's separation anxiety into the three distinct categories of protest, despair, and detachment. He contended that fear of separation or actual separation from the attachment figure activated attachment behaviour, whereby a child will use all available resources to maintain close proximity to their caregivers, most notably clinging, crying, calling, and angry coercion (protest).

Drawing on the principles of **homeostasis** (attempting to regulate distress by maintaining a stable psychological constant condition), Bowlby (1975) proposed that over time, should the child be unsuccessful at maintaining the close proximity of their attachment figure, the protest phase of separation anxiety is followed by despair, categorized by the child searching for the attachment figure.

If unresolved, despair turns to detachment with the child withdrawing psychologically from their attachment figures and other caregivers who attempt to take their place. Robertson's film showed the child crying and calling before she searched for her mother by looking through windows and at doors. Eventually, the child became quiet, and the staff thought she was happy. Unfortunately, as her care-seeking behaviour remained ungratified, she had become psychologically detached from her mother and the nurses who sought to take her mother's place; hence the term detachment. This means that her psychological attachment to her mother was broken (detached).

It may seem bizarre to even consider asking parents to leave their children alone in hospital, but you will also experience times when parents cannot stay with their children. They often have other children and other commitments that mean some children will spend a considerable amount of time on their own. The effects of this should be clearly understood to avoid deleterious effects on individual children, particularly children younger than five years of age.

Subjective evidence in support of Bowlby and Robertson's work is apparent in the personal stories told by many adults admitted to hospital as children; one 40-year-old man who had been in hospital as a child recalled how: 'I endured many discomforts of weekly aspiration of pus … but this has not left a mark … I remember my mother's first and only visit far more vividly … I returned home an alien. I held a passport but it had ceased to be valid' (Cleary, 1992, p 11).

Bowlby's and Robertson's seminal work was fundamental in the campaign for better standards of hospital care for children and for bringing about major changes to the visiting arrangements for children in hospital. Since then numerous government reports have explicitly stated that parents should be allowed to accompany their child, have unrestricted visiting, and that hospitals should provide adequate accommodation so that parents can stay overnight (Commission for Healthcare Audit and Inspection, 2007b; Department for Education and Skills, 2004).

Effects of hospitalization on the child and family

In light of the previous discussion, it is understandable that hospitalization can be a very stressful and frightening experience for most children. In the UK, children account for 19% of the total population and many are admitted to hospital. For example each year, 28% of children attend an Accident and Emergency department, 700,000 have at least one overnight stay, and 300,000 attend for day surgery (National Statistics, 2006).

In addition, many children admitted to hospital have complex healthcare needs with a significant proportion requiring complex interventions. Regardless of the appropriateness of the hospital environment, some children will stay in hospital wards for lengthy periods of time, for instance in 2005–2006, 65 children living in Northern Ireland had hospital stays that exceeded three months.

Given this, it is very important that nurses understand the potential effects hospitalization may have on children and their families. There are contributing factors, such as the age of the child (younger children are far more likely to suffer adverse effects of hospitalization), length of stay (stays of longer duration are more disruptive), number of invasive procedures, and lack of support from attachment figures. Even short periods of hospitalization can have adverse effects on children, their siblings, and their families (Shields, 2001).

Children are potentially a vulnerable group because they have limited autonomy and are dependent upon others for physical and emotional care and protection. A child's physical and cognitive development is different from that of an adult; their physiology is different, their intellect is developing, and they have specific psychosocial and emotional needs. Children who are hospitalized are particularly vulnerable because of their illness, their limited understanding, and because they have so little control over what is happening to them.

Consideration

- Try to imagine yourself as a child entering hospital for the first time.
- How would you feel?
- What kind of concerns would you have?

Children's fears and concerns

Hospitalization generates a range of anxieties for many children, such as fears about the unknown, unfamiliar faces, separation from significant others, hospital environment, possibility of pain, immobility, restricted activity, disruption, and loss of control. Research with hospitalized children in England revealed an expressed range of fears about the hospitalization; in particular dislikes about the ward environment (Battrick & Glasper, 2004; Coyne, 2006b). The children reported disliking several aspects of the ward environment, such as: noisy wards, constant bright lights, hot 'stuffy' environment, lack of privacy, and inadequate play facilities.

The bright lights and noise (for example phones ringing, babies crying) caused children difficulty with resting and sleeping. Older children, and particularly adolescents, disliked the lack of privacy and found the ward décor too 'babyish' and the play facilities and toys geared towards younger children (Coyne, 2006b). Similar dislikes about the ward environment have been reported in recent research with children (n = 255) from three hospitals in the UK (Curtis et al., 2007). The children aged seven

and older reported hospital as being geared towards very young children. They universally disliked the clown motifs in all three sites, with even the older children regarding them as frightening. This latter finding is interesting considering the trend towards employing clowns to provide humour and diversion on certain wards in the UK.

The children in this study also reported disliking dull, dirty, disordered, and crowded spaces. They liked clean, tidy, colourful, bright, comfortable, and well-maintained areas. Similar findings were revealed in one Irish study (Coyne & Conlon, 2007). Children and young people (n = 18) aged 7 to 16 years in Ireland expressed their dislikes, which were categorized in terms of two main themes: fears/dislikes of ward environment and fears about procedures. These are further outlined in **Table 2.1**. These study findings clearly indicate that separation from significant others is not the only factor to consider in children's experiences of hospitalization.

In keeping with earlier reports in the literature, children perceive intrusive procedures such as blood tests and other painful procedures as particularly threatening and very stressful (Coyne & Conlon, 2007). It is of concern to note that perceptions of *alien hospital environment*,

Table 2.1 Children and young people's experiences of hospitalization

Being in an unfamiliar environment	**Fears:** Scary environment The unknown—lack of information Unfamiliar health professionals Risk of infections (MRSA) **Dislikes:** Noisy ward Bright lights at night Seeing other sick children Lack of privacy Busy wards 'Babyish' play facilities
Receiving investigations and treatments	**Fears:** Needles Blood tests Pain Operations Harm to body

strangeness of staff, and *fear of the unknown* prevail despite reported improvements in hospital décor, better information exchange, and unrestricted parental participation. It is also striking that many children, even those over 14, reported feeling unsafe in the hospital setting. The range of fears was surprising considering that most of the children had their parent staying or spending long periods with them.

Thus despite many advances in children's healthcare and approaches to children's nursing, there are many pervasive concerns, which you as a nurse ought to be mindful of. The individual fears and concerns of both child and family could be outlined and addressed during the admission procedure (Chapter Five) and addressed within the plan of care if possible. As you will learn in Chapter Five, assessing, planning, implementing, and evaluating nursing care delivery is cyclical. As a result your assessment and other phases of care are ongoing. Thus should you learn of a child's difficulty sleeping due to noise, for example, a simple plan could be further implemented (e.g. moving beds). Similarly if teenagers consistently appear to be in an environment that is unsuitable (walls adorned with clowns), the ward could consider alternative décor or simply holding a range of pop star posters for display.

Possible interventions will be further discussed later in the chapter. However, it is important to remember that continued effects of hospitalization often manifest after discharge. This can include behavioural problems such as separation anxiety, sleep disturbance, bed-wetting, and general regression in physical and cognitive development. For some, the deleterious effects of hospitalization may continue through to adulthood, as highlighted earlier (Cleary, 1992; Jolley, 2004).

It is therefore important to identify any potential effects of hospitalization within the nursing care plan, through identification of needs and good planning to address these. Often, rather than complex interventions, very small gestures can make the difference (Timmins *et al.*, 2005). Timmins *et al.* (2005) reported that a friendly smile or wave made all the difference to parents of babies being nursed in Neonatal Intensive Care. There are also interventions such as use of analgesic cream and distraction that can be effectively utilized to lessen the effect and perceived effect of painful procedures, and these will be discussed later.

Nursing Alert

Sometimes children experience pain during needle insertion because anaesthetic cream is not used to numb the area, or they had to endure repeated insertions due to failed attempts, or they were not prepared adequately. Sometimes nurses/doctors view needle insertion as a quick and relatively painless procedure. But children say otherwise, so never underestimate the impact of needles/injections, and prepare the child carefully and appropriately. Be aware that children never forget a bad experience of painful needles, with some developing needle phobia that can cause major problems with further hospitalizations.

Effects on siblings and other family members

It should be remembered that it is not only the ill child who may suffer adverse effects of hospitalization; careful attention should also be given to their siblings' experiences and needs. Siblings can often feel neglected or isolated because other relatives are caring for them rather than their parents, they may be unable to attend after school activities, and their parents are spending large periods of time away from home. When parents are at home they may be so preoccupied with concerns about the hospitalized child that they fail to consider the needs of their other children. Also, siblings may often feel wrongly that they are to blame for their brother or sister's illness and display this misconception by being tearful or withdrawn. The hospitalization of a child affects the whole family because it is a worrying time and represents a major disruption to family members and family routines.

Standards for children in hospital

Prior to considering ways in which you can reduce the adverse aspects of hospitalization for children and families, it is important to be aware of the recommendations and principles available. The National Service Framework (NSF) (Department of Health, 2003a) has identified ten core principles that are fundamental to better health and social care services for children and families both in hospital and in the community. It would be useful for you to read the documents that fully outline the NSF standards on the website: **http://www.doh.gov.uk/ nsf/children.htm**.

The NSF have developed standards for children in hospital that aim: 'To deliver hospital services that meet the needs of children, young people and their parents, and provide effective and safe care, through appropriately trained and skilled staff working in suitable, child-friendly, and safe environments' (Department of Health, 2003a, p 8). This aim is translated into standards of care that are listed in **Table 2.2** and which are fully explicated in a document for parents and carers (Department of Health, 2003b). They are based on a more detailed version that has been produced for the NHS and local authorities (see **http://www. doh.gov.uk/nsf/children/gettingtherightstart**).

The drive to improve the provision of services for children in hospital continues. More recently, a common core set of knowledge and skills for all people who work with children has been identified (Children's Workforce Development Council, 2005). These centre on six key areas that link closely with the NSF standards and which are listed in **Table 2.3**.

Table 2.2 Standards for children in hospital: a guide for parents and carers (Department of Health, 2003, p 1–20)

1. Children should receive care that is integrated and coordinated around their particular needs and the needs of their family.
2. They and their parents should be treated with respect and should be given support and information to enable them to understand and cope with the illness or injury, and the treatment needed.
3. They should be encouraged to be active partners in decisions about their health and care, and, where possible, be able to exercise choice.
4. Children and young people and their parents will participate in designing NHS and social care services that are readily accessible, respectful, and empowering, follow best practice in obtaining consent, and provide an effective response to their need.
5. Children and young people should receive appropriate high quality, evidence-based hospital care, developed through clinical governance and delivered by staff who have the right skills.
6. Care will be provided in an appropriate location and in an environment that is safe and well-suited to the age and stage of development of the child or young person.

Table 2.3 Common core set of knowledge and skills (Children's Workforce Development Council, 2005)

- Effective communication and engagement with children, young people, and families.
- Child and young person development.
- Safeguarding and promoting the welfare of children.
- Supporting transitions.
- Multi-agency working.
- Sharing information.

In Europe the EACH organization (European Association for Children in Hospital), which is made up of eighteen associations from sixteen European countries and from Japan, promotes the care of hospitalized children through the EACH Charter. This Charter contains a list of ten rights for all children, before, during, and after a stay in hospital (**http://www.each-for-sick-children.org/ each-charter**). The EACH Charter links closely with the UN Convention and the hospital standards outlined by the NSF. Other voluntary organizations such as Action for Sick Children, UK (**http://www.actionforsickchildren. org/news.asp**) and Children in Hospital Ireland (**http://www.childreninhospital.ie/aintro.html**) have made significant efforts to promote better standards of hospital care for children and their families and to safeguard children's rights. Visit these websites and you will notice how the key principles, although sometimes worded differently, are recommending the same approach for children.

Unacceptable standards

Unfortunately, it is apparent that legislation and policy directives alone are insufficient to ensure that effective care in hospital takes place. Kendrick and Taylor (2000) define this as 'programme abuse', whereby standards fall below normally acceptable standards. Evidence of unacceptable standards is listed below:

- Shortage of appropriately qualified staff to meet the needs of children admitted to hospital.
- Admission of children to adult wards.
- Failure to meet the needs of adolescents.
- Inadequate intensive care facilities.
- Under-treatment of pain in children.

It is every nurse's responsibility to speak out against unacceptable standards so that children's welfare is protected. Nurses not only need to work within policy and legislative frameworks, they also need to influence those policies and legislative frameworks. While policy has the power to change priorities through legislation and the allocation of resources, what really matters to children is what impacts on their health and well-being and what happens to them while they are in hospital (Little *et al.*, 2003).

Strategies for reducing the adverse aspects of hospitalization

Bearing in mind the hospital standards, efforts should be made to reduce the need for hospitalization of children through increased use of day surgery, outpatient care, and community care, with tertiary care only used as a last resort. There should be regular reviews of children's care so that hospital stays are kept to a minimum. As discussed earlier, hospitalization remains a stressful experience for many children despite unrestricted parent participation and considerable improvements in hospital environments. There are several strategies that can be used to reduce the threatening aspects of hospitalization and to make the experience easier for children and their families, as listed in **Table 2.4.** Think about how you could use some of these strategies before you begin a procedure, for example, using a child's favourite toy to explain a procedure.

Ensuring the child has contact with family and friends

Supporting parents to be with their child in hospital, allowing siblings to visit, and providing appropriately qualified nurses are significant steps towards reducing the adverse effects of hospitalization. Parental presence is thought to reduce levels of pain, reduce the duration of stay, and reduce infection rates and emotional disturbance on discharge (Shields, 2001).

Parents play a significant role in reassuring their children and providing security and normality. Therefore nurses

Table 2.4 Strategies for reducing the adverse aspects of hospitalization

1. Children should not be in hospital unless it is absolutely necessary.
2. Children should be discharged as soon as appropriate and full support should be given for aftercare.
3. Ensure care is family centred through recognition of child and family members' needs and circumstances.
4. Support parents to be with their child in hospital through adequate provision of accommodation and facilities.
5. Ensure children have continued contact with siblings, family members, and friends through open visiting policies.
6. There should be no age restriction for visitors to children.
7. Promote use of dim lights and coordination of activities at night-time so that children can rest and sleep.
8. Ensure children can continue with schoolwork if able to do so.
9. Ensure children have opportunities for play and adequate play facilities.
10. Prepare children prior to procedures and surgery through the use of hospital tours, videos, role-play, books, leaflets, computer games, and toys.
11. Allow children to express their views and feelings as this will provide guidance in anticipating the types of events that children may find stressful.
12. Promote a safe environment in the hospital.
13. Encourage children to bring in familiar items from home to personalize their bed space.
14. Encourage young children to bring a transitional object (i.e. teddy bear or special toy) with them to all events and procedures throughout their hospitalization.
15. Ensure that hospital décor is kept simple and clean with areas clearly signposted.
16. Try to meet children's preferences for accommodation, in that some may prefer single rooms whilst others prefer sharing bed space for the company.
17. Accommodation, facilities, and staffing should be appropriate to the needs of children.
18. Children's right for privacy, confidentiality, and autonomy should be respected.

should facilitate parent participation and provide parents with accurate information so that they can help relieve children's anxieties. Nurses need to remember to take special note of children who may spend time on their own and those children whose parents may be unable to provide the necessary emotional support that is needed (Livesley, 2005).

Children who are on their own in hospital are those who are most vulnerable to adverse effects of hospitalization. Children dislike disruption to their normal routines, and separation from family and friends. Along with their parents' presence, making friends, being with their peer group, and knowing the nurses/doctors are factors that help reduce children's fears and ameliorate the adverse aspects of the hospitalization (Coyne & Conlon, 2007). Efforts should be directed towards maximizing children's continued contact with siblings, family members, friends, and school, and minimizing the adverse aspects of the hospital environment.

Parents should keep siblings informed of what is happening to their brother or sister and encourage siblings to maintain contact with the ill sibling in the hospital. You may need to gently remind parents that although it is important to be with their hospitalized child, they must try to ensure that their other children's needs are not forgotten. Parents could be advised to take turns being in the hospital so that at least one parent is able to spend time with their other children.

Dealing with children's fears and dislikes

Understanding how children can feel threatened and fearful about many aspects of the hospitalization will help you to use different strategies to help reduce children's anxieties, increase their understanding, and facilitate overall coping. The presence of parents will not fully mitigate children's concerns and fears. Thus a better effort needs to be made by hospital management and health professionals to promote a safe environment in the hospital.

Health professionals need to see the ward environment from the child's perspective and take measures to make it more appropriately child-centred in relation to décor, appearance, and facilities. Children seek order and security in an environment that is alien to them. Therefore nurses can encourage children to bring in familiar

items from home to personalize their bed space. Encouraging young children to bring a transitional object (i.e. teddy bear or special toy) with them to all events and procedures throughout their hospitalization helps provide security and reassurance. Such a simple action can have a significant effect on a child's overall experience in hospital. Young children as well as adolescents value personal space and privacy so their preferences should be accommodated where possible, bearing in mind that some children may prefer single cubicles whilst others prefer sharing bed space for the company.

Reducing adverse aspects of the hospital environment

Children themselves recommend that hospitals need to be clean, tidy, bright, colourful, spacious, welcoming, comfortable, and quiet (Curtis *et al.*, 2007). Like adults, children too desire order and consistency in their surroundings, so décor should be kept simple and clean and areas clearly signposted. Ensuring quiet times are scheduled during the day and that professionals minimize loud interactions in spaces occupied by children could reduce constant traffic of staff.

Dim lights and coordination of activities could reduce the disruption at night-time and promote children's efforts to obtain rest and sleep. High noise levels, cloying heat, and bright lights are factors that could be easily minimized by both hospital and ward managers. Hospital environments should not only be geared to health professionals' requirements and comfort levels. There is increasing interest in soliciting children's views on hospital décor, environments, and hospital services (Coad & Coad, 2008; Curtis *et al.*, 2007; Eisen *et al.*, 2008), which is commendable and should lead to healthcare environments and spaces tailored more to children's preferences rather than what adults assume children like. Children's and families' satisfaction with these elements of their hospital stay could be incorporated into ongoing quality reviews, thus contributing to further development of the environment if required.

Preparing children for procedures

As seen earlier, children have fears about unfamiliar routines, procedures, and health professionals, which indicates the importance of preparatory procedures and preadmission programmes for children. It is vital that children are provided with age-appropriate information tailored to their specific needs. Intervention studies that used preparation strategies reported lower levels of anxiety in children both preoperatively and postoperatively (Brewer *et al.*, 2006). Thus, providing children with clear explanations prior to procedures potentially lessens the stress caused by fear of the unknown, enhances their coping abilities, and promotes cooperation.

There are numerous ways to prepare children prior to procedures and surgery through the use of hospital tours, videos, role-play, books, leaflets, computer games, and toys (O'Connor-Von, 2000). Children who are prepared for surgery and who have support throughout their hospitalization are more likely to recover more quickly and have fewer emotional problems (Justus *et al.*, 2006).

Helping children to express their fears and concerns and responding to those concerns is essential for successful outcomes. It is important to allow children to express their views and feelings as this will provide guidance in anticipating the types of events that children may find stressful. Ensuring that the views of children are taken into account in matters affecting them is a key principle of the National Children's Strategy in Ireland (Department of Health and Children, 2000a) and the National Service Framework for Children, Young People and Maternity Services—Standards for Hospital Services (Department of Health, 2003a).

Research with 92 children (57 of whom were consulted in hospital wards and outpatient departments) in the UK highlighted the importance of communication, relationships, environment, courtesy, and respect as fundamental aspects of what worked well and what needed to be improved in the care of hospitalized children (Curtis *et al.*, 2004). You can read more about preparing children for procedures in Chapter Four, about distraction techniques in Chapter Five, and preparation prior to performing each skill in Chapters Eight through to Sixteen.

Nursing Alert

It is important that you try to establish a trusting relationship with children and parents as it is easier for them when they feel they know nurses as people rather than as detached professionals or strangers.

Family centred care philosophy

Family centred care has been promoted as the ideal way to structure the nursing care of sick children and their families and is seen as an essential principle in children's healthcare provision globally, for example in Ireland (Hughes, 2007), the UK (Coyne & Cowley, 2007), USA (Daneman *et al.*, 2003), Canada (Espezel & Canam, 2003; MacKean *et al.*, 2005), Sweden (Ygge & Arnetz, 2004), and Australia (Kelly, 2007; Shields & Nixon, 2004).

In the UK, the National Service Framework (Department of Health, 2003a) has explicitly emphasized the importance of partnership with parents and promoting the role of families in the care of their hospitalized children. The promotion of this core principle has been driven by evidence spanning a 50-year period that highlighted the adverse effects of hospitalization for children, siblings, and parents. Children have a strong need for their familiar caregivers and the involvement of parents in the delivery of care is seen as leading to positive outcomes both for the child and family.

Definition of family

In today's society it is difficult to define the term 'family' as it can often mean different things to different people. Frequently, family is defined as the immediate relatives of an individual. However, this definition may be too narrow and exclude other family configurations. There have been enormous changes in the structure of families in the past 20 years and consideration needs to be given to 'non-traditional' families such as single parents, cohabitating couples, separated couples, divorced and reconstituted families, and gay and lesbian couples.

Clearly these changes in contemporary social life highlight a need to question the traditional model of the family (a married couple and their children) in relation to the reality of many people's lives. Therefore viewing the family in terms of a nuclear family (two parents and child) alone may result in several significant individuals not being included or acknowledged in the healthcare setting. Likewise family may include anyone related, by birth or not, who is significant to the patient and parents.

Therefore, in consideration of the wide variety of family types and structures that currently exists, we should incorporate a broader definition of family. The family may be viewed as a self-identified group of individuals whose association is characterized by special terms, who may or may not be related by bloodlines or law, but who function in such a way that they consider themselves to be a family. With this definition of the family at the forefront, the family centred care philosophy will be discussed.

Nursing Alert

Try drawing a **genogram** of your own family (diagram showing relationships between family members) and then think about the assumptions that you may hold about what makes up a family. Sometimes we are unaware of our own belief systems, such as views on lone parenthood or lesbian parents, and how these beliefs can influence our clinical practice.

Definition of family centred care

The term family centred care can mean different things to different people in different environments. Hence it is not surprising that different interpretations exist within the literature and it is usually defined as a complex concept. Other terms associated with family centred care include: parent involvement, parent participation, partnership-in-care, care-by-parent, and mutual participation. Parent participation may be seen as the care-giving activities performed by a parent/guardian for a child in the hospital setting. Thus parent participation is an important element of family centred care, which is a broader concept that focuses on the whole family.

Family centred care is defined as 'a way of caring for children and their families within health services which ensures that care is planned around the whole family, not just the individual child/person, and in which all the family members are recognized as care recipients' (Shields *et al.*, 2007, p 1318). This definition emphasizes that families need support and care while a child is hospitalized and that parents' and siblings' needs should not be forgotten. There are several key elements to family centred care and these are outlined in **Table** 2.5.

Table 2.5 Key characteristics of family centred care

- The family must be viewed as the constant in the child's life.
- The hospital is a disruption to normal family life and routines.
- Parents/primary carers want to provide emotional support for their child.
- Children have a strong need for their parents' emotional support.
- Parental/primary carer preferences for participation may vary considerably.
- Families from different cultures have unique social, cultural, and linguistic needs.
- Families have diverse needs and different forms of coping.
- Respecting families' individuality involves understanding and negotiating how parents will be involved in the care-giving activities.
- Listening and sharing information is essential for optimum parent/professional collaboration.
- Families' situations may alter daily therefore assessment and negotiation of care should be ongoing and not a singular event.
- Families need assurances that nurses will provide the care for their child when they are unable to be there.
- Some families may be reluctant to perform technical nursing care and their preferences should be accommodated.
- Families will require emotional, physical, and financial support.
- Siblings have needs that should not be neglected.
- The hospital system and policies need to be flexible and responsive to the need of families to avoid disruption to the family unit.
- Services should be designed and delivered around the needs of children and their families, not around organizations or professionals.
- The impact of resident parents on nurses' workload needs to be acknowledged by hospital management.
- Supporting families has significant resource consequences.
- Staffing levels need to be optimum so that nurses have time to support parents' participation adequately and appropriately.
- Nurses need to be aware of the importance of being there as a caring human presence for children and parents.

Family centred care frameworks

Several frameworks have been developed in different countries to guide nurses in the facilitation of family centred care, and you should try to read some of these (Cisneros-Moore *et al.*, 2003; King *et al.*, 2004; Smith *et al.*, 2002). However, there is some indication that these models, while ideals, are difficult to implement. Research studies have found that nurses frequently assume that every parent will be involved actively in their child's care and leave parents to do the care, whilst parents struggle to understand what care they are allowed to do and lack information on how their roles interact with nurses' roles (Coyne, 2003; Shields & Nixon, 2004). As a result some parents can feel abandoned by nurses and feel responsible for the provision of their child's usual child-care as well as aspects of nursing care (Coyne & Cowley, 2007).

The philosophy of family centred care is to be commended, as it seeks to empower and promote respect for parents and families. The underlying principle is for parents to be able to be present, to love and emotionally support their child, and to reduce separation anxiety. It is essential that parents be allowed to provide emotional care and support for their sick children. But the philosophy of family centred care means that parents *have a choice* about their contribution to their child's care and that they can determine their level of involvement in negotiation with nurses. It means that parents and nurses *work together* in the delivery of care. It does not mean that parents will substitute for nurses in providing nursing care. This principle is the same regardless of nursing care being delivered in hospital or at home. To achieve this, you need to think about what it is that you can do to help parents.

What nurses can do to support families

Parents have three principal needs, which are: (1) to be with their child in hospital; (2) to receive information about their child's care and their role in the care-giving activities; and (3) support from nurses. Currently many hospitals provide a variety of accommodation to enable parents to stay nearby their child if they so wish. These include beds beside the child's bed, rooms within the hospital, and accommodation in a separate building in close proximity to the hospital. It is important that facilities are also available for parents to meet their hygiene needs, have access to a quiet area for rest, and meet their nutritional needs.

Parent participation can also be stressful for parents and lead to additional financial, social, and personal costs for families, and it is important that the nurse take cognisance of this when dealing with the family. Staying throughout a child's hospitalization and staying overnight for long periods can often cause parents to incur financial costs (e.g. cost of food and drink, travel expenses, loss of income), personal costs (e.g. disruption to routines and distress), and social costs (in that they have to rely on family and neighbours for help with family activities and normal routines, e.g. school runs, siblings' after school activities, care of elderly parents, housework, etc.) (Callery, 1997; Coyne & Cowley, 2007). Hence maintaining a constant presence in hospital and delivering care on a daily basis can have considerable impact on families and may adversely affect parents' welfare in the long term. This may have relevance when, for example, families may be unable to sustain staying with the child for long periods due to stress, other essential commitments, and financial reasons. It is important that nurses are sensitive to this situation, for example, if the family have been involved in essential care of the child they should be reassured about this continued care delivery.

Nursing Alert

Try to imagine what it is like for parents living in the hospital for long periods and how their spirit and well-being could be adversely affected. Sometimes parents can be at breaking point but do not want to show that to the nurses, as they want to be seen as capable parents. In such cases a simple act such as offering a cup of tea, or offering to stay with the child so that the parent can go outside and get some time away and fresh air, can make a huge difference to a parent's welfare.

Negotiating with parents

Nurses are in a pivotal position to help alleviate parents' potential distress and anxieties by maintaining constant contact with parents and negotiating care with them.

Many parents are willing to help but need guidance and information from nurses, so nurses should clearly outline what care they can be involved in and provide support accordingly. To avoid making assumptions about parents' involvement, nurses need to make an accurate assessment of parents' wishes for involvement and negotiate care accordingly.

This could be accomplished if all nurses made a conscious effort to sit down with parents on admission or when they first meet the family in the community and document what role parents would like to perform. Such assessments should be ongoing, especially for admissions lasting more than three days or when working with children who have lifelong illnesses, as parents' expectations may alter depending on circumstances. Most parents are willing to provide childcare and continue their parenting role while in hospital or at home. However, nurses should not assume that when parents are by the child's bedside that they are obliged or wish to take full responsibility for performance of fundamental nursing care. This is within the nurses' domain of responsibility, and assistance to parents is often welcome. Similarly it must not be assumed that parents wish to undertake nursing interventions when their children are ill at home; families' needs and abilities need to be assessed on a case-by-case basis.

Many parents would welcome help from nurses at a time when they are feeling vulnerable and unsure about their child, whether in hospital or at home. In any context, parents may prefer to provide emotional support, being there as a caring presence rather than performing childcare activities.

Parents helping with nursing procedures

Some parents, depending on their child's illness, may help with nursing activities, for example, feeding (via nasogastric tubes or gastrostomy devices), administering medications, recording vital signs, and monitoring fluid balance. Sometimes parents of chronically ill children become competent in performing certain nursing procedures traditionally done by nurses and many prefer to do so in order that their children can be discharged or stay at home. However, this does not mean that you should assume that such parents prefer to continue performing these procedures forever. On occasion it may become

very necessary that they have a break and receive respite from their care-giving role.

Take some time to consider when you last asked a parent about the extent to which they wished to be involved, or if they would welcome a break from performing nursing interventions. Parents generally dislike inflicting pain on their children and therefore are reluctant to be involved in interventions that are painful. In such instances parents performing nursing care may harm the parent-child relationship, rather than reduce anxieties. How many times have you intervened to make sure that they do not need to be responsible for interventions that cause pain? As can be seen from the above, parents' expectations, abilities, and preferences for participation in care may vary considerably throughout their child's stay. This emphasizes the importance of nurses using clear communication and active negotiation of care in partnership with parents on a daily basis, so that parents and families are adequately supported.

Respecting families' cultures

Effective negotiation is fundamental to family centred care and you must remember that families and their children may have very different cultural understandings of health and illness to your own. People from diverse ethnic groups have unique social, cultural, and linguistic backgrounds that profoundly influence their perceptions of health and illness. Families also carry, from generation to generation, cultural beliefs and traditions associated with health and illness.

Families from different cultures may also lack knowledge of what is considered appropriate behaviour in healthcare interactions, and this can result in misunderstandings and conflict. Valuing families' cultural and ethnic identity is central to the provision of culturally competent care and culturally specific information and advice. Therefore nurses need to understand and respect families' belief systems and learn about their help-seeking behaviours so that they can help prepare parents for the care their child requires in hospital and for when care needs to be continued at home. Taking time to communicate effectively with families will result in increased understanding of their worldviews, which will shape healthcare interactions and interventions according to families' individual needs.

Linguistic services and bilingual healthcare workers can help reduce language barriers, thereby enhancing the communication process. It is important in both the hospital setting and in the home that you approach the family as unique, respect their cultural beliefs, and carefully assess their preferences for participation. Doing this will ensure that you avoid making generalizations and assumptions about parents' preferences and willingness to participate in care-giving activities for their child in hospital and at home. You could make a special attempt to find out about different cultural groups and reflect on how easy it is for the families to accommodate the nursing needs of their child into their cultural practices.

Nursing Alert

Be aware that children from different cultures are usually bilingual and may speak and understand English words and phrases better than their parents. In such instances you will need to use simple words to communicate with parents and where they have no comprehension of English you should use interpreters to explain what is happening. Sometimes the child may be able to explain terms to their parents but you should not rely upon the child as most healthcare settings employ interpreters.

Discharge planning within family centred care

The continued trend towards care delivery in outpatient and community settings means that parents are increasingly expected to care for children with complex healthcare needs at home. With shorter hospital stays and more children surviving with chronic conditions, parents often have to perform procedures such as catheterizations, artificial tube feeding, administering medications/injections, wound care, and wound dressings. Discharge planning is also discussed further in Chapter Five.

In most instances it is much better for the child to be discharged home quickly, reducing risk of infection and disruption to family life. But families need good support, especially if they have to continue the complex care procedures at home, as this can be stressful for many parents. Often parents are fearful of taking on skills that they see as nurses' responsibility in case they make mistakes and harm their child. Other parents may have difficulty learning

all the steps in a procedure and feel frustrated with their progress. It is so important that parents are not made to feel that their learning styles or pace of learning are a 'problem', as this will cause unnecessary distress and lead parents to question their abilities to cope at home.

The hospital admission represents but a sub-set in the world of the families. Nurses, therefore, need to be vigilant to ensure that parents are treated with respect and dignity, since their welfare affects the family's welfare. The preparation and education process should begin at an early stage of the hospitalization to ensure that parents can practise the procedures many times under supervision. The teaching should be documented and parents' questions and concerns clarified. The nurse should ensure that the parents are capable of performing the procedure safely, and know what to do in case of an adverse event occurring.

Discharge planning should begin early so as to ensure that community support services are tailored to meet the family's and child's needs. Expecting parents to learn procedures quickly and be responsible for care at home may threaten the stability of the family unit and consequently be detrimental for overall family functioning. Therefore nurses need to acknowledge the family context and assess its support system, so that parents are prepared to care for their child safely and shown how to incorporate the care so that family life and routines experience minimal disruption.

A full assessment of the parents' understanding of the illness, their ability to cope with the demands of the illness, and their support network is important. Clear identification of the family's current resources and requirements will enable nurses to identify needs quickly and so provide options and referrals effectively, so that nursing interventions can be tailored to the individual's needs. Nurses can provide a valuable link between the family system and the social system with which they interact by securing support for families within the primary care sector, such as community children's nursing teams (CCNs).

In the UK, the CCN services provide vital support and care for the child and family, whilst in Ireland the Public Health Nurse (PHN) provides similar support. Professionals working in the community (e.g. CCNs, PHNs, health visitors, district nurses, school nurses, and family doctors) need to be aware of the challenges facing families and children, particularly those with chronic illnesses, life-threatening conditions, and palliative care needs, and provide support and understanding of their special needs. With families increasingly assuming more responsibilities in the care of the chronically ill child both in hospital and at home, it is essential that nurses work with families in achieving a satisfactory balance of care for all concerned, so that families and children receive the best possible care.

Consideration

List all the professionals in the community that can provide support for families with a chronically ill child. Think about how some healthcare professionals' roles can overlap and identify ways in which they can work together to support families.

Communicating with children

The past decade has seen a growing recognition of the importance of children's rights and the need to listen to and consult with children both at a national (Department of Health and Children, 2000a; Department of Health & Children, 2000b) and international level (Department of Health, 2003a; Royal College of Paediatrics and Child Health, 2000; Spinetta *et al.*, 2003; United Nations, 1989). The United Nations Convention on the Rights of the Child (UNCRC) (United Nations, 1989), which was ratified by the UK in 1991 and Ireland in 1992, clearly stated the right of every child to **self-determination**, dignity, respect, non-interference, and the right to make informed decisions. Changes in how children are viewed and how childhood is understood are exerting powerful influences on how adults work with children. **Social agency** simply means being able to act on behalf of yourself or in your own self-interest. Consultation with children is now a key policy issue that is recognized and actively promoted by many non-government and voluntary organizations such as Action for Sick Children, Barnardo's, Carnegie Young People Initiative, National Youth Agency, National Children's Bureau, and Save the Children. The view of children as social agents is clearly evident in the current policy directing the care of children in hospital (Commission for Healthcare Audit and Inspection, 2007b).

Both the National Children's Strategy (2000) for Ireland and the National Service Framework (NSF) for England (Department for Education and Skills, 2004) directs healthcare services to give children greater choice and participation in decisions about their health and care. The Children's NSF explicitly states that: 'Children and young people should receive care that is integrated and coordinated around their particular needs, and the needs of their family. They, and their parents, should be treated with respect, and should be given support and information to enable them to understand and cope with illness or injury, and the treatment needed. They should be encouraged to be active partners in decisions about their health and care, and, where possible, be able to exercise choice' (Department of Health, 2003a, p 9). The central tenet of these policies is that all children, regardless of ability, race, or ethnic background, have the right to express their views on what happens to them and to have those views taken seriously by the adults delivering services. This means that health professionals have a responsibility to listen to children's views and involve them in discussions that directly affect them. The rights of the child are discussed again in Chapter Four in relation to consent and legal matters.

Children's views on communication

Children and young people want to be heard, listened to, and allowed to participate in healthcare matters (Cavet & Sloper, 2005). They have expressed strong desires to have their voices heard in relation to everyday decisions about their care and treatment (Alderson *et al.*, 2006; Coad & Houston, 2007; Coyne *et al.*, 2006). Many children like receiving information because it helps prepare them for what to expect and thus reduces their worries and provides reassurance. Receiving information and having their views respected enhances children's understanding and adaptation to the hospitalization. Children report feeling valued, comfortable, less anxious, and more prepared when they are involved in communication (Coyne *et al.*, 2006). Conversely, children who are excluded from the communication process report feeling disappointed, sad, confused, angry, rotten, worried, misled, shocked, betrayed, lonely, and ignored. The range and depth of these feelings clearly illustrate the impact of non-consultation on many children. Likewise avoidance of children's questions and children's suspicion of health professionals withholding information from them potentially undermines their trust in the health professionals' good intentions and adds to anxiety levels. However, you need to be aware that some children may cope with the stress of hospitalization and ill health by using an '**information-limiting strategy**', which can be quite effective in managing the stress of anticipated hospitalization or illness.

Children's experiences of communication interactions

Although there is increasing recognition within children's nursing of the need to consult with children and the importance of obtaining children's views, this is not reflected in healthcare. The research studies that have been conducted with children in hospital indicate that children have varying experiences of being consulted and involved in their care and that children experience less than optimal communication (Beresford & Sloper, 2003; Coyne, 2006a; Coyne et al., 2006; Curtis et al., 2004; Hallstrom & Elander, 2004; Savage & Callery, 2007). Children have identified several factors that may constrain them from actively participating in consultations. These include: not knowing health professionals; not wanting to hear bad news; fear of causing 'trouble' by asking questions; lack of time with health professionals; being ignored; being disbelieved; difficulty contacting health professionals; health professionals not listening; difficulty understanding medical terminology; and parents' actions. Although there are many factors that obstruct children's participation, the key factors appear to be health professionals' communication styles, attitudes, and behaviours (Coyne et al., 2006). Children generally report that health professionals tend to 'do things' to them with very brief explanations or no explanations. Children have reported being unable to ask questions during their interactions with health professionals due to being rushed. They speak about being afraid to ask questions due to fear of inconveniencing or annoying health professionals because they are busy and important adults. It is obvious that children's ability to participate effectively in communication interactions may be hindered by health professionals' attitudes and behaviour.

Nursing Alert

Many children, particularly younger children less than seven years old or children that are shy or quiet, are afraid to ask questions, voice concerns, or seek help. You can play a really important advocacy role by eliciting their feelings and understandings, and supporting them to ask any questions or, if that is not possible, asking the questions on the child's behalf.

Parents' role in the communication process

Children frequently rely on their parents to act as advocates and interpreters in the communication process. Children of different ages (pre-school and adolescents) often prefer their parents to be their advocates and/or interpreters in the communication process because of fear of hearing bad news, or difficulty understanding health professionals' style of communication (Coyne et al., 2006). Using parents as 'buffers' to limit exposure to potentially worrying information has been reported by other sick children (Young et al., 2003). Parents can help explain and clarify information received from health professionals. However, sometimes parents can inhibit their children's attempts to participate in the communication process by answering questions on their behalf, telling them to stay quiet, reprimanding them for interrupting discussions, and/or withholding information (Coyne et al., 2006). Parents' actions may reflect their need to protect their children's well-being and thus are well intentioned. Alternatively parents may hold the belief that children should be seen and not heard and thus discourage children's active participation. Parents may experience difficulty balancing their need to protect their children with the need to also encourage children's participation. Therefore parents may need help to consider how their children's interests might best be served, and encouragement from health professionals to facilitate children's participation in the communication process.

What nurses can do to ensure children's voices are heard

Nurses, as the child's advocate, can play a key role in ensuring that all children are encouraged to express their views and receive information according to their preference. Information provided should be tailored so that it is accessible and appropriate according to individual children's level of understanding. Written information should be designed and presented in a way that ensures it is easy to read and relevant to children. Children need sufficient time to be given to them to consider the information provided and also to be able to talk to health professionals and others so that clarifications can be sought. Where children cannot be provided with their first choice, they should be given an explanation of why their preference cannot be met and offered alternatives where possible. Children need time to feel able to ask questions, express their concerns, express preferences, share information, and have their views heard. Children's preferences for communication are listed in **Table 2.6**. Children find it easier to ask questions when the person they are in contact with is more familiar to them. Knowing the doctors and nurses helps children to feel confident in their good intentions and thereby provides reassurance (Coyne, 2006a). This suggests that children need to feel comfortable with health professionals in order to ask questions, which is not unusual when one considers the powerful position that adults hold in relation to children's subordinate status. Health professionals who are approachable and willing to chat encourage children's participation in the communication process. But children often experience difficulty knowing health professionals due to lack of time, lack of frequent contact, and lack of continuity due to health professionals' shift work. They can be greatly assisted by the allocation of a primary carer (nurse) so that a relationship can develop. Making an effort to know

Table 2.6 Children's preferences for communication

- Having sufficient time to ask questions.
- Asking questions.
- Receiving information in simple words.
- Being asked questions.
- Expressing a view.
- Being listened to.
- Being heard.
- Being allowed to take part in discussions.
- Contributing preferences in decisions.
- Sharing in the decision making process.
- Not having full responsibility for medical decisions.

the child as a person and sharing information on oneself can assist in the development of a trusting relationship, which will encourage children to communicate.

Ensuring communication is tailored to children's preferences

Each child should be treated as an individual and given information in a manner that is accessible and appropriate according to his or her level of understanding. As mentioned earlier, some children may not want to receive information for various reasons and consequently prefer their parents to receive the information. This suggests that sensitivity is required to ensure that children are not overwhelmed with information, particularly if they use an information-limiting strategy to cope. Parents' advice should be sought on how best to involve children. It may also be necessary to work with parents to enable them to help their children become more actively involved in the decisions that affect them. Children should be kept as fully informed as they wish about their care and treatment and provided with enough information so that they feel prepared adequately for procedures. Acknowledging children's rights to be listened to and to be informed is not the same as giving them sole responsibility for making decisions. Instead health professionals need to view children's involvement not as all or nothing, but as a process that evolves over time according to the circumstances and needs of the children.

Assumptions about children's cognitive immaturity need to be challenged and addressed and health professionals need to re-evaluate their practices to ensure that they embrace a more flexible approach to children's participation in consultations and decisions (Coad & Houston, 2007; Coyne, 2008; Zwaanswijk et al., 2007). All professionals have an ethical and clinical obligation to communicate with children in a way that facilitates their participation in issues that affect them. The benefits for children include: better provision of information; having an opportunity to express feelings; developing confidence; increasing skills in decision making; and enhancing self-esteem and overall coping with hospitalization. It is imperative that efforts are directed towards facilitating and supporting children's involvement because it will improve the quality of care provided for children and families. Furthermore, it is an important investment with immense future potential benefits for children, staff, and the health service.

To summarize, effective communication with children requires you to be cognisant of verbal and non-verbal communication. Your posture, **body language**, and positioning will indicate the amount of respect you have for the child and family. You need to actively listen and build empathy; summarize, explain, consult, and negotiate (see **http://www.everychildmatters.gov.uk/deliveringservices/commoncore/communication/**).

Safety and safeguarding children

Concern for the safety of children in healthcare is an international phenomenon. Many countries have produced a series of policy documents to improve the overall safety and well-being of children, and healthcare is no exception. Children receive healthcare in many settings including clinics, hospitals, schools, and their own homes. Regardless of the setting there can be a significant risk of harm. The CHAI (Commission for Healthcare Audit and Inspection, 2007a) identified that in developed countries, one in ten patients suffer some form of harm from healthcare. One third of these suffer severe morbidity (disability caused by an accident or error) or die. In all, accidents (such as falls) account for most harm, followed by medication errors, misuse of equipment, poor record keeping, and inadequate communication. Many incidents are avoidable if appropriate safety measures are maintained. There is a discernible shift in healthcare practice from a culture of blame when something goes wrong to one of openness, transparency, and learning from adverse events (Vincent, 2006). Hence it is essential that all incidents are clearly documented so that lessons are learned from errors and action taken to prevent such incidents from re-occurring. Nurses play a key role in promoting a safe environment for children and families in the hospital by adhering to the key principles of safety as listed in **Table 2.7**.

As already discussed, hospitals can be frightening and alien environments for many children, whether it is their first admission or part of a series of admissions. Children's wards are often busy environments with many people (e.g. nurses, doctors, patients, families, teachers, play

Table 2.7 Broad principles of safety

- Know the local policies and procedures.
- Be aware of the principles of safety for children.
- Attend risk management training days.
- Keep up to date with best practice.
- Carry out risk assessment if concerned.
- Report all potential hazards, otherwise you are contributing to the possibility of adverse events.

therapists, social workers, support workers, volunteers, ward clerks, cleaners, kitchen staff etc.) congregating in a confined area and all focused on different activities. It can be quite bewildering and disorientating for a small child to be exposed to such a busy environment peopled by strangers. It can be easy for a small child to 'wander off' even with numerous adults in the vicinity. Or for a child to experience harm from the immediate environment. Nurses need to be aware of the potential hazards associated with the hospital environment so that safety measures are maintained to a high standard. Children should not incur any harm from the hospital environment and as such are the responsibility of the health professionals whilst hospitalized. The main aim should be to keep the child free from injury or harm throughout their stay in hospital and this requires extra vigilance and observational skills in nurses caring for children.

Nursing Alert

Small children are naturally inquisitive and love to explore, and toddlers who are learning to walk have high safety needs, so you need to be extra vigilant. Always check the environment for potential hazards and take action to minimize the possibility of accidents occurring.

Safety hazards in the environment

Safety is essential for all patients and visitors, and particularly so for children who have characteristics that require a greater concern for safety. Children are a particularly vulnerable group because of their age, cognitive immaturity, size, development, and natural inquisitiveness. Children and young people are not merely little adults;

they are different from adults and have different needs. Childhood is a time of rapid growth and development and children's cognitive and intellectual development increases with age. Due to cognitive immaturity, young children below the age of seven years are often unaware of the dangers within their environment. Toddlers from the age of eight months upwards are eager to explore their environment as displayed by crawling, using objects to pull themselves up, and attempts to walk. In a busy hospital ward it is very difficult for toddlers to exercise their natural instinct to explore because of equipment, staff, and general lack of safe spaces. Young children with special needs and/or sensory deficits are particularly vulnerable to potential harm because of their potential communicative deficits (Rabiee *et al.*, 2005). Ensuring that every child has an identity bracelet or name band attached is a standard safety procedure. Often small babies are provided with two identity bracelets, one on each arm, in case one identity bracelet is lost or is accidentally removed in carrying out a procedure. There are many actions nurses can use to safeguard children from environmental hazards and these are listed in **Table 2.8.**

As mentioned earlier, the environment where children are cared for, i.e. the building, people, and equipment, can potentially pose many risks or dangers for children (Stower, 2000). It is important that you are aware of local policies and procedures, know the principles of safety for children, and attend risk management training regularly. Nurses should keep up to date with best practice and most importantly report all concerns, otherwise they are contributing to the possibility of adverse events occurring.

The importance of play

Play is an integral aspect of childhood and child development and a basic need of all children. It is an activity that assists in their normal development, as children learn physical, mental, and social skills through play. It is a universal activity in all cultures. Consequently the child's freedom to play must be preserved in hospital. All children, irrespective of gender, culture or racial origin, background, or individual ability, should have equal access to play experiences while in hospital (Department of Health and Children, 2004; Department for Education and Skills, 2004). Play serves an important function for hospitalized children in that it restores a sense of normality, reduces anxieties, serves as an outlet for tensions and conflicts, facilitates communication, and enhances recovery (Children in Hospital Ireland, 2000). As seen earlier, hospitals are alien environments for many children because they encounter unfamiliar people, treatments, medical equipment, and language. Play helps reduce the adverse effects of hospitalization by acting as a diversion and refocusing attention away from stressors and the unfamiliar environment. In recognition of the essential role of play for children, hospitals in Ireland and the United Kingdom increasingly employ the services of a play specialist and provide play facilities and play equipment. Play specialists play a key role in facilitating and encouraging children's opportunities for play. These professionals frequently play a valuable role in advising and educating nursing and medical staff in the use of play for therapeutic purposes.

Table 2.8 Nursing interventions to maintain safety

- Familiarize yourself with safety policies on your unit.
- Report any potential hazards, e.g. slippery floors, poor lighting, uneven flooring, broken equipment, unprotected windows, doors not closing properly, latches missing on windows or doors, or missing cot sides.
- Keep potentially hazardous items and equipment out of children's reach.
- Do not leave breakable items within children's reach.
- Dispose of hazardous waste as per hospital policy.
- Use safety harnesses in highchairs, prams, strollers, and wheelchairs.
- Transport infants and children appropriately.
- Keep cot sides up and securely fastened.
- Use bedrails for older children if at risk of falling.
- Keep exit routes free from obstruction.
- Ensure the ward exit is secure as per hospital policy.
- Electrical outlets should be covered to prevent fingers being inserted into wall sockets or accidental burns.

Resources for play

Although play is an important and fundamental right for all children, play provision is often overlooked or given low priority in the healthcare setting. In England the National Association of Hospital Play Specialists (see **http://www.nshps.org.uk**) was only established in 1975, 28 years after the first staff were employed to play with children admitted to a London hospital. These developments have been mirrored in other countries, for instance in New Zealand (see **http://www.hospitalplay.org.nz/history.html**). Inadequate play facilities have been reported in studies of children in hospital (Cross & Gregory, 2002), and inadequate numbers of play specialists have been identified in the National Play Policy Report, Ireland (Department of Health and Children, 2004). Similarly in the UK, a national survey of play services in hospitals admitting children reported that five hospitals had no play provision available for children (Walker, 2000). There was also great variability in the number of play specialists employed to work with children. Even where play specialists are employed, they often work only between 9am and 5pm, Monday to Friday. It is not possible for one play specialist to be able to fulfil the play needs of all the children on any unit. This means that children's nurses need to advocate for the necessary time, space, and equipment for play to take place, and to play with children. It is essential that all health professionals incorporate play into their daily care provision for hospitalized children. The Irish National Play Policy (Department of Health and Children, 2004) specifically states that the therapeutic value of play should be recognized and actively promoted by health boards and hospitals.

Therapeutic value of play

In addition to being a fun activity for children, play is of immense therapeutic value for children in hospital and has many functions that are listed in **Table 2.9**.

Play is a very useful method for forming a therapeutic alliance with a sick child in that it can assist the nurse in getting to know the child as an individual. Likewise for a child, shared play helps establish the nurse as a person rather than a professional. Knowing that nurses are willing to play and share humour helps children feel secure and contributes towards a trusting relationship. Using expressive arts with children encourages them to express and master their feelings about being ill (Wikstrom, 2005). It also provides insight into their experiences and this knowledge can help nurses to provide appropriate support. Play therefore is a valuable tool in enhancing children's emotional welfare.

Table 2.9 Functions of play

- Fun activity for children.
- Provides mental, physical, and social stimulation.
- Integral to child development and acquisition of skills.
- Provides opportunity for self-expression.
- Encourages creativity and imagination.
- Provides outlet for emotion.
- Allows children to practise roles and situations.
- Helps provide or restore normality.
- Helps nurses to build a relationship with the child.
- Helps the child to adjust to and gain control over a potentially frightening environment.
- Helps the child assimilate new information.
- Prepares the child psychologically for procedures and interventions.
- Assists in coping with painful procedures.
- Helps provide distraction.
- Aids assessment of the child's condition and developmental level.
- Stimulates the senses for children with special needs.

Play can help prepare children for admission to hospital, the ward environment, and illness trajectory. Children find intrusive procedures and blood tests particularly threatening and very stressful, as has been noted earlier. Play can be extremely beneficial in preparing children for painful procedures and gaining their cooperation. Nurses can use play material such as dolls as props to explain procedures beforehand and allow children time to express their fears and concerns. Parents can play a significant role in preparing their child, and therefore nurses should involve parents in play sessions to impart information. In addition to toys there are numerous play interventions that can be used, such as creative materials, music, dance, dressing-up clothes, puppets, clown therapy, computer games, play stations, online discussion forums, and pet therapy. Recent research has found that pet therapy programmes are useful aids for enhancing well-being and promoting normalcy while a child is hospitalized (Kaminski et al., 2002). Play enhances a child's overall coping abilities by allowing them the time and opportunity to assimilate information and accommodate to new experiences. Using play to explain procedures lessens the stress caused by fear of the unknown, enhances the child's coping abilities, and promotes cooperation (Brewer et al., 2006).

Nursing Alert

It is important to remember that play interventions designed to reduce children's stress during hospitalization are not only likely to decrease their stress at the time, but are also likely to influence how future experiences are appraised and managed by the child in any healthcare encounter.

Maximizing a child's opportunity for play

Intrusive events and medical treatments are obvious sources of stress for hospitalized children, but nurses may not be aware of other events that are stressful for children such as disruption to normal routines and loss of self-determination (Coyne, 2006b). Play can help children to gain control and authority over frightening healthcare experiences by allowing them some choices and involvement in the process, thus lessening the impact of the experience (Alderson, 2008). Keeping occupied through play is an important strategy that children use to cope with their hospitalization, and inadequate play facilities will hamper children's abilities to deal with the hospitalization.

Inhibiting children's ability to play deprives them of one of their most important coping mechanisms. Play should be an integral part of a child's daily care plan. Nurses have a responsibility to ensure that children are provided with the opportunity to play, have adequate space to play safely, and are provided with age-appropriate play materials. Children with disabilities will require access to adapted play equipment, and children from different cultures may require written material translated into a number of different languages. Although many hospitals have dedicated playrooms, too many playrooms are used for alternative purposes (i.e. storage of beds and equipment) or have strict opening times, making them inaccessible to children when needed. Where such facilities exist it is important that the toys are clean and unbroken and that the facilities cater for both young children and adolescents, as frequently there is a lack of play materials suitable for adolescents and young people (Curtis et al., 2007).

Conclusion

This chapter has explored the key concepts of attachment and loss, effects of hospitalization, family centred care, communication skills, safety, and play. All of these principles are equally important in the performance of skills and procedures. It is suggested that you explore these issues further by obtaining some of the papers referenced and follow up on the suggestions for further reading.

Working through the scenarios with this chapter will help you to link theory and practice. The importance of involving the family in delivery of care and respecting a family's culture are key themes that are threaded through all of the chapters in this textbook. The trend towards reduced hospital stay and parents caring for children in their own homes means that increasingly hospital nurses play a key role in educating parents and community nurses play an equally important role in supporting parents in the delivery of care. The key principles discussed in this chapter underpin the entire set of core skills required by students at the point of registration as detailed in the Essential Skills Clusters document (Nursing and Midwifery Council, UK) and the clinical skill competency requirements (An Bord Altranais, Republic of Ireland). All of these essential principles are applied to the knowledge, skills, and procedures in the proceeding chapters. Using these principles in the development of your knowledge and performance of skills will enhance your practice and ensure that high quality care is delivered for children and their families.

Online resource centre

You may find it helpful to work through our online resources including interactive scenarios intended to help you to develop and apply the skills in this chapter. Where material referenced below is available electronically, we're pleased to provide active web links to the source via *(w)* **http:// www.oxfordtextbooks.co.uk/orc/coyne/**

References

Ainsworth, M. (1989) Attachments Beyond Infancy. *American Psychologist* **44**, 709–716.

Alderson, P. (2008) *Young Children's Rights: Exploring beliefs, principles and practice*. London: Jessica Kingsley.

Alderson, P., Sutcliffe, K. & Curtis, K. (2006) Children as partners with adults in their medical care. *Archives of Disease in Childhood* **91**, 300–303.

Battrick, C. & Glasper, E.A. (2004) The views of children and their families on being in hospital. *British Journal of Nursing* **13**, 328–338.

Beresford, B.A. & Sloper, P. (2003) Chronically ill adolescents' experiences of communicating with doctors: A qualitative study. *Journal of Adolescent Health* **33**, 172–179.

Bowlby, J. (1952) *Maternal Child Care and Mental Health*. Geneva: World Health Organization.

Bowlby, J. (1975) *Attachment and Loss*. London: Penguin.

Bowlby, J. (1980) *Attachment and Loss, volume 3*. London: Penguin.

Bowlby, J., Ainsworth, M., Boston, M. & Rosenbluth, B. (1956) The effects of mother-child separation:

A follow-up study. *British Journal of Medical Psychology* **29**, 211–247.

Brewer, S., Gleditsch, S.L., Syblik, D., Tietjens, M.E. & Vacik, H.W. (2006) Pediatric anxiety: Child life intervention in day surgery. *Journal of Pediatric Nursing* **12**, 13–22.

Callery, P. (1997) Paying to participate: Financial, social and personal costs to parents of involvement in their children's care in hospital. *Journal of Advanced Nursing* **25**, 746–752.

Casey, A. & Mobbs, S. (1988) Partnership in practice. *Nursing Times* **84**, 67–68.

Cavet, J. & Sloper, P. (2005) *Children and young people's views on health and health services: A review of the evidence*. London: National Children's Bureau, pp. 1–83.

Children in Hospital Ireland (2000) *Update on play facilities report*. Dublin: Children in Hospital Ireland.

Children's Workforce Development Council (2005) *Common core of skills and knowledge*. **http://www.everychildmatters.gov.uk/ deliveringservices/commoncore/**

Cisneros-Moore, K.A., Coker, K., DuBuisson, A.B., Swett, B. & Edwards, W.H. (2003) Implementing potentially better practices for improving family-centered care in neonatal intensive care units: Successes and challenges. *Pediatrics* **111**, 450–460.

Cleary, J. (1992) *Caring for Children in Hospital: Parents and nurses in partnership*. London: Bailliere Tindall.

Coad, J. & Coad, N. (2008) Children and young people's preference of thematic design and colour for their hospital environment. *Journal of Child Healthcare* **12**, 33–48.

Coad, J. & Houston, R. (2007) *Voices of Children and Young People: Involving children and young people in the decision-making processes of healthcare services. A review of the literature*. London: Action for Sick Children.

Commission for Healthcare Audit and Inspection (2007a) *Meeting of the Healthcare Commission November 22nd 2007. Safety—programme of work*. London: Healthcare Commission.

Commission for Healthcare Audit and Inspection (2007b) *Improving Hospital Services for Children*. London: Commission for Healthcare Audit and Inspection.

Coyne, I.T. (2003) A grounded theory of disrupted lives: Children, parents, and nurses in the children's ward. London: King's College University of London.

Coyne, I. (2006a) Consultation with children in hospital: Children's, parents' and nurses' perspectives. *Journal of Clinical Nursing* **15**, 61–71.

Coyne, I.T. (2006b) Children's experiences of hospitalization. *Journal of Child Healthcare* **10**, 326–336.

Coyne, I.T. (2008) Children's participation in consultations and decision-making at health service level: a critical review of the literature. *International Journal of Nursing Studies* **45**, 1682–1689.

Coyne, I.T. & Conlon, J. (2007) Children's and young people's views of hospitalization: 'It's a scary place'. *Journal of Children's and Young People's Nursing* **1**, 16–21.

Coyne, I.T. & Cowley, S. (2007) Challenging the philosophy of partnership with parents: A grounded theory study. *International Journal of Nursing Studies* **44**, 893–904.

Coyne, I.T., Hayes, E., Gallagher, P. & Regan, G. (2006) Giving children a voice: Investigation of children's experiences of participation in consultation and decision-making in Irish hospitals. Dublin: Office of the Minister for Children.

Cross, R. & Gregory, S. (2002) Giving children a 'voice'. *Emergency Nurse* **10**, 11–15.

Curtis, K., Liabo, K., Roberts, H. & Barker, M. (2004) Consulted but not heard: A qualitative study of young people's views of their local health service. *Health Expectations* **7**, 149–156.

Curtis, P., James, A. & Birch, J. (2007) *Space to Care: Children's perceptions of spatial aspects of hospitals. Full Research Report. ESRC End of Award Report, RES-000-23-0765*. Swindon: ESRC, pp. 1–25.

Daneman, S., Macaluso, J. & Guzzetta, C. (2003) Healthcare providers' attitudes toward parent participation in the care of the hospitalized child. *Journal for Specialists in Pediatric Nursing* **8**, 90–98.

Department for Education and Skills (2004) *Ill Child Standard, National Service Framework for Children, Young People and Maternity Services*. Nottingham: Department for Education and Skills.

Department of Health (2003a) *Getting the Right Start: The National Service Framework for Children, Young People and Maternity Services—Standards for Hospital Services*. London: Stationery Office.

Department of Health (2003b) *Standards for Children in Hospital: A guide for parents and carers*. London: Department of Health, pp. 1–20.

Department of Health and Children (2000a) *The National Children's Strategy: Our Children—Their Lives*. Dublin: Department of Health and Children.

Department of Health and Children (2000b) *Report of the Public Consultation for the National Children's Strategy*. Dublin: Department of Health and Children.

Department of Health and Children (2004) *Ready, Steady, Play. National Play Policy*. Dublin: Department of Health and Children.

Eisen, S.J., Ulrich, R.S., Shepley, M.M., Varni, J.W. & Sherman, S. (2008) The stress reducing effects of art in pediatric healthcare: Art preferences of healthy children and hospitalized children. *Journal of Child Healthcare* **12**, 173–190.

Espezel, H.J.E. & Canam, C.J. (2003) Parent-nurse interactions: Care of hospitalized children. *Journal of Advanced Nursing* **44**, 34–41.

Hallstrom, I. & Elander, G. (2004) Decision making during hospitalization: Parents' and children's involvement. *Journal of Clinical Nursing* **13**, 367–375.

Howe, D. (2005) *Child Abuse and Neglect: Attachment, Development and Intervention*. Basingstoke: Palgrave Macmillan.

Hughes, M. (2007) Parents' and nurses' attitudes to family-centred care: An Irish perspective. *Journal of Clinical Nursing* **16**, 2341–2348.

James, A. & James, A. (2004) *Constructing Childhood: Theory, policy and social practice*. Houndmills: Palgrave.

Jolley, J. (2004) *A Social History of Paediatric Nursing 1920–1970*. Hull: The University of Hull.

Justus, R., Wyles, D., Wilson, J., Rode, D., Walther, V. & Lim-Sulit, N. (2006) Preparing children and families for surgery: Mount Sinai's multidisciplinary perspective. *Pediatric Nursing* **32**, 35–43.

Kaminski, M., Pellino, T. & Wish, J. (2002) Play and pets: The physical and emotional impact of child-life and pet therapy on hospitalized children. *Children's Healthcare* **31**, 321–335.

Kelly, M.T. (2007) Achieving family-centred care: Working on or working with stakeholders? *Neonatal, Paediatric and Child Health Nursing* **10**, 4–11.

Kendrick, A. & Taylor, J. (2000) Hidden on the ward: The abuse of children in hospitals. *Journal of Advanced Nursing* **31**, 565–573.

King, S., King, G. & Rosenbaum, P. (2004) Evaluating health service delivery to children with chronic conditions and their families: Development of a refined measure of processes of care (MPOC-20). *Children's Healthcare* **33**, 35–57.

Little, M., Axford, N. & Morpeth, L. (2003) Children's services in the UK 1997–2003: Problems, developments and challenges for the future. *Children and Society* **17**, 205–214.

Livesley, J. (2005) Telling tales: A qualitative exploration of how children's nurses interpret work with unaccompanied hospitalized children. *Journal of Clinical Nursing* **14**, 43–50.

MacKean, G.L., Thurston, W.E. & Scott, S.M. (2005) Bridging the divide between families' and health professionals' perspectives on family-centred care. *Health Expectations* **8**, 74–85.

Mayall, B. (2002) *Towards a Sociology for Childhood: Thinking from children's lives*. Buckingham: Open University Press.

National Statistics (2006) *Children*. Available at: **http://www.statistics.gov.uk/CCI/nugget.asp? ID= 348&Pos=2&ColRank=1&Rank=326**

O'Connor-Von, S. (2000) Preparing children for surgery—An integrative research review. *AORN Journal* **71**, 334–343.

Rabiee, P., Sloper, P. & Beresford, B. (2005) Doing research with children and young people who do not use speech for communication. *Children & Society* **19**, 385–396.

Robertson, J. (1958a) *Going to Hospital with Mother*. London: Tavistock.

Robertson, J. (1958b) *Young Children in Hospital*. London: Tavistock.

Robertson, J. (1989) *Separation and the Very Young*. London: Free Association Books.

Royal College of Paediatrics and Child Health, Ethics Advisory Committee (2000) Guidelines for the ethical conduct of medical research involving children. *Archives of Disease in Childhood* **82**, 117–182.

Savage, E. & Callery, P. (2007) Clinic consultations with children and parents on the dietary management of cystic fibrosis. *Social Science & Medicine* **64**, 363–374.

Shields, L. (2001) A review of the literature from developed countries relating to the effects of hospitalization on children and their parents. *International Nursing Review* **48**, 29–37.

Shields, L. & Nixon, J. (2004) Hospital care of children in four countries. *Journal of Advanced Nursing* **45**, 475–486.

Shields, L., Pratt, J., Davis, L.M. & Hunter, J. (2007) Family-centred care for children in hospital. *Cochrane Database of Systematic Reviews*, Art. No. CD004811. DOI 10.1002/14651858. CD004811.pub2.

Smith, L., Coleman, V. & Bradshaw, M. (2002) Family-centred care: Concept, theory and practice. Hampshire: Palgrave.

Spinetta, J.J., Masera, G., Jankovic, M., *et al.* (2003) Valid informed consent and participative decision-making in children with cancer and their parents: A report of the SIOP Working Committee on psychosocial issues in pediatric oncology. *Medical Pediatric Oncology* **40**, 244–246.

Stower, S. (2000) Keeping the hospital environment safe for children. *Paediatric Nursing* **12**, 37–42.

Timmins, F., McCabe, C., Griffiths, C., Gleeson, M. & O'Shea, J. (2005) *Lessons from Practice—Reflection on Communication across the Disciplines*. International Conference Symposium Presentation: Royal College of Nursing of the United Kingdom Research Society Annual International Nursing Research Conference, 9–11 March 2005, Belfast, UK.

United Nations (1989) *Convention on the Rights of the Child*. Geneva: United Nations.

Vincent, C. (2006) *Patient Safety*. Edinburgh: Elsevier.

Walker, J. (2000) Background and preliminary findings of a national survey of play services in hospitals admitting children in the UK. Middlesex: National Association of Hospital Play Staff.

Wikstrom, B.-M. (2005) Communicating via expressive arts: The natural medium of self-expression for hospitalized children. *Pediatric Nursing* **31**, 480–485.

Ygge, B.M. & Arnetz, J.E. (2004) A study of parental involvement in pediatric hospital care: Implications for clinical practice. *Journal of Pediatric Nursing* **19**, 217–223.

Young, B., Dixon-Woods, M., Windridge, K.C & Heney, D. (2003) Managing communication with young people who have a life threatening chronic illness: A qualitative study of patients and parents. *British Medical Journal* **326**, 305–309.

Zwaanswijk, M., Tates, K., van Dulmen, S., Hoogerbrugge, P., Kamps, W. & Bensing, J. (2007) Young patients', parents', and survivors' communication preferences in paediatric oncology: Results of online focus groups. *BMC Pediatrics* **7**, 35.

Further reading and URLs

Alderson, P. (2008) Young children's rights: Exploring beliefs, principles and practice. London: Jessica Kingsley.

John, M. (2003) Children's rights and power: Charging up for a new century. London: Jessica Kingsley.

Mayall, B. (2002) *Towards a Sociology for Childhood: Thinking from Children's Lives.* Buckingham: Open University Press.

Pound, L. (2005) *How Children Learn from Montessori to Vygotsky.* London: Step Forward Publishing.

Smith, I., Coleman, V. & Bradshaw, M. (2002) *Family-centred Care: Concept, theory and practice.* Basingstoke: Palgrave.

Action for Sick Children: **http://www. actionforsickchildren.org/news.asp**

CAPT—Child Accident Prevention Trust: **http:// www.capt.org.uk/**

Children in Hospital Ireland: **http://www. childreninhospital.ie/aintro.html**

Child Safety Awareness: **http://www.hse.ie**

EACH charter: **http://www.each-for-sick-children. org/each-charter**

Every Child Matters: **http://www. everychildmatters.gov.uk/**

National Safety Council: **http://www.nsc.ie/**

National Safety Kids Campaign: **http://www. safekids.org/index.cfm**

NSF Report: **http://www.doh.gov.uk/nsf/ children.htm**.

Child development

3

CAROL BARRON

Skills

Introduction

Child development can be described as the biological and psychological changes that occur in human beings between birth and the end of adolescence. There are many different factors that influence child development, such as biology/genetics, the personal experiences we undergo throughout our childhood, and the influence of the environment. Child development is often categorized into five **domains**: cognitive (development of the ability to think and reason); social/psychosocial (the process by which a child learns to interact with others); emotional (the child has to learn how to recognize and control their own differing emotional states and to recognize emotions in others); language (how children acquire language); and finally physical development (the physical changes that occur from birth to adolescence). It is important to remember that development occurs simultaneously in all domains and that they are interrelated and interdependent, for example a delay in physical development may hamper the child's social and emotional development. It is imperative that nurses have a sound understanding of 'normal' child development before they can begin to appreciate deviations in any aspect of development. On completion of reading this chapter you will begin to link your knowledge of child development to the preparation, implementation, and aftercare involved in clinical nursing procedures such as measuring a baby's head circumference, as outlined later on in the chapter.

Learning outcomes

It is anticipated that you will be able to do the following once you have read and studied this chapter:

- Understand the main influences on child development and the **nature versus nurture** debate.
- Understand normal child development so you can apply this knowledge to the key nursing skills required to care for a child and their family.
- Understand the importance of developmental assessment throughout childhood, such as the development checks undertaken by health visitors/public health nurses, as a means to assess 'normal development' as well as delays in the achievement of expected developmental **milestones**.

What is child development?

Child development refers to the biological and psychological changes that occur in human beings between birth and the end of adolescence, as the individual progresses from dependency to increasing autonomy (**see Figure 3.1**). The term 'milestones' is used frequently in relation to child development and this means the changes in

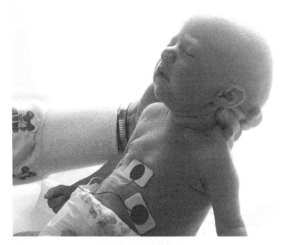

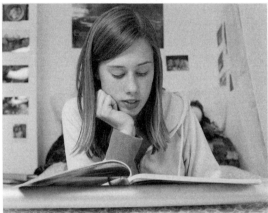

Figure 3.1 Birth to adolescence
above © Corbis/Digital Stock, below © Valueline

specific physical and mental abilities (such as walking and understanding language) that mark the end of one developmental period and the beginning of another. However, there is considerable variation in the achievement of milestones, for example some children walk at 12 months, and others not until 16 months. A common concern in child development is developmental delay, involving a delay in an age-specific ability such as walking or talking. Prevention of and early intervention in developmental delay are significant topics in the study of child development and this is predominantly the role of the health visitor/public health nurse, who carries out nationally agreed developmental assessments on all children at specific chronological age groupings, normally up to the age of five or the commencement of school (different countries have slight variations in the timing of their assessments).

Influences on child development

The history of child development or developmental psychology has had many important debates, such as: is development due more to genetics or environment (nature versus nurture)? Does development occur slowly and smoothly, or do changes happen in stages? Do early childhood experiences have the greatest impact on development, or are later events equally important?

Nature versus nurture

The nature vs. nurture debate is one that has been argued and debated for decades. To what degree is a child's development governed by a pattern built in at birth (i.e. nature)? Or to what degree is a child's development moulded by experiences after birth (i.e. nurture)? Different **theorists** have come to different conclusions in relation to these questions. Studies have consistently shown that as much as 50% of all temperamental and behavioural tendencies are determined by genetics (Glass, 1999). These traits include extroversion, agreeableness, conscientiousness, and openness to experience. Studies of twins separated at birth and raised in different environments show that the twins still end up more alike than many would predict, supporting the argument that genetics play a large role in personality development (Glass, 1999). However, twin studies have also revealed differences in twins reared in the same environment, e.g. one twin may be shy while the other is extroverted, and thus there are factors other than our genes that determine our personality. Most clinicians and psychologists now agree that both nature and nurture influence our development.

Experiences and their impact on development

A second important consideration in developmental psychology involves the relative importance of early experiences versus those that occur later in life. Are we more affected by events that occur in early childhood, or do later events play an equally important role? Two common terms are used in this debate; the first is '**critical period**', which is a period of time during development when the human is especially responsive to and learns from a specific type of stimulation. In foetal development there are clear critical periods, for example if a pregnant mother contracts rubella within the first three months of pregnancy, the foetus may develop cardiac defects. However, if the mother contracts rubella later on in pregnancy, no such defects occur. The second term used in this debate, and one that has been widely adopted, is that of the '**sensitive period**', which is a period of time in development when a particular type of stimulation is particularly important or effective. So, for example, the period from six to twelve months of age may be a sensitive period for the formation of core attachments to parents (Bee & Boyd, 2006), and different time periods may be very important for the development of language.

'Stages' versus 'continuous' development

Does childhood growth occur continuously and gradually, or is it instead a series of distinct stages? People often think of childhood as a sequence of age-related stages (such as infancy, toddler, early childhood, middle childhood, adolescence), and many developmental theories portray childhood growth in this manner (Jean Piaget would be a good example of a stage theorist). Such a view recognizes that each period of growth has its own distinct characteristics. But many aspects of childhood development are more gradual and continuous, such as the development of physical skills, social abilities, and emotional understanding (Bee & Boyd, 2006). Even some milestones that seem to denote a new stage of growth—such as a child's first word or their first step—are actually the outcome of a more gradual developmental process. Some theorists believe that children develop smoothly and continuously, but other theorists believe that children develop more discretely in a series of stages, each of which is fairly stable. Theorists who believe children grow continuously believe that children grow at a steady, uniform speed, adding new knowledge and skills to those already existing. On the other hand, theorists who believe children grow discontinuously believe children grow in

stages, as they seem to develop groups of abilities and to experience events at certain set times in life. Both views of child development, as continuous development and staged development, are correct in their own way. While it is true that development is a continuous process that never stops, it is also true that there are stages to growth and that developments unfold at predictable times across the life span.

Environment

The importance of the environment in relation to child development is recognized as early as the gestational stages of life (Feldman, 2000), for example pregnant women are advised not to smoke or drink as this can have a negative effect on the developing foetus. Our environment affects our behaviour even in the early stages of our lives. Some aspects of development are distinctly biological such as puberty, yet the onset of puberty can be affected by environmental factors such as nutrition and diet.

Introduction to child development theories

We will now examine differing theories of child development from a cognitive, physical, social/psychosocial, and emotional perspective. The theories discussed below are only an introduction to one theoretical perspective on each aspect of development; there are many more, but the theories and theorists selected have stood the test of time and are most often discussed in the literature relating to child development. While each aspect of development is discussed separately, it is vitally important to remember that development continues in each domain simultaneously (whether in continuous development, staged development, or a combination).

Cognitive development

Jean Piaget (1896–1980) was one of the twentieth century's most influential researchers in the area of developmental psychology. He was predominantly interested in **cognitive development** and coined the phrase '**genetic epistemology**', which is the study of the development of knowledge or how we come to know what we know (intelligence). Piaget believed that biological maturation establishes the preconditions for cognitive development; his **theory** of cognitive development is a stage theory, i.e. development occurs in distinct stages throughout childhood. Piaget (1963; 1970) believed that the child is constantly trying to adapt to the world around them, and that this process of adaptation is in turn made up of several key concepts.

Schemas

The concept of a **schema** is one of the most central concepts of this theory. A schema describes both the mental and physical actions involved in understanding and knowing. Schemas are categories of knowledge that help us to interpret and understand the world. In Piaget's view, a schema includes both a category of knowledge and the process of obtaining that knowledge. As experiences happen, this new information is used to modify, add to, or change previously existing schemas. For example, a child may have a schema about a type of animal, such as a dog. If the child's only experience has been with small dogs, they might believe that all dogs are small, and have four legs. Suppose then that the child encounters a very large dog. The child will take in this new information, modifying the previously existing schema to include the new information. How does the child get from simple sensory and motor schemas to the more internalized and complex mental schemas that we see in later childhood? Piaget proposed three basic processes to account for this change.

Assimilation: The process of taking in new information into our previously existing schemas is known as assimilation. The process is somewhat subjective, because we tend to modify experience or information somewhat to fit in with our pre-existing beliefs. In the example above, seeing a dog and labelling it 'dog' is an example of assimilating the animal into the child's dog schema.

Accommodation: Another part of adaptation involves changing or altering our existing schemas in light of new information, a process known as accommodation. Accommodation involves altering existing schemas, or ideas, as a result of new information or new experiences. New schemas may also be developed during this process. For example, a baby who grasps a toy block for the first time will accommodate their grasping schema, so the next time the baby grasps the same block their hand will be more appropriately bent to grasp it. Thus through accommodation we reorganize our thoughts, improve our skills (in this case motor skills), and change our strategies.

Equilibration: Piaget believed that all children try to strike a balance between assimilation and accommodation, which is achieved through a mechanism Piaget called equilibration. As children progress through the stages of cognitive development, it is important to maintain a balance between applying previous knowledge (assimilation) and changing behaviour to account for new knowledge (accommodation). Equilibration helps explain how children are able to move from one stage of thought into the next. Piaget saw three significant points of equilibration during childhood. The first occurs at roughly 18 months when the child shifts from using predominantly sensory and motor schemas to the first truly mental schemas; Piaget called these 'internal representations'. The next shift occurs around the ages of five to seven when the child adds a new set of powerful schemas called 'operations', which are more abstract. The third major equilibration occurs at adolescence, when the child is able to 'operate on' ideas as well as objects or events. The development of these differing forms of equilibration led Piaget to his four-stage theory of cognitive development. Piaget felt that the order of these stages was invariant and that they were associated with approximate ages. He also felt that children in different cultures go through the same stages, thus claiming 'universality' for his theory.

Sensor motor stage, 0–2 years

The first stage of Piaget's theory lasts from birth to approximately age two and is centred on the infant trying to make sense of the world. During the sensor motor stage, an infant's knowledge of the world is limited to their sensory perceptions and motor activities; therefore they use sensory and motor schemas. Children utilize skills and abilities they were born with, such as looking, sucking, grasping, and listening, to learn more about their environment. Piaget divided the sensor motor stage into six sub-stages that are all characterized by the development of a new skill:

- Reflexes (0–1 month): The child understands the environment purely through inborn reflexes such as sucking and looking.
- Primary Circular Reactions (1–4 months): This sub-stage involves coordinating sensation and new schemas. For example, an infant may suck their thumb by accident and then later intentionally repeat the action because the infant finds it pleasurable.
- Secondary Circular Reactions (4–8 months): The infant begins to intentionally repeat an action in order to trigger a response in the environment. For example, a child will purposefully pick up an object in order to put it their mouth.
- Coordination of Reactions (8–12 months): The child starts to show clearly intentional actions. The child may also combine schemas in order to achieve a desired effect. Children begin exploring the environment around them and will often imitate the observed behaviour of others. The understanding of objects also begins during this time and children begin to recognize certain objects as having specific qualities. For example, a child might realize that a rattle will make a sound when shaken.
- Tertiary Circular Reactions (12–18 months): Experimentation by the infant begins; for example, a child may try out different sounds or actions as a way of getting attention from a caregiver.
- Early Representational Thought (18–24 months): Internal representation is now apparent. The infant can use words to stand for objects. During this sub-stage the infant begins to move towards understanding their world through mental operations rather than purely physical actions. This final sub-stage is really the beginning of the next major stage, preoperational thought.

Preoperational stage, 2–6 years

The preoperational stage occurs between ages two and six. Language development is one of the hallmarks of this period. Piaget noted that children in this stage do not yet understand concrete logic, cannot mentally manipulate information and are unable to take the point of view of other people, which he termed egocentrism. During the preoperational stage, children become increasingly adept at using symbols, as evidenced by the emergence of pretend play, for example, a child is able to use an object to represent something else, such as pretending a stick is a wand or a pen. Role-playing also becomes important during the preoperational stage. Children often play the roles of 'mummy', 'daddy', and many others. Reality and fantasy can be indistinguishable to the child, and there is evidence of animistic thinking (attributing feelings to inanimate objects), e.g. if a child hits their head on the table and hurts themselves, they may hit the table back in the belief that they are hurting the table. Piaget focused more on the negative aspects within this stage, i.e. on what children still cannot do as opposed to what they now can do.

Concrete operational stage, 6–12 years

The concrete operations stage lasts from about six or seven years to about eleven or twelve years. The word operations refers to logical operations or principles we use when solving problems. In this stage, the child not only uses symbols representationally (uses one object to represent another) but can manipulate those symbols logically. By six or seven, most children develop the ability to conserve number, length, and liquid volume. Conservation refers to the idea that a quantity remains the same despite changes in appearance. If you show a child four chocolate buttons in two a rows, then spread out one of the rows the preoperational child will focus on the spread, and tend to believe that there are now more chocolate buttons than before (see Figure 3.2).

The concrete operations child, on the other hand, will know that there are still four chocolate buttons. By seven or eight years old, children develop conservation of mass: if I take a ball of play dough and roll it into a long, thin rod, the child knows that there is still the same amount of clay. And they know that, if you rolled it all back into a single ball, it would look quite the same as it did—a feature known as reversibility (see Figure 3.3).

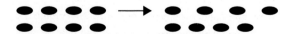

Figure 3.2 Conservation of number experiment

© Barron 2008

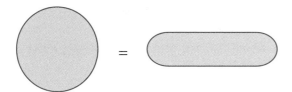

Figure 3.3 Conservation of mass experiment (equal amount of play dough in both shapes)
© Barron 2008

Figure 3.4 Formal operations experiment
© Barron 2008

Another aspect of reversibility is being able to reverse the order of relationships between mental categories. If we use the example of the dog we used earlier, a child might be able to recognize that their dog is a Springer spaniel, that a Springer spaniel is a dog, and that a dog is an animal. If all this sounds too simple to be such a big issue, test your friends on conservation of mass: which is heavier, a billion tons of cement, or a billion tons of feathers?

Formal operational stage, 12 years–adulthood

The formal operational stage begins at approximately age twelve and lasts into adulthood. Children tend to think very concretely and specifically in earlier stages according to Piaget and the ability to think about abstract concepts emerges during the formal operational stage. Instead of relying solely on previous experiences, children begin to consider possible outcomes and consequences of actions. Skills such as logical thought, deductive reasoning, and systematic planning also emerge during this stage. During this stage, the ability to systematically solve a problem in a logical and methodical way emerges. Children at the formal operational stage of cognitive development are often able to quickly plan an organized approach to solving a problem. Here's a simple example of a task that a concrete operations child couldn't do, but which a formal operations teenager or adult could—with a little time and effort. Consider this rule about a set of cards that have letters on one side and numbers on the other: 'If a card has a vowel on one side, then it has an even number on the other side'. Take a look at the cards in **Figure 3.4** and tell me, which cards do I need to turn over to tell if this rule is actually true? You'll find the answer at the end of this chapter.

Piaget's contribution to our understanding of child development

While Piaget did not specifically apply his theory to education, many educational programmes are built upon the belief that children should be taught at the level for which they are developmentally prepared. Look at child development assessments that are held at set age intervals during the child's life span, which assess for normal and abnormal development in a staged/chronological format. Much of the criticism of Piaget's work (see Matusov & Hayes, 2000; Seltman & Seltman, 2006) relates to his research methods. Piaget conducted research on his own three children, which calls into question his subjectivity; also, the other children in Piaget's small research sample were all from well-educated, professional, middle class, white European families. Because of this unrepresentative sample, it is difficult to generalize his findings to a larger population. Most researchers agree that children possess many of the abilities at an earlier age than Piaget suspected. Recent research on theory of mind has found that children of four or five have a sophisticated understanding of their own mental processes as well as those of other people. For example, children of this age have some ability to take the perspective of another person, meaning they are far less egocentric than Piaget believed. Piaget has also been criticized for underestimating the impact of culture (Keenan, 2002). While few would agree with all of Piaget's theory, there is no questioning his massive influence and legacy. His work generated interest in child development and had an enormous impact on the future of education and developmental psychology. What are the implications of cognitive development in relation to the undertaking and performance of clinical nursing skills? Nurses should regard children who are ill as capable of understanding their illness (depending on age and cognitive development) and the need for nursing (Inagaki & Hatano, 1999) and medical treatment.

Physical development: gross and fine motor skills

Overview

Physical growth in height and weight occurs throughout childhood. As the child's height and weight increase their body proportions also change, from the relatively large head and small torso and limbs of the neonate, to the adult's relatively small head and long torso and limbs. Physical development and growth is most rapid in the first few years of life, then proceeds at a slower rate until shortly before puberty (between about nine and fifteen years of age), when another period of rapid growth occurs. Development occurs in a cephalocaudal and a proximodistal progression. Cephalocaudal is an organized pattern of physical growth and motor control that proceeds from head to tail (Bee & Boyd, 2006); in other words, growth of the head and chest occurs before that of the trunk and legs—see Figure 3.5.

Proximodistal (near to far) is a pattern of physical growth and motor control that proceeds from the centre of the body outward, or growth of the arms and legs occurs before that of the hands and feet.

Principles of physical development

- Development is orderly, not random.
- Development is a continuous and gradual process.
- Development is most rapid during the early stages of infancy.

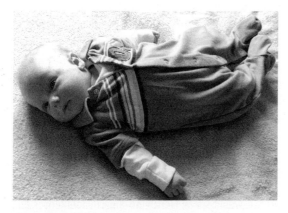

Figure 3.5 Cephalocaudal growth and development
© Barron 2008

- There are critical periods for growth and development.
- Rates and patterns of growth are specific to certain parts of the body.
- Wide individual differences exist in growth rates.
- Growth and development are influenced by a multitude of factors, e.g. nutrition, genetics.

Acquisition of motor skills

Motor skills are actions that involve the movement of muscles in the body. They are divided into two groups: gross motor skills and fine motor skills. Gross motor skills are the abilities required in order to develop control and coordination of the large muscles of the body necessary for developing head control, rolling, sitting, crawling, standing, and walking; movements that primarily require the larger, more proximal muscle groups. Fine motor skills generally refer to the small movements of the hands, wrists, fingers, feet, toes, lips, and tongue, which are smaller actions, such as grasping an object between the thumb and a finger or using the lips and tongue to taste objects. The acquisition of gross motor skills precedes the development of fine motor skills and both processes occur in a cephalocaudal fashion, that is head control preceding arm and hand control then followed by leg and foot control. Any delay or dysfunction in the acquisition of gross and/or fine motor skills may limit the behaviours (walking, grasping etc.) that a child can perform (Keenan, 2002). Observe in **Figure 3.6** a ten-week-old baby in a chair; at this stage he has head control (can hold his head unsupported) but he does not have the gross motor skills to support his upper body yet.

Gross motor skills

- Head control: At birth the newborn is barely able to lift their head; by six months, however, they can easily lift their head, chest, and upper abdomen and can bear weight on their arms.
- Sitting up: At two months of age the baby requires assistance to sit upright; by six months of age they can sit alone in the tripod position and by eight months old they can sit without support and engage in play.

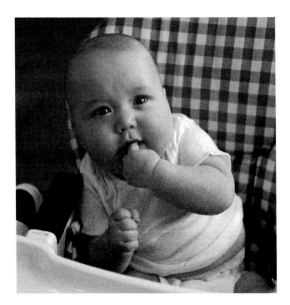

Figure 3.6 A ten-week-old baby sitting up with support
© Photodisc

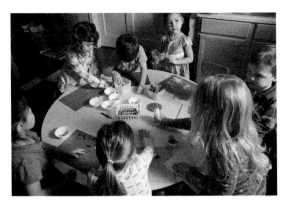

Figure 3.7 Fine motor skills
© Image Source

- Ambulation: Most babies begin to crawl around nine months of age; by one year they can stand independently from a crawl position. By 13–14 months they can walk and toddle quickly and by 15 months they can run. It is important to note that there is wide variation in the time spans in which children acquire these skills.

Fine motor skills

- Voluntary reaching and grasping: At birth the newborn has little control over fine motor skills. The newborn has a grasp reflex at birth that is soon replaced by the ulnar grasp, and the pincer grasp develops towards the end of the first year. Voluntary reaching appears at about three months and gradually improves; this skill is vital for overall child development as this is how the baby explores and learns about the world around them.
- First year of life: The newborn has very little control. Objects will be involuntarily grasped and dropped without notice. By two to three months the baby can hold a rattle or toy but will not reach for it; they play predominantly with their fingers and hands. By four to five months of age the baby starts to reach

for objects and will bring objects to their mouth. At around six to seven months of age the baby can reach for an object with one hand and can also transfer objects between hands. By eight months the baby can use a pincer grasp (pick up or grasp an object between two fingers) and further develops their reaching abilities. Finally, between 10 to 12 months the baby can hold a crayon or pencil to mark a piece of paper.

This development of fine motor skills continues throughout the next few years with children learning to draw, open and close buttons, cut paper, tie shoe laces, write, and much more (**see Figure 3.7**).

Hearing, speech, and language

Only humans acquire a communication system with the complexity and structure of language. Virtually all humans acquire it, so we can say that language is species (the human) specific. Although some non-human primates have been trained to use signs or other symbols after concentrated effort by humans, there appears to be little evidence that they have acquired **syntax** (Schaffer, 2006). All humans talk but house plants do not, so we can assume that heredity must be involved in language. However, a child growing up in China may speak Mandarin whereas the same child brought up in France would speak French, so the environment is also crucial to language acquisition. Both nature and nurture (genetics and the environment) have a role to play in language acquisition. The development of children's language is closely associated with cognition (thinking) and cognitive development. There is a 'critical period' in the acquisition of a first or second language. To learn language, children must be exposed to other people using language, and at some time between age five and puberty language acquisition becomes much more difficult and ultimately less successful (Keenan, 2002). There are five main components to the structure and acquisition of language (see below).

Five components of language

Phonology: refers to the basic units of sound or phonemes that are used in a language and the rules for combining these sounds.

Morphology: rules governing the formation of meaningful words from sounds.

Semantics: refers to the meanings expressed in words and sentences.

Syntax: the rules that specify how words are to be combined to form meaningful phrases and sentences.

Pragmatics: principles that underlie the effective and appropriate use of language in social contexts.

Theories of language development

Language is a complex skill learned by children. The sequence of acquisition seems stable; however, *how* it is learned is disputed, with differing theorists putting forward their differing perspectives. The three main perspectives on language development are briefly discussed below.

The learning (or empiricist) perspective: Language is learned through the processes of imitation and reinforcement (Skinner, 1950). Learning theorists propose that children acquire language as they imitate others' speech and are reinforced for grammatically correct utterances. However, research provides little support for the notion that parents shape grammatical speech or that children acquire language by mimicking the sentences they hear.

The nativist perspective: According to the nativists, language acquisition is natural and almost automatic, as long as children have linguistic data to process. Chomsky (1975) proposes that humans are equipped with a language acquisition device (LAD), which is an inborn linguistic processor that is activated by verbal input. According to Chomsky, the LAD contains a universal grammar, or knowledge of rules that are common to all languages. The approach is criticized, however, for focusing almost exclusively on syntax and ignoring the communicative role of language.

The interactionist perspective: This is a combination of both the learning and nativist perspectives (nature and nurture). From an interactionist perspective, then, language development is the product of a complex transaction between nature and nurture. Children are born with a powerful human brain that develops slowly and predisposes them to acquire new understandings that they are motivated to share with others (Bates, 1989; Tomasello, 1999).

Sequence of language development

The pre-linguistic period

Language acquisition occurs in a series of identifiable sequential stages. The first of these is the pre-linguistic phase of language development, which is the period before babies verbalize their first meaningful words. Within the first few days after birth, babies begin to discriminate different stress patterns, or rhythms, in two-syllable and three-syllable words (Sansavini *et al.*, 1997). The ability to discriminate speech from non-speech and to differentiate a variety of speech-like sounds is either: (1) innate or (2) acquired in the first few days and weeks of life. In either case, young babies are very well prepared for the task of decoding the speech they hear. During the pre-linguistic period there are several recognizable elements to babies' language acquisition (see below):

- Cooing—around two months babies begin to make cooing-like sounds that they repeat when content.
- Babbling—vowel/consonant sounds produced at four to six months.
- Vocables—patterns of sounds that represent objects/actions/events.
- By seven to eight months—vocal turn-taking.
- By eight to ten months—use of gestures and other non-verbal responses to communicate.
- By 12 to 13 months—receptive language (comprehension) is ahead of productive language (expression).

The holophrastic period

This is the first stage of meaningful speech, where infants use one word utterances that often seem to represent an entire sentence's worth of meaning. Most infants produce their first words between ten and fifteen months of age and first words typically include names for people, objects, and events from everyday life. By 18 months, infants typically have on average 50 words they can produce and 100 words they can understand. At around 18 months, language changes in two ways. Vocabulary growth increases; the child begins to learn words at a rate of one every two waking hours, and will keep learning at that rate or faster through to adolescence (Clark, 1993; Pinker, 1994). The young child also has a tendency to use relatively specific words to refer to a broader set of objects, actions, or events; this is known as 'over-extension', e.g. every man is called 'dada'.

The telegraphic period

Telegraphic speech consists of early sentences that contain content words and omit the less meaningful parts of speech, such as articles, prepositions, pronouns, and auxiliary verbs. Telegraphic speech reflects the child's understanding of syntax. Between the late twos and mid-threes, children's language acquisition blooms into fluent grammatical conversation rapidly; sentence length increases steadily, and because grammar is a combinatorial system, the number of syntactic types increases exponentially, doubling every month and typically reaching the thousands before the third birthday (Ingram, 1989; Pinker, 1994).

Grammar explosion

After age three, children experience a phase linguists refer to as the grammar explosion. During this period children employ 'over-regularization', which is the inappropriate application of the grammatical rules for forming plurals and past tenses to irregular nouns and verbs. The strongest support for the idea that young children are learning grammatical rules comes from their production of word endings. Parents play a role in children's grammatical development by modelling correct grammar and expanding incomplete utterances; however, parents are more likely to correct factually inaccurate statements than grammatically incorrect ones.

What are the implications of language development in relation to the undertaking and performance of clinical nursing skills? Explanations of nursing procedures need to be 'translated' into a language that the child is capable of understanding depending on their stage of language acquisition; the avoidance of technical terms is recommended. Thoughtful explanations of required nursing procedures may remove fear, frustration, and confusion (Inagaki & Hatano, 1999) and thus gain the child's cooperation and consent.

Social/Psychosocial development

One of the most widely cited models of **psychosocial development** is that of Erik Erikson. Erik Erikson's theory about psychosocial development has similarities to several others but with distinct differences. Like Freud, he believed that development came in specific stages, but rather than being sexually driven, he focused on the social aspects of development. Like Piaget, he saw advancements coming in a predetermined order, but he stressed the socialization aspect rather than cognitive development. Erikson divided the human life span into eight phases (see below for details), each with its own unique time frame and characteristics. We shall examine the first five phases only, as they relate to childhood.

The term 'identity crisis', which many of us are familiar with, originates from Erikson's idea that at each stage of our development, we face the possibility of a negative rather than a positive outcome, constituting a possible crisis. Each stage is regarded by Erikson as a 'psychosocial crisis', which arises and demands resolution before the next stage can be satisfactorily negotiated. Failing to complete one stage has a negative impact on being able to manoeuvre well through the remaining stages.

Trust vs. Mistrust: birth to 1 year—During the first year of life when a baby receives consistent care and love by the primary caregivers, trust and a sense of security develop. If this sense is not developed, anxiety, insecurity, and mistrust of the world are formed.

Autonomy vs. Shame and doubt: 1 to 3 years—The second psychosocial crisis, Erikson believes, occurs during early childhood. If a child's efforts at independent thinking are supported and encouraged at this stage then their self-confidence increases; they feel proud of themselves rather than ashamed. These first attempts by the child at decision making are important milestones according to Erikson, and if parents/primary caregivers criticize the child, or do not permit them to make simple decisions, then the child may feel inadequate and doubtful about their abilities. Low self-esteem and a tendency to be overly dependent on others can have their roots in an unsuccessful transition at this age.

Initiative vs. Guilt: 3 to 6 years—Erikson believes that during the third psychosocial crisis between the ages of three and six, the healthily developing child learns: (1) to imagine, and to broaden their skills through active play of all sorts, including fantasy; (2) to cooperate with others; and (3) to lead as well as to follow. If the child is not allowed to develop these skills or is criticized for their attempts then they: (1) become fearful; (2) tend to hang on the fringes of groups; (3) continue to depend unduly on adults; and (4) are restricted both in the development of play skills and in imagination.

Industry vs. Inferiority: 6 years to puberty—Erikson believes that the fourth psychosocial crisis occurs during what he calls 'school age'. Here the child learns to: (1) relate with peers according to rules; (2) take part in play with rules such as football; and (3) master social studies, reading, arithmetic, etc. The child who, because of their successive and successful resolutions of earlier psychosocial crises, is trusting, autonomous, and full of initiative will learn easily enough to be industrious. However, the mistrusting child will doubt the future. The child who unsuccessfully resolves this crisis experiences defeat and feelings of inferiority according to Erikson.

Identity vs. Role confusion: adolescence—During the fifth psychosocial crisis (adolescence, from about 13 or 14 to about 20) the child, now an adolescent, undergoes the transition from adolescent to adult and learns how to answer the question of 'Who am I?' and be happy with their own identity. But even very well balanced adolescents experience some role identity diffusion; most boys and probably most girls experiment with risk-taking behaviours and rebellion, and experience self-doubts, etc. An inability on the part of the adolescent to figure out their own identity, plans for the future, etc. may leave them confused and directionless.

Emotional development in children

Children learn about emotions through their interaction or relationships with others. Throughout childhood they learn an awareness of their own emotional state, the ability to control the expression of their own emotions (think of the clichéd 'temper tantrums'), and to accurately recognize emotions in others (Schaffer, 2006). The study of the emotional development of infants and children is relatively new, having been studied empirically only during the past few decades.

The emergence of emotions in babies and infants within the first year

Emotional development is a continuous process that starts soon after birth and continues throughout childhood and beyond. However, a discussion of this range is not possible within this chapter and therefore the author has focused on the first year of life. Between six and ten weeks, a social smile emerges, usually accompanied by other pleasure-indicative actions and sounds, including cooing and mouthing. This social smile occurs in response to interactions with adults. As infants become more aware of their environment, smiling occurs in response to a wider variety of contexts such as being given their favourite toy. The social smile is considered to serve a developmental function. Laughter, which begins at around three or four months, requires a level of cognitive development because it is usually elicited by actions that deviate from the norm, such as being kissed on the abdomen or a parent playing peek-a-boo. Because it fosters reciprocal interactions with others, laughter promotes social development. Between six and twelve months infants begin expressing fear, disgust, and anger because of the maturation of cognitive abilities. Anger, often expressed by crying, is a frequent emotion expressed by infants. As is the case with all emotional expressions, anger serves an adaptive function, signalling to parents the infant's discomfort or displeasure. Fear also emerges during this stage as children become able to compare an unfamiliar event with what they know. Unfamiliar situations or objects often elicit fear responses in infants. One of the most common is the presence of an adult stranger, a fear that begins to appear at about seven months. A second fear of this stage is called separation anxiety. Infants of seven to twelve months old may cry in fear if the mother or caregiver leaves them, particularly in an unfamiliar place, for example the first day in a crèche or hospital ward. (See Chapter Two for a more detailed discussion of attachment.)

Child Health Surveillance/Child Health Promotion Programme

Child Health Surveillance, more recently known as the Child Health Promotion Programme (Department of Health, 2008), is a programme of care initiated and provided by professionals with the aim of preventing illness and promoting good health and development. Social, emotional, physical, language, and hearing development are all assessed throughout childhood under this programme. Differing nations have variations on when and how this occurs and the following is one example only. Babies may be seen/examined by the midwife and/or paediatrician soon after birth. Checks are then conducted by the health visitor/public health nurse at approximately one week to ten days after birth, six to eight weeks, three months, seven to nine months, 18 to 24 months, 3.25 to 3.5 years, school entry, and finally school leaving. At each check the health visitor/public health nurse will focus on differing aspects of development, for example:

Soon after birth

- Physical examination (ideally within 24 hours) with particular emphasis on eyes (mainly to detect cataracts), heart, and hips. Also check weight, head circumference, tone, spine, genitals, testes, femoral pulse, palate. Look for hernias, jaundice, large organs, dysmorphic features.
- Administration of vitamin K (if parents choose vitamin K drops, these are administered during the first week after birth).
- Review any pregnancy or birth complications, feeding, risk factors for hip dysplasia (breech, family history, foot deformity, torticollis), and risk factors for hearing loss (family history of permanent deafness

starting in childhood, congenital infection, ototoxic drugs, dysmorphic craniofacial features).
- Health promotion:
  - breastfeeding
  - sleeping position and other advice to reduce risk of sudden infant death
  - dangers of passive smoking
  - assess need for BCG or hepatitis B immunization.
- Automated hearing screen (ideally within first seven days):
  - this test is likely to be phased in following pilot schemes in differing countries
  - it will eventually replace the distraction test that has been performed for many years at age eight to nine months.
- The Guthrie 'heel prick' blood screening test (at five to seven days):
  - for congenital hypothyroidism and phenylketonuria
  - screening for cystic fibrosis and haemoglobinopathies are likely to be phased in.

The 6–8 week review

- Physical examination:
  - main emphasis on heart, hips, eyes (cataracts), and testes
  - also check weight, head circumference, tone, spine, genitals, femoral pulse, palate
  - look for hernias, jaundice, large organs, dysmorphic features
- Review of general progress and delivery of key messages about parenting and health promotion.
- Identification of post-natal depression or other maternal health needs.
- Consider any other parental concerns.
- Health promotion:
  - immunization
  - breastfeeding and other advice on feeding and weaning
  - sleeping position and other advice to reduce risk of sudden infant death
  - dangers of passive smoking
  - dental health: sugar-free medicines, avoid sugary drinks, sugar on dummies, etc.
  - car safety and other injury prevention strategies.

Age 3–4 months

- Immunizations.
- Check weight.
- Health promotion as for 6–8 week check.

Developmental and health reviews at 7–9 months, 18–24 months, and 3.25–3.5 years

- These have been performed routinely in both the UK and Ireland for a number of years. However, they are no longer recommended as a routine part of the core programme for all children in the UK.
- It is thought that primary healthcare teams will take a flexible approach and offer health reviews and health promotion advice for children and families most in need, or most 'at risk'. Also, to respond to parents who have concerns about their child's development.

By the first birthday

- Systematic assessment of the child's physical, emotional, and social development and family needs by the health visiting team.
- The hearing distraction test at eight to nine months is likely to be phased out as the automated hearing screen in the newborn period is phased in.

Age 12–15 months

- Immunization.
- Take opportunity to discuss injury prevention: stair gates, fireguards, small toys, etc.

Age 3–4 years

- Immunization.

Age 4–5 years

A review at school entry provides an opportunity to:
- Check that immunizations are up to date.
- Check that children have access to primary and dental care.

- Carry out appropriate assessment and interventions for any physical, developmental, or emotional problems.
- Provide children, parents, and school staff with information about specific health issues.
- Check the child's height and weight.
- Administer the sweep test of hearing.
- National orthoptist-led programme for pre-school vision screening to be introduced.

Foundation stage profile

Assessment by the teacher to include a child's:
- Personal, social, and emotional development.
- Communication, language, and literacy.
- Physical development.
- Creative development.

School entry—about the age of five (by school nurse)

- Height and weight.
- 'Sweep' hearing test.
- Vision test is likely to be phased out as the pre-school vision check by orthoptist is phased in.
- Review of immunization status.

Ongoing support at primary and secondary schools

- Access to school nurse at open sessions/drop-in and clinics by parents, teachers, or through self-referral.
- Provision for referral to specialists for children causing concern.
- Children and young people with medical needs and disabilities may receive nursing care within the school environment according to their needs.
- Immunization when indicated.

The above information was adapted from *The Child Health Promotion Programme: Pregnancy and the first five years of life* (2008). Immunization schedules change periodically and vary from nation to nation. Therefore the following immunization schedule is for illustrative purposes only.

Table 3.1 Sample immunization schedule in Ireland

Age to Vaccinate	Type of Vaccination
At birth	BCG tuberculosis vaccine (given in maternity hospitals or a HSE clinic)
At 2 months Free from your GP	**6 in 1** Diphtheria Tetanus Whooping cough (Pertussis) Hib (Haemophilus influenzae B) Polio (Inactivated poliomyelitis) Hepatitis B **PCV** (Pneumococcal Conjugate Vaccine)
At 4 months Free from your GP	**6 in 1** Diphtheria Tetanus Whooping cough (Pertussis) Hib (Haemophilus influenzae B) Polio (Inactivated poliomyelitis) Hepatitis B **Men C** (Meningococcal C)
At 6 months Free from your GP	**6 in 1** Diphtheria Tetanus Whooping cough (Pertussis) Hib (Haemophilus influenzae B) Polio (Inactivated poliomyelitis) Hepatitis B **Men C** (Meningococcal C) **PCV** (Pneumococcal Conjugate Vaccine)
At 12 months Free from your GP	**MMR** Measles Mumps Rubella **PCV** (Pneumococcal Conjugate Vaccine)

Skills in monitoring physical growth

3.1 Measuring weight

As already indicated in these health checks, growth is a key indicator of normal health and development. The World Health Organization (2005) identifies growth assessment as the best single measurement for defining the nutritional status and health of children. Growth measurements encompass the measurement of height/ length, weight, and head circumference. All children admitted to hospital or attending any healthcare setting should have their weight measured and plotted on an appropriate **centile chart**. Accurate recording of babies'/ infants'/children's weight is vital for the calculation of medications and fluids. It is the responsibility of the nurse to correctly measure and record the weight of babies/ infants/children in his or her care. Differing clinical skills are required for weighing a baby and for measuring and recording the weight of an older child.

Procedure: Measuring and recording baby/infant weight

Equipment

Ensure all equipment is available and in good working order prior to commencing the procedure. All weighing equipment must be checked and calibrated prior to use for accuracy.
- Electronic baby scales
- Relevant centile chart and pen to record the measurement
- Another nurse or parent to assist with the procedure if necessary
- Antiseptic wipes or cleaning solution and cloth

Consent and communication

Explain the procedure and rationale to the parent(s) to ensure that they understand what will happen and to gain their consent and cooperation.

Step-by-step guide to measuring and recording baby/infant weight

Procedure   Rationale

	Procedure	Rationale
1	Wash hands and don gloves.	To prevent the spread of micro-organisms.
2	A child under the age of two years should be weighed naked or with a dry nappy on only.	For accuracy of measurement (Hall, 2000).
	Undress baby/infant as appropriate.	
	If for any reason clothing has not been removed or a child is weighed with additional equipment, e.g. splint or any medical equipment, this must be recorded in the infant's healthcare records.	For accuracy of measurement (Hall, 2000).
3	Ensure the digital readout is reading zero prior to placing the baby/infant on the weighing scales.	For accuracy of measurement (Hall, 2000). To minimize the time the baby/infant is exposed.
4	Place the baby/infant completely on the scales. Observe your local policy guidelines for moving and handling.	Safety issues for the baby/infant and nurse.
	The baby/infant must never be left on their own at any point.	
5	Record the measurement on the digital readout exactly. Always record the exact weight. Never round the figures up or down.	For accuracy.
6	Lift the baby/infant carefully off the scales and return to his/her parents as soon as possible following the procedure.	For the comfort of the baby/infant.
7	Ensure the baby/infant is dressed quickly.	To prevent the baby/infant getting cold.
8	The weight should be plotted on the relevant grid of the growth chart with a well-defined dot. Do not use a cross (x). The dot must not be circled.	To check that growth is normal. A normal growth curve is one that runs roughly on or parallel to one of the printed lines.
	It should also be recorded in the recording box.	
	The growth curve should be traced with a line that leaves the dots clearly visible.	Accurate documentation helps to track the baby's/infant's development.
	The measurements must be recorded in: • the child's parent-held record • the admission assessment record if applicable • a centile chart.	
	The date, time, and the name of the measurer must also be recorded.	

| Wipe down the measuring scales with an antiseptic wipe or antiseptic solution and a cloth. | To prevent the spread of micro-organisms. |
| Dispose of used equipment appropriately. | To prevent the spread of micro-organisms. |

Older children can have their weight recorded on digital scales in the upright position or sitting on digital chair scales.

3.2 **Measuring head circumference**

The aim of measuring a baby's/infant's head circumference is to determine the maximal head circumference. It is performed to monitor the growth of a child, particularly those under two years (Cox, 1993). However, it is still valuable to continue to record a child's head circumference after this period, as it may detect any abnormalities that may develop such as hydrocephalus, craniosynostosis, or microcephaly. All newborn babies should have their head circumference measured. It should be done after 36 hours after birth or preferably at seven to ten days to allow the effects of moulding and oedema from birth to settle (Lindley *et al.*, 1999). Any child who is admitted to hospital with a known or suspected neurological or craniofacial abnormality will need their head circumference recorded more frequently, for example, an increase in the volume of cerebrospinal fluid can result in an increasing head circumference.

Procedure: Measuring and recording a baby's head circumference

Equipment

Ensure all equipment is available. The following equipment is required:
- Non-cloth tape measure (Batrum & Baxter, 2005)
- Centile chart
- Pen

- Gloves and apron if applicable
- Another nurse or parent to assist with the procedure

A non-cloth tape measure is recommended for the recording of babies' head circumferences as they do not stretch with use and they are easily made into flexible loops (Batrum & Baxter, 2005; Fry, 1994). (See procedure 3.2)

Consent and communication

Explain the procedure and rationale to the parent(s) to ensure that they understand what will happen and to gain their consent and cooperation.

3.3 **Measuring length and height**

A healthy, adequately nourished, and emotionally secure child grows at an optimal rate (Stanhope, 1994). However, a slow rate of growth may suggest a pathological disorder requiring diagnosis and possible treatment, e.g. malabsorption, an eating disorder, hypertension, or psychosocial problems (Skuse, 1989). Many diseases do not cause obvious symptoms and poor growth may be the first or only indicator of a problem (Hall, 2000). Therefore regular measurement of children in the community setting can allow early diagnosis of these problems.

Procedure: Measuring and recording a baby's/ infant's length

Equipment

Ensure all equipment is available and check it for accuracy prior to commencing the procedure. For children

Step-by-step guide to measuring and recording a baby's head circumference

Procedure	Rationale
1 Wash hands and don gloves (this may vary depending on the context and your individual workplace policy).	To prevent the spread of micro-organisms.
2 With the assistance of another nurse or the parent, position the baby sitting up or lying down.	Correctly positioning the baby is essential for an accurate measurement.
3 If recording the head circumference on an infant or older child, remove any plaits, braids or hair adornments.	To avoid inconsistencies of measurements.
4 Loop the tape measure and place the tape measure over the child's head. The tape measure should be placed above the ears and from midway between the eyebrows and the hairline to the occipital prominence at the back of the head (Batrum & Baxter, 2005). Pull the tape measure so that any hair is compressed.	To ensure accuracy and consistency of measurement (Batrum & Baxter, 2005).
5 Read the measurement from the appropriately marked place on the tape measure. The measurement should be taken to the nearest millimetre.	To ensure accuracy and consistency of measurement.
6 Repeat points 4 and 5. • Differing healthcare providers will request the procedure to be conducted twice or perhaps three times, with the highest measurement being recorded. • Please follow your local policy guidelines.	To ensure accuracy of measurement.
7 Discard paper tape measures. Discard gloves and apron if applicable.	Tape measures are predominantly disposable and suitable for one use only. To prevent the spread of micro-organisms.
8 Perform hand hygiene.	To prevent the spread of micro-organisms.
9 The measurement must be recorded in the child's parent-held record and plotted on a centile chart. Ensure the correct centile chart is used. The date and time must also be recorded.	Accurate documentation helps to develop a growth curve of the baby's head circumference development.

under the age of two years the following equipment is required:

- A medically approved measuring mat
- Disposable gloves and an apron if appropriate
- Relevant centile chart and pen to record the measurement
- Another nurse or parent to assist with the procedure

See below for the step-by-step guide to measuring and recording a baby's/infant's length.

Consent and communication

Explain the procedure and rationale to the parent(s) to ensure that they understand what will happen and to gain their consent and cooperation.

The techniques and clinical skills required to obtain the length of a baby or infant differ from those required to measure and record the height of an older child.

Procedure: Measuring and recording a child's height

Equipment

Ensure all equipment is available and in good working order prior to commencing the procedure. For children over the age of two years, the following equipment is required:

Step-by-step guide to measuring and recording a baby's/infant's length

Procedure	Rationale
1 Wash hands and don gloves.	To prevent the spread of micro-organisms.
2 Ensure the measuring mat is lying perfectly flat on a solid, even surface.	To ensure accurate measurement and correct positioning of the baby.
3 With the assistance of another nurse or the parent, position the baby on the measuring mat: • They should be lying flat on their back with their head facing toward the ceiling but not hyper-extended. • The back of the baby's head should be touching the top of the mat. • The body should be in alignment—shoulders, hips, etc. in a straight line. • Feet must be flat against the bottom of the measuring mat.	Correctly positioning the baby on the measuring mat is essential for an accurate measurement.
4 Visually record the baby's length.	A visual record of the measurement must be taken by the nurse before a written record is documented.
5 Lift the baby carefully off the mat and return to his/her parents as soon as possible following the procedure.	For the baby's comfort.
6 Record the baby's length accurately on the correct centile chart.	Documentation is necessary to ensure continuity of care.

- A medically approved stadiometer
- Disposable gloves and an apron if appropriate
- Relevant centile chart and pen to record the measurement
- Another nurse or parent to assist with the procedure
- Antiseptic wipes or cleaning solution and cloth

Consent and communication

Explain the procedure and rationale to the parent(s) and the child to ensure that they understand what will happen and to gain their consent and cooperation.

Centile charts and assessing growth

As you will have noticed, all length/height, weight, and head circumference measurements are recorded on centile charts, but what are they? Centile charts show the position of a measured parameter within a statistical distribution. They are called centiles and not per centiles. If a parameter such as height is on the third centile, this means that for every 100 children of that age, three would be expected to be shorter and 97 taller.

Step-by-step guide to measuring and recording a child's height

Procedure	Rationale
1 Wash hands and don gloves.	To prevent the spread of micro-organisms.
2 The child may require preparation from a play specialist or nurse prior to measuring their height.	To prepare them psychologically for the procedure.
3 Prior to the procedure the child should normally have the following removed: • their shoes (some healthcare providers ask for children to be measured without socks; please follow your own local policy guidelines in this regard) • hair clips and braids, i.e. undo hair.	To ensure an accurate measurement of the child's height.
4 The child's body must be positioned with their: • feet together and both feet flat on the ground • heels touching the back plate of the measuring instrument • legs straight • buttocks against the backboard • scapula, wherever possible, against the backboard • arms loosely at their sides.	Correctly positioning the child is vital to obtaining an accurate measurement of height (Voss, 2000).
5 The child's head must be positioned with the lower margins of the orbit in the same horizontal plane as the external auditory meati, i.e. the corner of the eyes horizontal to the middle of the ear (Schlig & Hulse, 1997). This is know as the 'Frankfurt Plane'.	To obtain an accurate measurement.
6 Ensure the child is in the correct position and hold their mastoid processes (Voss, 2000; Schlig & Hulse, 1997).	To ensure accurate positioning of the child.

7	Ask the child to breathe in normally and as they inhale maintain the pressure on the mastoids.	To relax the muscles down the spine.
	Ask the child to breathe out normally and exert upward pressure on their mastoid processes.	To allow the spine to be straightened.
	Once the child has fully exhaled, record the measurement to the last complete millimetre, reading the instrument at eye level.	To obtain height of child and enable an accurate reading (Voss, 2000).
8	Lift the sliding scale up and away from the child's head.	To enable the child to move away from the equipment.
9	Wipe down the stadiometer with an antiseptic wipe or antiseptic solution and cloth. Dispose of used equipment appropriately.	To prevent the spread of micro-organisms.
10	The measurements must be recorded in the child's parent-held record and plotted on a centile chart. Ensure the correct centile chart is used. The date, time, and the name of the measurer must also be recorded.	Accurate documentation helps to develop a growth curve of the child's height.

If it is on the 97th centile, 97 would be shorter and three taller. Centile charts are very useful for plotting changing parameters such as a child's height, weight, or head circumference (see Figure 3.8). Because centile charts are usually used to assess a parameter over time, they are normally presented graphically. The parameter such as height, weight, or head circumference is shown on the y-axis and the age or gestation on the x-axis. The graph shows a number of lines representing important centiles. These would usually be the 50th centile (average), 25th and 75th centiles, as well as the 3rd and/or 10th centile and the 97th and/or 90th centile. These charts are purely to illustrate that presentation. There are different charts for boys and girls, which reflect the differences in their respective rate of growth.

Conclusion

This chapter introduced you to the topic of child development, which is the biological and psychological changes that occur in human beings between birth and the end of adolescence. Many differing issues can and do affect development; both nature and nurture contribute to and influence child development, and there are 'critical periods' in children's development such as the development of cardiac defects in the first trimester if the mother is exposed to rubella. Equally we have 'sensitive periods', which are periods of time in development when a particular type of stimulation is particularly important or effective. So, for example, the period from six to twelve months of age may be a sensitive period for the formation of core attachments to parents (Bee & Boyd, 2006). It is true to say that child development is a continuous process that never stops; it is equally true that there are stages to growth and that developments unfold at predictable times across the life span. Whether one is more important than the other (continuous versus stage) is yet to be determined. Theories of child development are normally divided into differing domains: cognitive; social/psychosocial; emotional; physical; and language acquisition. It is important to remember that while each aspect of development is discussed separately, all the domains are interrelated and interdependent as in the Child Health Promotion checks/Health Surveillance screening that is performed by many differing nations. Assessment of growth is a key indicator of normal health and development.

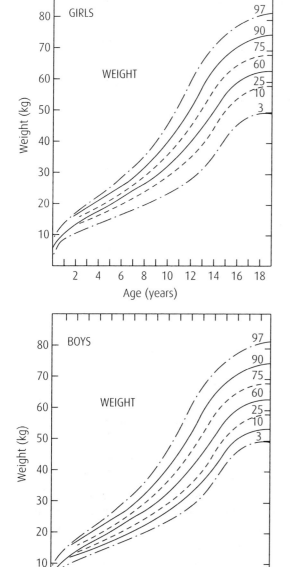

Cross-sectional standards of weight attained at each age (English girls and boys). The central line represents the mean. or 50th centile The two dashed lines above and below it represent the 75th and 25th centiles respectively. Other centile lines are also shown. This chart is intended as an approximate guide only.

Figure 3.8 Centile charts

© EMIS and PiP 2009

The World Health Organization (2005) identifies growth assessment as the best single measurement for defining the nutritional status and health of children. Therefore

the clinical skills of accurately measuring and recording babies'/infants' and children's head circumference, height, and weight are vital in both the community and clinical healthcare settings.

Answer to the card question

The A and the 3. The A must have an even number on the back—that much is obvious. The 3 is odd, so it cannot have a vowel on the other side—that would be against the rule. **But** the rule says nothing about what has to be on the back of a consonant such as the W, nor does it say that the 6 must have a vowel on the other side.

Online resource centre

You may find it helpful to work through our online resources including interactive scenarios intended to help you to develop and apply the skills in this chapter. Where material referenced below is available electronically, we're pleased to provide active web links to the source via 🌐 **http://www.oxfordtextbooks.co.uk/orc/coyne/**

References

Bates, E. (1989) Functionalism and the competition model. In B. MacWhinney and E. Bates (eds.) *The Cross Linguistic Study of Sentence Processing*. New York: Cambridge University Press.

Batrum, J.L. & Baxter, P.S. (2005) The Lasso-0 tape: Stretchability and observer reliability in head circumference measurement. *Archives of Disease in Childhood* **90** (8), 820–821.

Bee, H. & Boyd, D. (2006) *The Developing Child, 11th ed.* Boston, MA: Pearson International Edition.

Chomsky, N. (1975) *Reflections on Language*. New York: Random House.

Clark, E.V. (1993) *The Lexicon in Acquisition*. New York: Cambridge University Press.

Cox, L.A. (1993) *A Guide to the Measurement and Assessment of Growth in Children*. Ware: Castlemead Publications.

Department of Health (2008) *The Child Health Promotion Programme: Pregnancy and the first five years of life*. London: DH.

Feldmen, R. (2000). *Essentials of Understanding Psychology, 4th ed.* Amherst, MA: University of Massachusetts.

Fry, T. (1994) Introducing the new child growth standards. *Professional Care Mother Child* **4** (8), 231.

Glass, J. (1999). Nature vs. nurture. *Parenting* **13**, 156.

Hall, D. (2000) Growth monitoring. *Archives of Diseases in Childhood* **82** (1), 10–14.

Inagaki, K. & Hatano, G. (1999) Young children's understanding of mind-body relationships. In M. Siegal & C. Peterson (eds.) *Children's Understanding of Biology and Health.* Cambridge: Cambridge University Press.

Ingram, D. (1989) *First Language Acquisition: Method, description, and explanation.* New York: Cambridge University Press.

Keenan, T. (2002) *An Introduction to Child Development.* New York: Sage Publications.

Lindley, A., Benson, J. & Grimes, C. (1999) The relationship in neonates between clinically measured head circumference and brain volume estimated from head CT scans. *Early Human Development* **56** (1), 17–29.

Matusov, E. & Hayes, R. (2000) Sociocultural critique of Piaget and Vygotsky. *New Ideas in Psychology* **18**, 215–239.

Piaget, J. (1963). *The Psychology of Intelligence.* New York: Routledge.

Piaget, J. (1970). *Genetic Epistemology.* New York: W.W. Norton & Company.

Pinker, S. (1994) *The Language Instinct.* New York: Morrow.

Sansavini, A., Bertoncini, J., & Giovanelli, G. (1997) Newborns discriminate the rhythm of multisyllabic stressed words. *Developmental Psychology* **33** (1), 3–11.

Schaffer, H.R. (2006) *Key Concepts in Developmental Psychology.* New York: Sage Publications.

Schlig, S. & Hulse, T. (1997) *Growth Monitoring and Assessment in the Community: A guide to good practice.* London: Child Growth Foundation.

Seltman, M. & Seltman, P. (2006) *Piaget's Logic: A critique of genetic epistemology*. London: Routledge.

Skinner, B.F. (1950) Are theories of learning necessary? *Psychological Review* **57**, 193–216.

Skuse, D.H. (1989) ABC of child abuse. Emotional abuse and delay in growth. *British Medical Journal* **299** (6691), 113–115.

Stanhope, R., Wilks, Z. & Hamill, G. (1994) Failure to grow: Lack of food or lack of love? *Professional Care Mother and Child* **4** (8), 234–237.

Tomasello, M. (1999) *The Cultural Origins of Human Cognition.* Harvard: Harvard University Press.

Voss, L.D. (2000) Growth monitoring. *Archives of Disease in Childhood* **82**, 14–15.

World Health Organization (2005) *European Strategy for Child and Adolescent Health and Development.* Copenhagen: WHO.

Further reading and URLs

Bowlby, J. (1973) *Attachment and Loss, Vol. 2: Separation, Anxiety, and Anger.* London: Penguin Books.

Bowlby, J. (1980) *Attachment and Loss, Vol. 3: Loss, Sadness and Depression.* New York: Basic Books.

Bowlby, J. (1998) *Attachment and Loss, Vol. 1: Attachment.* New York: Basic Books.

Brown, R. (1973) *A First Language: The early stages.* Cambridge, MA: Harvard University Press.

Centre for Community Child Health, Royal Children's Hospital Melbourne (2002) *Child Health Surveillance and Screening: A Critical Review of the Evidence.* Melbourne, Australia: NHMRC.

Child Growth Foundation (1996) *Four-in-one growth charts.* London: Child Growth Foundation.

Department of Health (2004) *National Service Framework for Children, Young People and Maternity Services.* London: DH.

Erikson, E. (1971) *Identity: youth in crisis.* London: Faber.

Gerrig, R. & Zimbardo, P.G. (2002) *Psychology and Life, 16th ed.* Boston, MA: Allyn & Bacon.

Health Service Executive (2006) *Training Programme for Public Health Nurses and Doctors in Child Health Screening, Surveillance and Health Promotion.* Dublin: HSE.

Keenan, T. (2002) *An Introduction to Child Development.* New York: Sage Publications Ltd.

Mercer, J. (2009) *Child Development: Myths and misunderstandings.* New York: Sage Publications.

Mills, J. & Mills, R. (editors) (2000) *Childhood Studies: A Reader in Perspectives of Childhood*. London: Routledge.

Nadelman, L. (2004) *Research Manual in Child Development*. Mahwah, New Jersey: Lawrence Erlbaum Associates.

Pinker, S. & Bloom, P. (1990) Natural language and natural selection. *Behavioral and Brain Sciences* **13**, 707–784.

Schaffer, H.R. & Callender, W.M. (1959) Psychological effects of hospitalisation in infancy. *Pediatrics* **24** (4), 528–539.

Siegal, M. & Peterson, C. (eds.) (1999) *Children's Understanding of Biology and Health*. Cambridge: Cambridge University Press.

http://www.who.int/child-adolescent-health/
This page provides information about interventions concerning health, growth, and development outcomes from birth to 19 years. Main areas of work include: integrated management of childhood illness; child and adolescent rights; adolescent sexual and reproductive health; and HIV and AIDS.

http://www.eldis.org/go/topics/resource-guides/health/child-health/childhood-devel opment&id=17124&type=Document This web resource, produced by the World Bank, outlines what is meant by early child development (ECD) with further guidance on stages of development, healthy development, and the reasons for investing in ECD.

http://www.eldis.org/go/topics/resource-guides/health/child-health/childhood-development &id=1467&type=Organisation Operates a WWW service that includes information on UNICEF activities. Includes full text of the annual *State of the World's Children Report* and the *Progress of Nations Report*. Also available are: documentation on the World Summit for Children held in 1990; information on children's rights; information on child labour; and educational resources.

http://www.eldis.org/go/topics/resource-guides/health/child-health/trends-and-indicators
This web page provides links to papers on rates of improvement in child survival.

http://www.piaget.org/links.html
The Jean Piaget Society, established in 1970, has an international, interdisciplinary membership of scholars, teachers, and researchers interested in exploring the nature of the developmental construction of human knowledge. The Society was named in honour of the Swiss developmentalist, Jean Piaget, who made major theoretical and empirical contributions to our understanding of the origins and evolution of knowledge

http://www.kolar.org/vygotsky/
Online resources for Lev Vygotsky: essays, explanations, and links.

http://web.cortland.edu/andersmd/ERIK/ WELCOME.HTML This website was created by students and clearly explains Erik Eriskon's psychosocial theory of development.

http://embryology.med.unsw.edu.au/
This is an excellent website as an educational resource for learning concepts in embryological development.

http://embryology.med.unsw.edu.au/sysnote.htm
Part of the UNSW embryology website, this page links the reader to resources covering the different systems of the body. You can click on either the image or the link to open the specific topic. Each section has additional content pages listed in the left-hand menu under internal links.

Websites on immunization

UK
Health information provided by the NHS (Scotland): **http://www.fitfortravel.scot.nhs.uk**
Immunization for life (NHS) National Health Service: **http://www.immunization.nhs.uk**
The Meningitis Research Foundation: **http://www. meningitis.org/**
The National Meningitis Trust: **http://www. meningitis-trust.org/**

Irish
Immunization Guidelines for Ireland, 2008 edition: **http://www.hpsc.ie/hpsc/A-Z/ VaccinePreventable/Vaccination/Guidance/ File,3066,en.pdf**
Information on mumps: **http://www.ndsc.ie/hpsc/ A-Z/VaccinePreventable/Mumps/**

Influenza, information for health professionals:
**http://www.ndsc.ie/hpsc/A-Z/Respiratory/
Influenza/Guidance/Title,1214,en.html**
Influenza for healthcare workers, FAQs: **http://
www.ndsc.ie/hpsc/A-Z/Respiratory/Influenza/
Guidance/Title,992,en.html**
Influenza vaccine for healthcare workers, common myths:
**http://www.ndsc.ie/hpsc/A-Z/Respiratory/
Influenza/Guidance/Title,991,en.html**
Measles, mumps, rubella (MMR) vaccine
discussion pack. An information guide for health
professionals and parents: **http://www.
ndsc.ie/hpsc/A-Z/VaccinePreventable/MMR/
Publications/**

International
World Health Organization (WHO): **http://www.
who.int**
International travel and health is a WHO publication
and a reference book for doctors and nurses, giving
health advice: **http://www.who.int**

European
Euvac is a European surveillance network for vaccine-
preventable infectious diseases: **http://www.
euvac.net/graphics/euvac/index.html** (external
link)

4 Consent and legal/ethical matters

MOIRA McLOUGHLIN, CAROLE KING, AND HAZEL CHAMBERLAIN

Introduction

This chapter will explore contemporary **child protection** issues including safeguarding policies and laws currently in place for children, in order to provide a framework to guide your understanding and practice as a nursing student. We will also highlight the influence of other agencies in fulfilling their statutory responsibility for safeguarding children and the importance of inter-professional work.

It is important that student nurses can recognize the presentation of children who may have suffered abuse and so common scenarios are explored and discussed. Examples of the nature and range of abuse will be outlined as will the skills used for both recognition and identification. You may find some of the content disturbing, and it may be useful for you to seek support and guidance when reading the chapter.

The chapter commences with a discussion of the background literature in this area, which provides a definition and explanation of abuse and outlines related contributory factors. In order to provide a discussion of the legislation related to this topic, examples from the United Kingdom (UK) will be outlined. Legislation in this area varies between countries; therefore it is not possible to provide information on the scope of the law in individual countries. It may be useful to refer to your own country's legislation when considering the chapter content.

Learning outcomes

By reading this chapter and engaging with the various activities, you will have:

- A basic understanding of several aspects of child protection and safeguarding policy and law (examples are drawn from the UK and Ireland).
- An understanding of the nature of presenting abuse in children.
- An understanding of child protection/safeguarding guidelines that would enable you to act if you have concerns.
- An awareness of accountability and responsibility issues in relation to your role in nursing children.

Classification of child abuse behaviours

From preceding chapters you will have developed an understanding that children need to grow up in a nurturing environment that encourages their physical and emotional development. Sadly, however, abuse of children occurs. There is no definitive pattern for this deviation from the nurture and care that children require, and abuse take place in a wide variety of settings and can take a variety of forms. There are many underlying reasons for this and abuse can occur between families (inter-family abuse), within organizations (institutional abuse), or as a deliberate component of certain cultures or religions (ritual abuse).

Abuse can occur intentionally (commission) or through withholding essentials required for the child's physical and emotional development (omission). To a certain extent, abuse is also socially constructed, in that it occurs (or rather it is defined) within the cultural context it takes place in; therefore the interpretation of child abuse is dependent upon, and arises, because of values and beliefs of cultures. It can also be context dependent. That is, the interpretation of abuse is not only culturally dependent but also relevant to the time and place it occurs; for example, child labour in the UK in the 1800s. Elements of this may be defined as abusive in today's world, but were not at the time. As a result of these variations, there is no internationally agreed precise definition of child **abuse and neglect**, and attempts at definition prove elusive:

> *'[definitions are] complex, subject to constant change and realignment. They are highly contested concepts, underpinned by and subject to a range of political and cultural factors particular to the society in which they occur. For these reasons, therefore, child abuse and neglect are not phenomena that lend themselves to easy definition or measurement' (Corby, 2006, p 79).*

However, in spite of this lack of clear definitions, in practice children's nurses and other practitioners need guides to aid detection and intervention. Therefore the use of a classification system is a useful adjunct to clinical observation. Common classifications are neglect, physical abuse, sexual abuse, and emotional abuse (Department of Health and Children, 2006).

Neglect or deprivational abuse

Acts of omission, depriving a child of those basic provisions that are required for normal physical and emotional development, are otherwise known as neglect or deprivational abuse. Neglect of children can occur for a variety of reasons, including the presence of substance abuse or mental health issues in the caregivers, or simply through inadequate knowledge and parental readiness and preparation. It may be as a direct result of the care provided by the main caregiver, or there can be societal or cultural reasons.

Neglect by omission may be defined as follows:

> *'...where a child suffers significant harm or impairment of development by being deprived of food, clothing, warmth, hygiene, intellectual stimulation, supervision and safety, attachment to and affection from adults, medical care...*

> *[that] is likely to result in the serious impairment of the child's health or development' (Department of Health and Children, 2006, p 38)*

Physical abuse

Physical abuse, on the other hand, is usually an action of commission, thus deliberate, and may be defined as follows:

> *'Physical abuse is any form of non-accidental injury or injury which results from wilful or neglectful failure to protect a child.' (Department of Health and Children, 1999, p 32).*

There are many types of physical abuse and some examples are provided in **Box 4.1**.

Sexual abuse

When a child takes part in sexual activities, whether or not the child is aware or consents, this constitutes sexual abuse (Department of Health and Children, 1999). Sexual abuse occurs when another person uses a child for sexual 'gratification' or 'arousal' purposes (Department of Health and Children, 2006, p 38). It can occur through either force or enticement of the child, and includes the use of a child for prostitution purposes (Department of Health and Children, 2006). It is not simply the act of sexual intercourse that is under consideration here, but any activity that a child becomes involved in that may sexually gratify another person. Examples of range of offences that denote sexual abuse are provided in **Box 4.2**; however, this list is not exhaustive.

One anomaly with regard to the sexual abuse of children relates to age of consent to sexual intercourse, which

Box 4.1 Examples of physical injury

- Shaking, hitting, or throwing.
- Use of excessive force in handling.
- Deliberate poisoning.
- Suffocating.
- Munchausen Syndrome by Proxy (see definition on page 60).
- Allowing or creating a substantial risk of significant harm to a child.

(DHC, Ireland, 1999, p 32; DH/DfES, UK, 2006, p 37)

Box 4.2 Sexual abuse covers a wide range of offences

- Exposure of the sexual organs or any sexual activity intentionally performed in the presence of the child.
- Intentionally touching or molesting of the body of a child whether by a person or object for the purpose of sexual arousal or gratification.
- Masturbation in the presence of the child or the involvement of the child in the act of masturbation.
- Sexual intercourse with a child whether oral, anal, or vaginal.
- Sexual exploitation of a child including inciting, encouraging, propositioning, requiring, or permitting a child to solicit for, or engage in, prostitution or other sexual acts. Sexual exploitation also occurs when a child is involved in exhibition, modelling, or posing for the purpose of sexual arousal, gratification, or sexual acts, including its recording (on film, video tape, or other media) or the manipulation, for those purposes, of the image by computer or other means. It may include showing sexually explicit material to children, which is often a feature of the 'grooming' process by perpetrators of abuse.
- Consensual sexual activity involving an adult and an underage person.

can be at odds with the legislative definition of a child. In the UK, for example, a child is anyone up to the age of 18 (Department of Health 1989 and 2004b); whereas the legal age of *consent* to sexual intercourse is 16 years old.

For specific guidance about this issue it is best to refer to national guidelines within your own country. These laws, and the interpretation of these laws, are very influential in relation to nursing practice in this area, and you should familiarize yourself with these. See **http://www.childrenslawcentre.org** for Ireland and **http://www.childrenslegalcentre.com** for the United Kingdom.

Emotional abuse

Sexual abuse and all forms of child abuse can affect a child's emotional development and in some cases can be further classified as emotional abuse. Emotional abuse can occur within the context of a caregiver relationship, when emotional development is affected through 'persistent maltreatment' (Department of Health and Children, 2006, p 36). It is not related to a specific event,

but rather a pattern within the relationship and 'occurs when a child's needs for affection, approval, consistency, and security are not met' (Department of Health and Children, 1999, p 31). It can arise as a result of other types of abuse, but it can also occur in isolation. Unless there are other forms of abuse, it rarely results in physical signs or symptoms (Department of Health and Children, 1999). It may be defined as:

> '...the persistent emotional maltreatment of a child such as to cause severe and persistent adverse effects on the child's emotional development. Some level of emotional abuse is involved in all types of maltreatment of a child, although it may occur alone' (Department of Health and Children, 2006: 36).

Box 4.3 provides some examples of experiences that may result in emotional abuse. There are many other possible examples, although in some cases it may be difficult to quantify this type of abuse, as it is sometimes more subtle than the aforementioned abuses.

Box 4.3 Examples of emotional abuse of children

- The imposition of negative attributes on children, expressed by persistent criticism, sarcasm, and hostility or blaming—conveying to children that they are worthless or unloved.
- Under or overprotection of the child with limitation of exploration and learning.
- Conditional parenting in which the level of care shown to the child is made contingent on his or her behaviour or actions.
- Emotional unavailability by the child's parent/carer.
- Unresponsiveness.
- Inconsistent or inappropriate expectations of the child.
- Premature imposition of responsibility on the child.
- Unrealistic or inappropriate expectations of the child's capacity to understand something or to behave and control him or herself in a certain way.
- Failure to show interest in, or provide age-appropriate opportunities for, the child's cognitive and emotional development.
- Use of unreasonable or overly harsh disciplinary measures.
- Exposure to domestic violence.

(DHC, Ireland, 1999, p 32; DfES, UK, 2006, p 38)

Fabricated or induced illness (FII)

There are other less common forms of abuse that may present to nurses in the hospital or community setting, and this includes an abuse formerly known as Munchausen's Syndrome by Proxy (MSBP). This was named so after the original discovery of a condition in adults known as Munchausen's Syndrome whereby adults present to medical services with fake symptoms and conditions that are deliberately (physically) induced or simply fabricated (Asher, 1951). Where a caregiver presented a child in this way, this became known as a 'proxy' to the condition and hence the name. However, the latter syndrome is now more frequently referred to as factitious disorder or fabricated or induced illness (FII), with symptoms that are primarily fabricated or induced by the caregiver, so as to give an impression that the child is ill (Royal College of Paediatrics and Child Health, 2002).

Professor Roy Meadow (Meadow, 1977) first used this term to describe a spectrum of conditions in which parents or carers presented with a fabrication of illness in their children (using fabricated history and/or evidence). This form of abuse was also referred to by several other names including Meadow's Syndrome, Medea Complex, and factitious disorder by proxy (Parnell & Day, 1998). The most recent UK recommendation, following exploration of the history and controversy about term use, is that the description *fabricated or induced illness (FII)* is consistently used in all cases (Royal College of Paediatrics and Child Health, 2002, 2006). Examples of situations that may constitute fabricated or induced illness are outlined in **Box 4.4**.

However, there is a belief that the condition is not widely understood by staff and so raising awareness of its occurrence may be likely to increase detection. Children's nurses are in a unique position to detect child abuse due to their close proximity to and relationship with both child and family, and need to become adept at appropriate suspicion. In cases of suspicion, however, careful and thorough investigation of a child's history and presenting condition is of course required before judgements relating the presentation to the aforementioned condition (FII) are made. In keeping with the principles outlined in Chapter Two and Chapter Five, the family are an excellent source of information about the child's presenting condition, and need not only to be involved in the child's care, but also

Box 4.4 Examples of possible fabricated or induced illness

- The illness is unexplained, despite extensive medical investigation, or extremely rare.
- The reported symptoms and signs will only occur in the presence of the parents/carers.
- The treatment prescribed is described as ineffective and not tolerated positively by the parents/carers.
- There are multiple illnesses and a history of similar symptoms in other family members.
- Withdrawal of special treatment (e.g. naso-gastric feeds, IV lines) and 'getting better' is not viewed positively by the parents/carers.
- Parenting that may result in the following:
  - Causes an illness state in the child by administration of noxious substances.
  - Causes the child to have multiple (unnecessary) and at times dangerous investigations because of the parent's belief that the child is ill.
  - Leads to the child failing to thrive either through the active withholding of food or the giving of insufficient food.

Children First: National Guidelines for the Protection and Welfare of Children, DHC, Ireland, 1999, p 132; DfES, UK, 2006, p 146

need to be listened to. Simply because a child's diagnosis may initially be illusive, does not mean that the family have fabricated an illness, and as a nurse you will need to engage in a range of general physical observations and assessments (for example, those outlined in Chapter Five) to guide your judgements. Family anxiety at the time of a child's illness is common, and presenting features of this, for example a display of over-protectiveness or indeed aggression towards staff, is not uncommon and needs to be interpreted in context. Labelling or stereotyping of parents and family needs to be avoided and obviously prejudging FII without a full and thorough investigation (usually involving a multidisciplinary approach including a psychiatrist) would be ethically and morally incorrect.

As with all cases, specific examination by a physician may be required, and/or further investigative procedures, depending on the presenting condition, in order to rule out a real underlying illness. Once the child has been identified as having a clean bill of health, and depending on the circumstances and professional judgement of the health professionals, a thorough multidisciplinary investigation, including collaboration with a child psychiatrist, can take place to analyse the situation. In one case study a mother of a four-year-old girl was found to have contaminated a specimen of her child's urine with her own blood, and later through causing a local abrasion to the child's genitalia (see Chapter Sixteen). Once thorough investigation of the child's suspected urine infection (see Chapter Eleven) revealed no infection, local investigation, involving a psychiatrist, uncovered a diagnosis of FII. The psychiatrist and the community team in their subsequent care later supported both mother and child.

The role of the children's nurse with FII

Children's nurses are in a unique position to detect many types of child abuse due to their close proximity and relationship with both child and family. It is always important to raise concerns you may have, in an appropriate fashion, with a senior member of staff or the named nurse for safeguarding in your area. Nurses working in all areas of childcare need to become adept at *appropriate* suspicion, while at the same time respecting families and ceasing to prejudge. The children's nurse also has a unique role in relation to the child and the family, and must remain objective, professional, and non-judgemental in the delivery of care (Nursing and Midwifery Council (NMC), 2008).

It can also be difficult for nurses, faced with FII, to believe the emerging evidence and this can cause internal conflict (Powell, 2007), particularly in retaining this professional non-judgemental approach. For example, in the latter case study, the mother was very likeable and presentable and it came as a shock to staff that she could have committed such an abuse. It is important in such cases to seek appropriate counsel in the clinical environment (many organizations offer support such as counselling to staff should the need arise) and also to remain objective in the treatment of both carer and child.

Children's nurses working within a family centred care framework should work in partnership with the child and family, and advocate and link with the childcare team, both in the hospital and community settings. It is important that your responsibility here is clearly identified and understood (see Chapter Two). You should strive to build a professional and caring relationship on trust, respect, and open communication. This unique and special relationship

is vital and valued by nurses and parents and forms the cornerstone of evidence-based practice. Children's nurses may, therefore, experience internal conflict with this traditional role when faced with a suspected or presumptive diagnosis of child abuse or neglect. A new dimension of forensic nursing is introduced by virtue of the nurse's role in detection, suspicion, evidence gathering, and monitoring in cases of suspected and presumptive abuse. This role may, at times, be in direct conflict with the concepts of open communication, trust, and partnership within a family centred care framework. When working in this way, towards child protection, the nurse is said to have, at all times, a high suspicion index.

Consideration

Reflect on your understanding of what this means for your future practice as a qualified children's nurse. How will you ensure you safeguard and promote the welfare of children you encounter who may present with FII? How do you deliver family centred care in the presence of a presumptive diagnosis of child abuse?

Potential issues that you may have considered through your reflection could include:

- Familiarity with local procedures for promoting and safeguarding the welfare of children both in hospital and community settings.

- Alertness to the potential indicators of abuse and neglect when you are assessing the child and family.

- Understanding the principles of patient confidentiality and information sharing.

- Knowledge of the role of the named nurse for safeguarding in your local hospital or health setting.

Child protection policy and legal frameworks for the UK and Ireland

In the UK, identification of children in need is addressed through public health values and primarily universal access to professionals through a core child health promotion programme (Hall and Elliman, 2003). Targeted work with a child and family usually commences once a health need is identified during the standard health promotion approaches (for example, a health visitor suspects the need for family support during post-natal visits to a child). However, in spite of these safeguards, the nurse who comes into contact with children during routine medical procedures or in Accident and Emergency must always have a good awareness and understanding of child abuse, a high suspicion index, good recognition ability, and a fundamental understanding of the legal and ethical issues involved.

Child abuse is an emotional and complex area for all involved in the care of children, young people, and their families, because it involves emotive, sensitive issues and raises many ethical and legal concerns. The role of the children's nurse in child protection is in stark contrast to the philosophy of family centred care and the central role of negotiation and partnership in care (Coyne, 1995). The current child protection system in the UK is based around the legislative framework of the Children Act (Department of Health, 1989); this was introduced in an effort to reform and clarify the existing plethora of laws affecting children. The system in Ireland also has a framework relating to a number of Acts providing for the protection and welfare of children. Legislation covering safeguarding and child protection can therefore be divided into two main categories:

- **civil law** (further divided into *public law*, which puts in place systems and processes in order to minimize the risk of children coming to harm and lays out what action should be taken if children are at risk; and *private law*, which deals with family proceedings such as divorce and contact);

and

- **criminal law**, which deals with people who have offended or are at risk of offending against children.

In practice, some Acts of law may include both provisions that relate to *civil law* and provisions that relate to *criminal law*. For children's nurses, the Children Act (Department of Health, 1989) encapsulated a number of related principles including the paramountcy principle, which means that a child's welfare is paramount when making any decisions about the child's upbringing. In practice, the court must also ascertain the wishes and feelings of the child and shall not make an order unless this is better for the child than making no order at all.

Every effort should be made to preserve the child's home and family links.

Nursing Alert

When caring for children with a suspected or confirmed diagnosis of child abuse, professionals must work within the legislation and guidelines of both their local (healthcare setting) and national EU or non-EU jurisdiction. In each clinical placement, familiarize yourself with local policy, guidelines, and best practice.

The Children Act also introduced the concept of parental responsibility, which sets out the rights, duties, powers, and responsibilities of the parent or carer of a child (Department of Health, 1989). The Children Act (Department of Health, 1989) and the Children (Scotland) Act (1995) stipulate that local authorities (for example those with responsibility for education, health, and housing) must work together to safeguard and support the welfare of children in need. The later Children Act (Department of Health, 2004b) introduced a statutory framework for local cooperation to protect children in England and Wales. There is no single piece of legislation that fully covers child protection in the UK or Ireland, but rather a myriad of laws and guidance that are continually being amended and updated.

It should also be noted that not all laws cover all parts of the UK (England, Wales, Scotland, Northern Ireland, and the Channel Islands) and that the legal systems vary in the different areas (Walters, 2007). The child protection practices and the expectations of the professional with respect to safeguarding internationally will be reliant on legislation within their country (Farrell, 2004). In most countries the principles of safeguarding reflect the country's commitment to this cause. Professionals need to utilize national criteria and law at local level in order for the legal framework to be initiated.

However, legislation by itself is not enough; it needs to be part of a wider process of change. All organizations in the UK and Ireland with responsibility for services to children, including healthcare organizations, are now obliged to make arrangements to ensure that in discharging their functions they safeguard and promote the welfare of children. Government publications suggest that all public agencies work to ensure that all children living within the UK have the opportunity to experience five basic elements significant to child health and development (HM Government, 2006):

- **S**—Staying safe
- **H**—Healthy
- **E**—Enjoy and achieve
- **E**—Economic well-being
- **P**—Positive contribution to society

In the UK there is also a need for agencies (which includes hospitals) to assess whether the child is 'at risk of significant harm'. This concept was initially outlined in the Children's Act 1989 (Department of Health, 1989) and was updated in 2006 (Department of Health and Children, 2006). Significant harm is later described in *Every Child Matters* (HM Government, 2006) as the criteria that a professional must apply to assess whether intervention into family life is required. If the professional deems that a child's well-being would be harmed if that intervention did not occur then this is the criterion by which that intervention by agencies is compulsory. **Figure 4.1**

outlines some of the key principles from policy related to safeguarding children.

For children's nurses this means actively promoting the health and well-being of children and also protecting vulnerable children in collaboration with other organizations and authorities (HM Government, 2006). Child protection is closely linked to all aspects of children's well-being, and as the health and safety of children and young people are essential aspects of their overall well-being, therefore healthcare interventions should also equip children and young people to 'stay safe' (HM Government, 2006). Children's nurses are uniquely positioned to detect child abuse and nurses should maintain a high suspicion index at all times (**see Box 4.5**). Within the context of the high suspicion index that you need to develop as a nurse, it is also important to remember some simple guidelines related to this practice. These are outlined in **Box 4.6**.

A National Service Framework (Department of Health, 2004a) sets standards of care for children in all settings. The first standard addressed many of the issues raised in

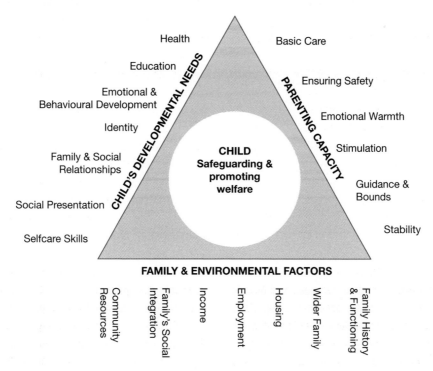

Figure 4.1 Working together to safeguard children

© Crown Copyright

Box 4.5 Children's nurses' role in detecting potential abuse

- Children's nurses spend a great deal of time with children and families and therefore are in a unique position to assess, evaluate, monitor, and detect abuse and protection issues (Powell, 2007).
- Children's nurses are experienced in caring for children at all phases of development and should therefore be able to recognize or detect unusual or strange behaviours.
- They are experienced in the recognition of family dynamics in a variety of settings and situations.
- They are in a position of forming a unique and caring relationship with both children and their families.
- They form an important part of the child protection/family support team and are in a position to draw on expert support and advice.

Box 4.6 Guidelines for suspicion of child abuse or neglect

DO:
- Report your concerns to your line manager or staff nurse.
- Seek advice from a named professional with expertise in child protection.
- Follow local child protection procedures and report your concerns to the appropriate authority. In Ireland refer to the National Guidelines and the notification process with the Irish Gardai.
- Keep records of your concerns and any action you take—defensible documentation is important.

DO NOT:
- Ignore your concerns and do nothing.
- Attempt to investigate your suspicions or allegations of abuse.
- Necessarily discuss your concerns with the suspected/alleged perpetrator until you have sought advice and guidance from someone senior, e.g. named nurse.

the Victoria Climbié Inquiry Report and her treatment in hospital (Lord Laming, 2003). In particular, it addressed the importance of continuity of care and how this should be achieved, as well as record keeping. *Every Child Matters: Change for Children* (HM Government, 2006), was a direct response to both the death of Victoria Climbié and the Laming Report, and sets out the national framework for local change programmes.

Nursing practice in this area is to be further developed in response to a recent follow-up publication to *Every Child Matters* (HM Government, 2006), which evaluates England's policy approach in this area (Lord Laming, 2009). There are several recommendations within this report aimed at further safeguarding children, which will have far-reaching consequences in the future. Children's services, for example, require that managers have experience in safeguarding children or that they appoint a senior manager with this experience. Strategic cooperation between local and national agencies is to be strengthened, which will outline specific targets for child protection, and these will also be supported by statutory targets at government level.

Nursing Alert

A suspicion index is formed from evidence-based knowledge in relation to all forms of child abuse. It is important to remember that it is usually a collection of several factors, rather than one single finding, which leads to a presumptive or proven diagnosis.

Childrens nursing skills for child protection

There are certain key skills required to ensure that the child health nurse is competent to safeguard and protect children, and these are summarized in **Box 4.7**. In addition to specific skills, there are also a number of broader skill clusters that are required, as well as specific behaviours, in order to ensure that you are best placed to accurately operate within this high level of suspicion. These include the ability to recognize inconsistencies; being able to avoid presumptions (jumping to conclusions); and good observational, communication, and documentation skills. You must also in all situations be prepared to act as child advocate and have a good understanding of the nurse's role in relation to both child abuse and protection, as well as an understanding of the concept of child protection. All of these skills will now be further discussed.

Recognition of 'inconsistencies'

Children's nurses, in normal circumstances, work in partnership with families/carers and would depend on the

Box 4.7 Children's nursing skills for child protection

- *Concentration* and active *listening* in order to understand what is being communicated and provide appropriate feedback.
- *Objectivity* in relation to what is being said and its implications for professional practice and ethical or legal conflicts that arise as a result.
- *Focusing* on the concerns and issues of the child and family during the communication process.
- *Respect* for culture and diversity and differing values between the parties involved in the communication process.
- *Confidence* in relation to interpersonal and communication skills with children and their families.

parental history and knowledge of the child in order to assist the team in reaching a diagnosis and planning the care the child requires. In cases of suspected abuse or presumptive diagnosis, it is important to reflect on what parents say and consider if what they say makes medical or logical sense. But it is also important to consider how you deal with this information.

Many children, for example, present with bruises. However, it is important to identify 'unusual' bruises in relation to location, pattern, and number (Hattfield, 2008). It may be unusual that a bruise appears older than the history given (i.e. the child is reported to have fallen accidentally today, but bruising appears older). However, systematic review evidence (Maguire *et al.*, 2005) suggests that clinical assessment is insufficient to determine bruise age (e.g. estimating the age of a bruise from its colour has no scientific basis), and therefore it should be avoided in child protection proceedings. Another example of an inconsistency could be an injury that does not 'fit' with the explanation given by the family/carer, such as a child who fell off an armchair onto a carpet but has multiple stab injuries and old fractures.

Unusual lesions that cannot be explained, such as a cigarette burn or fingerprint bruising, should also be investigated. The recognition of inconsistencies is an important skill for nurses working in the field of child protection as it could assist in early detection of cases and could 'break a lethal cycle' (Volz, 1995). The Royal College of Paediatrics and Child Health provide useful information for practice in this area (See Royal College of Paediatrics and Child Health, 2006, p 18).

Consideration

A child has presented to you in an Accident and Emergency department with an inconsistent injury. What are the first steps you need to take?

Avoid jumping to conclusions

The primary role of children's nurses is that of child protection/family support; however, a professional responsibility is to be objective and fair to those under suspicion (NMC, 2008; Hattfield, 2008). It is vital for the children's nurse to be objective and make no false assumptions or accusations. All evidence should be considered by the child protection/family support team and action agreed and planned within an agreed time frame. The evidence collection begins with clinical observation (Chapter Five) and may require investigations such as X-rays (to clarify the nature, age, and aetiology of a bone injury).

Skeletal surveys may establish the presence of old 'unexplained' injuries. Blood coagulation studies are helpful in ruling out blood disorders that may present with bruising. Toxicology studies may identify ingested substances presenting puzzling symptoms. Careful examination of skin lesions may identify unusual findings including shape and distribution; an example may be a cigarette burn.

A social worker's report may also highlight issues of concern, which may be related to the presumptive diagnosis. Jumping to conclusions threatens the child, family, carers, and nursing relationship. It will prevent the effective functioning of the childcare team and may, in some cases, present legal difficulties in securing a conviction in the future.

Careful analysis of the history given, times, dates, and findings may establish a pattern suggestive of abuse. Being objective raises many conflicts for the children's nurse, for example, the normal trusting partnership relationship between nurse, child, and family/carer may become strained and tense. The nurse may find it difficult to balance protection of the child with his or her relationship with the family/carers. The role of the nurse takes on a new dimension in relation to evidence gathering and prevention of further abuse. It is helpful to remember that it is possible to protect the child from further danger and accept the presumptive diagnosis of alleged abuse without making assumptions in relation to the innocence or guilt of the family/carer/perpetrator.

The role of the children's nurse also involves observation of both the child and family. Evaluation of these observations in light of evidence-based findings and clinical experience is then made. Observations need to be objective, professional, and non-judgemental (NMC, 2008). The interpretation and evaluation of observations should be guided by knowledge, evidence, and the expertise of the child protection and family support team. It is important to have knowledge of normal child development, the child, and family circumstances and structure in order to have a balanced and objective basis for intervention.

What may be considered as abnormal behaviour in children or indeed parents needs to be considered in relation to their lived experiences and the effects these have had on their lives and relationships. Children who have been abused have altered relationships with their parents but still love them; in fact their need for a loving family relationship is strong. Howe (2005, p 111) noted that 'neglected children tend to be passive' and that they may experience 'a feeling of inescapable anxiety' (Howe, 2005, p 110). Observation and any documentation of the child and family should be inclusive of all activities over the 24-hour time span and should include behaviour such as body language, posture, expression, level and frequency of interactions, and play activities.

> **Nursing Alert**
>
> When caring for children with a suspected, presumptive, or confirmed diagnosis of child abuse, children's nurses must work within the scope of practice and check the skills to be undertaken are within the guidelines of both their local (healthcare setting) and their national regulating nursing bodies (NMC, 2008). Students should always be aware of local policies and guidelines in this area and seek advice before making decisions.

The nurse's role in relation to both child abuse and protection

All health professionals in the inter-professional team who encounter children, parents, and carers in the course of their work need to be aware of their responsibility to safeguard and promote the welfare of children and young people. This is important even when the health professionals do not work directly with a child but may be seeing their parent, carer, or other significant adult. The children's nurse needs to be specifically aware of and fully understand the child protection policies and guidelines that apply to their area of practice. They form an important part of the overarching child protection team and usually have the most extensive contact with children and their families. They must work within their scope of practice and child protection policy and guidelines to contribute to prevention, detection, intervention, and monitoring of vulnerable children and their families in a holistic, caring, non-judgemental, and professional manner as advised in the Code (NMC, 2008). **Figure 4.2** outlines the referral process that a health professional can use if they are concerned about a child's welfare.

Communication skills

Communication, according to Arnold and Boggs (2003, p 25), is '...the foundation and basic tool of the nurse-client relationship'. The skills required in communicating with both children and their families are multidimensional and involve cognitive, affective, and psychomotor skills (further information is found in Chapter Two). Communication, therefore, is an active process involving listening, thinking, evaluating, responding, and encouraging dialogue. When English is not the first language of a child or family, translation services will be required.

Setting the scene

Communication will be facilitated by provision of space, time, and privacy. Meeting with children and families in relation to child abuse and protection issues is highly sensitive and may be perceived as very threatening; therefore, the children's nurse should first establish a relationship of openness and respect and introduce themselves if this is their first contact with either child or family. In order to facilitate effective communication a private, quiet area should be chosen and seating should be informal. Children and families may be more relaxed within their own home or may prefer a 'neutral' setting. As communication may be difficult until a flow is established, ensure there are no interruptions or high noise levels, if possible. If the location is in the community, the same guidelines apply.

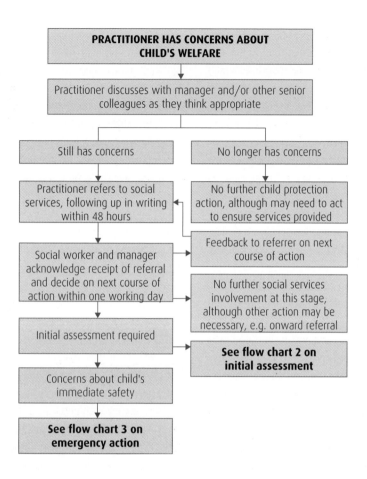

Figure 4.2 What to do if you worry a child is being abused
© Crown Copyright

Active listening

Active listening has been described as a process in which the nurse listens to what is being said and explores the values, attitudes, and meanings that underlie what is being said. It is a participatory process and should be non-judgemental. It is also described as 'really' listening to someone with undivided attention in order to fully 'hear' what they are saying. It is associated with eye contact, open posture, a caring atmosphere, and empathy.

Timing

As communication is a two-way process it is important to speak slowly, where appropriate, and allow time for understanding and assimilation of information to take place. Communication dealing with sensitive issues may be difficult as the participants in the communication may be fearful, anxious, emotional, and guarded in their responses. Rephrasing of questions may be required and the use of open-ended questions may help the flow of the communication. Silence also plays a role in communication and should not be dismissed or discouraged as it allows time for reflection and formulation of ideas and responses.

Probing may be a useful strategy; however, it should be used in an appropriate way and never to lead or influence responses. Take time to observe how an experienced practitioner or the named nurse for safeguarding uses this strategy to elicit information.

Understandable language is important in order to avoid misunderstanding and encourage participation in the communication process. Age-related appropriate language in relation to children and adults, as with any situation in children's nursing, is vital. When communicating with children the use of play, drawings, and sociodrama may yield important information, especially from children who lack language skills or who are reluctant to talk due to fear or anxiety. The formulation of non-threatening open-ended questions should be employed with both children and families.

Non-verbal communication

This involves the interpretation of posture, facial expression, gestures, and active listening. 'In a professional relationship, verbal and non-verbal components of communication are intimately related' (Arnold & Boggs, 2003, p 217). Non-verbal communication can convey meaning to the spoken word and reflect both caring and interest, but on occasion it may not match what is said and therefore cause misunderstanding and confusion; it may even convey the 'wrong' message. For example, if you are building a relationship with a family and tell them to take their time in answering questions, yet at the same time frequently look at your watch, you can see how these actions are inconsistent with the verbal communication process. Non-verbal communication should be used in order to build rapport with children and families and therefore it is important to ensure verbal and non-verbal communication processes match each other. The quality of the communication process requires the children's nurse to incorporate and put into practice the following skills: concentration, objectivity, listening, focusing, respect, and confidence (Arnold & Boggs, 2003, p 240).

> **Consideration**
>
> Consider how children and families may interpret your non-verbal communication. What might be some consequences of misinterpreting non-verbal communication?
>
> Consider cultural aspects of communication and how this may influence effective communication.
>
> Can you identify any of the recommendations from the Climbié Inquiry that related to good practice in this area?

Documentation skills

Documentation has always been an important part of nursing and should be factual, accurate, reliable, and clearly written. All documentation should be signed and dated by the writer (NMC, 2008). In relation to child abuse and protection, documentation may be required

and used in subsequent court proceedings. Lord Laming (2003) drew attention to the nurse's responsibility in recognition and reporting of suspected child abuse and their 'fundamental duty' to document suspicious lesions and injuries (p 9). It is important to document exactly what has been said or disclosed to you 'verbatim' and not to document your perceptions or impressions of such statements (Powell, 2007). The importance of documentation and record keeping is further outlined in Chapter Five.

Advocacy skills

The children's nurse has an important role in representing the child and family when they are unable to represent themselves, and in practice this is referred to as advocacy. An advocate is defined as one who pleads or acts for another. Recognizing that a crucial role for children's nurses is that of acting as the advocate for the child poses questions about how children's voices can be heard and how child health nurses know whose voice they represent when they act in an advocacy capacity.

Advocacy involves getting to know the child and family, and respecting their unique values and belief systems. It also involves not only the process of informing and empowering them to making choices, but also supporting the child and family during the process and in the pursuit of their chosen options. Speaking on their behalf, if requested, may be involved in this role; therefore, advocacy can be challenging, as you have to be objective and aware of your own value system and beliefs. Protection of clients is also an element within advocacy; however, this requires careful consideration as the protection of the child is of paramount importance in such situations.

> **Consideration**
>
> Can the child health nurse truly act as an advocate for the child? Discuss with your peers.

> **Nursing Alert**
>
> Children's nurses are required to have a clear criminal record (for example, Irish Garda vetting or UK Criminal Records Bureau (CRB) Police clearance), whilst working with children.

The concept of child protection

The concept of child protection and family support covers a wide spectrum of activities and can be considered under the following headings:

- Prevention prior to abuse or neglect occurring.
- Protection and support when abuse or neglect exists.
- Prevention of further abuse or neglect after the occurrence.

Child protection as a concept has been influenced by social change and the awareness of the risks to children and vulnerable persons in society. Modern thinking suggests that life is not more dangerous today than in the past, but rather there is increased awareness of known risks in today's society.

'In the context of the last 100 years of "modern" practices, child protection and welfare systems have never been as efficient as they are today, and probably more children are effectively protected in time than ever before' (Ferguson, 1997, p 228).

Child protection is sometimes considered to be mainly within the domain of social workers, and is often wrongly associated with a failure to protect vulnerable persons. These negative outcomes have gained much attention in the media. However, child protection actually requires professional multidisciplinary team input in order to be effective in the protection and support of vulnerable persons. Contemporary emphasis is on family support, and child protection now balances prevention and protection rather than being reactionary in nature.

However, educating and maintaining the child protection workforce presents a considerable challenge. Child protection education should include risk management but also raise awareness of the importance of reducing childhood adversity, because it has such negative impacts on children's health, growth, development, psychological well-being, behaviour, and relationships. Families require physical and practical support along with therapeutic interventions that meet their complex needs (Ferguson, 2001).

There have been many advances and evidence-based changes introduced into the child protection and family support process and as new issues emerge, it is important that these changes keep pace with the modern world and reflect the changing nature of society. In the Republic of Ireland a special Rapporteur on Child Protection has been appointed to review and advise the government on issues relevant to child protection and related family support issues. In his submission to the Oireachtas in November 2007, he recommended a range of new legislation in relation to the following issues:

- Police 'vetting' and the use of soft information.
- Criminal law in relation to sexual abuse.
- Grooming of children.
- The concept of *loco parentis*.

Other areas identified as needing review included: child trafficking in Ireland, the competency of minors to consent or refuse treatment, and parental authority in light of the Irish constitution (Shannon, 2007).

In May 2009, the Commission on Child Abuse (Ireland) reported its findings on an enquiry into institutional abuse of minors in Ireland; this report looked at the period of 1936 onwards. The report identified physical, emotional, and sexual abuse and its impact on the surviving victims, and the general lived experiences of children in residential care. Its recommendations are wide ranging and include alleviation of suffering of the surviving victims and reflecting on the past in order to reduce the incidence of such abuse occurring in the future. Issues identified included childcare policy being child centred, the frequent reviewing and evaluation of childcare services, the need for children in care to have a voice and be heard, and the importance of ensuring a caring environment for such children (Commission on Child Abuse, 2009).

As part of your daily contact in practice is with children and families in hospital or community settings, you should undertake to:

- Understand the risk factors and recognize children in need of support and/or safeguarding.
- Recognize the needs of parents who may need extra help in bringing up their children, and know where to refer for help.
- Recognize the risks of abuse to an unborn child.
- Contribute to enquiries from other professionals about a child and their family or carers.
- Liaise closely with other agencies including other health professionals.
- Play an active part, through the child protection plan, in safeguarding children from significant harm.

- Consider local protocols where they exist, particularly with respect to sexual health and contraceptive services, and comply with these other than in exceptional circumstances.

Nursing Alert

- What are the obligations on healthcare professionals in relation to safeguarding and protecting children and young people?
- What is the procedure for referral that you would be required to follow when you have reason to believe that harm has been done or is likely to be done to a child?

The current Child Health Promotion Programme (CHPP) in the UK is the early intervention and prevention public health programme that lies at the heart of a universal service for children and families. At a crucial stage of life, the CHPP's universal reach provides an invaluable opportunity to identify families that are in need of additional support and children who are at risk of poor outcomes. Providing a high-quality CHPP that is visible and accessible to families with children is a core health responsibility contributing to the goals of *Every Child Matters* (HM Government, 2006) and services provided in Sure Start children's centres (Department of Health, 2007).

Working together to safeguard children

In April 2006, the UK government updated its publication on inter-agency working. The statutory guidance on making arrangements to safeguard and promote the welfare of children under Section 11 of the Children Act (2004) sets out the key arrangements agencies should make to achieve this whilst carrying out their normal functions.

Consideration

What are the functions and responsibilities of the Social Services Child Protection Team in the UK after receiving a referral in relation to safeguarding children and young people?

Structures—Social Services

Social Services is the lead agency for safeguarding children in the UK, with statutory responsibility to make enquiries into all child protection issues, and is the principal point of contact for child welfare concerns. The police also have powers to intervene where there is concern about a child's welfare. The Children and Young Persons Act, 1933 is one of the older pieces of child protection legislation that has parts that are still in force today. These include a list of offences that constitute child abuse, which are referred to as Schedule One offences (Walters, 2007).

Rights of the child

Every child and young person has the right to a life free from abuse, and Article 19 of the United Nations Convention on the Rights of the Child (United Nations, 1989), to which the UK is a signatory, states that:

> *Parties shall take all appropriate legislative, administrative, social and educational measures to protect the child from all forms of physical or mental violence, injury or abuse, neglect or negligent treatment, maltreatment or exploitation, including sexual abuse, while in the care of parent(s), legal guardian(s) or any other person who has the care of the child.*

> *Such protective measures should, as appropriate, include effective procedures for the establishment of social programmes to provide necessary support for the child and for those who have the care of the child, as well as for other forms of prevention and for identification, reporting, referral, investigation, treatment and follow-up of instances of child maltreatment described heretofore, and, as appropriate, for judicial involvement.*

Every child must be protected from all forms of violence, abuse, neglect, and mistreatment. 'A particular priority must be effective protection of the rights of children, both against economic exploitation and all forms of abuse' (Commission of the European Communities, 2006). As a children's nurse it is important to ensure that the views of children are taken into account in matters affecting them, and this is a key principle of the National Service Framework (NSF) (Department of Health, 2004a).

What is parental responsibility?

Parental responsibility is a legal concept that consists of the rights, duties, powers, responsibilities, and authority that most parents have in respect of their children. It includes the right to give consent, on behalf of the child, to medical treatment. However, this right is not absolute, and in certain circumstances there is freedom to delegate some decision-making responsibility to others. In addition, in some cases, competent children can consent to diagnosis and treatment on their own behalf if they understand the implications of what is proposed. Those with parental responsibility also have a statutory right to apply for access to the health records of their child, although children who are mature enough to express views on the issue also need to be asked before parents see their records. Parental responsibility is afforded not only to parents, however, and not all parents have parental responsibility, despite arguably having equal moral rights to make decisions for their children where they have been equally involved in their care (British Medical Association (BMA), 2008).

The law in the UK has recently been revised. In relation to children born after 1 December 2003 (England and Wales), 15 April 2002 (Northern Ireland), or 4 May 2006 (Scotland), both of the child's parents have parental responsibility if they are registered on the child's birth certificate (irrespective of whether the parents are married or not). A child's biological parents are the child's legal parents (although legal parenthood does not necessarily confer parental responsibility), unless the child has been adopted or was born as the result of some methods of assisted reproduction. Where the child has been formally adopted, the adoptive parents are the child's legal parents and automatically acquire parental responsibility.

If a child has been born because of assisted reproduction, there are rules under the Human Fertilisation and Embryology Act (HFEA, 1990) that determine the child's legal parentage. If both parents have parental responsibility, neither loses it if they divorce, and responsibility endures if the child is in care or custody. It can, however, be restricted by court order and it is lost if the child is adopted. A person other than a child's biological parent can acquire parental responsibility by being appointed as the child's guardian (an appointment usually takes effect on the death of the parents) or by having a residence order made in his or her favour, in which case parental responsibility lasts for the duration of the order.

A local authority acquires parental responsibility (shared with the parents) while the child is the subject of a care or supervision order. In relation to children born before 1 December 2003 in England and Wales, 15 April 2002 in Northern Ireland, and 4 May 2006 in Scotland, both of the child's biological parents will only automatically acquire parental responsibility if they were married at the time of the child's birth or at some time thereafter. If the parents have never been married, only the mother automatically has parental responsibility. The father may acquire it in various ways, including by entering into a parental responsibility agreement with the mother, or through a parental responsibility order made by a court. In England, Wales, and Northern Ireland, parental responsibilities may be exercised until a young person reaches 18 years. In Scotland, only the aspect of parental responsibilities concerned with the giving of 'guidance' (Children (Scotland) Act, 1995) endures until 18 years, guidance meaning the provision of advice. The rest is lost when the young person reaches 16 years.

What are the limits to parental responsibility?

The moral authority behind parental responsibility depends upon parents acting in the best interests of their children. If it appears, however, that parents are following a course of action that is contrary to their child's interests, their decisions can be challenged. Where doctors believe that parental decisions are not in the best interests of the child, it may be necessary to seek a view from the courts, whilst meanwhile providing only emergency treatment essential to preserve life or prevent serious deterioration. The courts are required, in their decision making, to have regard to the rights given force by the Human Rights Act (1998), and to have the child's welfare as their paramount consideration (Department of Health, 1989; The Children (Northern Ireland) Order, 1995; Children (Scotland) Act, 1995; The Child Care Act (1991) Ireland). Child health professionals must take care to concern themselves only with the welfare of the child and avoid being drawn into matters such as marital disputes. Discussion aimed at reaching consensus should be attempted. If this fails, the clinician in charge must make a decision whether to go ahead despite the disagreement. The onus is then on the dissenting parent to take steps to reverse the doctor's decision. If the dispute is over a controversial and elective procedure, for example male infant circumcision for religious purposes (BMA, 2006), doctors must not proceed without the authority of a court (Re 'J', 2000). In Scotland, however, the Children Act imposes an obligation on any person exercising a parental responsibility or parental right to have regard to the views of any other person with the same rights and responsibilities (Children (Scotland) Act, 1995).

Consideration

- Can a parent who does not live with a child gain access to the child's medical records?

- How would you deal with this request if it occurred in your daily practice?

- Can a relative other than a parent give consent to medical treatment on behalf of a child?

Anyone with parental responsibility has a statutory right to apply for access to their child's health records. If the child is capable of giving consent, access may only be given with his or her consent. It may be necessary to discuss parental access alone with children if there is a suspicion that they are under pressure to agree. (For example, the young person may not wish a parent to know about a request for contraceptive advice.) If a child lacks the competence to understand the nature of an application but access to medical records would be in his or her best interests, it should be granted. Parental access must not be given where it conflicts with the child's best interests and any information that a child revealed in the

expectation that it would not be disclosed should not be released unless it is in the child's best interests to do so. Where parents are separated and one of them applies for access to the medical records, doctors are under no obligation to inform the other parent, although they may consider doing so if they believe it to be in the child's best interests.

Another exception to parental responsibility is Gillick competence. This is a term originating in England used to determine whether a child alone may consent to treatment. This is based on a House of Lords decision in the case Gillick v West Norfolk and Wisbech AHA (1985). This also applies in Australia, Canada, and New Zealand and there is similar provision in Scotland by The Age of Legal Capacity (Scotland) Act 1991.

Parents are also entitled to authorize another person to take over particular responsibilities. This might be because they have arranged for somebody else to look after their child while they are away. It is unlikely to be 'reasonable' in the terms of the Children Act (Department of Health, 1989) for a non-parent to give consent if he or she knows that the child's parents are likely to object, and treatment should only be given in such circumstances if the situation is an emergency and delay would lead to death or serious harm. In Scotland, the primacy of any known wishes of the parents in these situations has statutory force (Children (Scotland) Act, 1995). If a carer brings a child for treatment, steps should be taken to ascertain the parents' views, and if there is doubt about authority to proceed, doctors should seek legal advice.

Consideration

As a child health nurse, when may you need to consider whether parental responsibility is shared?

Competent children and the limits to parental responsibility

As children grow and mature, so their ability to make decisions on their own behalf increases until, on reaching adulthood (in UK law this is considered to be 18 years old vs. consent law, which is 16 years), they are presumed to be competent to take full responsibility for personal decision making. During this period of maturation, it is possible that children will disagree with their parents as to what constitutes their best interests, and there may be situations where doctors are confronted with disagreements over a proposed course of action. In England and Wales, no statute governs the rights of people under 16 to give consent to medical treatment, and there remains some uncertainty in the common law. In the landmark Gillick case, for example, the judges held that 'parental rights were recognised by the law only as long as they were needed for the protection of the child and such rights yielded to the child's right to make his own decisions when he reached a sufficient understanding and intelligence to be capable of making up his own mind' (Gillick v West Norfolk and Wisbech AHA, 1986).

Although this ruling appeared to clarify the decision making autonomy of competent young people, subsequent cases have retreated from this position, particularly where they have involved treatment refusal by the young person. For treatment decisions that are unlikely to have such grave consequences, however, a young person under 16 can consent to treatment provided he or she is competent to understand the nature, purpose, and possible consequences of the treatment proposed. However, the professional taking the consent of the young person needs to be able to demonstrate that they have made efforts to persuade the young person to share the information with their parents (NMC, 2008).

Clearly, children and young people are able to choose treatment options, in some cases, for themselves. However, what is the extent of this accountability and responsibility and are there any inherent challenges in permitting such freedom of choice in the youth?

Accountability and responsibility

In 2001 there were 14.8 million children aged less than 20 years living in the UK. In 2006, children and young people made up approximately a quarter of the total population in England and almost a third of the population in Northern Ireland. Therefore, there are 11.7 million dependent children in England and Wales (Office of the First Minister and Deputy Prime Minister, 2006; National Statistics Online, 2008). They hold specific legal rights as children, and their families have the autonomy to select an

individual lifestyle. The vulnerability of children and their related immaturity affects their ability to articulate what they feel or need; however, their emerging autonomy can also pose a challenge for health and social services in effectively planning their care.

Nursing Alert

Understanding what is happening to a child when there are concerns that the child's health and development are being impaired remains a core professional activity for those working with children and families (see Common Assessment Frameworks, Framework for the Assessment of Children in Need, Department of Health and Children, 2006).

If you accept the conviction embedded in the United Nations Convention that children have the right to have a voice, what is your responsibility as a child health nurse in relation to the voice of individual children and of communities of children? To fully respect the rights of the child, nurses need to grapple with the complex question of what qualifies as voice for the purposes of children's nursing care. Children express their thoughts and feelings and try to communicate their desires and needs in numerous ways.

Good practice in assessment

Nurses must look and listen for children's voices in many dimensions: audible sounds and words, artwork, facial expressions, body language, music, and even in silence. Within any cry, story, grimace, action, or grunt, there may be an important message about a child's wishes, opinions, or choices. Although the nature and form of these expressions may change considerably as the child develops from infant to child to adolescent, the complexities inherent in giving them voice may be equally challenging. It is the child health nurse's responsibility to observe and attend to the expressions and try to decipher their meanings.

Involvement in decision making

Although contemporary national policy and practice strongly encourage the involvement of children in decision making, little is known about this decision making process. For example, Morrow (1999) and Oates (2007) state that when eliciting children's views, child health professionals must confront their assumptions around whether they truly believe children and young people's accounts of their experiences. The UNCRC (United Nations, 1989) was developed to protect and promote the rights and welfare of children and young people, recognizing that these rights were separate from the rights of parents, families, and other adults involved in the care of children and young people. The UNCRC (United Nations, 1989) also promoted the idea that children and young people are capable of expressing a view and that they should be allowed to express this view freely and be taken seriously on all matters affecting them. This acknowledges that they are active social players who have the right to hold and express opinions and to assume responsibility for their actions (Coyne, 2006).

Healthcare professionals are required to observe the UN Convention rights in their decision making, and where they feel that their actions may possibly be in breach of the rights, they should take legal advice. Some of the recommendations from Lord Laming (2003) related to caring for children in healthcare settings are detailed at the end of this chapter.

> **Consideration**
>
> List the qualities required for effective working in partnership with children and their families. Specifically think about the areas of preparing children for procedures, gaining consent, and then keeping records.

Preparing children for clinical observations

There are ranges of procedures that may be undertaken in the case of a child where abuse is suspected. The type of procedures utilized depends on the case presenting and the physical and psychological needs of the child. The preparation for these is consistent with preparing children for any procedure in hospital or community settings and has to be undertaken in the context of their place within the family, their developmental status, and their level of understanding. Further discussions of communication are found in Chapter Two and preparation for procedures and distraction is outlined in Chapter Five. Open, clear

communication between the child, family, and nurse is vital in order to avoid misunderstanding (NMC, 2008). Demonstrations using toys may be helpful to promote a visual picture of the procedure being undertaken. The presence of the parents along with the emotional and psychological support given by the children's nurse may also help to alleviate anxiety and the use of 'rewards for bravery 'should be considered. Hattfield (2008) postulates that rewards should not be given for bravery but rather should be given in order to make the entire experience a pleasant one.

Consent prior to clinical observations

Children may consent to clinical observations if they demonstrate enough maturity to understand the significance of the ethical, social, and emotional aspects of their situation (Department of Health, 2002).

> **Consideration**
>
> How is this assessed or determined in your practice? How do you involve children in consent issues?

Conclusion

> *'It has been said that a measure of a society is how it treats its most vulnerable citizens. Amongst the most vulnerable in our society are children' (Shannon, 2007, p 11).*

Given the moral, ethical, and legal imperatives discussed in relation to the protection of children throughout this chapter, you must now recognize that child protection is the business of everyone at every level of society. Therefore, the fundamental objective of child protection is to ensure that all those with a duty to safeguard children recognize that duty, and are able to fulfil it. By revisiting the four learning outcomes detailed at the outset of the chapter and having worked through the activities and discussion points outlined, you should be able to explore your knowledge, attitudes, skills, and ideas about this sensitive area of child health nursing practice.

Online resource centre

You may find it helpful to work through our online resources including interactive scenarios intended to help you to develop and apply the skills in this chapter. Where material referenced below is available electronically, we're pleased to provide active web links to the source via @ **http://www.oxfordtextbooks.co.uk/orc/coyne/**

References

Arnold, E. & Boggs, K.U. (2003) *Interpersonal Relationships: Professional communication skills for nurses, 4th ed*. USA: Saunders.

Asher, R. (1951) Munchausen's syndrome. *Lancet* **1** (6), 339–341.

British Medical Association (2006) *The law and Ethics of Male Circumcision: Guidance for doctors*. London: BMA.

British Medical Association (2008). *Parental Responsibility: Guidance from the British Medical Association*. London: BMA.

Children and Young Persons Act (1933). Chapter 12. London: HMSO.

Children (Northern Ireland) Order (1995). Belfast: HMSO.

Children (Scotland) Act (1995). London: HMSO.

Commission of the European Communities (2006) *Communication from the Commission: Towards an EU Strategy on the Rights of the Child*. Brussels: Commission of the European Communities.

Commission on Child Abuse (2009) *The Ryan Report*. Dublin: Commission on Child Abuse.

Corby, B. (2006) *Child Abuse: Towards knowledge base, 3rd ed*. Berkshire: Open University Press.

Coyne, I. (1995) Partnership in Care: Parents' views of participation in their hospitalized child's care. *Journal of Clinical Nursing* **4** (2), 71–79.

Coyne, I. (2006) Children's experiences of hospitalization. *Journal of Child Health Care* **10**, 326.

Department for Education and Skills (2004) *Every Child Matters: Change for Children*. Nottingham, UK: HM Government.

Department of Health (1989) Children Act 1989 s3 (5). London: HMSO.

Department of Health (2004a) *National Service Framework for Children, Young People and Maternity Services: Standards for Hospital Services*. London: Department of Health.

Department of Health (2004b) Children Act c31. London: HMSO.

Department of Health (2007) *Delivering Health Services through Sure Start Children's Centres*. London: HMSO.

Department of Health and Children (1999) *Children First: National Guidelines for the protection and welfare of children*. Dublin: The Stationery Office.

Department of Health and Children (2002) *Our Duty to Care: The principles of good practice for the protection of children and young people*. Dublin: The Stationery Office.

Department of Health and Children (2006) *Ensuring the Safety and Welfare of Children/Young People: Child protection policy and code of behaviour for working with children/young people*. Dublin: Office of the Minister for Children.

Farrell, A. (2004) Child protection policy perspectives and reform of Australian legislation. *Child Abuse Review* **13** (4), 234–245.

Ferguson, H. (1997) Protecting children in new times: Child protection and the risk society. *Child and Family Social Work* **2**, 221–234.

Ferguson, H. (2001) Promoting child protection, welfare and healing: The case for developing best practice. *Child and Family Social Work* **6**, 1–12.

Gillick v West Norfolk and Wisbech AHA [1985] 3 All ER 402 (HL).

Gillick v West Norfolk and Wisbech AHA [1986] AC 112 at 113.

Government of Ireland (1991) Child Care Act. Dublin: Oireachtas Stationery Office.

Hall, D.M.B. & Elliman, D. (2003) *Health for all Children, 4th ed*. Oxford: Oxford University Press.

Hattfield, N.T. (2008) *Broadribbs Introductory Pediatric Nursing, 7th ed*. Philadelphia: Lippincott Williams & Wilkins.

HM Government (2006) *Every Child Matters: Working together to safeguard children*. London: The Stationery Office.

Howe, D. (2005) *Child Abuse and Neglect: Attachment, development and interventions*. Hampshire: Palgrave.

Human Fertilisation and Embryology Act (1990) Chapter 37. London: HMSO.

Human Rights Act (1998) Chapter 42. London: HMSO.

Lord Laming (2003) *The Victoria Climbié Inquiry*. London: The Stationery Office.

Lord Laming (2009) *The Protection of Children in England: A progress report*. London: The Stationery Office.

Maguire, S., Mann, M.K., Sibert, J., & Kemp, A. (2005) Can you age bruises accurately in children? A systematic review. *Archives of Disease in Childhood* **90**, 187–189.

Meadow, R. (1977) Munchausen Syndrome by Proxy: The hinterlands of child abuse. *The Lancet* **2**, 343–345.

Morrow, V. (1999) 'It's cool...'cos you can't give us detentions and things. Can you?!' Reflections on research with children. In P. Milner & B. Carolin (eds.) *Time to Listen to Children*. London: Routledge.

National Statistics Online (2008) *The Census in England and Wales 2001*. Available at: **http://www. statistics.gov.uk/census**

Nursing and Midwifery Council (2008) *The Code: Standards of conduct, performance and ethics for nurses and midwives*. London: NMC.

Oates, K. (2007) Can we believe what children tell us? *Journal of Paediatrics and Child Health* **43**, 843–847.

Office of the First Minister and Deputy Prime Minister (2006) *Our Children and Young People—Our Pledge. A ten-year strategy for children and young people in Northern Ireland 2006-2016*. Belfast: Children & Young People's Unit.

Parnell, D. & Day, D. (eds.) (1998) *Munchausen Syndrome by Proxy: Misunderstood Child Abuse*. Thousand Oaks: Sage Publications.

Powell, C. (2007) *Safeguarding Children and Young People: A guide for nurses and midwives*. Maidenhead: Open University Press.

Re 'J' (a minor) (prohibited steps order: circumcision) sub nom Re 'J' (child's religious upbringing and circumcision) and Re 'J' (specific issue orders: Muslim upbringing and circumcision) [2000] 1 FLR 571.

Royal College of Paediatrics and Child Health (2002) *Fabricated or Induced Illness by Carers*. London: RCPCH.

Royal College of Paediatrics and Child Health (2006) *Child Protection Reader: Recognition and response in child protection, 1st ed*. London: RCPCH.

Shannon, G. (2007) *Report of the Special Rapporteur on Child Protection: A report submitted to the Oireachtas*. Dublin: Government Publication Office.

United Nations (1989) *Convention on the Rights of the Child*. Geneva: United Nations.

Volz, A.G. (1995) Nursing interventions in Munchausen Syndrome by Proxy. *Journal of Psychosocial Nursing and Mental Health* **33** (9), 51–58.

Walters, H. (2007) An Introduction to the Child Protection System in the UK. London: NSPCC.

Further reading and URLs

Bristol Royal Infirmary (2001) *The Bristol Royal Infirmary Summary*. Bristol: BRI. Available at: **http:// www.bristol-inquiry.org.uk/final_report/ report/Summary.htm**

British Medical Association (2001) *Consent, Rights and Choices in Health Care for Children and Young People*. London: BMA.

British Medical Association (2004) *Medical Ethics Today: The BMA's handbook of ethics and law*, Chapter 4. London: BMA.

British Medical Association, Health Education Authority, Royal College of General Practitioners, Brook Advisory Centres, Family Planning Association (1993) *Confidentiality and People Under 16*. London: BMA.

Callery, P. & Smith, L. (1991) A study of role negotiation between nurses and the parents of hospitalized children. *Journal of Advanced Nursing* **16**, 772–781.

Casey, A. (1988) A partnership with child and family. *Senior Nurse* **8** (4), 8–9.

Casey, A. (1995) Partnership nursing: influences on involvement of informal carers. *Journal of Advanced Nursing* **22**, 1058–1062.

Department of Health (1994) *Shaping a Healthier Future: A strategy for effective healthcare in the 1990s*. Dublin: The Stationery Office.

Department of Health (1995) *Notification of Suspected Cases of Child Abuse between Health Boards and Gardai*. Dublin: Cahill Publications.

Department of Health (1996a) *Report of the Inquiry into the Operation of Madonna House*. Dublin: Government Publications.

Department of Health (1996b) *Putting Children First: Discussion document on mandatory reporting*. Dublin: Department of Health.

Department of Health (1997) *Putting Children First: Promoting and protecting the rights of children*. Dublin: Department of Health.

Department of Health and Children (2003) *Code of Good Practice: Child protection for the youth work sector*. Dublin: Department of Education and Science.

Department of Health and Children (2008) *Analysis of Submissions made on National Review of Compliance with Children First: National Guidelines for the protection and welfare of children*. Dublin: Office of the Minister for Children and Youth Affairs.

Eminson, D.M. & Postlethwaite, R.J. (1992) Factitious illness: recognition and management. *Archives of Disease in Childhood* **67**, 1510–1516.

European Commission's Communication (2008) *Towards an EU strategy on the Rights of the Child*. Available at: **http://ec.europa.eu/justice_home/fsj/privacy/workinggroup/consultations/index_en.htm**

Gibbons, J., Conroy, S., & Bell, C. (1995) *Operating the Child Protection System: A study of child protection practices in English Local Authorities*. London: HMSO.

Irish Catholic Bishops' Advisory Committee on Child Sexual Abuse by Priests and Religious (1996) *Child Sexual Abuse Framework for a Church Response*. Dublin: Veritas publications.

James, A., Jenks, C., & Prout, A. (1998) *Theorising Childhood*. Cambridge: Polity Press.

James, A. & Prout, A. (2001) *Constructing and Reconstructing Childhood: Contemporary issues in the sociological study of childhood, 2nd ed.* London: Routledge Farmer.

Lowden, J. (2002) Children's rights: a decade of dispute. *Journal of Advanced Nursing* **37** (1), 100–107.

McGuiness, C. (1993) *The Report of the Kilkenny Incest Investigation*. Dublin: Government Publications.

Punch, S. (2002) Research with children: The same or different from research with adults? *Childhood* **9** (3), 321–341.

Scottish Executive (1999) *Protecting Children: A shared responsibility*. Available at: **http://www.scotland.gov.uk/Topics/People/Young-People/children-families/17834/14723**

Turk, L.I., Hanrahan, K.M., & Weber, E.R. (1990) Munchausen Syndrome by Proxy: A nursing overview. *Issues in Comprehensive Paediatric Nursing* **13**, 279–288.

Western Health Board (1996) *Kelly—A Child is Dead: Interim Report of the Joint Committee on the Family*. Dublin: Government Publication Office.

http://www.isa-gov.org.uk/—The Independent Safeguarding Authority (ISA), created to help prevent unsuitable people from working with children and vulnerable adults. They do this by working in partnership with the Criminal Records Bureau (CRB), which gathers relevant information on every person who wants to work or volunteer with vulnerable people.

http://www.dcsf.gov.uk/—UK government department with responsibility for children's services, families, schools, 14–19 education, and the Respect Taskforce.

New guidelines for police, teachers, social workers, and health workers to protect children at risk from sexual exploitation can be found at: **http://www.dcsf.gov.uk/everychildmatters/safeguardingandsocialcare/safeguardingchildren/safeguarding/**

Safeguarding and promoting the welfare of children, including keeping children safe from sexual exploitation, is a key part of the UK Government's drive to improve outcomes for children and young people. In December 2007, the government published its *Children's Plan*, setting out its ambition to make England the best place in the world for children to grow up by 2020. The *Staying Safe: Action Plan*, published in February 2008, set out how the government would deliver a key strand of that ambition, including publishing this guidance.

Part Two

5 Essential skills

MARY NEVIN, JAMES MULKERRINS, AND AMANDA DRIFFIELD

Skills

Introduction

Children present to the health services with a variety of health needs. The Department of Health (DH) National Service Framework (2004) in the United Kingdom (UK) identifies that children with health needs should receive good quality care. Furthermore this care needs to be provided by staff that have adequate preparation to work with children and families (DH, 2004). In order to provide such care, the nursing student needs to develop and acquire the necessary knowledge and skills to gain an understanding and appreciation of the common needs of both family and child on hospitalization. This chapter aims to equip you with the knowledge and background skills to enable you to provide this quality care.

Learning outcomes

After reading this chapter you should be able to:
- Identify and outline the essential skills that are required during the child's admission to hospital.
- Understand the essential clinical observations that are performed upon the child's admission to hospital.
- Develop a further understanding of the basic elements of admission and discharge planning, including the nursing process and care planning.
- Understand the importance of good record keeping during care.
- Identify the means of transmission of infection and the specific precautions and practices that the nursing student can utilize to prevent such transmission.
- Understand the principles of distraction therapy.
- Understand the situations in which restraint may be required.
- Comprehend the principles of **last offices** and the nurse's role in providing bereavement care.

This chapter assists with your understanding of your nursing care by helping you to understand the skills that can be used during the child's admission to hospital. These skills develop with experience and education and enable you to develop a caring, family centred approach that makes the transition from home to hospital and vice versa a smooth one for both family and child. Crucially, the assessment process, in the initial phase, helps to set the scene in your relationship with both child and family and communication skills are vital. At the same time essential physical observations of the child are carried out and documented to support your overall assessment and these will be outlined in this chapter. In addition to the nursing process, a conceptual model of nursing often underpins the assessment process and the planning of the child and family's care. These too will be discussed. A crucial element of care planning is documentation and record keeping, the principles of which will be further outlined.

For a child, the hospital experience is often both strange and unique, and this can make them fearful. Parental anxiety may further compound the child's fear. This chapter will identify how strategies like distraction can be used to reduce the stress and anxiety of both family and child.

This chapter will also identify means of transmission of infection and the specific precautions and practices that the nursing student can utilize to prevent such transmission. Although less frequently observed, it is also essential that you familiarize yourself with skills and information required to perform the respectful last offices when caring for the deceased child.

Prior knowledge

For the first section, which discusses the observations required for the sick child, such as measuring a child's height, weight, and vital signs, you should have prior knowledge of the implications of these procedures and the importance of accuracy. It is essential to have knowledge of the equipment you are using and ensure it is in working order. It is important always to adhere to local policy regarding infection control and documentation. In all interactions with the child and family good communication and listening skills are essential. Reading Chapter Two is particularly important to develop a good understanding of family centred care, which underpins the nursing care provided by nurses to children.

Observation of the sick child

What is clinical observation?

Clinical observation is a process of 'systematic gathering of information about behavioural, physiological and psychological actions and reactions through the use of specific instruments or professional impressions' (Aylott, 2006, p 40). Clinical observations are key to providing appropriate treatment to a child that is sick, whether in the community or hospital setting. These observations assist with early identification of the child at risk of deterioration, and ultimately observation and assessment are fundamental aspects of the children's nurse role (Aylott, 2006). The possibilities for observation are unlimited and include the observation of physical characteristics and non-verbal behaviours, interactions with the child and family, and measurements of vital signs.

Clinical observation involves direct experience and skilled interpretation of the findings. In order to be effective it should be planned, executed, and recorded systematically. However, the active cooperation of the child is not always required; in some cases visual non-obtrusive observation rather than vital sign measurement may be more appropriate. For example, observing respiratory rate together with the general appearance and behaviour of a child may give a more reliable assessment of circulatory status than taking a blood pressure reading in an anxious, crying child who is responding to the intrusive intervention (Aylott, 2006).

Observational information must be interpreted and recorded. For information to be valid and reliable, it is best to combine several approaches to observation in order to fully interpret the findings (Moules and Ramsay, 2008). For example, an accurate assessment of a child's pain should include not only use of a pain score assessment tool, but also observations such as the child's appearance and vital signs measurements. Furthermore, repeating observations a number of times will provide a record and enable the nurse to ascertain baseline measurements and identify changes over a period of time (Aylott, 2006).

The frequency and timing of carrying out clinical observations is another factor that must be considered.

In principle, the frequency should be sufficient to detect possible changes early in order to initiate appropriate interventions. Therefore the frequency may be individual to the child's condition and potential for deterioration (Aylott, 2006). Also, in some clinical settings there are policies that state the frequency at which clinical observations need to be repeated, for example, following operative procedures or blood transfusion. Ensure you are familiar with policies relevant to your environment so that you are informed of the frequency of observations required. Remember:

- Plan your observation.
- Think about the frequency.
- Document your observations.
- Look at the results of all observations – does it mean anything?
- Observations can be informal and not intrusive.

Recording observations

Remember that the validity of clinical observations will depend on how competent and reliable the nurse is at carrying out and interpreting the observations. As a nursing student it will take time to develop your skills of clinical observation. You will find that the ability to interpret clinical observational findings will develop as you progress through your educational programme. One fundamental principle, however, that you can develop from the outset, is accuracy. It is essential that any clinical observation you carry out is measured and recorded accurately. If you are ever unsure, ask your preceptor/mentor to recheck your findings. Finally, when carrying out your clinical observations of the sick child it is vital that any changes in previous recordings or readings outside of the normal ranges are reported immediately to your preceptor/mentor or the medical team. Remember:

- Accuracy is very important.
- If you are unsure, ask a qualified member of staff.

Nursing Alert

Much of the observation and assessment of the sick child can be achieved by looking at and listening to the child. Where intrusive observations are required it is essential that the nurse develops good rapport and uses appropriate communication skills with both the child and the parents/carers.

Key points to consider when observing the sick child

- Plan your observation and collect the necessary equipment.
- Think about the appropriate frequency.
- Remember that observations can be informal and not intrusive.
- Accurately document your observations.
- Interpret observations holistically.
- Report relevant findings to your preceptor/mentor.

We will now move on to the principles of obtaining more specific measurements of height and weight in children.

5.1 **Measurement of height and weight**

Children come in different ages and sizes. A premature baby may weigh only a few hundred grams whilst an obese teenager may weigh many stones! Thus a child's height and weight are important clinical observations. Height and weight in a child are reliable indicators of the growth of the child and his or her general health and well-being. Hence great accuracy is needed in this measurement. **Table 5.1** outlines average height and weight information for children.

In everyday practice the weight of a child is used to calculate drug doses and intravenous fluids. The height and weight measurements are also useful to calculate **body surface area** (BSA). BSA is occasionally used to calculate some drug doses and intravenous (IV) fluids.

A newborn's weight may decrease by 10% below birth weight during the first week of life. Subsequently they enter a period of rapid growth, the most rapid growth occurring during the first year of life. An average birth weight of 3.5 kg would have doubled by five months and trebled to 10 kg by the age of one year. After that time weight increases more slowly until the pubertal growth spurt.

Length is rarely measured at birth. A term newborn baby normally measures about 50 cm at birth. They have a very rapid growth period up until the age of one year, by which time they will have increased their length to

Table 5.1 Average height and weight for children aged 2–10 years

Age	Height	Weight
2	87 cm	12.5 kg
3	96 cm	14.75 kg
4	102 cm	16.5 kg
5	109 cm	18.6 kg
6	116 cm	21 kg
7	122 cm	23 kg
8	128 cm	25 kg
9	133 cm	28 kg
10	138 cm	31 kg

(www.healthforallchildren.co.uk)

about 75 cm. After the age of two years growth slows to a steadier rate and usually averages 3–3.5 kg (7 lb) and 5–7.5 cm (2–3 inches) per year until the pubertal growth spurt at approximately 12 years for girls and 14 years for boys.

Babies and children attending hospital should have their height and weight taken and accurately recorded on an appropriate growth chart or documented in their nursing or medical notes. Children in the community setting should have their measurements recorded in their parent-held records or notes. Equipment should be fit for purpose, therefore the most appropriate for the environment in which you are working. It should be robust and reliable and regularly calibrated to ensure accurate recordings are obtained.

Obtaining weight measurements in children

Children and babies up until the age of two years should have all clothing and nappies removed prior to being weighed. If the child is fully weight-bearing and out of nappies before the age of two years then the same advice can be used as for older children. Children over the age of two years should be asked to remove outdoor clothing and shoes, and any other heavy garment. Digital scales should be used and the weight recorded accurately in the appropriate documentation. It is important at all times to explain the procedure clearly to both child and parent. Although it seems very straightforward and routine within the hospital, to a child and parent this could be an anxiety-provoking event. Preparing them for it will reduce this apprehension.

Measuring height of children under two years of age

When measuring the height of children, supine height is a measurement used for children under two years or for the child who is disabled or immobile. This measurement must be taken on a flat surface with equipment that has a headboard and a footboard. Two people are required in order to make an accurate measurement. One of these people may assist to keep the child's head positioned against the bed headboard with the head facing upwards and positioned in the **Frankfurt plane** position. The second person ensures the child is in an appropriate position, with straight legs and feet at a 90-degree angle to the footboard with toes pointing upwards, and that they lie still. The footboard is the movable part that will allow for the measurement to be taken. Again, explanation and information need to be given before, during, and after the procedure.

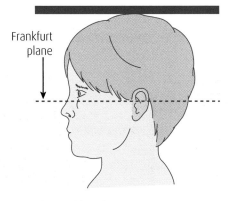

Figure 5.1 The Frankfurt plane position

Measuring height of children who are aged more than two years

Standing height is a suitable way to measure children over the age of two years, or younger once they are able to stand alone. This measurement is taken against

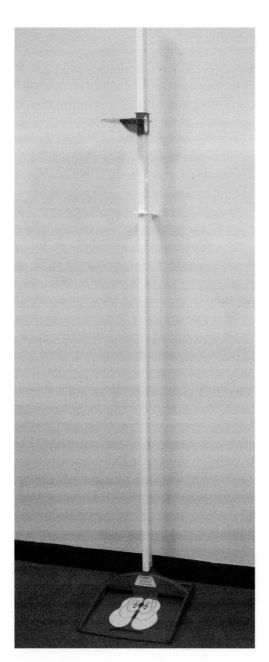

Figure 5.2 Leicester height measure

Box 5.1 How to calculate body mass index

$$\frac{\text{weight (kg)}}{\text{height (m)}^2}$$

(Department of Health, 2005)

a vertical height measure. The child's feet should be together with their heels, buttocks, and shoulder blades touching the vertical measure. The child's head should be positioned in the Frankfurt plane, which is used to ensure correct positioning when measuring height. This measurement can be carried out in the community setting with an appropriate rigid measuring device such as the **Leicester height metre**. Once a child's height has been taken by either of the above methods, the measurement should be plotted onto the growth chart or hand-held parent record, or written in the medical notes. Height and weight measurements are needed to calculate **body mass index** (BMI) (**see Box 5.1**).

Remember:

- Approaches to weight and height measurement vary according to age.
- Equipment needs to be in good working order.
- Use a family centred approach.
- Use good communication skills to inform child and family of what to expect.
- Document your observations accurately.

More commonly used clinical observations that a nurse may assess are known as the 'vital signs' or 'observations'. These relate to measurements commonly performed in hospital situations by nurses, consisting of body temperature, pulse, respiration, and blood pressure monitoring. Although commonly observed, they are far from being routine, as they provide vital information about the condition of the child. These will now be explained.

Assessing and recording vital signs

What are vital signs?

Included in the broader clinical observation and assessment of the health and well-being of the child are a range of physical measurements that may be carried out by the nurse—vital signs. The following measurements are commonly referred to as a child's vital signs: pulse rate, blood pressure, respiratory rate, and body temperature.

Visual observation, listening, palpation, and communication are key skills used when assessing and recording vital signs (Royal College of Nursing (RCN), 2007). Using a family centred approach and enlisting parental cooperation and participation while assessing the child's vital signs are important in order to keep the child as comfortable as possible. Vital sign observation of a frightened or crying child may not always be accurate. Vital sign measurement is a regular feature of nursing both children and adults, and for this reason can be perceived as part of the nursing routine, or indeed ritual. However, these are fundamental measurements in the establishment of reference points prior to procedures such as surgery, so that later alterations can be easily detected. They are also key tools in detecting subtle changes in the child's condition.

It is therefore essential that the principles of each vital sign are understood, and that you as a student are familiar with these underpinning principles and the reason why vital signs are recorded for each individual child. Accuracy in technique, measurement reading, and recording are paramount. During your education programme you will undoubtedly both observe and demonstrate a range of skills under the supervision of a qualified nurse. As you progress through your nursing career you will progress from novice to expert in this regard. It is very important that you always maintain your commitment to this accuracy and ensure that equipment used is of satisfactory quality. Never be tempted to estimate a measurement for recording purposes, as this would be false. As well as providing an inaccurate picture of the child's health, inappropriate recording of false information may be deemed contrary to your code of conduct as a nurse and result in a fitness to practice issue (Endacott and Conway, 2009). If you are unsure, it is always best to consult a qualified member of the nursing staff.

Nurses frequently rely on instruments and equipment, which are essential requirements of monitoring and recording many vital signs. However, visual observation and the nurse's touch are also integral components of the assessment process. One commonly used piece of equipment that you may need is an accurate watch. It is helpful if this displays seconds in time, so that you can accurately count one minute during measurements of pulse or respiration. Many hospitals have good quality clocks displayed that assist this process. Traditionally nurses would have worn a 'fob' watch, pinned to their uniform at the chest, in a position where they could easily view it during observations. This type of watch remains a useful adage for the modern nurse, as it provides a great advantage in permitting you free use of both hands, since one is not tied up acting as a hold for the watch. It is also extremely useful in avoiding cross infection, as the wearing of a wristwatch can become a focal point for germs. Remember:

- Vital signs, while commonly recorded in the hospital setting, are not routine. Each is giving crucial information on each child, and should be approached as such.
- Instruments and equipment support the nurse's assessment. Complete, accurate clinical observation also requires use of visual and other senses.
- Instruments and equipment should be in good working order.
- It is useful to invest in a watch that can be pinned to your uniform.

One vital sign that can give us a wide range of information about the physiological status of the child is the measurement and recording of the pulse.

5.2 **Pulse measurement**

The pulse can be palpated in an area where a large artery lies close to the skin, in particular where the artery passes across the bone. The pulse is felt when the artery is gently compressed against the underlying firm structures such as the bone. The radial, brachial, carotid, femoral, posterior tibial, and dorsalis pedis artery in the ankle are the main peripheral arterial pulses. The pulse of an older child is taken in a similar way to that of an adult, at the radial site at the wrist. In small children and neonates the pulse may be difficult to palpate in this area, so the heart rate is counted by listening over the heart (apex area) on the chest wall using a stethoscope (RCN, 2007).

Whilst counting the pulse, it is important that the child is at rest and you are required to count for one full minute. Ranges of pulse rates can vary from 90 to 160 beats per minute at birth, to 80 to 120 at one to three years of age, reducing to 65 to 100 beats per minute at 11 to 14 years of age (Glasper and Richardson, 2006). In addition to the heart rate you may also make an observation of the rhythm (is it regular or irregular?) and the depth (is it weak and thready or strong and bounding?). These latter observations may be relevant where a child is critically ill. However, it is important to begin to understand the broad range of measures associated with pulse measurement that are useful adjuncts to child assessment and care planning in the clinical environment.

Procedure for taking a child's pulse

Preparation

The child should be resting as a resting pulse is desirable.

Equipment

A watch with a second hand is required.

Consent and communication

Parents may be in attendance and can assist in distracting the child to reduce anxiety while obtaining measurements. Consent should be gained.

5.3 **Measuring respirations**

When assessing the respirations of infants the abdominal movement should be observed as this is where the effort of breathing is observed in this age group. However, in older children chest wall movements can be observed, in a similar way to adults.

This skill involves sitting in a chair or standing beside the child and looking at the rise and fall of either the abdomen or chest wall. The number of times that the child's chest (or abdomen) both rises and falls (one rise and fall is counted as one) is observed and counted for the duration of one minute. Respiratory rates will vary with age. Average respiratory rates for newborns are 30–50 breaths per minute, reducing to 20–40 breaths per minute in early infancy and childhood. In late childhood and adolescence this further reduces to approximately 15–25 per minute

Step-by-step guide to taking a child's pulse

Action	Rationale
1 Locate the site that will be used to obtain the pulse reading. The site may depend on the age of the child (sites are discussed above).	To allow you to carry out the reading.
2 Using the first and second fingertips, press firmly but gently on the site until you feel a pulse (except with the apical pulse where a stethoscope is used).	To palpate the artery.
3 Count the pulse for 60 seconds, noting the rate, rhythm, and depth.	To allow sufficient time in order to obtain the rate, rhythm, and depth.
4 Accurately record the finding in the relevant documentation.	Provides evidence of care and should be recorded as per local policy.
5 Report any abnormalities.	To ensure any problems are identified and acted upon quickly.

(Velasco-Whetsell *et al.*, 2000). Accuracy in monitoring and recording of the respiration rate is crucial.

The pattern and effort of the child's respirations should also be noted by looking and listening for signs of distress, such as grunting, wheezing, nasal flaring, recession, and use of accessory muscles (such as those in the neck). Depending on the condition of the child, specific recording and reporting of these latter signs may be required on an ongoing basis to observe for early signs of deterioration in condition or response to specific treatment.

The importance of such observations cannot be underestimated, as the presence of any of these signs may indicate significant respiratory problems. As an adjunct to the monitoring and recording of the respiratory rate, the child's colour should be noted. In a Caucasian child the skin is expected to have a pink hue. Cyanosis (lack of oxygen to the tissues) often manifests as blue-tinged skin, which needs to be immediately recorded. In black children the mucous membranes (inside the lips) may be observed. Pink indicates a good oxygen supply; blue-tinged may indicate a lack thereof. These observations need immediate reporting and action by the healthcare team. Recording is also essential, and this element of vital sign monitoring will now be discussed. Remember:

- Assessment of respiratory status requires multiple measurements and recordings.

- These measurements require the use of the senses of touch, sight, and hearing.
- Accurate readings and recording are essential.

Procedure: Assessing a child's respirations

Preparation

The child should be resting.

Consent and communication

Parents may be in attendance and can assist in distracting the child to reduce anxiety while obtaining measurements. Consent should be gained.

5.4 **Measuring body temperature**

Body temperature should be recorded in degrees Celsius. The temperature of normal children is between 36.5 and 37.5°C. Temperature can be recorded in different sites (axilla, sublingual, rectal, tympanic) using different

Step-by-step guide to assessing a child's respirations

Action	Rationale
1 Look at the child's chest/abdomen for 60 seconds, counting how many times it rises and falls (Trigg and Mohammed, 2006).	To allow sufficient time to identify the rate per minute.
2 Observe the child's general appearance and colour, and any signs of distress, grunting, wheezing, nasal flaring, recession, and use of accessory muscles.	Any of these signs may indicate respiratory problems.
3 Accurately record the findings in the relevant documentation.	Provides evidence of care and should be recorded as per local policy.
4 Report any abnormalities immediately to your preceptor.	To ensure any problems are identified and acted upon quickly.

devices. Body temperature will vary slightly between different sites in the body and is most often taken in the axilla (armpit) area. Axillary temperatures are accurate in neonates for detecting **pyrexia**. However, axillary temperatures are less accurate in older children. One degree Celsius must be added to the axillary temperature for any child older than a month of age. For safety reasons, oral (mouth) and rectal (rectum) routes should not be routinely used in children up to the age of five years (National Institute for Health and Clinical Excellence (NICE), 2007). In order to accurately take the child's temperature, a thermometer is required. Although frequently used in the past, mercury thermometers are considered hazardous and are not recommended for use. Instead electronic, chemical, or infra-red dot thermometers are recommended to assess children's temperatures and should be left in position for sufficient time to gain an accurate reading. Specific times vary between devices and advice is always sought from the manufacturer's

Table 5.2 Temperature norms in children

Method	Range in degrees Celsius
Oral	36.4–37.4
Tympanic	36.9–37.5
Axillary	35.8–36.6
Rectal	37.0–37.8

guidelines in each case (NICE, 2007; Nursing and Midwifery Council (NMC), 2007b). Normal body temperature ranges for children are displayed in **Table 5.2**.

5.5 **Measuring blood pressure**

The term blood pressure generally applies to the pressure exerted on the walls of the arteries by the blood and is measured in millimetres of mercury (**mmHg**) using a sphygmomanometer. This equipment (which can be either manual or electronic) provides a material cuff that is secured around the child's arm. This fills with air (either automatically or through manual pumping of a fitted balloon) and the pressure is later gradually reduced so that the maximum (systolic) and minimum (diastolic) pressure exerted on the arterial walls by the blood (once restricted and now free flowing) are recorded. This may be either automatically or by listening across the artery for the sound of a heart beat once it begins (systole) and ends (diastole). A child's blood pressure reading varies with age and on average the readings rise as the child gets older. **Table 5.3** outlines the normal ranges of blood pressure in children. More detail and the step-by-step procedure for this skill are provided in Chapter Nine.

In manual readings, listening (auscultation) is done in the same way as with adults (with a stethoscope and cuff) except that a smaller (paediatric) stethoscope and cuff are used. It can be very difficult, however, to obtain an accurate manual (stethoscope and cuff) blood pressure reading in infants and young children as they are often

Table 5.3 Normal ranges for physiological variables in children

Age (years)	Respiratory rate (breaths per minute)	Heart rate (beats per minute)	Systolic blood pressure (mmHg)
<1	30–40	110–160	70–90
1–2	25–35	100–150	80–95
2–5	25–30	95–140	80–100
5–12	20–25	80–120	90–110
>12	15–20	60–100	100–120

not willing to cooperate with the procedure or remain still for a sufficient period of time for measurement to take place. Measuring blood pressure in children can be done in several arterial sites including the radial, brachial, and popliteal arteries. It is important to ensure that the width of the cuff covers two-thirds of the extremity and is long enough to encircle the extremity (NICE, 2007). Too small a cuff will produce a falsely elevated reading.

Nursing Alert

While electronic automated blood pressure recording devices are very useful, particularly with young children and infants, it is important that the nurse is also proficient with a manual sphygmomanometer and stethoscope.

Putting the skills together to complete the clinical observation

The frequency of recording vital signs will be determined by the condition of the child (**see** Figure 5.3) and local

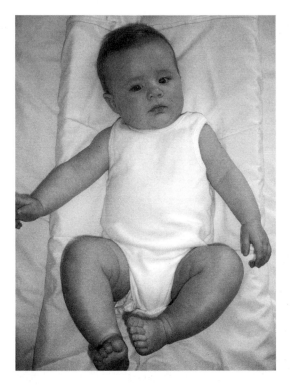

Figure 5.3 Emily is six months old—how would you assess her vital signs?

policy. It is generally advisable to consult with the qualified nurse if you are unsure of the requirements. Vital signs measurements should be accurately and clearly recorded at the time the measurements are taken in the appropriate documentation and in accordance with local policies or guidelines. The record should also include the sites and methods or devices used (RCN, 2007). The relationship between the vital signs and other clinical observations also needs to be taken into account when making a judgement about the child's condition (Leifer, 2007).

One example of this is the relationship between the pulse rate, respiratory rate, body temperature, and blood pressure. Raised readings in some or all of these may indicate infection. It is, however, essential to discuss your observations with a qualified nurse, particularly any change in a child's vital signs from that which was previously recorded. The nurse may explain to you that minor variations are acceptable (you would not expect the pulse rate to be identical each time). More sinister variations may need further action by the nurse, which you may seek to understand by observing the course of a child's care (reading about specific conditions in other chapters in this book will also aid your understanding).

All variations and assumptions will of course be considered in light of the child's overall condition, and not as isolated recordings. In the case of an emergency where, for example, you find that the child's colour is quite blue and they may not be breathing or are unresponsive and no pulse is found, the appropriate emergency call procedure should also be followed according to local policy, which you should familiarize yourself with each time you visit a new placement. It is important as you gain experience in different clinical sites that you familiarize yourself with the emergency response procedures and the position of the relevant equipment that may be used (NMC, 2007b).

Vital signs and measurements of weight and height are frequently observed and recorded upon a child's admission to hospital. This allows the healthcare team to: (a) gain an insight into the child's own normal range; (b) assess for abnormalities related to the child's condition and use these for comparison with future readings, to direct treatment or monitor response to treatment; (c) perform a health assessment related to weight and height and make comparisons with expected targets; (d) accurately prescribe and deliver medication according to the child's weight. Other factors to consider when admitting and discharging children are now discussed.

Patient pathway

When considering the admission to and discharge from hospital process you need to be knowledgeable of local hospital policy relating to admission and discharge procedures. This will ensure that you are able to complete all relevant details and documentation relating to a child's admission and discharge correctly. Other key prior knowledge includes an awareness of the admission and discharge processes and an understanding and working knowledge of national guidelines for record keeping, which will be later discussed. A good understanding of services available for children in the local community area, such as the public health nurse, community children's nurse, health visitor, and school nursing service, is beneficial for discharge.

Admission

The admission to hospital can be associated with a number of fears and anxieties experienced by both the child and family. More recently those involved in healthcare have recognized the need to make the hospital experience for a child much less daunting, through the close inclusion of family in care delivery and the use of distraction and play techniques (you can read about these concepts in more detail in Chapter Two). The admission process will therefore involve the nurse using strategies to ease the child's and family's anxiety. Another central and fundamental nursing task at this point is the observation, measurement, and recording of vital signs, weight, and height (as appropriate to the child's condition) and the collection and recording of specific biographical details related to their age, address, next of kin, past medical history, and medications.

During admission the nurse will need to obtain details relating to names of the child and parents, relevant addresses, telephone numbers, age of the child, and cultural/religious background details. This provides essential information relating to the contact details of parents, next of kin in case of emergency, preferred name of child, and identification of cultural needs of child and family.

A disposable identification band is also applied (to the wrist) and double checked with another nurse for accuracy. This identification band permits easy official identification for the purposes of procedures and medication delivery, rather than relying upon simply calling the child's name on each occasion, which could prove unreliable and thus unsafe. The nurse also establishes the child's previous medical and nursing histories including diseases and illnesses, surgical procedures, allergies, immunizations, and current medications. This information can be obtained from previous nursing notes and will be useful in formulating and providing nursing care.

The nurse establishes, from consulting with both parents and child in a family centred way, the reasons for admission, including events, symptoms, and duration of complaint that occurred prior to admission (Muscari, 2005). The admission procedure includes assessment of the child's health status, establishing everyday activities and how the reason for admission has affected these, and ultimately the requirements needed while in the healthcare setting. An example of this would involve asking about family practices in relation to nutrition, meal times, cultural food practices, problems with feeding, and how the reason for admission has affected these, when reviewing the child's nutritional health status.

The nurse also reviews psychosocial considerations including play activities, hobbies, interests, cultural activities, and schoolwork. The nurse should also observe the child's facial expression, general appearance, posturing, hygiene, and behaviour throughout this process (Price and Gwin, 2008). The admission process also includes a recording of baseline observations (for later comparison) including blood pressure, temperature, pulse, respirations, weight, height, and oxygen saturations. Specimen collection may also be required, such as urine or respiratory secretions, depending on the child's condition. All details relating to the admission process should be recorded using best-established national and local guidelines on record keeping and documentation.

The whole family can be affected by a child's admission to hospital (Shields et al., 2007). Resulting from an increased awareness of this fact, the concept of family centred care addresses the care of children and family in a more holistic and responsive way. Chapter Two provides more detailed information on this approach, which should underpin the admission procedure. One example is that you can aim to provide family centred care by being friendly and welcoming, calm, proficient, and professional during all aspects of nursing care provision. This will help to reduce or even alleviate the child and family's anxiety and develop a trusting relationship between you as a nursing student and the family. The process of admission also involves you as a nursing student in conjunction with the qualified nurse, listening, communicating openly, and conveying the importance of the parents' continued involvement in their child's care, which will also enhance the child's and family's well-being.

It is important that you smile, introduce yourself by name, and give the family the essential information that is required at this time. This will vary from family to family, depending on the circumstances of the child's condition and their individual family needs. However, letting families know that they are welcome to stay with their child while in hospital, and alerting them to facilities that support this, is one very useful support at this time. Ultimately, in addition to the nursing care that the child requires upon admission, it is important that parents' needs are addressed. As key people in the child's life, their well-being affects the child's in-hospital and post-hospital experience.

Meeting parents' needs

Family centred care begins on admission. Meeting parents' needs firstly begins with open communication. Central to this is the creation of a warm, friendly, professional environment upon admission. This immediately creates an environment that is conducive to alleviating the fears and anxieties of both child and family. The physical environment within which the child is nursed is also important and you will notice that the walls of hospitals are adorned with bright children's paintings, and that many toys are available, all making this extraordinary experience a tolerable one for the child. Becoming distracted by these decorations enables quite basic, but essential, elements of admission to begin, almost unnoticed.

It is also essential to use language appropriate to the child's developmental level so as not to appear confusing to a younger child or disrespectful to an adolescent, and also to aim information at the understanding level of the parents. Parents really value it when healthcare providers are able to openly share information, listen to them,

and work with them to meet their needs and those of their child (Mackean, Thurston, & Scott, 2004). However, it is important that this information is tailored according to individual understandings.

Information leaflets are useful in this situation. They support verbal communication by confirming what has already been said, and they are often also available in a range of different languages. Communication, whether verbal or written, is a key skill at this point in the journey of the child and family. It is essential that the nurse always includes and encourages parent questioning and prepares parents and child for any healthcare activities that are undertaken on admission. It is helpful to find out, during assessment, what names both child and family prefer, and to use these consistently, as these too can vary.

The nurse is also required to listen, communicate openly, and encourage and convey the importance of parents' continued involvement in their child's care. These are essential elements of partnership with family and will facilitate a smooth, composed, and unperturbed admission process. The use of these principles will enable a rapport to develop that will alleviate anxieties and gain the trust of both the child and family. The importance of utilizing these skills during a child's admission cannot be undervalued, as it is the continual basis on which all information will be gathered. As you observe nurses in practice you will become increasingly aware of these skills. Remember:

- Introduce yourself and be friendly.
- Find out how parents and child wish to be addressed.
- Try to provide an atmosphere that is calm.
- Ensure you communicate openly, giving simple explanations supported by written material.

Communication about the hospital experience includes not only information about the child's condition and proposed treatment but also practical information aimed at supporting the child and family towards a comfortable hospital experience. It is crucial to communicate the outline of the ward area and hospital to the family and child, so that they know the layout and where essential services are.

As nurses we become so accustomed to hospitals that the importance of these details can be easily underestimated. It is important to explain about parking, regulations about other visitors, dining arrangements, public phones, ward phone numbers, family sleeping arrangements, and the location of the playroom. It is also important for the nurse to identify what activities parents would like to perform during their child's hospital stay (Coyne and Cowley, 2007). Again, written material may be available to support this type of information and this can be useful for consultation by parents, as verbal information can be easily forgotten. Further information about communication with families can be found in Chapter Two.

Nursing Alert

To alleviate children's and families' anxieties and facilitate a calm and efficient admission process, the nurse should obtain information about the child's admission prior to arrival on the ward. The nurse should have all relevant admission documentation, including observation charts, fluid balance charts, and height/weight charts. The bed area should also be prepared to include relevant monitoring equipment and checking of all equipment including oxygen points and suctioning equipment is a mandatory requirement.

Discharge planning

Upon admission it is also useful to begin to plan for discharge. Good discharge planning begins upon admission. That is not to say that you continuously mention going home, but rather that you begin to make practical plans, with the parents, for the specific needs that will arise after the discharge period. During assessment, the children's nurse, family, and child need to identify and consider the services that they may require on discharge home; this will assist with planning and management of these. The early identification of these and initiation of communication between community nurses, health visitors, public health nurses, and other members of the multidisciplinary team will ensure timely and successful discharge. This inclusion and appreciation of the family as a continuous feature within a child's care from assessment to discharge is an essential element of family centred care.

Nursing Alert

Always remember that discharge planning is a very complex process that cannot be arranged hurriedly, and if flawed, a failed discharge may result, and ultimately readmission.

Another element of effective discharge planning is the extent of family and child education. The quality of discharge teaching, particularly the nurse's skills in the delivery of parent teaching, has been found to be associated with increased parental readiness for discharge (Weiss *et al.*, 2008). Weiss *et al.*'s (2008) study of 135 parents of hospitalized children found that good discharge teaching led to less coping difficulty during the first three weeks after discharge. Throughout any day, the nurse is given ample opportunities to educate family and child about their diagnosis and/or skills and procedures that may need to be acquired. Every conversational interaction is an opportunity for teaching (London, 2004). There are formalized teaching times, for example during completion of admission and discharge, and these are essential, but every nurse should be observing for additional patient and family teaching opportunities (London, 2004).

Consider the newly diagnosed diabetic child. Formal teaching on admission may involve teaching about the nature of the disease. Later, when monitoring the blood glucose level of the child, the astute nurse may observe the family's level of interest in the procedure and then reinforce earlier teaching by reiterating the importance of continued monitoring of blood sugars. The absolute importance of patient and family education is highlighted by London (2004), who states that after interventions have ensured a child's recovery, education may be the single most important work that nurses do, as it impacts on the rest of the child's life. Remember:

- Teaching is vital to successful discharge.
- There are many opportune moments for teaching during the hospital experience.

The importance of multidisciplinary team coordination with inclusion of family and child cannot be underestimated when considering discharge planning. Discharge planning involves all members of the in-hospital multidisciplinary team, in addition to supporting teams such as hospital specialties, social services, community specialties, and general practitioners. Best practice indicates that the decision to discharge is best taken following careful multidisciplinary assessment that includes the family (Jaimovich *et al.*, 2004). Jaimovich *et al.* (2004) also identify that while overall responsibility for patient care remains with a named consultant, various local policies can indicate that a named member of staff may take responsibility for organization of discharge, and this responsibility in some areas lies with the nurse.

All members of the multidisciplinary team and family should be aware of who is actually coordinating the discharge. This role will involve the children's nurse arranging the integration of many relevant disciplines in order to discuss and identify the medical, nursing, and social needs of the family and child, both before and after discharge. It is also essential within this process to ensure that documentation and record keeping are included and up to date, both to avoid repetition of tasks and to review progress. This information should be readily available to both staff and family.

Finally, another essential element to successful and effective discharge planning is timely and effective communication. Discharge planning is only as effective as the communication used within the process (Ramsay, 2008). The importance of developing good communication links between multidisciplinary team and family during assessment, when planning discharge, and during education and health promotion activities ensures the timely and effective discharge of child and family. Consideration will now be given to the conceptual frameworks that specifically underpin the delivery of nursing care of the child from admission to discharge, namely conceptual models of nursing and the nursing process.

Nursing Alert

The use of discharge checklists and provision of written discharge guidelines and contact details of the hospital to the family in case of further enquiries and concerns will aid in the process of discharge of a child and family from hospital.

The nursing process and conceptual models of nursing are fundamental tools that supplement the nursing care that is given to the child and family. There are many conceptual models of nursing that may be used as a framework for the assessment, planning, implementation, and evaluation of care given. Within this chapter we discuss the principles of nursing theory and those conceptual models that are more commonly used.

Conceptual models of nursing and the nursing process

The nursing process

The nursing process is a problem-solving framework that enables the nurse to plan care for a patient on an individual basis (Hogston and Simpson, 2002). It is a straightforward model, used easily by nurses across a range of healthcare settings. It helps nurses to apply a more logical and systematic approach to the care that they provide. It is often used in conjunction with conceptual models of nursing, which will be briefly described later. As a qualified nurse you will need to be able to document a comprehensive, systematic, and accurate nursing assessment of the physical, psychological, social, and spiritual needs of patients (DH, 2000). The nursing process comprises four distinct phases that provide for this documentary process (see Box 5.2).

In the first phase, assessment, you need to gain relevant information from many sources such as the patient, relatives, friends, and nursing and medical notes. You need good verbal and non-verbal communication skills, which include listening, and the skills to take baseline observations and record these accurately, as previously discussed. You will also need to develop specific skills in order to observe the child in the way that the aforementioned vital sign assessment and other specific measurements require. However, the assessment is more far reaching than these measurements, or indeed the admission process. Most commonly staff utilize the nursing process in conjunction with a conceptual model of nursing and this guides specific questioning related to the individual's health needs and problems.

Box 5.2 The nursing process

1. Assessment (identification of the child's problems/ nursing diagnosis).
2. Planning of care.
3. Implementation of care.
4. Evaluation of care.

Once assessment information has been identified from relevant sources and observations, this forms the basis of identifying what the child's needs or problems are whilst in your care. It may lead to the formulation of a nursing diagnosis if this is a local requirement. In any case, regardless of particular conceptual model usage or indeed in the absence of one (using simply a nursing process approach), the assessment phase creates sufficient information to create an individualized care plan for the child. If all the relevant information has not been obtained and documented accurately, then the patient may not receive all the care they require.

Following the assessment (and recording of this), specific nursing care is planned. Intended outcomes or goals are identified and these must be realistic and achievable. In keeping with the principles of family centred care, the child and family actively participate in the plan. The plan can be outlined as a series of nursing actions required to resolve problems or address specific needs while in hospital or in the community (Hogston & Simpson, 2002). The plan can be kept close to the child, if appropriate; perhaps in long-term settings this may be supported with the child's drawings or photographs, to personalize it.

Implementation is the action phase. The nurse delivers the nursing care that was identified in the planning stage. With children, the involvement of the family is encouraged to help deliver this care. Most children welcome the involvement of their family members, but it is important to assess this on an individual basis. Communication with both child and family is required at all stages of this process. It is important to carry out planned care and to record implementation accurately.

Evaluation is the final phase of the process, and one that is key. Evaluation is one of the most important stages of the whole process, as it is here that the care you have been giving is monitored to ensure that it has been effective. This is where the process becomes cyclical. If the care has not achieved its goal then the nursing care will need to be reassessed and may have to be altered, whereas if the required outcome has been achieved a positive outcome needs to be documented in the nursing notes.

Completing this final phase of the process can sometimes prove to be a challenge, and it may be difficult to accommodate in practice, say for example during short hospitalizations, such as day surgery. However, it is crucial that the four phases are completed in a timely fashion, and that evaluation of the initial goals and plans takes place. The identification of realistic, measurable, achievable goals in the planning phase assists greatly with this stage. Remember:

- The nursing process has four key phases.
- Nursing care that is underpinned by a process approach may be more systematic.
- Documentation is important.

Conceptual models of nursing

There are many conceptual models of nursing that are used in conjunction with the nursing process. Models are used to provide a framework upon which nurses may assess, plan, and implement patient care. The model directs the thinking of the nurse in relation to how the child or client is viewed in the healthcare situation. The model also directs the nursing interventions, the way these are done, and the way the nurse views their role in the situation. Two are outlined below that you may be familiar with.

Orem's self-care model (Pearson *et al.*, 2005)

This model of care identifies through assessment what care the patient or family can do for themselves. This model of care is based on the premise that individuals are orientated towards self-care, and alterations occur in their ability to perform this care due to their developmental level or medical condition. If they are unable to provide a certain aspect of care due to illness or their developmental level then this is identified as a self-care deficit. This deficit may be provided by someone else such as a nurse or a family member, the manner of which is incorporated into the plan of care. The self-care requisites Orem identifies are listed in **Box 5.3**. Care planning for the child using this model may incorporate assessment of the level of self-care in these key areas and planning for support of the child or the family with regard to facilitating self-care.

Box 5.3 Orem's self-care requisites

- Air
- Water
- Food
- Elimination
- Activity and rest
- Solitude and social interaction
- Hazard prevention
- Promotion of normality

(Orem, 2002)

Roper, Logan, and Tierney activities of living (ALs) model (2000)

The Roper, Logan, and Tierney activities of living (ALs) model (2000) is a model of care that is based upon the notion that each individual carries out 12 essential activities of daily living (ALs). These are: eating and drinking; mobilizing; breathing; eliminating; cleansing and dressing; communication; sexuality; dying; working and playing; sleeping; controlling body temperature; and hygiene. Problems or needs in each of the 12 areas are identified upon assessment, and this assessment is used as the basis for care planning.

The RLT model is widely used in general nursing, although it has received criticism for being overly medically orientated. However, many theorists devising nursing models, and Roper, Logan, and Tierney (2000) in particular, emphasize that their conceptual model is not intended to fit all situations, and that it is very useful to adapt the model for local use.

There are many examples in the published literature of successful adaptations of RLT that are in use in nursing practice. This adaptation process seeks to firstly ascertain staff's views on the philosophy of care, then find a suitable model and adapt it to integrate the staff philosophy. This approach has been used in children's nursing. As a result the RLT model has been successfully adapted for use with children, and incorporates more specific psychological intervention and a greater emphasis on family centred care (Smith, 1995). This latter adaptation is termed the 'Nottingham model', and you may see this used in practice. This retains the essential elements of the original model, including assessment, planning, intervention, and evaluation within the 12 ALs, and planning care on this basis.

Use of conceptual models of nursing care

Conceptual models affect the way that a nurse thinks about and carries out the nursing care that children receive. A conceptual model is often previously agreed within a particular hospital or region, and it is usually implemented using a nursing process approach. Once deficits or problems or needs have been identified and a plan of care put in place, this may be documented and subsequently implemented and evaluated. In addition to these global concepts of nursing and nursing care delivery, those involved in nursing children are also required to examine the evidence base that informs particular areas of practice.

An increasingly important element of nursing process, care planning, and conceptual model use is documentation. Documentation of care provides evidence of care given. This evidence needs to be accurate and complete, and principles of good record keeping apply across the whole spectrum of nursing interventions, not just care planning. All assessments (including the vital signs and other measurements mentioned earlier in the chapter) and all care planned, implemented, and evaluated needs to be clearly documented in the child's notes. Commonly the framework upon which this documentation is based closely relates to a conceptual model of care, or at least to the nursing process. Care pathways are also becoming increasingly common, as multidisciplinary agreed processes for all hospital interventions for specific conditions. Regardless of the form, in today's healthcare environment it is essential that good records are written and maintained appropriately. The principles of this will now be described.

Principles of good record keeping

Prior knowledge

The NMC (2007a) have produced guidelines for records and record keeping in the UK and An Bord Altranais (ABA) (2002) have provided guidelines on keeping and writing nursing notes in the Irish Republic. These guidelines provide practical and essential information that should be adhered to when writing and documenting in nursing practice. A summation of these two documents is provided within this chapter of the book. It is also important that you familiarize yourself with the code of professional conduct for nurses and nursing students (if relevant) that pertain to the country where you are studying.

Good record keeping

Dent (2005) states that keeping good records is 'providing the best for our patients and their families'. A health record contains information recorded by a healthcare professional about the health status of an individual in their care (Data Protection Act, 1998). The quality of that record is a reflection of the quality of the care provided by nurses and midwives to patients/clients (ABA, 2002).

The health record is a prerequisite for effective communication between multidisciplinary team and family and should provide clear evidence of care planned, decisions made, and care delivered (NMC, 2002). The keeping of health records therefore is quite extensive and includes recording of admission and assessment details, plans of care, evaluation of care given, patient condition, and details of discharge planning. National nursing regulatory bodies often provide good guidelines on effective record keeping, such as the NMC (2007) and ABA (2002). However, nursing practitioners must also use their own professional judgement and consider local policy when writing records (McGeehan, 2007).

Nursing Alert

There are times when carrying out nursing care duties and activities that it can be difficult to write down full comprehensive details, so it can be beneficial to note down short key points, times, dates, and actions and ensure that these are then transcribed in an appropriate and logical order as soon as possible after the event.

Below is a simple mnemonic, using the term good records, which you might find helpful to use as a visual or verbal prompt for record keeping. This represents a summation of a number of the main points identified in various guidelines (ABA, 2002; NMC, 2007). It describes the principles of good and effective record keeping:

- **G**ood linguistic style, with avoidance of jargon, abbreviations, irrelevant speculation, witticisms, or derogatory remarks.
- **O**bservable and understandable to the patient and other parties involved in the patient's care.
- **O**wnership of healthcare records is a right of the patient.
- **D**uty to protect confidentiality of healthcare records is a prerequisite of every practising nurse.
- **R**ecord details as soon as possible after an event has occurred.
- **E**xact in terms of being factual and consistent.
- **C**orrect, accurate, clear, legible, and written in such a manner that text cannot be erased.
- **O**bservable and legible following photocopying.
- **R**evision of details including alterations or additions are dated, timed, and signed with original entry remaining clearly readable.
- **D**ated, timed, signed, and in chronological order.
- **S**killed and safe nursing, midwifery, and community health nursing practice includes good record keeping.

Good record keeping is said to aid continuity of care, improve communication between nurses, and help in early detection of patient problems (McGeehan, 2007). The skill of accurate record keeping is fundamental within nursing and is therefore a skill that you, the nursing student, will need to master, but that you may be unfamiliar with initially. To aid your understanding of this process, examine patient records during your next practice placement and consider them in light of the principles of good record keeping. It may also be helpful to practise drafting recordings with your preceptor/mentor and then compare these with the principles of good record keeping. Remember:

- Record keeping is vital.
- You must ensure that you learn and develop the principles of best practice.

A common experience of children in hospital is the need for surgical intervention. This requires meticulous record keeping, as well as the incorporation of many of the other principles and skills addressed throughout this chapter. Although a component of the holistic care of a child and family, this phase of a child's care is often represented as a distinct entity from a teaching and learning perspective. The next section describes fundamental principles related to the care of the child before and after surgical intervention (commonly known as pre and postoperative care).

Table 5.4 Factors that will influence care of the child undergoing a surgical procedure

Elective or emergency surgery	Less time to prepare the child psychologically if they must undergo an emergency procedure.
Day procedures	A shorter stay in hospital means fewer negative effects of hospitalization, although higher parental involvement in care is needed and community care structures should be in place to facilitate this after discharge.
Age of the child	Younger children may experience more separation anxiety and will have shorter attention spans, so information and education is mainly directed at the family. Older children are more able to be involved in their own care and will require more information (Trigg and Mohammed, 2006; O'Conner-von, 2000).

The child undergoing a surgical procedure

Undergoing a surgical procedure, regardless of the age of the child, can evoke feelings of stress and anxiety related to separation from parents, a strange environment, physical harm, and loss of control (Justus *et al.*, 2006). When caring for a child before and after surgery it is crucial to consider the needs of the family too, as they often experience levels of anxiety at this time (O'Conner-von, 2000). Parents who are kept fully informed and feel included in their child's care are less inclined to experience this and can thus better assist staff in caring for their child through the hospitalization and recovery process (Justus *et al.*, 2006; O'Conner-von, 2000). Listed in **Table 5.4** are a number of factors that will have an influence on the pre and postoperative care that a child receives.

5.6 **Preoperative care**

Key components of effective preoperative preparation include not only the physical preparation but also providing adequate information, encouraging expression of concerns, and establishing a trusting relationship with the nurse (O'Conner-von, 2000). Some hospitals offer preadmission programmes, which involve the child and family visiting the theatre area prior to the day of surgery. They can gain familiarity with the environment and this reduces the anxiety associated with hospitalization (Glasper and Richardson, 2006).

Procedure: Preoperative care (see next page)

5.7 **Postoperative care**

There are three main stages in the postoperative period: the immediate phase; the intermediate phase; and the discharge phase. The immediate care following surgery is carried out in the recovery unit, which is situated near the operating theatres. The length of time the child stays here will depend on the type of surgery and the reaction to the anaesthetic. During this time the child is monitored very closely for potential complications associated with the surgery and anaesthetic. Hospitals may or may not permit parents to see the child at this stage. The child is transferred to the ward once staff are satisfied that the child is sufficiently stable and the specific discharge criteria (according to local policy) have been met.

The intermediate postoperative care takes place when the child arrives on the ward. The frequency of observations will depend on the child's general condition and can be increased or decreased accordingly. Close postoperative observation of the child can detect complications such as potential hypoventilation and asphyxia, shock, haemorrhage, nausea and vomiting, urine retention, and wound complications (Moules and Ramsay, 2008).

Step-by-step guide to preoperative care

Action | Rationale

Action	Rationale
1 Complete the appropriate admission procedure and nursing documentation including baseline observations and weight and consult with the medical staff as to any particular investigations that need to be performed.	To ensure the necessary preoperative preparation is complete. Baseline observations will allow for comparison in the postoperative period.
2 The child should be hygienically clean; assist the parents in carrying out this care where necessary. Ensure if a surgical site has been marked that this is still visible. Encourage the child to empty their bladder or put on a clean nappy prior to administering pre-medication.	To reduce the risks of post-operative infections.
3 Ensure pre-medication is given at the correct time as per the prescription.	Adherence to safe drug administration practices and local policies (NMC, 2007b).
4 Check and record whether the child has any loose teeth and inform the anaesthetist.	Loose teeth may become dislodged during intubation.
5 Nail varnish, jewellery, any prostheses, and hearing aids are removed. The latter two can be left until immediately before the child is anaesthetized to avoid excess stress. Jewellery should be returned to the parents or stored as per hospital policy.	Anything that may cause injury or that will make monitoring of the child difficult postoperatively has to be removed. These will be identified in the preoperative checklist.
6 Children may be allowed to wear their own clothes or a suitable theatre gown should be worn (refer to hospital guidelines for appropriate clothing). Babies and neonates lose much of their heat through their head so a cap may be worn. Local policies will dictate what may be appropriate.	Allowing a child to wear their own clothes may reduce fear and anxiety.
7 Ensure and document that the child has been fasting for the required duration. Local policies may dictate fasting times.	To minimize the risk of vomiting.
8 Ensure the child has the correct identification and that all information is clear and legible.	For the easy identification of the child.
9 Check that all documentation to accompany the child is ready, i.e. medical notes, X-rays, laboratory results, signed consent.	So the necessary documentation is available during the surgery.
10 Complete the preoperative checklist immediately prior to departure for theatre as per local policy.	To make a final check that all aspects of the preoperative preparation of the child have been carried out prior to leaving the ward.
11 The child and parents should be accompanied to the theatre reception area. Toys may also be brought.	To help reduce anxiety and distract the child where appropriate.

(Dougherty and Lister, 2008; Glasper and Richardson, 2006)

Accurate assessment of the degree and severity of pain using a pain score assessment tool is vital in order to effectively administer analgesia and control postoperative pain (Glasper and Richardson, 2006). There is a greater risk of respiratory depression in children than in adults so close observation is required if the child has been administered narcotic analgesia. Parents are an integral part of the child's postoperative experience and should be kept fully informed and included in aspects of the postoperative care that they are comfortable participating in.

Finally, the discharge phase (which is discussed in detail in the previous section of this chapter) should begin when the child is admitted to the ward so that when the child is ready to be discharged the necessary support structures are in place. The aim of care is for the child to be discharged home as soon as possible following surgery. This has implications for the family, so any decisions must be made with the cooperation of the parents or carers. Essential information needs to be given at this point, particularly in relation to care of dressings to surgical wounds and suture care and removal (if appropriate), as well as any other specific discharge advice related to the particular condition.

Children in hospital are at risk of developing infections. Those with surgical incisions are obviously at risk. The next section will discuss some of the key points relating to infection control.

5.8 **Infection control**

Prior knowledge

Throughout hospital admission up to the point of discharge, and also within all community settings, the fundamental importance of implementing and adhering to principles of infection control cannot be underestimated. It is essential that nursing students have background knowledge of the principles of microbiology, including how infection is spread and the growth of bacteria, fungi, and viruses. It is also essential that you attain knowledge of local infection control policies relating to such diseases as methicillin-resistant *Staphylococcus aureus* (MRSA), in order to ensure that you practise in accordance with best practice and established guidelines.

The term **healthcare-associated infections** (HCAIs) refers to any infection that is associated with healthcare-associated activities. Infection control involves a range of nursing and medical care delivery systems, methods, and techniques that prevent the transmission and spread of infection during healthcare-associated activities. Between 5% and 10% of patients admitted to hospitals in developing countries acquire healthcare-associated infections, and they are also associated with over 5000 deaths a year in England (World Health Organization, 2006). Posfay-Barbe *et al.* (2008) state that children are at increased risk of HCAI due to immaturity of their immune system and this requires the adoption of infection control measures that are specific to paediatric settings rather than a transposition of adult recommendations. Whether young or old, HCAIs can result in a delayed recovery, loss of income, longer period of hospitalization, and disability.

Chain of infection

The chain of infection provides detail of how infection, including HCAI, spreads, and the rationale for interventions used to prevent the spread of these infections. The chain of infection has several stages (see Figure 5.4). The chain or spread of infection involves an infectious agent, which can be bacteria, fungi, or viruses. The reservoir is the environment where the organism can survive and includes medical equipment, toys, stethoscopes, and the actual hospital environment. The portal of exit is the route where the organism leaves the reservoir, such as secretion of body fluids. The means of transmission is the

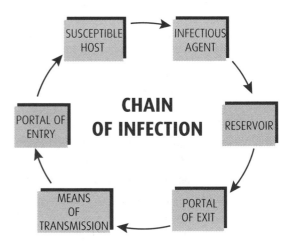

Figure 5.4 Chain of infection

way in which the organism is acquired and includes contact with the hands of healthcare workers and inanimate objects like bedding or toys.

Infection can also be transmitted by airborne pathogens, for example by sneezing and coughing. This is the easiest link to break in the chain and therefore is the key to infection control in the healthcare setting (Damani, 2003). The portal of entry is the entry point of infection and includes the mouth (e.g. chewing on various objects), eye, urethra, and entry points for various devices such as urinary catheters and intravenous devices. The final part of the chain is the susceptible host, a child, who is already at greater risk than most other individuals due to immunity immaturity (Storr & Clayton-Kent, 2004).

Principles of infection control

Breaking the chain of infection and preventing the development of HCAIs is accomplished by partaking in principles of infection control and standard precautions. Pratt *et al.* (2007) outline national evidence-based guidelines including standard precautions for preventing HCAIs in National Health Service hospitals. These standard precautions include performing hand hygiene measures, using **personal protective equipment (PPE)**, safe use and disposal of sharps, and safe handling and disposal of waste, all of which can break the chain of infection. There are also other measures relating to laundry and linen handling, maintenance of a clean environment, aseptic technique, and isolation precautions.

Hand hygiene practices in children's nursing are the same as in other branches of nursing and ought to follow usual local and national recommendations (Posfay-Barbe et al. 2008). During any care activity involving children, pathogens (germs) that can cause HCAIs may come into contact with the hands of nurses or other staff and remain there. These can then be inadvertently transferred to other persons, thus enacting the chain of infection. It is therefore essential to remove these in order to prevent the spread of infection during routine care activities. In the primary or community setting, NICE (2003) guidelines state that hands must be decontaminated immediately before each and every episode of direct patient contact or care and after any

activity or contact that could potentially result in hands becoming contaminated. It is important to know that hand hygiene is the single most important intervention in the prevention of infection (**Strategy for Antimicrobial Resistance in Ireland (SARI)**, 2005; World Health Organization, 2006).

All healthcare staff, including nursing students, must strictly adhere to hand hygiene principles and the nursing student also has a role in educating parents and children on the importance of meticulous hand washing. Hand hygiene can be achieved with soap and water, antimicrobial detergent and water, or alcohol-based hand rub. There are a number of authors who provide guidelines on hand hygiene technique. One excellent overall view of both hand washing (**Box 5.4**) and alcohol hand rub technique (**Box 5.5**)

 Box 5.4 Hand washing technique

PREPARATION

1. Remove hand and wrist jewellery (wedding band allowed). N.B. keep nails short.
2. Wet hands thoroughly under running water.
3. Apply 5 ml of soap/**antiseptic** soap to cupped hand by pressing dispenser with heel of hand (do not use fingertips on the dispenser).

HANDWASHING

4. Wet hands and rub palm to palm five times.
5. Rub right palm over back of left hand up to wrist level five times. Do the same with the other hand (see **Figure 5.5**).
6. With right hand over back of left hand rub fingers five times. Do the same with the other hand.
7. Rub palm on palm with the fingers interlaced.
8. Wash thumbs of each hand separately using a rotating movement.
9. Rub the tips of the fingers against the opposite palm using a circular motion. Also ensure nail beds are washed.
10. Rinse hands thoroughly under running water to remove all traces of soap.
11. Turn off taps using elbows.
12. Dry hands completely using a disposable paper towel.
13. Discard paper towel in waste bin. Open bin using foot pedal only, to avoid contaminating clean hands.

(SARI, 2005)

Box 5.5 Alcohol hand rub technique

1. Remove hand jewellery (wedding band allowed).
2. Apply 3 ml of alcohol and rub into palm of hand.
3. Rub palm to palm to spread alcohol over entire hands and fingers.
4. Rub the back of your left hand with the palm of your right hand. Reverse and repeat action.
5. Open fingers and rub the finger webs. Reverse and repeat action.
6. Rub palm to palm with fingers interlocked.
7. Rub thumb of each hand using a rotating movement.
8. Rub the tips of the fingers against the opposite palm using circular movements.
9. Rub the wrists of both hands.
10. Allow hands to dry completely.

(SARI, 2005)

is outlined in SARI (2005). This identifies all the areas of the hand that need to be considered when performing hand hygiene techniques. **Figure** 5.5 outlines the correct hand washing technique. When applying alcohol hand rub, take off any rings, apply the rub, and follow steps (b) to (f) of **Figure 5.5**, also applying it to your wrists, and leave to dry. You will find colour photos demonstrating how to apply alcohol rub in more detail online at 🌐 **http://www. oxfordtextbooks.co.uk/orc/coyne/**.

Nursing Alert

When performing hand washing, follow an exact procedure as outlined by local and national policies and always remember the areas of the hands that are frequently missed in hand washing, such as nail beds, webs of fingers, and the thumbs.

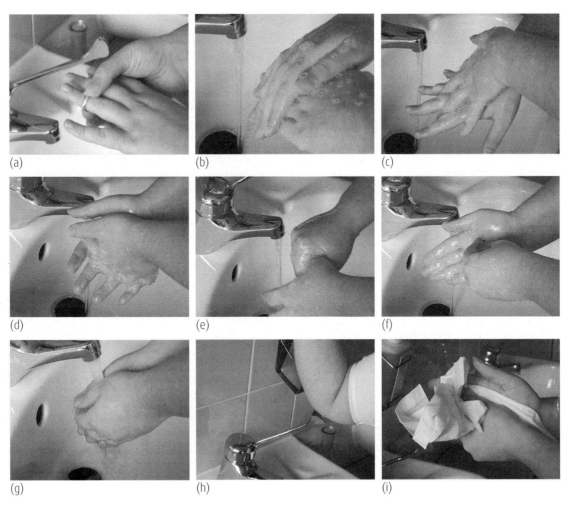

(a) (b) (c)
(d) (e) (f)
(g) (h) (i)

Figure 5.5 Alcohol hand rub technique

Before any nursing activity such as attending to patient hygiene needs, the nursing student will need to assess the need for use of PPE including gloves, aprons, and face and eye protection. All these items aim to protect staff and patients from the risk of exposure to potential pathogens or body fluids. NICE (2003) guidelines on infection control in primary and community settings state that selection of protective equipment should be based on an assessment of the risk of transmission of **micro-organisms** to the patient, and the risk of contamination of the healthcare practitioner's clothing and skin by the patient's blood, body fluids, secretions, or excretions. Gloves are but one example of personal protective equipment and are worn for invasive procedures, contact with sterile sites and non-intact skin or mucous membranes, all activities that have been assessed as carrying a risk of exposure to blood, body fluids, secretions, and excretions, and when handling sharp or contaminated instruments (Pratt *et al.*, 2007).

Plastic aprons are single use items (Dougherty and Lister, 2008) and provide protection for clothing such as nursing uniforms from pathogens or body fluids. It must be noted that gloves are not considered a substitute for hand hygiene and hands must be washed before and after use of gloves (Damani, 2003). If there is a risk of body fluid splashing then facial protection for eyes, nose, and mouth is essential.

Nursing Alert

When you are considering which PPE to use, consider the pathogen and how it is transmitted to aid your decision of what equipment to use. It is imperative that you read and become aware of all local infection control guidelines and procedures in relation to use of PPE. It may also be useful to liaise with the infection control team in relation to use of PPE and if there are any uncertainties relating to specific procedures.

The children's nurse should avoid the use of sharps unless absolutely required; however, when they are used, responsibility for their safe use and disposal lies with the user. Chalmers and Straub (2006) state that where sharps are used, safe handling and disposal includes never re-sheathing a needle and disposing of sharps as soon as possible after use. The importance of proper assembly and storing of sharps containers, away

from vulnerable patients including children, cannot be overstated. In cases of inoculation injury, such as being injured by a needle, the wound should be encouraged to bleed, washed under running water with soap, and covered with a waterproof dressing, and the incident should be reported immediately to relevant parties and dealt with according to local and national policy (Chalmers and Straub, 2006). All types of injuries sustained in relation to work activities need to be reported to the most appropriate persons.

Nursing Alert

Nursing students may be asked to dispose of equipment used during invasive procedures by other healthcare professionals, but you should not dispose of such equipment as you may be unaware of all sharps used.

When dealing with potentially infectious materials such as wound dressings, these should be placed in a clinical waste bag, while household waste such as packaging and children's magazines, which are not contaminated with potentially infectious substances, should be placed in a household bag. When carrying out bed making, the nursing student must place all linen in the linen bag when at the bedside, with contaminated linen placed in a water-soluble bag. When dealing with waste and laundry, it is also essential that the nursing student considers and uses personal protective equipment as appropriate. All hospital environments or equipment are potential reservoirs of HCAIs.

Due to a child's close proximity to and interaction with the environment and equipment including toys, games consoles, and communal areas, they are at particular risk of HCAIs. The children's nurse has a crucial role in seeing that cleaning schedules are adhered to, ensuring systematic decontamination of all equipment including bedside lockers, tables, and toys, and also dealing with any potential environmental contamination. It is therefore vital that you are aware of hospital policy relating to such procedures. This not only promotes best practice but also maintains the appearance of the hospital environment and public confidence in health service provision, which is a cornerstone of healthcare provision. Other measures that break the chain of infection and prevent HCAIs are aseptic technique and isolation procedures.

Nurses have a duty to provide safe and competent care (ABA, 2002; NMC, 2004) and there are usually codes of professional conduct issued by national regulatory bodies that identify these principles. This duty extends to all care practices, including those that prevent the transmission of HCAIs. The NMC (2007b) states that newly registered nurses must maintain effective standard infection control precautions for every client. The children's nurse must therefore always implement standard precautions procedures during healthcare activities in order to provide evidence-based nursing care and also fundamentally abide by the ethical principle of beneficence (doing no harm); thus infection is prevented.

Distraction and restraint

When you visit a children's hospital or operating theatre for the first time you may be struck by the cartoons and other images that may adorn the walls. These additions are a more modern feature of children's nursing where there is a deliberate, planned, often successful attempt to distract children from that which they may find daunting. Distraction is an interesting concept that is frequently used as a technique in other areas of children's nursing and it will be discussed now in more detail.

One issue that is of particular interest to the nurse is the issue of the restraint of children. Understandably, even in the presence of distraction or play techniques (Chapter Two), children will sometimes resist medical or nursing interventions that they perceive to be painful or difficult. This is also age dependent; a very young child may simply not be physically capable of holding their arm straight to have blood taken (venepuncture). Obviously with an older child, the essential skills that have been addressed within this chapter such as good communication, education and explanation to both child and family, in addition to family centred care, are key to creating a situation whereby a child understands the procedure and complies voluntarily. However, where this is not the case, or where the child is too young, the issues of distraction and, less frequently, restraint come into focus. These will now be discussed.

Prior knowledge

Distraction is an important part of children's nursing and can make a child's experience of hospital a much more acceptable one. You need to have prior knowledge of the developmental stages of children so that appropriate toys, books and so on can be used. This is particularly relevant when caring for the child who must undergo a surgical procedure. Important reading can also be found in Chapter Two: Introduction to core principles in children's nursing and Chapter Three: Child development.

5.9 **Distraction**

Distraction or distraction techniques are strategies employed by healthcare professionals to focus a child's attention away from pain or an unpleasant clinical procedure that may need to take place, for example, blood sampling or suturing. The benefits of preparation and diversion therapy as mechanisms of pain control have been well documented (Burgess, 2001). These are usually developed around play and the role of the play specialist is invaluable in developing a trusting relationship with the child (Iles, 2007; Weaver *et al.*, 2007). Play is essential for the normal growth and development of a child and is further discussed in Chapter Two. In the hospital setting play has a different focus and can be used to reduce stress and anxiety (Weaver *et al.*, 2007). There are several different methods that can be used and these are dependent upon the age and cognitive ability of the child. Some examples are included in **Table 5.5**.

If a child is having planned surgery or there is time to plan for a procedure, the child can be assessed by the play specialist and a specific plan of intervention can be designed for that child's needs. If suitably qualified staff and facilities are available many children undergoing clinical procedures in the hospital or community setting can benefit from this. Consent needs to be obtained from the parent/carer or from the child prior to any intervention. Involvement of the family is encouraged but only if it has a positive impact on the process; children can feel the fear from a close relative and this could be detrimental (Weaver *et al.*, 2007).

Good communication skills are essential and telling the truth about the procedure will build a good rapport for the future. As a nursing student there is a role for you in distracting

Table 5.5 Distraction methods

Age	Methods
0–2 years	Touching, stroking, patting, rocking, playing music, using mobiles over the cot.
2–4 years	Puppet play, storytelling, reading books, breathing, blowing bubbles.
4–6 years	Breathing, storytelling, puppet play, talking about favourite places, TV shows, activities.
6–11 years	Music, breathing, counting, eye fixation, thumb squeezing, talking about favourite places, activities, TV shows, humour.

(www.childcancerpain.org)

a child. Simple interventions such as reading stories, using age-appropriate toys, and bubble blowing can help in diverting the child's attention from a clinical procedure. You could also encourage parents to be involved with these.

Some distraction techniques such as guided imagery need to be practised by appropriately trained staff. Parents need to be informed fully about these procedures and medical staff made aware of them. Guided imagery has been described as 'engaging the child's imagination and concentrating on a specific event to modify a particular response' (Doody *et al.*, 1991). Guided imagery has also been likened to hypnotherapy and is therefore only suitable for children of certain cognitive abilities (two years and over). Furthermore, it needs to be tailored to the individual child's needs. Routine use of an intervention could prove less than satisfactory, as it could provoke a reaction in the child due to past fears or allergies. Burgess (2001) suggests, for example, that the visualization of a hot, sunny day in the garden could exacerbate an underlying condition such as an asthma attack.

Key points related to distraction techniques

- Distraction techniques have been proven to reduce pain levels of children undergoing clinical procedures.
- Consent needs to be obtained from the child and family.

- Nurses and parents can participate in distraction techniques.
- More advanced techniques need to be carried out by appropriately trained healthcare professional such as hospital play specialists.
- Children can be offered distraction techniques in both the hospital and community setting as long as appropriately trained staff are present.

5.10 **Restraint in children's nursing**

Restraint or clinical holding can also sometimes have a part to play in the care of a child, although this is used much less frequently in modern nursing. Techniques such as distraction, play, and guided imagery in addition to advances in care and treatment have lessened the requirement for such techniques. Nevertheless there are still some situations where clinical holding may be required in the best interest of the child. This must be done in an informed way based on best practice and there are usually local policy guidelines to support this. You need to ensure you have familiarized yourself with the local policy before involving yourself in this procedure. Inappropriate use of restraint is not recommended and Chapter Four outlines consent and legal/ethical issues concerning such matters. You may find the Royal College of Nursing website useful for further information (**http://www.rcn.org.uk**).

What is restraint?

Restraint is often termed clinical holding, therapeutic holding, or immobilization. It may be defined as 'restricting someone's liberty or preventing them from doing something they want to do' or 'the forcible confinement or control of a subject' (RCN, 2004; Dorland's Medical Dictionary, 2007). It is recognized that there may be occasions when children may need to be held in a safe and controlled manner in order to carry out clinical procedures safely and effectively. This can take the form of physical restraint such as preventing a child from moving for a period of time in order to carry out a clinical procedure.

Procedure: Clinical holding

Considerations when restraining children

The decision to restrain a child is not taken lightly and is dependent upon many factors. It is important to take into account the necessity of the procedure, the child's safety, the type of procedure, the child's level of agitation, the child's age, the parents' opinion, the child's consent, and staff safety (Brenner *et al.*, 2007). These areas can also be influenced by legal and ethical issues surrounding restraint, especially the morality of restraining a child regardless of the urgency or necessity of the procedure (Graham and Hardy, 2004). Holding of the child should be with the minimum force or pressure (RCN, 2003). As healthcare professionals we have a duty of care to our clients, and the more dependent the client both physically and psychologically, the greater the duty to provide care (NMC, 2008). Mindful of this, clinical holding is not the first choice option for children, but may be necessary to carry out an emergency or urgent intervention.

One of the key areas that has been identified in relation to whether a child will need to be restrained is the age of the child. Children who are aged up to five years old are the most likely to need restraining. For children between the ages of five and eleven it is only occasionally used, and rarely in those aged 12 and over (Graham & Hardy, 2004; Brenner *et al.*, 2007). This is due to the increasing cognitive development of the child and their ability to understand reasoning. Children with learning disabilities will need to be assessed on an individual basis regarding this. It is important to consider using a combination of techniques to prevent the need for restraint, such as distraction techniques with the support of a play specialist, local anaesthetic cream prior to the procedure, and discussion and explanation of the procedure.

Parental/Carer involvement in restraint

Rather than performing restraint themselves, it is common now for healthcare professionals to suggest that parents do this task. The parent holding their child for a procedure has an added benefit that support and reassurance can be given. However, not all parents or carers are comfortable with this and may feel unskilled, lack confidence, or be anxious themselves about the procedure (Brenner *et al.*, 2007). Obviously their stance on the matter and their decision must be respected (RCN, 2003). It is vital, regardless of who performs the restraint, to give clear explanation to the parent about the methods that are to be used and gain parental agreement (RCN, 2003). There should be a local policy regarding the use of restraint, so familiarize yourself with the local policy in your health service.

Key points related to restraint

- Consider whether the procedure is necessary or whether an alternative could be used such as distraction or de-escalation techniques. Involve members of the multidisciplinary team such as play therapists.
- Give adequate and appropriate information to the child and parents/carer.
- Obtain consent or assent from the child. For young children or infants this needs to be obtained from the parent/carer.
- Agree with the child and family what is to take place and document this.
- Use minimum pressure/force to restrain or hold the child and examine other potential methods such as wrapping.
- Prepare both child and family and utilize appropriate adjunctive drug therapy, if necessary, such as local anaesthetics, sedation, or analgesia.
- If restraint is required for a child this needs to be documented.

Step-by-step guide to clinical holding

		Action	Rationale
Pre-procedure	1	Give information to child and carer.	To ensure full understanding of procedure and to ensure that informed consent is obtained.
	2	Listen to child and carer's concerns. Answer any questions.	To help reduce anxieties and avoid misconceptions.
	3	Discussion as to presence/involvement of carer.	To ensure parents' and child's wishes are catered for.
	4	Obtain consent.	Legal requirement.
	5	Preparation by play specialist.	To reduce stress and anxiety and prevent future fears of hospitals and procedures.
	6	Application of local anaesthetic cream if needed.	To limit pain.
	7	Agree procedure and process with child and carer and agree a time limit.	To help both child and family feel that they have some control.
Procedure	8	Involve play specialist.	To reduce stress and anxiety and prevent future fears of hospitals and procedures. MDT approach.
	9	Consider distraction techniques appropriate to child's developmental stage. Guided imagery. Play.	Individualized planning of care for each child so the child receives the best possible care.
	10	Hold child still with minimal force enabling procedure to take place. Aim for success at first attempt.	To reduce exposure to unpleasant and stressful situation.
Post-procedure	11	Comfort and reassure child. Debrief carer.	To reduce trauma and stress and prevent fear of future situations.
	12	Document procedure in notes.	Part of documenting child's care. Legal requirement.

Last offices

While it is common for children to become ill and require nursing care, in modern society the death of a child is much less common. This is a sad time for the nurse, other staff in the hospital, and especially the family. It is a time of sensitivity, where the nurse employs a range of skills to support the family through the bereavement. Conceptual model use can provide for effective care planning at this time; however, there are specific skills required by the nurse, to prepare for the performance of specific and essential duties that are required.

Prior knowledge

You should be familiar with local and national policies relating to carrying out last offices on a deceased child. Knowledge of communication strategies and coping skills, not only for the grieving family but for you the student as well, are also important.

5.11 **Skills required for performing last offices**

A last office is a term that describes the care given to someone who has died. In order to effectively perform respectful last offices the nurse requires an understanding of the procedure of how to prepare the child's body and an awareness of cultural preferences. Knowledge regarding current legislation and the ability to support and care for the family in a sensitive manner is also essential (Henderson, 2006).

There are a number of legal and ethical issues that pertain to a range of circumstances associated with the procedure for carrying out the last offices that you may need to be alerted to. You must be familiar with local and national policies relating to situations that will influence when the procedure for last offices is performed. In **Box 5.6** are some examples of situations where the nurse must consult with the medical team.

Cultural and religious needs are of essential importance at this time, and it is vital that the nurse is culturally sensitive to both the child's and family's needs. While all the relevant information may not be personally known by the nurse, using assessment information gleaned earlier in the process and communication with the family the relevant information about the child's culture or faith may be gathered. This helps to understand particular procedures that may need to be performed at last offices and is done with a high level of communication skills and using a family centred approach (Smith *et al.*, 2002). This can also be supported by an evidence-based approach. A range of information and evidence can be elicited to assist the nurse to gain the required level of knowledge. Listed in **Table** 5.6 are a number

Box 5.6 Last offices—special situations where medical team should be consulted

- The death has occurred within 24 hours of a surgical procedure.
- Sudden or unexpected death where the cause is unknown.
- Parents wish to donate the child's organs.
- Child who dies following insertion of radioactive material.
- Child who is brought into hospital already deceased.

Table 5.6 Last offices—information for a range of diverse religions

Buddhism	www.nbo.org.uk
Catholicism	www.catholic.org
Christianity	www.ccj.org.uk
Greek Orthodox	www.goarch.org
Hinduism	www.hinducounciluk.org
Islam	www.mcb.org.uk
Jehovah's Witness	www.watchtower.org/
Judaism	www.bod.org.uk
Presbyterian	www.pcanet.org
Sikhism	www.sikhs.org

of websites that can provide information relating to the last offices procedure for various religions. This list is not exhaustive and there may be subtle changes needed for individual families so close consultation with parents is needed.

Procedure: Last offices

Preparation

The preparation and procedure for last offices is particularly important. The procedure outlined below may be carried out in a number of settings such as the hospital, hospice, or the child's home.

Equipment

Ensure that all equipment for washing the child, mouth care, covering wounds, and removing and disposing of devices is gathered. Discuss with the parents what they would like the child to wear. Documentation according to local policy, such as identification label and notification of death cards, should also be obtained.

> **Nursing Alert**
>
> All infection control principles and local policies regarding safe handling and disposal of equipment must be strictly adhered to when in contact with the deceased child's bodily fluids.

Impact of a child's death on the family

It is important to take cognisance at all times, and at all stages of care, of the impact that the death of a child may have on the family. For a parent who has lost a child, bereavement is a long, complex, and very individual process. Children who have lost a sibling will also grieve; however, a child's perceptions of death will vary according to their stage of cognitive development and their individual experience. It is important that supportive services for bereaved families are in place, not only through the initial period after the child has died, but also long after the death of the child (Woodgate, 2006). There are a wide number of support services and voluntary organizations who offer support to bereaved families who have lost a child. Nurses caring for these families in hospital or

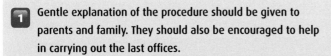

Step-by-step guide to last offices

Action	Rationale
1 Gentle explanation of the procedure should be given to parents and family. They should also be encouraged to help in carrying out the last offices.	The wishes of the family need to be respected and honoured. Participating in the last offices can help to facilitate the grieving process (Woodgate, 2006).
2 All mechanical aids and external devices such as catheters or intravenous cannulae are removed. Remove items as per local policy guidelines. No devices should be removed if post mortem is required.	Any external devices that leak bodily fluids pose a risk to staff in contact with the body.

3 Wounds are redressed. Exuding wound should be covered with a waterproof dressing. Existing dressings are left undisturbed if a post mortem is required.

To prevent leakage that may pose a health hazard to staff.

4 It is optimal to consider straightening the limbs and washing and laying out the body within two hours of death.

Rigor mortis will begin at this stage and handling the body can be difficult once rigor has commenced (Trigg & Mohammed, 2006).

5 Wash and carefully dry the child. Any unusual marks or bruising should be documented.

For hygiene purposes and to record and report any unusual findings. Draws to a conclusion the care given to the child.

6 Clean the child's mouth. The jaw can be supported with a small towel if it will not remain closed. Gently clean and close the eyes. Tape may be needed but only use a type that will not cause trauma to the skin.

A gaping mouth can be very distressing for parents to see and also there is a risk of leakage of bodily fluid.

7 If required a small lock of hair can be cut from the back of the child's head where it will not be seen. Hand/footprints may also be taken.

Parents may wish to keep some mementos of their child.

8 Any jewellery is removed (unless parents wish otherwise) in the presence of two witnesses, accurately documented, and given to the parents.

To meet with parents' wishes and legal requirements.

9 The bed or cot is made up with fresh linen. The child's hair is combed and they are dressed in whatever the parents wish. Cover the child with a sheet. A toy or flowers may be placed with the child where appropriate. Photographs may be taken with parents' consent. Parents may want to hold or cuddle the child at this time and should be allowed plenty of time and encouraged to do so (Glasper & Richardson, 2006). If they are unsure about photographs it can be explained that they can be taken and placed in the medical notes for retrieval later if they wish.

The child should look peaceful in order to provide some comfort for the family.

10 Ensure child has clearly legible identity name band. Generally two are required, on the wrist and ankle.

To ensure correct identification.

11 Ensure all documentation relating to the procedure is completed such as nursing notes and notification of death certificate.

To meet with legal and local policy requirements.

12 Safely dispose of all equipment in accordance with infection control guidelines.

To prevent cross infection.

13 For transfer to the mortuary/funeral home the body should be wrapped in a secure clean white sheet or placed in a body bag where required.

To avoid excess distress for those around and to avoid possible damage during transfer.

Box 5.7 Some helpful tips for nursing students following the death of a child

- Recognize that caring for children and families facing death may be extremely stressful and anxiety provoking for you.
- Do not be afraid to show grief or cry with a family after a child has died; however, do not let this affect your ability to care for the family or make them feel that they must comfort you.
- All staff involved in caring for a child who has died will be affected in different ways because we all have different coping mechanisms. Do not be afraid to speak to your preceptor/mentor about your fears and avail of appropriate staff counselling services (NMC, 2007b).
- Seek appropriate assistance within the health service or college if you have been affected by your experience.

the community setting should ensure that they have the necessary information regarding local support services and voluntary organizations to assist families in their grief. Box 5.7 provides an outline of some helpful tips for nursing students following the death of a child.

Conclusion

This chapter has hopefully provided you with an insight into the knowledge and skills required by a nurse caring for children. We have highlighted the importance of essential skills required to undertake the initial assessment when admitting a child and family to hospital, including the use of the nursing process and some of the nursing models you may encounter during your educational experience.

Discharge planning was also discussed and it was emphasized that good discharge planning starts from the moment the child is admitted. A nurse also has to comply with legal requirements such as record keeping and this important area was discussed. Clinical skills relating to the care of the sick child including vital signs and height and weight measurement and specific care for a child undergoing a surgical procedure were discussed. Within this the area of infection control was highlighted, including the principles and methods of reducing hospital acquired

infections. Distraction and restraint were also discussed, which require planning and negotiation and adherence to local policies and guidelines before commencement.

Bereavement care and last offices were outlined. This is an emotive topic to cover, but an essential area of nursing. As a nursing student you would never be expected to carry out this procedure without the appropriate support, but you need to be aware of local policies and the cultural and religious needs of the family. Further essential care of the child will now be discussed in Chapter Six.

Online resource centre

You may find it helpful to work through our online resources including interactive scenarios intended to help you to develop and apply the skills in this chapter.

Where material referenced below is available electronically, we're pleased to provide active web links to the source via 🕲 **http://www.oxfordtextbooks.co.uk/ orc/coyne/**

References

An Bord Altranais (2002) *Recording Clinical Practice: Guidance to Nurses and Midwives*. Dublin: An Bord Altranais.

Aylott, M. (2006) Developing rigour in observation of the sick child: Part 1. *Paediatric Nursing* **18** (8), 38–44.

Brenner, M., Parahoo, K., & Taggart, L. (2007) Restraint in children's nursing: Addressing the distress. *Journal of Children's and Young People's Nursing* **1** (4), 159–162.

Burgess, C.A. (2001) Complementary therapies: Guided imagery and infant massage. *Paediatric Nursing*, **13** (6), 37–41.

Chalmers, C. and Straub, M. (2006) Standard principles for preventing and controlling infection. *Nursing Standard* **20** (23), 57–65.

Coyne, I. & Cowley, S. (2007) Challenging the philosophy of partnership with parents: A grounded theory study. *International Journal of Nursing Studies* **44**, 893–904.

Damani, N. (2003) *Manual of Infection Control Procedures, 2nd* ed. London: Greenwich Medical Media.

Data Protection Act (1998) Available at: **http:// www.opsi.gov.uk/acts/acts1998/ ukpga_19980029_en_1**

Dent, K. (2005) Record keeping—just for the fun of it? *Paediatric Nursing* **17** (1), 18–20.

Department of Health (2000) *National Health Service Plan*. London: Stationery Office.

Department of Health (2004) *The National Service Framework for Children, Young People and Maternity Services*. London: Department of Health.

Department of Health (2005) *The National Child Measurement Programme*. London: Department of Health.

Doody, S.B., Smith, C. & Webb, J. (1991) Non-pharmacological intervention for pain management. *Critical Care Nursing Clinics of North America* **3** (1), 69–75.

Dorland's Medical Dictionary for Health Consumers (2007) Philadelphia: Saunders.

Dougherty, L. & Lister, S. (2008) *The Royal Marsden Hospital Manual of Clinical Nursing Procedures. Student Edition, 7th ed.* Oxford: The Royal Marsden Hospital NHS Trust Foundation: Blackwell Publishing.

Endacott, R. & Conway, N. (2009) The patient pathway. In: R. Endacott, P. Jevon, & S. Cooper, S. (eds.) *Clinical Nursing Skills: Core and Advanced*. Oxford: Oxford University Press.

Glasper, A. & Richardson, J. (2006) *A Textbook of Children's and Young People's Nursing*. London: Elsevier.

Graham, P. & Hardy, M. (2004) The immobilisation and restraint of paediatric patients during plain film radiographic examinations. *Radiography* **10**, 23–31.

Henderson, N. (2006) Communicating with families about post-mortems: Practice guidance. *Paediatric Nursing* **18** (1), 38–40.

Hogston, R. & Simpson, P.M. (2002) *Foundations of Nursing Practice. Making the difference, 2nd ed.* Hampshire: Palgrave Macmillan.

Iles, P. (2007) *Oxford Handbook of Children's and Young People's Nursing*. Chapter Two. Oxford: Oxford University Press.

Jaimovich, A.D., Committee on Hospital Care, & Section on Critical Care (2004) Admission and Discharge Guidelines for the Pediatric Patient Requiring Intermediate Care, *Pediatrics*, **113** (5), 1430–1433.

Justus, R., Wilson, J., Walther, V., Wyles, D., Rode, D., & Lim-Sulit, N. (2006) Preparing children and

families for surgery: Mount Sinai's multidisciplinary perspective. *Paediatric Nursing* **32** (1), 35–42.

Leifer, G. (2007) *Introduction to Maternity and Pediatric Nursing, 5th ed.* Canada: Elsevier.

London, F. (2004) How to prepare families for discharge in the limited time available. *Paediatric Nursing* **30** (3), 212–214.

MacKean, G.L., Thurston, W.E., & Scott, C.M. (2005) Bridging the divide between families and health professionals' perspectives on family-centered care. *Health Expectations* **8** (1), 74–85.

McGeehan, R. (2007) Best practice in record keeping. *Nursing Standard*, **21** (170), 51–55.

Moules, T. & Ramsey, J. (2008) *The Textbook of Children's and Young People's Nursing*. Oxford: Blackwell Publishing.

Muscari, M. (2005) *Pediatric Nursing*. Philadephia: Lippincott Williams and Wilkins.

National Institute for Clinical Excellence (2003) *Infection Control: Prevention of healthcare-associated infection in primary and community care*. London: Oaktree Press.

National Institute for Health and Clinical Excellence (2007) *Feverish Illness in Children. NICE Guideline 47*. Available at: **http://www.nice.org.uk/CG47**

Nursing and Midwifery Council (2002) *Code of Professional Conduct*. London: NMC.

Nursing and Midwifery Council (2004) *Code of Professional Conduct: Standards for conduct, performance and ethics*. London: NMC.

Nursing and Midwifery Council (2007a) *Guidelines for Records and Record Keeping*. London: NMC.

Nursing and Midwifery Council (2007b) *Essential Skills Clusters*. Available at: **http://www.nmc-uk. org/aDisplayDocument.aspx?documentID=3192**

Nursing and Midwifery Council (2008) *The Code*. London: NMC.

O'Conner-von, S. (2000) Preparing children for surgery—an integrative research review. *Association of Operating Room Nurses* **71** (2), 334–343.

Pearson, A., Vaughan, B., & Fitzgerald, M. (1998) *Nursing Models for Practice, 2nd ed.* Oxford: Butterworth-Heinemann.

Posfay-Barbe, K., Zerr, D., & Pittet, D. (2008) Infection control in paediatrics. *The Lancet* **8**, 19–31.

Pratt, R.J., Pellowea, C.M., Wilson, J.A., *et al.* (2007) Epic 2: National evidence-based guidelines for preventing healthcare-associated infections in NHS hospitals in England. *Journal of Hospital Infection* **65S**, S1–S64.

Price, D.L. & Gwin, J.F. (2008) *Pediatric Nursing: An introductory text. 10th ed.* USA: Saunders Elsevier.

Ramsay, J. (2008) Discharge planning. In T. Moules & J. Ramsay. *The Textbook of Children's and Young People's Nursing*. Oxford: Blackwell Publishing.

Roper, N., Logan, W., & Tierney, A. (2000) *The Roper-Logan-Tierney Model of Nursing: Based on activities of living*. Edinburgh: Churchill Livingstone.

Royal College of Nursing (2003) *Restraining, Holding Still and Containing Children and Young People. Guidance for nursing staff*. London: RCN.

Royal College of Nursing (2004) *Restraint Revisited—Rights, Risks and Responsibility. Guidance for nursing staff*. London: RCN.

Royal College of Nursing (2007) *Standards for assessing, measuring and monitoring vital signs in infants, children and young people*. Available at: **http://www.rcn.ork.uk/development/publications**

Shields, L., Pratt, J., Davis, L., & Hunter, J. (2007) Family-centred care for children in hospital. *Cochrane Database of Systematic Reviews*, Issue 1. Art. No.: CD004811. DOI: 10.1002/14651858. CD004811.pub2.

Smith, F. (1995) *Children's Nursing in Practice: The Nottingham Model*. Oxford: Blackwell Science.

Smith, L., Coleman, V., & Bradshaw, M. (2002) *Family-centred Care: Concept, theory and practice*. Hampshire: Palgrave.

Storr, J. & Clayton-Kent, S. (2004) Hand hygiene. *Nursing Standard* **18** (40), 45–51.

Strategy for Antimicrobial Resistance in Ireland (2005) *Guidelines for Hand Hygiene in Irish Health Care Settings*. Dublin: Health Protection Surveillance Centre.

Trigg, E. & Mohammed, T.A. (2006) *Practices in Children's Nursing. Guidelines for hospital and community, 2nd ed.* London: Elsevier.

Velasco-Whetsell, M., Coffin, D.A., Lizardo, L.M., *et al.* (2000) *Pediatric Nursing*. London: McGraw-Hill.

Weaver, K., Battrick, C., & Glasper, E.A. (2007) Developing a hospital play guideline and protocol for sick children with debilitating fears. *Journal of Children's and Young People's Nursing* **1** (3), 143–149. Available at: **http://eprints.soton.ac.uk/48720/**

Weiss, M., Johnson, N.L., Malin, S., Jerofke, T., Lang, C., & Sherburne, E. (2008) Readiness for discharge in parents of hospitalized children. *Journal of Pediatric Nursing* **23** (4), 282–295.

Woodgate, R.L. (2006) Living in a world without closure: Reality for parents who have experienced the death of a child. *Journal of Palliative Care* **22** (2), 75–82.

World Health Organization (2006) *The WHO Guidelines on Hand Hygiene in Healthcare (Advanced Draft)*. Switzerland: World Health Organization Press.

Further reading and URLs

Callaghan, C. (2007) Infection control in the neonatal intensive care unit. *Nursing Standard* **22** (1), 35–41.

Cooper, J. & Barnett, M. (2005) Aspects of caring for dying patients which cause anxiety to first year nursing students. *International Journal of Palliative Nursing* **11** (8), 423–430.

Hall, D. & Elliman, D. (2000) *Health for all children, 4th ed.* Oxford: Oxford University Press.

Ho Cheung, W.L. & Lopez, V. (2006) Assessing children's emotional responses to surgery: A multi dimensional approach. *Journal of Advanced Nursing* **53** (5), 543–550.

Kelsey, J. & McEwing, G. (2006) Physical growth and development in children. In: E.A. Glasper & J. Richardson. *A Textbook of Children's and Young People's Nursing*. London: Churchill Livingstone.

Nursing and Midwifery Council (2006) *Registrant/client Relationships and the Prevention of Abuse*. London: NMC.

For information on infection control and hand hygiene:

http://www.who.int/patientsafety/ information_centre/ghhad_download_link/ en/ http://www.who.int/patientsafety/ information_centre/Last_April_versionHH_ Guidelines%5b3%5d.pdf

http://www.cdc.gov/mmwr/PDF/rr/rr5116. pdf

http://www.nice.org.uk/nicemedia/pdf/ CG2fullguidelineinfectioncontrol.pdf

http://www.nmc-uk.org/aDisplayDocument. aspx?documentID=3192

Further reading in relation to infection control procedures can also be found in: Dougherty, L. & Lister, S. (2008)

The Royal Marsden Hospital Manual of Clinical Nursing Procedures. Student edition, 7th ed. Oxford: The Royal Marsden Hospital NHS Trust Foundation: Blackwell Publishing.

Advice sheets on record keeping can be found at:

http://www.nmc-uk.org/aFrameDisplay. aspx?DocumentID=4008&Keyword=

For information on grief relating to families who have lost a child visit: **http://www.healingheart.net**

http://www.healthforallchildren.co.uk

http://www.childcancerpain.org

http://www.nahps.org.uk

http://www.rcn.org.uk

http://www.childgrowthfoundation.org

http://www.nursingtheory.net

Essential care

6

DENISE JONAS, YVONNE MULDOWNEY, ISOBEL BYRNE, AND HILARY SOUTHERN

Skills

Introduction

This chapter examines the principal skills of assessment and management of pain and wounds. It provides information on the assessment of a child's skin and the management of eye and ear care, skin care, and mouth care. It also provides information on mobility and the moving and handling care of children. The care discussed is applicable to a variety of nursing settings such as the hospital or in the community and family participation and cultural needs are incorporated in keeping with the philosophy of family centred care (Chapter Two).

Learning outcomes

It is anticipated that you will be able to do the following after you have read and studied this chapter:
- Discuss the importance of pain assessment to the child's overall pain management.

- Understand different pain relief medications used to manage pain in children.
- Identify the factors affecting wound healing and discuss assessment of a wound.
- Develop an awareness of the importance of cleaning eyes and ears in children.
- Understand the general principles of maintaining mouth care in the child.
- Appreciate differences in the child's care and needs at different developmental stages.
- Be aware of general principles of maintaining skin care for the child, including: relating anatomy and physiology of skin to skin care; carrying out an assessment of child and skin; and ensuring child safety and dignity.
- Develop a greater understanding of parent participation and cultural needs of the child in skin care.
- Understand the principles of moving and handling, describing the carrying and supporting of infants and children.

You can review your knowledge in some of these areas using the online resource feature that accompanies this book.

Pain assessment and management

Pain assessment is an essential first step in the relief of pain. It forms a major part of overall pain management and provides a foundation on which future care is based.

Prior knowledge

Prior to considering pain assessment for the child you should be familiar with the related anatomy and physiology of the child's condition, an outline of which you should find in a chapter of this book. Revision of your core textbook in anatomy and physiology would also be useful. Other information that would be helpful as prior knowledge when reading this chapter is: communication skills used with children (Chapter Two); child development and behaviour (Chapter Three); assessing and measuring vital signs and record keeping (Chapter Five); and drug administration (Chapter Seven).

Pain in children

A commonly used definition of pain is provided by the International Association for the Study of Pain (IASP, 2007), who refer to seminal works on the topic and define pain as:

> *'...an unpleasant sensory and emotional experience arising from actual or potential tissue damage or described in terms of such damage'.*

McCaffrey & Beebe, on the other hand, considered pain to be whatever the experiencing person says it is, existing whenever they say it does (McCaffrey & Beebe, 1994).

Young children communicate their pain using a number of different behaviours and verbal prompts but for whatever reason may deny that they have pain. Children may say that they have no pain because they fear that saying yes may lead to something unpleasant happening. This may simply be the health professional moving the child or administering medicine.

Nursing Alert

Unrelieved pain can lead to long-term physical and psychological problems including anorexia, delayed wound healing, poor mobilization, social withdrawal, and developmental delay (Franck, 2003). Infants undergoing surgery without adequate **analgesia** can produce a pain memory, which may result in an exaggerated response to pain later in childhood (Howard, 2003).

Pain assessment

Pain assessment in children should consider child behaviours, the child's stage of development, their age, physiological indicators (for example their heart rate), and their

social background. All these factors influence the way an individual child may present their pain. For example, for social or cultural reasons the child may not verbally demonstrate pain, but their heart rate may be increased as a result. Similarly an older child will be able to give specific answers regarding pain site and severity upon direct questioning, whereas a baby will not. Thus the interpretation of various elements is required, and can present a challenge. Ultimately good pain assessment requires knowledge of child development and age-related behaviour, a summary of which you will find in Chapter Three.

Pain assessment tools

A variety of pain assessment tools are available to help you obtain a greater understanding of the pain the child is experiencing and document the pain (Royal College of Nursing, 2001). There are over 30 published pain assessment tools for use in children; however, as pain is such a complex multidimensional experience there is currently no agreement on which tool is the best (Franck, 2003). Infants and children with neurological impairment are especially vulnerable to poor pain assessment (Carter *et al.*, 2002).

Nursing Alert

The assessment tool that is used should be appropriate to the child's age, development, and level of understanding as there is no one assessment tool that applies to all children. Pain assessment tools that allow you to assess a variety of behaviours and physiological signs are most effective in children who cannot yet speak or those with cognitive impairment.

Carter *et al.* (2002), suggest that pain assessment is complicated and difficult, especially when assessing pain in children, and that using a pain assessment tool can assist with this assessment. For children who can talk a verbal questioning tool may be more appropriate (Franck, 2003). Some available tools within these two categories are as follows.

Behavioural tools

Self-report pain measurement tools are used when children can speak; however, for a number of children behaviour is a useful measure by which they let us know about their pain. There are specific distress behaviours such as crying, facial grimaces, or body posture, which have been associated with pain in young children. These behaviours have been put into pain scales to help with the assessment of pain when self-report is difficult. To assess a child's behaviours for pain you would stand and observe them from a short distance and use the cues written on the pain tool to help you decide what the child's level of pain is. The higher the score, the more likely the infant or child is in pain.

Examples of behavioural assessment tools containing cues are as follows.

FLACC pain assessment

The Faces, Legs, Activity, Cry, and Consolability (FLACC) pain assessment scale (Merkel *et al.*, 1997; Willis *et al.*, 2003) is based on a mnemonic of five behavioural categories. The health professional assesses the child's behaviours by examining these five factors:

1 Facial expression.
2 Leg movement.
3 Activity.
4 Cry.
5 Consolability.

Each category receives a score of zero, one, or two. Based on this assessment the maximum score that can be reached is ten and this indicates severe pain.

CRIES Pain Scale

The CRIES Pain Scale (Krechel & Bildner, 1995) is another behavioural tool used in neonates and infants that incorporates the assessment and integration of information about oxygen saturation, vital signs, and sleep. This tool also consists of five categories associated with the mnemonic title:

1 Cries.
2 Requires increased oxygen saturation.
3 Increased vital signs.
4 Expression.
5 Sleepiness.

Following assessment in each category, the child's pain is given a score between zero and two. Thus the maximum score that can be reached is ten, again indicative of severe pain.

The Liverpool Infant Distress Scale

The Liverpool Infant Distress Scale (LIDS) (Horgan *et al.*, 2002) is a behavioural assessment tool for infants following surgery and consists of eight categories:

1 Facial expression.
2 Sleep pattern.
3 Cry quantity.
4 Cry quality.
5 Spontaneous movement.
6 Spontaneous excitability.
7 Flexion of fingers and toes.
8 Tone.

Assessment within each category requires a score from zero to five. The higher the score the more pain the baby has. This is a very detailed scoring system, which may take time to undertake on a regular basis, but the cues can help you to identify pain in an infant.

The Paediatric Pain Profile

The Paediatric Pain Profile (PPP) (Institute of Child Health, University College, & Royal College of Nursing Institute, 2003) is a 20-item behaviour rating scale for assessing pain in children with cognitive impairments. The initial record is created by parents and provides the health professional with a number of behavioural cues applicable to the individual child. Parents have a great deal of expertise with their child and can often understand their behaviours more accurately than nursing staff, therefore they have a valuable contribution to make towards the assessment of their child's pain and should be involved wherever possible (Simons *et al.*, 2001).

Nursing Alert

Pain causes a physiological response, which leads to a rise in heart rate and blood pressure. Observing these vital signs on their own should not be used routinely for pain assessment as heart rate and blood pressure may be raised by other means. However, they form a useful contributory diagnostic to the assessments listed above.

Self-report tools for children over the age of four years

Self-report pain tools are classed as the gold standard of pain assessment; this means that they are the preferred choice when considering pain assessment, and so they are used in older children from four years upwards (Franck, 2003). Examples are as follows.

Faces scale

The Faces scale (Wong *et al.*, 2001) consists of a series of six cartoon-type faces that express a range of emotions from happy to sad. The Faces scale is explained to the child by telling them that the happy face means no pain at all whilst the sad/distressed face means the worst pain ever. The child then points to the face that best describes how much pain they are feeling.

Visual analogue or number scales

These visual analogue scales consist of a ladder or straight line ranging from zero up to five or ten. The child associates higher levels of pain with a higher score.

The Oucher scale

The Oucher scale uses a series of photographs (Beyer *et al.*, 1990). Again, for this tool the child chooses the face that corresponds with their pain level.

The Adolescent Pediatric Pain Tool

Franck *et al.* (2002) undertook a study assessing pain in children using the Adolescent Pediatric Pain Tool (APPT). This tool consists of three parts:

1 A body outline chart.
2 A visual analogue scale with five pain intensity words along the scale.
3 A list of words describing pain quality.

In children and young people suffering from sickle cell pain this provided a good mechanism to describe their pain and a more objective method in assessing if their pain medication was effective or not (Franck *et al.*, 2002).

There are other innovative methods of pain assessment described in the literature such as using a 'temporary tattoo' of the Faces scale on children's arms. This approach has been used in studies and while parents and children liked the method, the results did not reveal that this was any more effective than using a chart with the Faces scale on (Franck *et al.*, 2007).

Both behavioural and self-reporting tools can help the child, parent, and health professional to make an accurate pain assessment. However, Carter *et al.*

(2002) suggest that the best evidence for evaluating pain comes from the child themselves and nurses should take every opportunity to talk to the child about their pain.

Documentation of pain

The area where you are working should have specific pain tools in use for pain assessment. It is important to always assess the child's pain on admission using the appropriate pain tool and to obtain a history of past painful experiences. You can then document what pain management has been used previously, what worked, and what didn't work. Write down the words the child uses for pain (translations for the Faces scale are available (Wong, 2000)) or what behavioural signs the child uses to indicate they have pain. This will provide other nurses caring for the child with a good prompt for pain recognition.

Once pain has been assessed, a pain management plan can be made. It is important to ensure that the child's pain is reassessed frequently (this may be decided according to the child's condition) to check if the pain medication or other techniques are working. Write this information in the child's notes or care plan. Simons and Moseley (2009) found that nurses were more likely to document pain scores alongside vital signs when they used a single chart rather than multiple forms.

Nursing Alert

Standardized charts that incorporate pain assessment alongside other assessments (such as temperature and pulse) are particularly useful to prompt nurses to document pain.

Pain management and pharmacology

The use of pain medication has been referred to, and this is commonly known as analgesia. This term describes a range of medicinal preparations available to treat pain. **Acute pain** is usually managed using more than one preparation to maximize the effects of the analgesia (Lönnqvist & Morton, 2005). The choice of analgesia in children depends on the child's age, severity of the pain, type of pain, and the availability of the pain medication and must take into account any underlying disease.

The World Health Organization analgesia ladder can easily be adapted for acute pain management (WHO, 2008) and gives a guide to what medication should be used according to the type of pain.

> **Nursing Alert**
>
> All analgesic drugs are calculated according to the child's weight; however, care must be taken in infants as they are at increased risk of side effects due to accumulation in their bodies of some pain medications.

Simple analgesia

Paracetamol, **local anaesthetics**, and non-steroidal anti-inflammatory drugs (**NSAIDs**) are simple analgesia, considered as the first step in pain relief as they help reduce the need for stronger, morphine-based preparations (**opioids**) (Williams, 2006). These medications will now be briefly explained. Further understanding of these may be gleaned by consulting a pharmacological textbook.

Paracetamol (acetaminophen) is a commonly used analgesic, which is available for oral, intravenous, or rectal use. Intravenous paracetamol provides immediate and effective pain relief. Paracetamol has very few side effects and this means it is a suitable analgesic for most children, but lower doses will be needed in children with renal and liver impairment.

Non-steroidal anti-inflammatory drugs (NSAIDs) are another group of medicinal preparations given to children. Examples of these are ibuprofen or diclofenac. These drugs block the formation of a pain transmitter called prostaglandin, thus reducing pain and inflammation.

There is not enough research available in children regarding use of NSAIDs and bone healing but most orthopaedic surgeons avoid their use in limb-lengthening procedures (Association of Paediatric Anaesthetists of Great Britain and Ireland, 2008).

Local anaesthetic preparations

Local anaesthetics can also be used. For example, topical local anaesthetic creams such as Emla (eutectic mixture of lidocaine and prilocaine) or Ametop (tetracaine) can be

> **Nursing Alert**
>
> - NSAIDs should be avoided in children under three months old and in those with coagulation disorders, renal dysfunction, liver impairment, dehydration, or history of stomach ulcer. Children with unstable asthma should also avoid NSAIDs as they can increase allergic responses.
>
> - Aspirin is classed as a NSAID but is not recommended routinely in children under 16 years as there is a risk of developing a rare disorder known as Reye's syndrome (Harrop, 2007).

used and certainly should be considered before the taking of blood (venepuncture). Local anaesthetic injections can also be given by the anaesthetist to localized areas in the body; these are commonly known as 'blocks' and they provide excellent pain relief for a number of hours, for example after surgery, thus reducing the need for stronger morphine-based preparations.

> **Nursing Alert**
>
> These 'blocks' can cause considerable numbness of the area. If a child is sent home the same day, parents must be given written and oral discharge advice about when the child can be up and about again and also about care of the specific area if necessary.

Local anaesthetic infusions can also be given spinally, in the epidural space or along a specific nerve such as the sciatic or femoral nerve. These are specialist techniques that require close observation and monitoring in the ward area. Many hospitals have acute pain services, so seek advice from these specialist teams.

Opioids

Another group of medications is known as opioids. These include codeine and morphine, which act directly on the pain centres in the brain and spinal cord to reduce pain transmission. Codeine is more effective when combined with paracetamol (Moore *et al.*, 2003); however, recent evidence suggests that its use as a pain medication in infants and children is limited due to a variation in metabolism (Williams *et al.*, 2001, Williams *et al.*, 2002).

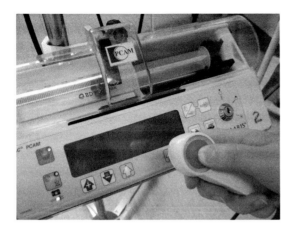

Figure 6.1 PCA machine

Morphine may be given orally, rectally, intravenously, or by means of patient controlled analgesia (PCA). Pain is always subjective and therefore difficult for others to control, so PCA uses a device that can be programmed to deliver a set amount of strong pain medication such as morphine when the child needs it by the child pressing a button on the machine. A programmed 'lockout' period prevents the child from receiving excess amounts of morphine.

PCA is usually recommended in children from age eight years upwards. The child needs to be able to understand that if they feel pain they need to press a button to activate the machine and give themselves a dose of pain relief. This means that the child manages to control their pain and does not have to wait for the nurse to give them medication. This also provides the child with an element of control over their pain and can reduce anxiety.

Nursing Alert

It is important that the child is the only one who presses the PCA device as this reduces the development of respiratory depression or excessive sedation.

Continuous infusions or nurse controlled analgesia (NCA) provide a steady rate of pain relief; they are useful for children following major surgery or during sickle cell crisis. Intramuscular (IM) analgesia should be avoided in children as it is painful and the uptake into the muscle can be variable. Intranasal diamorphine is useful for immediate pain relief prior to procedures or for fractures. A very

small amount of diamorphine is squirted up the child's nostril through a small tube. The drug is quickly absorbed into the blood supply of the nose and provides strong pain relief without the need to give the child an injection or insert a cannula. Studies have compared the use of intranasal diamorphine with intravenous morphine and found that it was more effective in relieving the child's acute pain and distress (Kendall *et al.*, 2001).

Nursing Alert

Side effects of opioids include increased sedation, respiratory depression, nausea and vomiting, confusion or hallucinations, reduction in gastric motility leading to constipation, itching, urine retention, and occasional muscle spasm. Therefore all infants and children receiving opioids must be monitored according to local guidelines

Other pain medications

Some other drugs are used for procedural pain. Nitrous oxide and oxygen (Entonox) is an inhaled gas and the child breathes the gas using a mask or mouthpiece. It works within a few breaths and is very effective for brief painful episodes (Jonas, 2008). This could be used in the Accident and Emergency Department, for example, for short-term use in painful procedures, or on the ward for changing a wound dressing.

Sucrose is sometimes used prior to painful procedures in infants up to three months (Association of Paediatric Anaesthetists of Great Britain and Ireland, 2008). The sweet solution is put onto the infant's tongue or in the cheek and the infant is encouraged to suck using a dummy; this activates the body's natural endorphins and provides short-term pain relief (Stevens *et al.*, 2004).

Chronic/cancer pain

The principles of pain assessment remain the same in children with cancer pain or those receiving palliative care; however, the management of treatments may be more complex as each child will have medication prescribed on an individual basis. Increased doses of opioids and use of sedation may be required (Hockenberry-Eaton *et al.*, 1999). Tricyclic antidepressants or anticonvulsants such as gabapentin tend to be used in children with neuropathic pain commonly associated with **chronic pain** conditions or cancer pain; this is a more complex area of pain management, which usually requires advice and support from a specialist pain service.

Non-pharmacological measures

Use of alternative methods of managing pain are also common in childcare, such as massage, distraction, and guided imagery, and provide a useful addition to pain relief medicines. These techniques do not remove pain but dull the pain perception, making it easier for the child to cope. A further discussion of distraction techniques is provided in Chapter Five.

Pain relief at home

Day surgery procedures are increasingly common and it is important that guidelines are in place for ensuring that parents receive adequate written and verbal information on how to manage their child's pain in the home (Jonas, 2003). Enough analgesia, appropriate to the type of operation, must be given or prescribed upon discharge to allow parents to give regular pain relief. Parents should be given contact numbers so they know whom to contact should problems arise. Further discussion of the central role of the family in children's care and essential components of this are discussed in Chapter Two.

Key learning points to be gleaned from this discussion are:

- Regular use of an agreed, appropriate pain assessment tool for managing pain assessment in children is needed. This assessment needs to be repeated regularly and used to effectively monitor and manage the child's pain and pain relief.
- Pain needs to be treated promptly where appropriate with suitable analgesia.
- Assessment, evaluation, and medication delivery need careful documentation and local policies and guidelines need to be adhered to at all times, but especially when administering pain relief.
- When undertaking wound dressings, remember that if pain has been poorly managed before then any future dressing changes may be difficult to manage and thus distressing to the child. Wound assessment and management will now be more fully explored.

Wound assessment and management

Prior to undertaking wound care for the child you should be familiar with communication skills and child play and distraction (Chapter Two); consent (Chapter Four); principles of infection control (Chapter Five); and the integumentary system (Chapter Fifteen).

Most wounds in healthy children heal quickly requiring little intervention; however, chronic wounds can be more complex and challenging.

Nursing Alert

If the wound is complex then advice should always be secured from the child's doctor or the tissue viability specialist within the organization.

Common wounds

The following are common wounds that children present with:

- Dog bites, cuts, burns/scalds.
- Accidental or non-accidental injuries.
- Nappy dermatitis.
- Surgical wounds.
- Congenital abnormalities, e.g. **epidermolysis bullosa**.
- Skin stripping caused by adhesive tape removal.
- Extravasation injuries.
- Pressure related—e.g. saturation probes left in same place for too long.
- Pressure sores in children who are immobile for significant periods or children in casts or splints (Chapter Fifteen) or 'shearing' injuries caused by the child being inappropriately moved up the bed.

Wound healing

Wounds in children follow the same healing process as in adults but are as individual as children themselves; therefore care must be planned according to their individual needs. There are four phases to wound healing: inflammation, regeneration, epithelialisation, and maturation (Johnstone *et al.*, 2005). Each of these phases overlaps and with chronic wounds the phases may move backwards and forwards between the stages of healing. The phases of wound healing can be affected by many different factors (Enoch, 2006).

The inflammation phase is a cellular process that prepares the wound for healing by removing dead or foreign cells. Clotting factors and platelets are activated and form a clot to stop bleeding. White blood cells also invade the area to protect against infection. At this stage redness and swelling are due to increased blood flow and may not be a sign of infection. Any pain is usually due to pressure on the nerve endings from increased fluid and swelling.

During the regeneration phase **fibroblast** activity leads to formation of new tissue that strengthens the wound. Tissue at this stage is called granulation tissue and is usually red or pink in colour. The fibroblasts contract and pull the wound together. Collagen strands produced by fibroblasts help rebuild the wound.

The epithelialisation phase involves the movements of cells across the surface of the wound, making it look paler. This process can be delayed if there is necrotic or sloughy tissue present. During the maturation phase the wound gains strength as the collagen grows. This stage can be impaired by poor nutrition, which slows down the healing process. Maturation can take many months.

In primary healing the wound edges are brought together and may be secured using sutures (stitches) or special glue preparations. Healing is usually rapid with minimal tissue loss and granulation is hidden. In secondary healing there is damage to the epithelium tissues, for example, in the case of burn injuries. Granulation here is visible as part of the healing process, and a fuller discussion of this process is provided in Chapter Fifteen. There are ranges of factors that affect wound healing such as poor nutritional status, lack of sleep and rest, pain, anxiety, pressure, foreign bodies, or infection. Diseases such as diabetes or anaemia can cause impaired perfusion and decreased oxygenation.

> **Nursing Alert**
>
> Children with poor immune systems such as children with cancer may have a tendency for their wounds to take longer to heal.

Assessment of a wound

Wound assessment provides a measurement of how good the treatment is and evaluates the rate of healing. Wound assessment also provides information to others involved in the child's care.

> **Nursing Alert**
>
> ■ If possible the wound should be assessed by the same health professional at each dressing change; this ensures consistency and can avoid unnecessary changes in treatment.
>
> ■ Be aware that some wound dressings contain animal-derived products that may conflict with the child's cultural needs.

In the UK, assessment of competence in wound assessment, dressing, and asepsis is undertaken within nursing training as a basic component of infection prevention and control. This fulfils the requirements laid down by the Nursing and Midwifery Council (NMC) essential skills clusters (NMC, 2008).

When assessing a wound ensure that you consider previous wound care treatment.

- Assess the cause, location, type, and size of wound.
- Use disposable measuring guides, drawings, or photographs.
- Examine the wound bed; check for granulating, infected, sloughy, or necrotic tissue.
- Document the amount and consistency of any **exudate** and presence of any odour.
- Examine the surrounding skin for swelling, bleeding, or dryness.
- Ensure that the patient has been assessed for signs of pain or existing infection.
- Also consider the child's nutritional status, their weight for their age, and their current mobility.
- You will need to take into account the child's current diagnosis and any medication they are taking.

Preparing to undertake a dressing change

When undertaking a change of dressing, firstly prepare the child and family by providing information on what you are about to do and how long the dressing will take.

This helps reduce anxiety and increases cooperation (see the discussion in Chapter Two on family centred care). Ensure parents are active participants in the dressing if they choose to be.

> **Nursing Alert**
>
> It is important to explain to parents what to expect from the wound that they will see, especially if it is for the first time. They could be very distressed by the sight of the wound, particularly if the wound is a result of an injury, where feelings of guilt and shock can overwhelm the parent.

Ideally the dressing should be performed by two health professionals, one to support the child and the other to undertake the dressing. However, depending on the type of dressing the parent may be adequately prepared to support their child. It is also important to prepare all equipment beforehand and away from the sight of the child as this minimizes delay, reduces anxiety and limits wound exposure.

Pain relief

Most wounds are painful and therefore analgesia should be given before the dressing takes place. Timing of the dressing is important to ensure analgesia has reached its maximum effect. If sucrose is being used this should be given five minutes before the dressing. Entonox should be breathed for one to two minutes before the dressing begins. Most oral analgesia takes approximately 90 minutes to be effective, and this must be taken into consideration in the plan of care. If a distraction technique is to be used, these need to be age appropriate and take into account the length of time the dressing will take. Many children can only sustain distraction techniques for short periods, not for long time spells. It may be necessary to provide little breaks for the child, in the form of negotiated episodes of 'time out', if the dressing is lengthy (see Chapter Five with regard to distraction techniques).

Reducing infection

If the child is in hospital, ideally the dressing should take place away from the child's bed to protect their personal space.

- Ensure doors and windows are closed and fans switched off to reduce airborne contamination.
- Close curtains or lock the door to maintain privacy and dignity.
- Ensure that the child is positioned comfortably and covered, but that there is easy access to the wound.
- Check that the dressing package is intact and check the expiry date. Ensure that all instructions on wound products are followed.
- Always wash your hands (National Patient Safety Agency, 2008).

> **Nursing Alert**
>
> The dressing should be undertaken using an aseptic non-touch technique (ANTT).

The aim is to minimize the introduction of infection into the wound. ANTT is used in many organizations and the procedure can be modified for use in the community (Randle & Clarke, 2007). The overriding principle of ANTT is that the wound should not come into contact with any item that is not sterile.

Removal of dressing

When removing the dressing it is essential to explain clearly to the child and parent what you are doing, and reinforce this throughout the whole dressing procedure. This education is particularly important if parents are to continue the dressing care in the home themselves. Firstly you remove the soiled dressing using gloves, taking care to address the child's needs.

> **Nursing Alert**
>
> Many children report that the removal of the old dressing is the most painful part of the dressing process.

It is important to follow the manufacturer's guidelines for removal of specialist dressings to avoid damaging new tissue. Depending on the age of the child and the position of the dressing, most children like to assist with removal of the top layer of the dressing. If a transparent dressing has been used, remove by stretching parallel with the skin. If the dressing has adhered to the child's skin then use warm saline to loosen the dressing.

Assessing the wound

Upon each dressing change it is important to observe the outside of the dressing for any exudates (weeping of fluid). This dressing is then removed and put into a clinical waste bag. You then make a thorough assessment of the wound to determine what cleaning method or final dressing is to be used. It is essential to examine for early signs of wound infection such as redness, heat, swelling, pus, black tissue, excessive exudates, or presence of an offensive odour. The child may also have a raised temperature, supporting suspicions of infection.

If a wound is considered infected, a sample of the wound exudates is retrieved and sent to the laboratory to detect infecting organisms. This is known as a wound swab, and special sterile implements are available for use in this task. They include a cotton-tipped swab that is contained within a sheath or capsule. The swap is undertaken before wound cleaning by gently rotating the cotton-tipped swab across an area of the wound.

Cleaning the wound

Cleansing a wound is dependent upon the size, site, and type of wound and the type of exudates. A clean, granulating wound does not need cleaning (Watret & McFarlane, 2004). Clean the wound using warm saline or sterile water depending on hospital policy.

Nursing Alert

- Routine use of antiseptics and disinfectants are not recommended (Taquino, 2000; Blunt, 2001).

- Do not rub the wound as this can increase tissue damage. Do not use cotton wool as the fibres can easily adhere to the wound.

The procedure is to clean the wound from top to bottom, or from the inside to the outside, by using a single stroke with each piece of moistened gauze. Ensure that the same process is followed when drying the wound.

Putting on a new dressing

The choice of new dressing is based on many factors; however, it should be safe and effective for the intended child but trauma free on removal and application. Also, the dressing should provide high humidity and thermal insulation, remove exudates, and not allow bacteria to enter (Casey, 2001). It is better to use a high performance dressing that requires fewer changes, especially in the community setting. A wound with exudates may need more than one dressing to absorb the bodily fluid and a wound near the perineum will need an impermeable dressing to avoid contamination by faeces or urine (Benbow, 2008).

Nursing Alert

Always use sterile scissors to modify dressings.

Securing the dressing

Securing the wound will depend on the age of the child and the position of the wound. Use tape, clear film, or stretch gauze netting. Use a full hand bandage for infants with finger/hand injuries to prevent them 'sucking off' the bandage (Mölnlycke Health Care, 2004).

Documentation

It is important to record the dressing change in the child's notes or care plan, ensuring that any changes in the wound are documented. This is especially important in chronic wounds to ensure evidence of a decision making trail and prevent repeating of past errors (Casey, 2001) (see Chapter Five for more information on record keeping).

Key learning points from these discussions are:

- Assess skin integrity on the child's admission to identify children at risk.
- Allow time for analgesia to reach its optimum effect.
- Follow manufacturers' instructions on all wound care products.
- Always observe child and wound for early signs of infection.

Eye and ear care

Prior to considering eye and ear care for the child you should be familiar with the anatomy and physiology of the ear and recording temperature using a tympanic thermometer. Other chapters in this book that may be helpful are: Chapter Two (communication skills and play); Chapter Three (child development and behaviour); Chapter Four (record keeping); and Chapter Seven (administering eye and ear drops).

6.1 Eye care

Generally eyes are kept moist naturally by blinking and the production of tears, thus eye care may only involve cleaning the skin around the eye area (Furze & Pearson, 2006). The majority of children should be encouraged to do this for themselves; however, some may need assistance. Some children may experience dry, sore, or infected eyes that require additional nursing interventions including eye swabbing, eye irrigation, or the instillation of prescribed eye drops/ointment to ease discomfort and/or treat infection. Eye care also includes the care of artificial eyes and the care of contact lenses. Others who require eye care include the unconscious child and children after surgery.

'Sticky' eyes are a common complaint among newborn babies and infants because their lacrimal drainage systems are immature at this stage (Ulyatt, 2007). The frequency of performing eye care is based on each individual child's needs and circumstances and should be assessed accordingly (Ulyatt, 2007). The use of a strict sterile (aseptic) technique is suggested only for use in certain circumstances; an example of this is where there may be damage to the eye after ophthalmic surgery (Dougherty & Lister, 2008). The nurse must be aware that on occasion children of any age, including infants, may harbour infectious organisms in their eyes, so infection control policies and/or guidelines should be adhered to.

It may be necessary to demonstrate the eye care procedure in a form of play, as a means of explanation as to what the procedure entails and to gain the child's cooperation (see Chapter Two). The nurse may need to consider frequent shorter periods of eye care intervention for the sick child, to lessen distress and aid recovery. In some cases the child themselves or the parent may carry out the procedure. It must be remembered that the eye is a very sensitive organ, which may be easily damaged. Therefore, gentle intervention is always required to ensure that it does not cause unnecessary discomfort or damage to the eye (Furze & Pearson, 2006).

> **Nursing Alert**
>
> Some eye conditions are more treatable if they are identified early (Health Service Executive, 2005). This highlights the importance of early detection and prompt treatment of eye conditions, thus maintaining optimum eye care.

Procedure: Eye care

Preparation

Babies/infants may be swaddled in a blanket and positioned with either the head or back supported, in either a sitting or lying position (Mallett & Bailey, 2004). Swaddling promotes a feeling of comfort and a sense of security, and restricting movement aids the procedure.

Equipment

Gather the necessary equipment before beginning eye care:
- Prescribed medication.
- Sterile cotton wool/gauze.
- Sterile water.
- Basic dressing pack.
- Alcohol hand rub.
- Gloves (if indicated).

(Mallett & Bailey, 2004)

Assessment

Before you begin find out if the patient is required to take eye drops or ointment. If so, read the doctor's prescription and manufacturer's instructions carefully before you begin the procedure.

Eye care

Step-by-step guide to eye care

Procedure	Rationale
1 Wash hands (see Chapter 5). Put on disposable gloves (or sterile gloves if required).	To minimize the risk of cross infection. (Ulyatt, 2007; Dougherty & Lister, 2008).
2 Open the dressing pack and prepare the equipment required. Dip the cotton wool/gauze into the sterile water and gently wipe the closed eye lid from the inner aspect of the eye to the outer. Discard the cotton wool/gauze as per hospital guidelines and repeat as necessary. It is essential that a new cotton wool/gauze piece is used each time (Mallett & Bailey, 2004).	To clean the eye and minimize the risk of cross infection.
3 Wash hands and repeat the procedure on the other eye (Mallett & Bailey, 2004).	To minimize the risk of cross infection.
4 If eye drops/ointment are required please refer to the doctor's prescription and manufacturer's instructions and carry out the correct procedure—refer to clinical skills policies/guidelines.	To ensure optimum healing of the eye (Ulyatt, 2007; Dougherty & Lister, 2008).

Consent and communication

Explain the procedure to the patient (Mallett & Bailey, 2004), demonstrating through play, for example on a doll, if necessary. This will alleviate the patient's anxieties, and will enable you to gain the consent and cooperation of the patient (Ulyatt, 2007; Dougherty & Lister, 2008).

Key learning points are: know your limitations; work within your scope of practice; and never attempt to undertake a task for which you have not yet received training (Furze & Pearson, 2006).

Ear care

Ear care, although generally minimal, should be encouraged as part of a child's daily personal hygiene routine.

The two main functions of the ear are hearing and balance (Waugh & Grant, 2007). **Cerumen** (wax) produced in the ear canal is usually honey-coloured and darkens in colour as it is exposed to air, and small amounts are visible at the entrance to the ear canal (Furze & Pearson,

> **Nursing Alert**
>
> The use of cotton buds to clean the inner ear should be discouraged as anything inserted into the ear may cause damage or pain (Furze & Pearson, 2006).
>
> Nurses must remember this when using tympanic thermometers, as they too can inflict pain and cause damage to the ear.

2006). Although some wax is normal, discreet observation by the nurse/parent is essential to ensure that there is not a build-up of wax in the child's ears, which may lead to discomfort or attribute to loss of hearing (Dougherty & Lister, 2008). Observe for any signs of pain or discomfort and listen to the child, as they may complain of earache. A young child may become irritable if they experience earache, rubbing the affected ear to gain relief (Furze & Pearson, 2006). Other signs that indicate earache are that the infant/child may be crying, there may be redness on the cheek on the affected side, or there may be elevation of temperature.

Occasionally signs of teething may mask the signs of earache. Therefore vigilance is required not to misdiagnose; the doctor should be contacted if the infant/child appears unwell or has a high temperature (Wilson, 2007). On occasion children may push items into their ears, and the removal of these foreign bodies and/or syringing of the ears should only be performed by experienced/trained staff (Furze & Pearson, 2006). Patients with pierced ears may also experience problems and should be observed for signs of infection at the points of entry of the earring with the skin (Mallett & Bailey, 2004). If there are signs of inflammation or oozing, inform the patient and report your findings to the nurse-in-charge and/or doctor (Furze & Pearson, 2006).

It is vital that prompt action is taken to alleviate pain and discomfort, as earache can cause the patient excruciating pain, which increases anxiety, so vigilance and prompt action by the nurse is essential (Furze & Pearson, 2006). If analgesia and/or ear medication is required, refer to the doctor's prescription and manufacturer's instructions.

The following are ear problems commonly experienced by children: deafness, otitis media, foreign bodies, wax or glue ear, perforated ear drum, conditions requiring surgical intervention (Furze & Pearson, 2006, p 201).

Nursing Alert

The nurse must also be alert for signs of otorrhoea (discharge) or bleeding from the ears. A clear discharge may be indicative of cerebral spinal fluid (CSF) leakage, which may indicate a more serious condition, for example, a head injury; this patient needs urgent attention (Furze & Pearson, 2006; Dougherty & Lister, 2008). If a child is prone to ear problems try to keep children's ears dry when washing their hair, showering, or swimming, and do not spray anything into the ears (Williams, 2007).

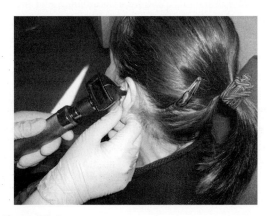

Figure 6.2 Ear exam

All newborns should have a neonatal hearing screening test and further hearing screening at developmental check-ups and periodically throughout their school years (Health Service Executive, 2005). A child communicates from birth, so any concerns regarding a child's hearing ability or their speech and language development should be reported as soon as possible. A prompt referral should be made to the speech and language therapist.

Nursing Alert

It is vital that if it is suspected that a child has a hearing problem or speech defect that this is investigated (Health Service Executive, 2005)

Key learning points from these discussions are:
- Carry out the correct procedure according to the clinical skills handbook or procedure manual.
- Remember to work within your scope of practice and do not undertake a task for which you have not yet received training (Furze & Pearson, 2006).

Skin care

Skin care is the actual act of cleaning the body to ensure that the skin, hair, and nails are kept in optimum condition (Dougherty & Lister, 2008). The principles of providing good skin care for the child are important basic caring needs and the primary mechanism for reducing transmission of infectious agents.

Prior knowledge

Prior to attending to skin care for the child you should be familiar with: the anatomy and physiology of the skin; normal childhood skin development; common skin diseases; and recognizing skin abnormalities and mechanisms of skin repair (Chapter Fifteen). Other chapters that may provide useful reading for this section are Chapter Two (principles of maintaining child safely, children's play, and communicating with children).

Skin anatomy and physiology

The anatomy and physiology of the skin, including skin functions, should be reviewed in order to gain a deeper understanding of their influence on health (Chapter Fifteen).

Preventing infection

One of the skin's functions is to prevent the introduction of micro-organisms to the body. The outer layer of the epidermis acting as a barrier to micro-organisms achieves this. If the skin is not kept clean and moist, micro-organisms build up and the skin becomes dry and broken. This results in the protective barrier breaking down, allowing the entrance of micro-organisms that can lead to infection. It is thus necessary to keep the skin clean and moist in order to maintain this function of the skin. Good skin care therefore prevents infection and promotes comfort. In the sick child the nurse either carries out the activity of skin care or acts as a facilitator for the parents in the participation of this activity.

> **Nursing Alert**
>
> Keep skin clean and moist to prevent the build-up of micro-organisms. A build-up of micro-organisms results in dry skin and thus skin breakdowns and skin infections.

Preventing dry skin

It is important to be aware that over-washing can result in dry skin (Nichol, 2004). Another skin function is the secretion of sebum through sebaceous glands (Chapter Fifteen). Sebum provides lubrication that keeps the skin moist; excess washing results in dry skin that can lead to compromising the skin's natural protection from micro-organisms. A balance between keeping the skin clean but not over-washing and choosing the correct products is therefore best practice.

> **Nursing Alert**
>
> Do not over-wash or under-wash as it can lead to skin breakdown. Choose products with a pH value of 3.8–4.2.

Skin assessment

While the performance of skin care provides an ideal opportunity for assessing the general condition of the child's skin (Moules & Ramsay, 2008), it also provides an opportunity for visual assessment of issues related to height and weight (Chapter Five), signs of malnutrition (Chapter Three), respiratory and cardiac function (Chapter Nine), and signs of abuse (Chapter Three). Premature and sick babies should have minimal physical interaction and be touched as little as possible during assessment. Therefore whilst carrying out a skin assessment, or when considering performing skin care, consideration should be given to what other aspects of care can be combined and done at the same time. For example, the baby's weight, blood pressure, pulse, respiratory rate assessment, and other clinical observations may be carried out just prior to bathing, rather than disturbing the baby again at a different time.

Different skin types

Points to bear in mind when assessing the child's skin include differences in skin type. For example, children with olive skin are more at risk of skin breakdown than those with darker skin (Suddaby et al., 2005), while darker skin is more prone to developing keloids (Prenzer, 2002).

Skin impairments

It is essential to observe for skin impairments such as nappy dermatitis. Nappy dermatitis is one of the most common skin disorders in infants and toddlers. It usually occurs due to irritation by urine, faeces, moisture, or friction and can become secondarily infected (Borkowski, 2004). It is vital that you identify the cause of any skin impairment, document an accurate description, and treat accordingly, and that a regular re-evaluation also takes place. Your main goal should be the prevention of skin impairments such as nappy dermatitis. This is achieved by preventing dry skin, changing the nappy frequently, carrying out hand hygiene, and providing parent education. Other skin disorders to observe for include: fungal infection, pressure sores, and rashes. For risk of pressure sore development use a standardized tool in accordance with local policy. For specific assessment of skin disorders and skin impairments please see the suggested reading list and **Table 6.1**.

Table 6.1 Normal skin conditions

Normal skin condition	Features	Causes	Treatment
Milia	Tiny white spots on face and nose.	Blocked sebaceous glands; may be related to hormonal stimulus of the sebaceous glands.	Never squeezed or pinched. Document.
Erythema toxicum	Develops within a day or two of birth; non-infective rash. Whitish/yellowish papules <3 mm in size.	Unknown origin.	Document.
Ictercus neonatorum (physiological jaundice)	Appears a few days after birth. Skin yellowish in colour; resolves spontaneously.	Quite normal break-down of excess red blood cells that were needed *in utero*.	Document.
Pathologic jaundice	Appears 24 hours post-birth. Skin yellowish in colour.	Rhesus or ABO incompatibilities.	Document.
Mongolian blue spot	Present at birth. Blue-black colour on lower back; may be mistaken for bruising caused by non-accidental injury. Disappears as the child grows older, though some remain into adulthood.	Baby of East Asian or Afro-Caribbean parents.	No treatment—usually document.
Naervus flammeus (port wine stain)	Port wine stains are located just below the epidermis, generally not elevated, and often appear on the face. In Afro-Caribbean skin they are jet black in colour. In Caucasian skin they are red and tend to increase or decrease in size with time.	By capillary angioma.	Document.
Telangiectatic naevus (strawberry birth mark)	Red in colour, usually resolve spontaneously as the child matures.	Vascular lesions due to the dilation of a group of small blood vessels.	None.
Freckles	Brown lesions over sun-exposed areas; not present in newborn infants. They are harmless (however, children's exposure to sun may result in skin cancers in later life).	Sun exposure. (approx. 80% of sun damage occurs during childhood).	Prevention: Babies under the age of 6 months should be kept out of the sun altogether. Dress children in densely woven cotton t-shirts when in sun and wide-brimmed hats. Keep children out of the sun from 11.00 to 13.00. Apply high factor sunscreen as part of their normal routine.

(Continued)

Table 6.1 *Continued*

Acne	Nearly all teenagers suffer acne to varying degrees (mild to severe). Can be stressful leading to isolation and low self-esteem depending on severity on face, chest, and back.	Stimulation of the androgens due to increased sebum secretion.	Access coping mechanisms and referral to a dermatologist. NICE (2001) provides guidelines regarding referral. Provide reassurance. Provide practical advice.

Nursing Alert

When providing skin care, use the opportunity for both an overall health assessment of the child and assessment of the child's skin. Any skin impairments observed should be documented and described in detail, the cause should be identified, and skin treated accordingly.

Child considerations and developmental needs

It is important to be conscious of the child's changing needs at various developmental stages when attending to hygiene needs.

The newborn

Babies are born with a skin surface pH of 6.34; within four days the skin surface changes to a pH of 4.95. This is due to the normal process of skin being colonized by micro-organisms known as **normal flora**. The normal flora act as a protective barrier against **pathogenic micro-organisms**. Pathogenic organisms are disease-causing micro-organisms. The introduction of chemical products during this time can disrupt this process and lead to problems such as eczema.

The umbilical cord

During the baby's first weeks of life, hygiene of the umbilical cord is also important. The umbilical cord starts to dry out, harden, and turn black in preparation for separation. There is a high risk of infection until separation is complete due to blood flow to the area for several days. The risk of infection increases if good skin care and hand hygiene are not maintained appropriately (Trotter, 2004). The use of antiseptics around the cord area can result in a prolonged healing process and hinder cord separation due to the destruction of normal flora around the umbilical cord (Trotter, 2004).

Therefore, when bathing during this time, correct hand hygiene techniques should be maintained (Chapter Five) and skin cleansing should be performed using sterile water with cotton wool only (Trotter, 2004). Refer to your local policy for specific care of the umbilical cord.

Nursing Alert

Do not introduce products or use antiseptics during the baby's first few days; this can disrupt the process of developing normal flora, which can lead to problems such as eczema. Skin cleansing should be performed using pure water with cotton wool.

6.2 **Washing a baby**

Procedure: Daily cleansing of a baby

Preparation

To encourage participation, facilitate education, and reduce parental separation it is important to involve the parents where possible (Smith *et al.*, 2002; Coyne & Cowley, 2007). Find out when the parent/s are going to be available and accommodate them where possible.

Ensure adequate room temperature with no draught. This promotes comfort and will help prevent illness.

Nursing Alert

A sick baby, for example a baby with respiratory problems, should not be bathed. This exposure can lead to the infant losing heat. The infant produces heat through shivering. Shivering requires both oxygen and glucose, so the cold infant is at risk of hypoxia and hypoglycaemia (Johnston *et al.*, 2003).

Equipment

To ensure adequate preparation and avoid leaving the baby and parent/s during the procedure, gather all the equipment before you begin (Dougherty & Lister, 2006).

- Two bowls of warm, clean water.
- Clean, warm, soft towels.
- Cleaning device: cotton wool balls/clean, soft flannel. Avoid baby wipes for babies under four weeks old (Trotter, 2004).
- A clean nappy.
- Disposal bag or bucket for soiled nappy and clothes.
- Soft baby hairbrush.
- Clean clothes.
- Mild cleansing agent if baby is over four weeks old.
- Baby's own nail scissors.

(Use plain water only for premature babies under eight weeks old and all babies under four weeks (Trotter, 2004; Hale, 2007).

Assessment

Assess the baby's needs (physical and religious) and parent participation level.

Consent and communication

Introduce yourself, confirm the baby's identity, and explain the procedure.

6.3 Bathing a baby, infant, toddler, or pre-schooler

Toddler and pre-schooler

When bathing a toddler or pre-schooler you can never leave them alone due to a high risk of drowning. Age-appropriate play for the toddler and pre-schooler during bath time is another consideration. This promotes comfort and play

Step-by-step guide to daily cleansing of an infant or baby

Procedure	Rationale
1 Wash hands (Chapter 5).	To prevent cross infection.
2 Place the dressed baby on the towel.	To ensure safety.
3 Attend to eye care (see earlier section).	To prevent cross infection.
4 Gently wash the baby's face and around the mouth and nose with cleaning device and gently pat dry.	To maintain skin integrity (Trotter, 2004).
5 Wash baby's hands and dry.	To maintain skin integrity.
6 If nails are long, snip them with baby's own blunt-ended baby scissors.	To prevent scratches to baby's skin from overgrown nails.
7 Gently brush scalp and hair with soft baby brush.	To prevent cradle cap (Trotter, 2004).

8	Expose nappy area and take off nappy. If the nappy is wet, clean with warm water using separate bowl of water. If soiled, wipe excess faeces away with cotton wool balls then clean from front to back.	To prevent nappy dermatitis (Borkowski, 2004; Hale, 2007). To prevent contaminating the urethra with faeces.
9	Observe for nappy dermatitis. If present, clearly document description of rash and identify cause. Treatment will depend on severity and etiology (Borkowski, 2004).	To maintain skin integrity.
10	Wash baby's bottom and dry. Clean visible area of genitalia only. Do not retract a boy's foreskin or clean inside labia of a girl.	To maintain skin integrity. To avoid injury as foreskin is not fully retracted until 18 months.
11	Ensure all creases of skin are dry.	To prevent rash or infection.
12	Position clean nappy beneath the umbilical cord if cord still attached (separation usually takes two weeks).	To prevent umbilical cord infection.
13	Observe umbilical cord for signs of infection.	To facilitate early treatment of infection.
14	Dress baby in clean clothes.	To promote comfort.
15	Dispose of used nappy according to local policy.	To prevent cross infection.
16	Clear away equipment according to local policy.	To prevent cross infection.
17	Wash hands and document care provided. Document and report any skin defects.	To prevent cross infection. To facilitate interdisciplinary communication.

and reduces anxiety (Glasper *et al.*, 2007). It also associates bath time as being pleasurable, which leads to good habits later in life. Please refer to Chapter Two for more information on play and safety.

The procedure for bathing a baby, infant, toddler, or pre-schooler is outlined below.

Procedure: Bathing a baby, infant, toddler, or pre-schooler

Preparation and equipment

Follow the instructions for *Daily cleansing of a baby* above. In addition to the equipment listed you will need a baby bath and stand if carrying out the procedure for a baby or infant. If for an older child, prepare the bathroom ensuring an adequate room temperature and that the floor is not wet.

Assessment

Assess the baby/child's needs (physical and religious) and parent participation level.

Consent and communication

Introduce yourself, confirm the baby/child's identity, and explain the procedure.

Nursing Alert

Never leave a baby or young child alone when bathing.

Young people

Young people's need for privacy heightens as sexual awareness develops. When assisting with bathing, young people should be covered until entering the water and

Step-by-step guide to bathing a baby, infant, toddler, or pre-schooler

Procedure	Rationale
1 Add cold water then hot water to baby bath/bath to fill bath to no more than 10 cm in depth. Water out of hot taps should be no more than 46 degrees Centigrade.	This reduces the risk of the water not mixing properly.
2 Test water temperature at intervals by dipping an elbow into water or using an individual water thermometer. It ought to feel warmer than tepid.	To prevent scalds and ensure the water is a comfortable temperature.
3 If using a baby bath, place on floor or stand.	To ensure a comfortable height of bath and facilitate manual handling technique.
4 Kneel or stand.	To ensure comfort and appropriate manual handling techniques.
5 Undress the child. If a nappy area is very soiled, clean off faeces with cotton wool balls.	To expose skin. To prevent nappy dermatitis.
6 Wrap child securely with a towel.	To promote comfort.
7 Prior to bathing, clean child's eyes, face, and mouth (see earlier section on eye care and next section on mouth care).	To prevent cross infection.
8 Hold baby's head over bath and gently rinse water over their hair, avoiding the eyes. For older children follow usual routine. Shampoo is not required for babies under one year (Trotter, 2004).	To wash hair.
9 For an older child unwrap their towel and assist into bath tub, ensuring they cannot reach the hot taps. **Never leave a child alone in a bath**. A non-slip mat or cradle can be used to prevent an accidental slip.	To prevent scalds.
For baby, unwrap their towel. Hold the baby securely, with one hand grasping the farthest upper arm, and the baby's neck and shoulders supported on the foreman.	To prevent accidental submerging.
For an infant learning to sit, support them in the water with a hand around the back. Never leave the infant unsupported.	
10 Gently wash with free hand, under the arms, back, and nappy area. Pay particular attention to the skin creases.	To maintain skin integrity.
Allow age-appropriate play (Chapter One).	To facilitate fun and reduce anxiety.
If there are any signs of distress, remove from bath as soon as possible.	To maintain safety.

11	When finished washing, remove child from water. Do not let the child become cold. Wrap them in a towel.	To keep warm and promote comfort.
12	Dry hair first.	To prevent child from getting cold as head loses warmth fastest.
13	Dry and dress in clean clothes.	To promote comfort.
14	If nails are long, snip them with child's own blunt-ended baby scissors.	To prevent scratches to child's skin from overgrown nails.
15	Clean and dispose of equipment as per local policy. Wash hands, document care, and document and report any skin defects.	To prevent cross infection. To facilitate communication and promote early treatment.

the bathroom door should be closed. This maintains the dignity of a young person (Nichol, 2004). However, a young person who is sick should never lock himself or herself into a bathroom alone. If a young person is bathing independently, ensure a bath mat is in place, they can reach the call bell, the floor is not slippery, and the door is not locked but a sign is on the door. This maintains both their safety and dignity. Also, young people experience embarrassment when they cannot attend to their own hygiene needs. In this situation the young adult will require assistance in the bathroom or require the nurse to perform a bed bath. It is recommended that this sensitive nursing care is same gender specific and sensitivity is vital in this regard.

Nursing Alert

When caring for a young person always maintain their dignity. It is recommended that the same gender carry out skin care.

Procedure: Giving a bed bath

Preparation

It is important to carry out this procedure in a safe and comfortable environment. Make sure you also keep your health and safety in mind, adhering to manual handling principles throughout the procedure (Smith *et al.*, 2002). See the section later in the chapter on manual handling for more information.

Assess the child's toileting needs and offer facilities appropriate to the child's needs.

To prepare the environment:

- Ensure bed brakes are on and adjust the bed to the appropriate height.
- Move furniture to allow easy access to the bed.
- Close any windows and ensure an adequate room temperature. Preventing draughts promotes patient comfort and reduces the spread of micro-organisms (Dougherty & Lister, 2008).

Equipment

Gather equipment before you begin to ensure adequate preparation and avoid leaving the child/parent during the procedure.

- Clean bed linen.
- Clean clothes.
- One bath towel.
- Soft towels.
- Wash bag containing child's own wash products, toothbrush and paste, brush, deodorant, and clean, dry washcloth.
- Laundry skip.
- Yellow bags.
- Alginate bags for soiled items.
- Disposable wipes.
- Manual handling aids as required.
- Clean washbowl and warm water. Ensure water remains hot enough; it might require changing.

Step-by-step guide to giving a bed bath

Procedure	Rationale
1 Wash hands and put on a plastic apron.	To prevent cross infection (SARI, 2001).
2 Close door/curtains.	To ensure privacy.
3 Remove top cover leaving top sheet in place, then place bath towel over child and top sheet. Gently remove top sheet leaving bath towel over child, ensuring you do not expose child's body.	To maintain privacy, dignity, and warmth (Pegram *et al.*, 2007).
Place bed covers on rail at end of bed or over two chairs.	To prevent cross infection.
Place linen in linen skip if dirty. (Two nurses is preferable if available for this step.)	
4 Assist child to sitting position if appropriate. Undress/assist undressing under the bath towel. Ensure child's body remains covered at this time (Pegram *et al.*, 2007). If there are intravenous lines or injuries, remove clothes from unaffected side first.	To facilitate washing and maintain dignity. To promote comfort.
5 Attend to eye care (see earlier section) and dental care (see later section). Check water temperature and adjust if necessary. Wash and dry face.	To ensure safety and comfort (Pegram *et al.*, 2007).
6 Prior to washing each limb, expose limb and place a dry towel under it. Once limb is fully dry re-cover, ensuring limbs are not exposed for prolonged periods.	To ensure dignity and comfort.
7 Wash, rinse, and dry arms. Start by rinsing washcloth in warm water and applying product. Use appropriate mild product (Gelmetti, 2001) according to care plan/preference. Wash hand and arm furthest away from you, ensuring specific attention to axillae and nails. Rinse washcloth and rinse cleanser off skin. Pat skin dry and re-cover arm. Repeat for other arm. Assess nails and trim using child's own scissors if necessary.	Washing arm furthest away ensures that spills will not moisten parts of the body that would have been previously washed (Pegram *et al.*, 2007).
8 Remove bath towel from torso leaving lower body covered. Wash, rinse, and dry torso. Re-cover torso.	To promote cleanliness and maintain dignity.
9 Check water temperature and change if cold or if very soapy or dirty (Pegram *et al.*, 2007; Dougherty & Lister, 2008).	To promote comfort and prevent cross infection (Dougherty & Lister, 2008).

10	Washing genitals: ask child if he/she wants to wash this area. If not expose area, put on gloves, and with clean disposal cloths wash genitals from front to back. (For post-pubertal boys, ensure the foreskin is pulled back and the penis underneath is washed). Dispose of disposal cloths in yellow bag. Rinse and dry genitals. Remove gloves and dispose of in yellow bag. Decontaminate hands, re-cover child, and **change water.**	To promote cleanliness. To prevent cross infection.
11	Repeat steps 6 and 7 for lower limbs. Assess heels and ankles for pressure sores. Attend to toe nail care (consider need for chiropodist). Pay particular attention to washing and drying between toes.	To maintain skin integrity and prevent/ facilitate early treatment of pressure sores (Butler, 2006). To avoid fungal infections.
12	Assist/roll child onto side facing away from you, using moving and handling principles and taking extra care of any intravenous lines, catheters, or drains.	To ensure safety.
13	Place a towel under child's back and wash, rinse, and dry back. Assess for pressure areas on occipital region, sacral region, and ear lobes. Assess for bruises or swellings and signs of skin infestations such as rashes or signs of scratching (Moules & Ramsay, 2008).	To maintain skin integrity and prevent/ facilitate early treatment of pressure sores (Butler, 2006), child abuse, or skin infestations (Moules & Ramsay, 2008).
14	Put on gloves and wash and rinse bottom using a disposable cloth. Dispose of cloth in yellow bag. Pat skin dry. Remove and dispose of gloves in yellow bag. Decontaminate hands and re-cover patient. Under-sheet can be changed at this point if required in accordance with local policy. (See suggested reading for bed making procedures.)	To promote comfort, maintain skin integrity, and prevent cross infection.
15	Dress child in clean clothes.	To promote comfort and safety.
16	Position child comfortably and appropriately according to care plan. Ensure bed rails are in place if required. Brush hair with child's own brush and assess scalp for dryness or infestations.	To promote comfort and safety. To facilitate early treatment.
17	Assess need to wash hair and if required wash hair (using children's specific shampoo) in bed using specialist equipment according to local policy. Seek specific guidance from parent/child regarding preferences and religious rituals.	To promote cleanliness. To ensure wishes of child and parents are respected.
18	Clear away equipment and return any moved furniture.	To maintain clear working environment (Dougherty & Lister, 2008).
19	Wash hands, document care, and document and report any abnormalities such as infestations, rashes, or pressure sores.	To facilitate early treatment and interdisciplinary communication.

Assessment

Assess the child's needs (physical and religious), preferences, independence, and parent participation level. Before you begin it is also important to assess the child for any signs of pain. If they are in pain, administer prescribed analgesia as required (see earlier section on pain assessment). This promotes comfort and reduces the possibility of disruption.

Consent and communication

Before you begin, introduce yourself and explain the procedure to parent/s and child. This ensures you have the correct patient, and that they have given you their consent (Dougherty & Lister, 2008).

Safety, comfort, and dignity

When bathing a child of any age, ensure that the water is not too hot. This prevents scalds and ensures child safety. Ensure that the room temperature and water are not too cold. This promotes comfort and prevents **hypothermia** (low body temperature) (Nichol, 2004). Correct manual handling techniques are imperative to ensure both the nurse's and child's safety (this will be discussed later in this chapter).

Other factors to consider

Maintaining normal routines and independence

A child in poor health either in hospital or at home should have their normal routines, individuality, and level of independence maintained as far as possible. Normal routines can be maintained by: negotiating care between nurse, parent, and child (depending on developmental stage); providing support; and providing encouragement. Negotiation of care may include timing of skin care (timing should be planned to maintain normal routines and for when the child is awake and content), type of hygiene activity (bath/shower/bed bath; individual preference should be maintained as much as possible), and parental participation (this should be discussed with parent and child). This reduces anxiety, promotes comfort, and maintains dignity.

> **Nursing Alert**
>
> Maintain the child's normal routines, individuality, and level of independence as far as possible when attending to hygiene needs.

Parent participation and cultural differences

Parent participation is another concept that is important to consider when attending to a child's skin care. When a parent participates in childcare it decreases parental separation issues and promotes child comfort (Coyne, 2007). Parent participation level can range from unavailability (e.g. due to other family commitments), through physical presence for emotional support, to full participation in skin care. It is best that the level of participation in skin care is established and negotiated when first meeting a parent. Ensure that you continue to assess, reassess, and document the desired participation level of the parent. Important aspects of parent participation include: establishing a good nurse-parent relationship; providing encouragement and support; and providing guidance on specific child hygiene needs (Coyne & Cowley, 2007).

It is also important to be culturally sensitive when carrying out skin care. For example, in some cultures body odour is socially acceptable, while in Western cultures body odours are socially unaccepted. This can create a dilemma for health carers. While the norms of the society a person lives in should determine practice and the way in which care is delivered, this should also be in accordance with cultural values (Hollins, 2006). For example, the cultural value of washing rituals around prayer time for Muslim and Hindu religions should be adhered to (Hollins, 2006). Some cultures are not generally tactile (e.g. Muslim), while others are highly tactile (e.g. French and Jewish). Same gender care delivery is imperative for some cultures (Arab and Muslim) and is further recommended for all children (Goldbloom, 2003). Developing a good relationship with the child and family should help you to identify cultural needs. Careful assessment, using the nursing process and models of care, will also aid delivery of culturally sensitive care (see Chapter Five).

Cultural differences also present language barriers on occasions and many hospitals provide interpreters for this reason. In addition, it is also recommended that hospitals develop a repertoire of healthcare information leaflets in the languages that are commonly required. It can also be useful, on the ward or in the hospital, to have a list of greeting phrases from different cultures to assist with greeting children and their families if English is not their first language. This can later be supported by the interpreting services (if available). Attempting to greet families in their own language and having a patient centred, authentic, and friendly approach (see Chapter Two) will hopefully ease anxiety in both parents and children under your care, as it signifies cultural appreciation (Goldbloom, 2003). In order to provide cultural sensitivity when attending to skin care you need to gain awareness of different cultural aspects related to skin care (Hollins, 2006). This is just a very basic introduction to cultural aspects that relate specifically to skin care. Cultural appreciation and sensitivity are fundamental to contemporary nursing care practice; therefore a more in-depth knowledge of this topic is essential. Further reading of texts such as Hollins (2006) will provide good information on this topic.

6.4 **Bed making**

Procedure: Bed making

Key learning points from this discussion are that children are dependent on others for skin care and are vulnerable to skin impairments. Skin should be kept clean, moisturized, and free from infection. The amount of nursing input will depend on the child's developmental stage, level of independence, self-care abilities, and willingness/availability of parent/s to participate. Therefore assessment prior to activity should also include level of independence, normal routine, developmental stage of child, and parent participation.

Step-by-step guide to bed making

Procedure	Rationale
1 Put on a plastic apron.	To prevent contamination of uniform (Parker, 2004).
2 Take linen skip to bed.	To avoid bedclothes touching uniform, thus preventing uniform contamination (Parker, 2004).
3 Strip the bed by folding each item of bedding separately.	To prevent contamination of uniform and avoid items touching floor, thus preventing cross infection (Parker, 2004).
4 Place soiled items into a dissolvable bag and then colour coded skip as per local policy. Prevent bedding from touching floor.	Bedclothes must not touch floor to prevent pathogens from transferring to or from floor (Parker, 2004).
5 Clean sheets must not touch floor and must have come from a linen cupboard used solely for linen that is dust free.	To adhere to infection control policies and prevent cross infection.
6 Do not shake bedclothes to freshen them or to lay them on the bed.	Shaking bedclothes helps large numbers of pathogens to spread throughout the environment (Parker, 2004).

Mouth care

Caring for a child's first teeth is as important as the care of their adult teeth. When good habits are formed from an early age, it is easier to keep teeth healthy throughout life. Parents should bring the child for a visit to their dentist regularly for normal checks of their dental and oral health, and early assessment by the child's dentist can identify if the child might develop problems (Health Service Executive, 2008). Attractive, healthy teeth promote self-esteem and contribute to physical well-being (Price & Gwin, 2008). Mouth care is an essential element of daily hygiene and should be carried on in the hospital. Infants and sick children need the nurse or a family member to perform mouth care; although young children can

manage a toothbrush and should be prompted to use it, most may require help to perform a satisfactory job. Procedures for cleaning teeth are outlined below.

6.5 Cleaning teeth

Procedure: Cleaning teeth

Equipment

- Disposable gloves.
- Soft toothbrush.
- Fluoride toothpaste (if the child is two years old or above).
- Running water.

Step-by-step guide to cleaning teeth

Procedure	Rationale
1 Explain procedure to child.	To gain consent (Dougherty & Lister, 2008) and cooperation.
2 Wash hands (Chapter 5). Put on disposable gloves.	To prevent cross infection (Dougherty & Lister, 2008).
3 Brush child's teeth with a soft toothbrush and tap water (Dental Health Foundation Ireland, 2008).	To maintain oral health. The most important plaque control method is tooth brushing (Dental Health Foundation Ireland, 2008).
4 Do not use toothpaste when child is very young. Fluoride toothpaste can be used twice a day from two years of age; supervise brushing up to age seven years. Make sure only a smear or small pea-sized amount is placed on the brush and teeth are brushed properly for three minutes (Health Service Executive, 2006; Dental Health Foundation Ireland, 2008).	To prevent child from swallowing toothpaste and developing white stains on their mouth, which may happen when fluoride toothpaste is swallowed (Dental Health Foundation Ireland, 2008). The more frequently and the longer teeth are cleaned, the greater the probability of effective plaque removal.
5 Repeat twice a day (Health Service Executive, 2006; British Dental Association, 2003).	To prevent dental caries and periodontal (gum) disease (Wong et al., 1999).

Consent and communication

Before you begin, explain the procedure to the child to ensure cooperation and consent.

Nursing Alert

Even when the child is not eating, such as when they are unconscious, regular and thorough mouth care is vital.

Some children have teething problems, including red, swollen gums, red cheeks, dribbling, and disturbed sleep. Certain teething rings that can be cooled in the fridge may help. However, teething may not always be the cause of the above symptoms, so further medical investigations may be required.

Mobility and moving and handling

Prior to considering mobility and moving and handling of a child you should be familiar with: communication skills (Chapter Two); child development and behaviour (Chapter Three); consent prior to procedures (Chapter

Box 6.1 Caring for a child's teeth

Do not give sugary foods and drinks in between meals (Health Service Executive, 2006; Dental Health Foundation Ireland, 2008) to prevent dental caries. Early childhood caries is associated with significant adverse physical, functional, and behavioural consequences that can greatly impair quality of life (Finlayson *et al.*, 2007).

From the age of one year, the child should be drinking from a beaker or cup. If the child uses a soother, avoid dipping it into sugar or sweet-tasting syrups (Health Service Executive, 2006; Health Service Executive, 2005). Only give the child a bottle at feed times. Do not allow the child to sleep with a bottle in their mouth (Health Service Executive, 2006; Dental Health Foundation Ireland, 2008) to prevent dental caries.

Encourage the child to eat foods that have a lot of calcium such as milk, cheese, and yogurt (Health Service Executive, 2005; Trigg & Mohammed, 2006). Calcium helps build strong teeth (Health Service Executive, 2005).

Four); and the musculo-skeletal system (Chapter Thirteen). You could also reflect upon episodes of moving and handling that you have come across during your nursing practice. To undertake moving and handling of children and infants, it is also important to have participated in locally arranged moving and handling training, and satisfied the requirements of your local health service in this regard.

Mobility is a term commonly used in nursing practice and relates to all forms of body movements (Workman & Cooper, 2003). Moving and handling, which is also referred to as manual handling, is the movement of an animate/inanimate object by a person either by hand or force, including pushing/pulling, lifting up/putting down, carrying, moving, or supporting (The Manual Handling Operations Regulations 1992 (amended in 2002), cited in Harrison, 2007). Prior to moving/repositioning a patient the nurse must carry out a risk assessment on the child's mobility, paying particular attention to the child's age, stage of development, understanding, previous mobility, and current health status (Dougherty & Lister, 2008). In healthcare, the main aim of any moving and handling manoeuvre is to move a patient safely from one position/place to another, without causing the patient undue discomfort/injury, and while reducing the risk of injury to the carer.

Moving and handling-related injuries are common among healthcare workers worldwide, with a high percentage of nurses sustaining back injuries (Retsas & Pinikahana, 2000; Mallett & Bailey, 2004). In Ireland, for example, a high incidence of workplace injuries was noted by the Health, Safety and Welfare at Work Act in 2005. As a result there is greater emphasis on reducing work injuries and initial moving and handling training is now mandatory for healthcare workers, with updates required every two years (Health, Safety and Welfare at Work Act (General Application) Regulations, 2007).

In healthcare settings, emphasis is placed on teamwork for moving and handling manoeuvres. Remember, always inform the child of your intent, as it helps to alleviate fears and gain their cooperation. The use of equipment, for example, hoists, roller boards, or pedals to raise/lower a bed or trolley is encouraged. However, children when immobilized may resist nursing interventions and show signs of aggression, or become quiet and withdrawn (Hockenberry & Wilson, 2007).

In children's nursing, the use of play to demonstrate your intent or to demonstrate how equipment works also helps to gain patient cooperation. In both hospital and community settings each situation requires careful planning, based on the principles of safe handling and minimizing risks to the patient and carer. Use of the acronym TILE (Task, Individual, Load, and Environment) can help the nurse consider all necessary factors before moving and handling, and careful consideration should be given to each of these areas before the manoeuvre is commenced (Rideout, 2006; Harrison, 2007; Intelligent Health Systems, 2007).

Some healthcare settings promote a 'no lifting' approach to moving and handling; however, in caring for children this may not be practical and alternative solutions and policies are required (Sales & Utting, 2002). The children's nurse may need to consider safely bending down and giving a crying child a hug rather than lifting the child up (Harrison, 2007). If the nurse has a toddler in his/her arms, the nurse should be aware that the child may be unpredictable and not wish to stand when the nurse puts the child down on the floor, possibly jolting the nurse's back. To help prevent injury it is essential that the nurse supports their own back and the child's head and back when lifting/moving the child (Health Service Executive, 2005).

Nursing Alert

- Back injuries are often caused from repetitive strain (Intelligent Health Systems, 2007); look after your back.
- Ensure that you receive moving and handling training.
- Wear appropriate footwear and clothing.
- Familiarize yourself with current local moving and handling policies.
- Never use equipment that you are not competent in operating.
- Never use faulty equipment.
- Report faulty equipment.
- Do not take risks.
- Report and document all accidents/injuries of patient/nurse in accordance with policies/guidelines.

The children's nurse in a ward or community setting should be vigilant at all times, ensuring that, for example, toys and empty bottles have not been left on the floor as obstacles that may result in injury (Sales & Utting, 2002). As in the hospital setting, the nurse in the community must also work closely with the multidisciplinary team to ensure overall continuity of care, in accordance with the child's specific needs.

It is imperative that nurses attend moving and handling training and implement changes in practice, thus reducing the theory-practice gap and reducing the risk of discomfort/injury to the patient/carer.

Conclusion

In this chapter you will have gained knowledge in the assessment and management of the skin and wounds and should understand the importance of pain relief to children prior to any potentially painful procedure. Pain assessment is a key component of pain management and necessary for the child's overall care. Incorporating regular pain assessment alongside recording of vital signs will ensure that any pain is acknowledged and treated quickly. A brief overview of the pain medication available for children has been provided to help you decide which pain relief is best suited to the child. Further reading of a children's pharmacology text will increase your knowledge of the side effects of these drugs.

A wound assessment provides the basis on which wound care is planned and implemented and this chapter has provided you with information on the key signs to look for when examining a wound. You have been given step-by-step information to enable you to provide a child's basic hygiene needs, and information on what abnormalities to look for when caring for the child's skin, eyes, ears, and mouth. Mouth care is an important part of a child's daily care and should not be overlooked if the child is being fed by other methods than by mouth. Plaque and dental decay can build up quickly and may result in unnecessary pain and discomfort for the child. The principles of moving and handling have been discussed; however, always follow your hospital's policies and protocols and do not be tempted to copy poor practice. The information within this chapter has been applied to the care of the child in the home and where possible provides advice on how to involve parents in the child's care, especially within the home environment.

Online resource centre

You may find it helpful to work through our online resources including interactive scenarios intended to help you to develop and apply the skills in this chapter. Where material referenced below is available electronically, we're pleased to provide active web links to the source via 🅦 **http://www.oxfordtextbooks.co.uk/orc/coyne/**

References

Association of Paediatric Anaesthetists of Great Britain and Ireland (2008). *Good Practice in Postoperative and Procedural Pain*. London: Association of Paediatric Anaesthetists of Great Britain and Ireland.

Benbow, M. (2008) Best practice—application of dressing products. *Journal of Community Nursing Online* **22** (3), 36. Available at: **http://www.jcn.co.uk/journal.asp?MonthNum=03&YearNum=2008&ArticleID=1156**

Beyer, J.E., McGrath, P.J., & Berde, C.B. (1990) Discordance between self-report and behavioral pain measures in children aged 3–7 years after surgery. *Journal of Pain and Symptom Management* **5**, 350.

Blunt, J. (2001) Wound cleansing, ritualistic or research based practice? *Nursing Standard* **16** (1), 33–36.

Borkowski, S. (2004) Diaper rash: Care and management. *Paediatric Nursing*, **30** (6), 467–470.

British Dental Association (2003) *Frequently Asked Questions: Children's teeth*. Available at: **http://www.dentalhealth.org.uk**

Butler, C.T. (2006) Pediatric skin care: Guidelines for assessment, prevention, and treatment. *Paediatric Nursing* **32** (5), 443–450.

Carter, B., Lambrenos, K., & Thursfield, J. (2002) A pain workshop: An approach to eliciting the views of young people with chronic pain. *Journal of Clinical Nursing* **11**, 753–762.

Carter, B., McArthur, E., & Cunliffe, M. (2002) Dealing with uncertainty: Parental assessment of pain in their children with profound special needs. *Journal of Advanced Nursing* **38** (5), 449–457.

Casey, G. (2001) Wound dressings. *Paediatric Nursing* **13** (4), 39–42.

Coyne, I. (2007) Disruption of parent participation: Nurses' strategies to manage parents on children's wards. *Journal of Clinical Nursing* **17** (23), 3150–3158.

Coyne, I. & Cowley, S. (2007) Challenging the philosophy of partnership with parents: A grounded theory study. *International Journal of Nursing Studies*, **44**, 893–904.

Dental Health Foundation Ireland (2008) Available at: **http://www.dentalhealth.ie**

Dougherty, L. & Lister, S. (2008) *The Royal Marsden Hospital Manual of Clinical Nursing procedures, Student Edition*. UK: Wiley Blackwell.

Enoch, S. (2006) ABC of wound healing—wound assessment. *Student BMJ* **14**, 89–132. Available at: **http://student.bmj.com/issues/06/03/education/98.php**

Finlayson, T.F., Siefert, K., Ismail, A.I., & Woosung, S. (2007) Psychosocial factors and early childhood caries among low income African-American children in Detroit. *Community Dentistry and Oral Epidemiology* **35** (6), 439–448.

Franck, L.S. (2003) Nursing management of children's pain: Current evidence and future directions for research. *NT Research* **8** (5), 330–353.

Franck, L.S., Allen, A., & Oulton, K. (2007) Making pain assessment more accessible to children and parents: Can greater involvement improve the quality of care? *Clinical Journal of Pain* **23** (4), 331–338.

Franck, L.S., Treadwell, M., Jacob, E., & Vichinsky, E. (2002) Assessment of sickle cell pain in children and young adults using the Adolescent Pediatric Pain Tool. *Journal of Pain and Symptom Management* **23** (2), 114–120.

Furze, C. & Pearson, B. (2006) Hygiene. In E. Trigg & T.A. Mohammed (eds.) *Practices in Children's Nursing Guidelines for Hospital and Community, 2nd ed.* London: Churchill Livingstone.

Gelmetti, C. (2001) Skin cleansing in children. *Journal of European Academy of Dermatology and Venereology* **15** (1), 12–15.

Glasper, E.A., McEwing, G., & Richardson, J. (2007) *Handbook of Children's and Young People's Nursing*. Oxford: Oxford University Press.

Goldbloom, R.B. (2003) *Pediatric Clinical skills, 3rd ed.* USA: Elsevier Science.

Hale, R. (2007) Protecting neonates' delicate skin. *British Journal of Midwifery* **15** (4), 231–235.

Harrison, M. (2007) Manual handling and children. In E.P. Glasper, G. McEwing, & J. Richardson (2007) *Oxford Handbook of Children's and Young People's Nursing*. Oxford: Blackwell.

Harrop, J.E. (2007) Management of pain in childhood. *Archive of Diseases in Childhood Education Practice* **92**, 101–108.

Health Service Executive (2005) *Caring for your Child: Six months to two years.* Dublin: Health Service Executive.

Health Service Executive (2006) *Food for Young Children.* Dublin: Health Service Executive.

Health Service Executive (2008) *Looking after your Child's Teeth: 0–8 years.* Dublin: Health Service Executive.

Health, Safety and Welfare at Work Regulations (2007). Dublin: Government Publications.

Hockenberry, M.J. & Wilson, D. (2007) *Wong's Nursing Care of Infants and Children, 8th ed.* St. Louis: Mosby.

Hockenberry-Eaton, M., Barrera, P., Brown, M., Bottomley, S., & Brace-O'Neill, J. (1999) *Pain Management in Children with Cancer. Texas Cancer Council.* Available at: **http://www. childcancerpain.org/contents/childpainmgmt.pdf**

Hollins, S. (2006) *Religions, Culture and Healthcare: A practical guide for use in healthcare environments.* Abingdon: Radcliffe Publishing.

Horgan, M.F., Glenn, S., & Choonara, I. (2002) Further development of the Liverpool Infant Distress Score. *Journal of Child Health Care* **6** (2), 33–42.

Howard, R.F. (2003) Current status of pain management in children. *Journal of American Medical Association* **290** (18), 2464–2469.

Intelligent Health Systems Ltd (2007) *Manual Handling Instructor Course.* Dublin. University College Dublin.

International Association for the Study of Pain (2007) *International Association for the Study of Pain—Pain terminology.* Available at: **http://www.iasp-pain.org/AM/Template.cfm?Section=General_Resource_Links&Template=/CM/HTMLDisplay.cfm&ContentID=3058**

Institute of Child Health, University College, London, & Royal College of Nursing Institute, Oxford (2003) *Paediatric Pain Profile.* Available at: **http://www.ppprofile.org.uk/index.htm**

Johnston, G.B.P., Flood, K., & Spinks, K. (2003) *The Newborn Child, 9th ed.* Edinburgh: Churchill Livingston.

Johnstone, C.C., Ferley, A., & Hendry, C. (2005) The physiological basics of wound healing. *Nursing Standard* **19** (43), 59–66.

Jonas, D.A. (2003) Parents' management of their child's pain in the home following day surgery. *Journal of Child Health Care* **7** (3), 150–162.

Jonas, D.A. (2008) The management of procedural pain in children using self-administered Entonox. In J. Kelsey & G. McEwing (eds.) *Clinical skills in Child Health Practice.* London: Churchill Livingstone.

Kendall, J., Reeves, B.C., Latter, V.S. (2001) Multicentre randomised controlled trial of nasal diamorphine for analgesia in children and teenagers with clinical fractures. *British Medical Journal* **322** (7281), 261–265.

Krechel, S.W. & Bildner, J. (1995) CRIES: a new neonatal postoperative pain measurement score. Initial testing of validation and reliability. *Paediatric Anaesthesia* **5**, 53–61.

Lönnqvist, P.A. & Morton, N.S. (2005) Postoperative analgesia in infants and children. *British Journal of Anaesthesia* **95** (1), 59–68.

Mallett, J. & Bailey, C. (2004) *The Royal Marsden NHS Trust Manual of Clinical Nursing Procedures, 6th ed.* Oxford: Blackwell Science Ltd.

McCaffrey, M. & Beebe, A. (1994) *Pain: Clinical manual for nursing practice. UK Edition.* Aylesbury: Mosby, Times Mirror International Publishers.

Merkel, S., Vopel-Lewis, T., Shayevitz, J., & Malviya, S. (1997) The FLACC: A behavioural scale for scoring postoperative pain in young children. *Pediatric Nursing* **23** (3), 293–297.

Mölnlycke Health Care (2004) *Issues in Paediatric Wound Care: Minimising trauma and pain. Report from an Independent Multidisciplinary Advisory Group.* Mölnlycke Health Care Wound Academy. Available at: **http://www.molnlycke.co.uk/item.asp?id=12809&si=14**

Moore, A., Edwards, J., Barden, J., & McQuay, H. (2003) *Bandolier's Little Book of Pain.* Oxford: Open University Press.

Moules, T. & Ramsey, J. (2008) *The Textbook of Children's and Young People's Nursing, 2nd ed.* Oxford: Blackwell Publishing.

National Institute for Clinical Excellence (2001) *Referral Advice. A guide to appropriate referral from general to specialist services.* National Institute for Clinical Excellence. Available at: **http://www.nice.org.uk/nicemedia/pdf/Referraladvice.pdf**

National Patient Safety Agency (2008) *Introduction to Hand Hygiene* (Videos series). Available at: **http://www.npsa.nhs.uk/cleanyourhands/resource-area/hand-hygiene-video/**

Nichol, M. (2004) *Clinical Nursing Skills.* London: Mosby.

Nursing and Midwifery Council (2008) *Annexe 2— Essential Skills Clusters (ESCs) for Pre-registration Nursing Programmes.* Available at: **http://www.nmc-uk.org/aArticle.aspx?ArticleID=2914**

Parker, L. (2004) Infection control: Maintaining the personal hygiene of patients and staff. *British Journal of Nursing* **13** (8), 474–478.

Pegram, A., Bloomfield, J., & Jones, A. (2007) Clinical skills: Bed making and personal hygiene needs of patients. *British Journal of Nursing* **16** (6), 356–358.

Prenzer, R. (2002) *Nursing Care of the Skin.* UK: Elsevier Science Ltd.

Price, D.L. & Gwin, J.F. (2008) *Paediatric Nursing, 10th ed.* Dublin: Saunders.

Randle, J. & Clarke, M. (2007) *RLO Aseptic Non-touch technique (ANTT).* University of Nottingham. Available at: **http://www.nottingham.ac.uk/nursing/sonet/rlos/placs/antt/index.html**

Retsas, A. & Pinikahana, J. (2000) Manual handling activities and injuries among nurses: An Australian hospital study. *Journal of Advanced Nursing* **31** (4), 875–883.

Rideout, S. (2006) Positioning, handling and exercises. In E. Trigg & T.A. Mohammed (eds.) *Practices in Children's Nursing Guidelines for Hospital and Community, 2nd ed.* London: Churchill Livingstone.

Royal College of Nursing (2001) *The Recognition and Assessment of Acute Pain in Children. Implementation Guide.* London: Royal College of Nursing. Available at: **http://www.rcn.org.uk/development/practice/clinicalguidelines/pain/2000_guideline**

Sales, R. & Utting, J. (2002) Manual handling and nursing children. *Paediatric Nursing* **14** (2), 36–42.

Simons, J., Franck, L., & Roberson, E. (2001) Parent involvement in children's pain care: Views of parents and nurses. *Journal of Advanced Nursing*, **36** (4), 591–599.

Simons, J. & Moseley, L. (2009) Influences on nurses' scoring of children's post-operative pain. *Journal of Child Health Care*, **13** (2), 101–115.

Smith, L., Coleman, V., & Bradshaw, M. (2002) *Family-centred Care: Concept Theory and Practice.* Hampshire: Palgrave Publishers Ltd.

Stevens, B., Yamada, J., & Ohlsson, A. (2004) Sucrose for analgesia in newborn infants undergoing painful procedures. *Cochrane Database of Systematic Reviews.* Issue 3. Art. No.: CD001069. DOI: 10.1002/14651858.CD001069.pub2.

Strategy for the Control of Antimicrobial Resistance in Ireland (2001) *Guidelines for Hand Hygiene in Irish Health Care Settings.* Ireland: Health Service Executive. Available at: **http://www.hpsc.ie/hpsc/Publications**

Suddaby, E.C., Barnett, S., & Facteau, L. (2005) Skin breakdown in acute pediatrics. *Dermatology Nursing* **18** (2), 155–161.

Taquino, L.T. (2000) Promoting wound healing in the neonatal setting: Process versus protocol. *Journal of Perinatal Nursing*, **14** (1), 104–118.

Trigg, E. & Mohammed, T. (eds.) (2006) *Practices in Children's Nursing: Guidelines for Hospital and Community, 2nd ed.* London: Churchill Livingstone.

Trotter, S. (2004) Care of the newborn: Proposed new guidelines. *British Journal of Midwifery* **12** (3), 152–157.

Ulyatt, J. (2007) Eye care. In A. Glasper, A. McEwing, & J. Richardson (eds.) *Oxford Handbook of Children's and Young People's Nursing.* New York: Oxford University Press.

Watret, L. & McFarlane, D. (2004) Audit of wound management practice. *Journal of Community Nursing Online.* Available at: **http://www.jcn.co.uk/journal.asp?MonthNum=07&YearNum=2004&Type=backissue&ArticleID=705**

Waugh, A. & Grant, A. (2007) *Ross and Wilson: Anatomy and Physiology in Health and Illness, 10th ed.* Edinburgh: Churchill Livingstone.

Williams, D.G., Hatch, D.J., & Howard, R.F. (2001) Codeine phosphate in paediatric medicine. *British Journal of Anaesthesia* **86** (3), 413–421.

Williams D.G., Patel, A., & Howard, R.F. (2002) Pharmacogenetics of codeine metabolism in an urban population of children and its implications for analgesic reliability. *British Journal of Anaesthesia* **89** (6), 839–845.

Williams, G. (2006) *Perioperative Analgesic Pharmacology in Children*. Anaesthesia UK. Available at **http://www.frca.co.uk/article. aspx?articleid=100635**

Williams, J. (2007) In A. Glasper, A. McEwing & J. Richardson. *Oxford Handbook of Children's and Young People's Nursing*. Oxford: Oxford University Press.

Willis, M.H.W., Merkel, S.I., Voepel-Lewis, T., & Malviya, S. (2003) FLACC Behavioral Pain Assessment Scale: A comparison with the child's self-report. *Pediatric Nursing* **29** (3), 195–198.

Wilson, D. (2007) In M.J. Hockenberry & D. Wilson. *Wong's Nursing Care of Infants and Children, 8th ed.* St. Louis: Mosby.

Wong, D.L. (2000) *Translations of Wong-Baker FACES Pain Rating Scale*. Available at: **http://www3.us.elsevierhealth.com/ WOW/facesTranslations.html**

Wong, D.L., Hockenberry, M.J., Wilson, D. Perry, S., & Lowdermilk, D.L. (1999) *Maternal Child Nursing Care*. St. Louis: Mosby.

Wong, D.L., Hockenberry-Eaton, M., Wilson, D., Winkelstein, M., & Schwartz, P. (2001) *Whaley and Wong's Essentials of Pediatric Nursing, 5th ed.* St Louis: Mosby.

Workman, B.A. & Cooper, N. (2003) Beginning the assessment process. In B.A. Workman & C.L. Bennett. *Key Nursing Skills*. London: Whurr Publishers Ltd.

World Health Organization (2008) *WHO's pain ladder*. Available at: **http://www.who.int/cancer/ palliative/painladder/en/**

Further reading and URLs

Cole, A. (1994) Staff hide back pain for fear of dismissal. *Nursing Times* **90** (16), 9.

Howard, R., Carter, B., Curry, J., *et al.* (2008) Good practice in postoperative and procedural pain management. *Pediatric Anesthesia* **18**, 1–81. Available at: **http://www.blackwell-synergy. com/toc/pan/18/s**

Swain, J., Pufahl, E., Williamson, G.R. (2003) Do they practice what we teach? A survey of manual handling practice amongst pre-registration student nurses. *Journal of Clinical Nursing* **12**, 297–306

Drug administration

CAROL BARRON AND ELEANOR HOLLYWOOD

Skills

Introduction

By the end of this chapter you will be introduced to the concepts of **pharmacokinetics** and pharmacodynamics with specific emphasis on the infant, child, and young person. You will be presented with the current evidenced-based practice in relation to differing routes of drug administration in children and young people, underpinned by a firm rationale throughout. The key points to consider when administering medications via differing routes to children will be explored. Throughout this chapter the importance and method of drug calculations and mental mathematics will be highlighted, as befits their

importance in the safe preparation and administration of all medications.

Learning outcomes

It is anticipated that you will be able to do the following once you have read and studied this chapter:
- Discuss pharmacokinetics and pharmacodynamics as they relate to drug administration with children.
- Understand the mathematical calculations required to accurately prepare and administer medications in children.
- Understand the key nursing skills required to administer medications to children and young people via differing routes.

Drug development, children, and young people

Historically, drug development specifically for children was only conducted for common disorders/diseases where medication was part of the accepted treatment. Examples are medicines for epilepsy or asthma, antibiotics, or vaccines (Rose, 2005). Because the numbers of children are small in comparison with adults, and the child population is subdivided into age groups from neonates to teenagers, pharmaceutical companies are governed by the commercial market. Consequently they assign limited resources to drug development in the child population because of more limited profit margins. However, this situation is changing, as the European Union established a European Network for Drug Investigation in Children in 1998, with a commitment to improve both clinical use and research into drugs for children (Van den Anker & Choonara, 1999). An international meta-register of controlled clinical trials has been created where particular emphasis is placed on paediatric aspects (Bonati *et al.*, 2001). All of these initiatives serve to change the prevailing view of children as 'therapeutic orphans' to an acknowledgement that children are consumers of healthcare services and as such have the right both ethically and morally to medications that are designed and trialled for them specifically.

General principles of pharmacology: Pharmacokinetics

Pharmacokinetics is the study of the movement of a drug through the body over time, and addresses the absorption from the site of administration, **distribution** throughout the body, **metabolism** of the drug, and its **elimination** from the body (Kanneh, 2002a). In other words, what the body does to a drug after it is taken. As identified by Kanneh (1998b; 2002b), a drug must leave its site of administration, enter into the bloodstream, and reach and be present in an appropriate concentration at its site of action before producing the desired effect. The pharmacokinetics of many drugs varies with age (Kearns, 1998). The underlying principles of pharmacokinetics—absorption, distribution, metabolism, and elimination—will now be discussed in more detail.

Absorption

Absorption is the movement of drugs from their site of administration into the vascular bed. Drugs must have the ability to penetrate cell membranes. For a drug to move through one cell requires that it first move across the cell membrane into the cell, pass across the cell, and then cross the cell membrane again in order to leave the cell. This is true whether the cells are in the skin, the lining of a blood vessel, or an internal organ such as the liver. In many cases, in order for a substance to reach its site of action, it must pass through several membrane barriers. The process is influenced by the **formulation** of the drug, its chemical

properties, the patient's blood flow, the surface area exposed to the drug, contact time of the drug with the absorption site, and route of administration (Kanneh, 2002b).

The selected route of administration is critical in determining the drug dosage and influences the rate and even the extent of drug absorption because of an important pharmacokinetic concept known as **bioavailability**, which is the fraction of the drug dose that is absorbed into the systemic circulation following an extra-vascular administration. Orally administered drugs pass through the liver twice, first after absorption from the intestine via the hepatic portal vein, and second for final metabolism in readiness for excretion from the body. **First-pass metabolism** describes the metabolism of a drug in the liver after oral administration, before it enters the systemic circulation (Kanneh, 2002a). Consequently, the amount of drug that reaches the site of action after this first-pass effect is reduced. Examples of drugs that undergo extensive first-pass metabolism are paracetamol and morphine.

Distribution

Distribution refers to the movement of the drug into the body tissues. The Volume of Distribution (VD) is the pharmacological concept that addresses drug distribution (Schmalbach & Hoekelman, 1997). After a drug enters the systemic circulation it is distributed throughout the body in the blood, passing across various barriers to reach its site of action. The rate at which drug molecules enter specific body tissue depends on two factors. The first is the rate of blood flow through the tissue. Drugs become diluted by the plasma volume of the entire cardiovascular system after gaining access to the bloodstream, the rate being dependent on the route of administration. As the total body water is higher in infants and young children, they will have a higher volume of distribution of water-soluble drugs. Secondly, the ease with which molecules pass through the capillary membranes also affects this mechanism.

The movement of drugs in and out of capillaries is influenced by each drug's chemical properties. Passive transfer is the most common way for drugs to cross cell membranes. Passive diffusion means the movement of substances down a concentration gradient, and the process does not require energy. For example, if the drug is present in the gastrointestinal tract in a greater concentration than it is in the bloodstream, then a concentration gradient is said to exist. A concentration gradient exists when there is more of a substance in one area than in another area. When the drug starts moving out of the gastrointestinal tract it is moving from an area of higher concentration to an area of lower concentration, i.e. it is moving down its concentration gradient. The presence of the concentration gradient will carry the drug through the cell membrane and into the circulation. The drug will be transported until the concentrations of drug are equal on either side of the cell membrane.

The volume of distribution of drugs in children changes with age because of changes in body composition (especially the extracellular and total body water spaces) and plasma protein binding. Higher doses (per kilogram of body weight) of water-soluble drugs are required in younger children because a higher percentage of their body weight is water. Conversely, lower doses are required to avoid toxicity as children grow older because of the decline in water as a percentage of body weight.

Metabolism or biotransformation

The primary organ for drug metabolism or **biotransformation** is the liver. Other important metabolic sites include the lungs, kidney, blood, gastrointestinal tract, and the skin. Drugs are metabolized by metabolic and enzymatic reactions within the liver. The cytochrome P-450 (CYP450) enzyme system is the most important known system for drug metabolism. The enzymatic breakdown of a medication usually results in partial or complete loss of its therapeutic effects. Enzyme maturation occurs at varying rates, with neonates metabolizing drugs at a rate several times lower than that seen in adults. This immaturity of drug-metabolizing enzyme activity may account for the marked toxicity of drugs in the very young (Kearns et al., 2003). Important developmental changes in the biotransformation of drugs in neonates and infants prompts the need for age-appropriate dose regimens for many drugs, such as the methylxanthines, third-generation cephalosporins, and morphine.

Excretion

Drug excretion describes the movement of drugs or their metabolites from tissue cells back into the systemic circulation. The kidneys play a major role in the excretion of drugs following hepatic biotransformation. Because drugs are small particles, they are filtered into the kidneys and then reabsorbed into the bloodstream. As the drug becomes concentrated inside the nephrons, the drug itself is reabsorbed into the plasma. The kidneys alone cannot eliminate drugs from the body. Some other mechanism must overcome the problem of re-absorption, and this is biotransformation, where the drug is enzymatically 'transformed' in the liver into a compound that is less fat soluble and therefore less capable of being reabsorbed. Hepatic biotransformation results in the conversion of fat-soluble into water-soluble metabolites that are poorly reabsorbed once they are filtered into the renal tubules. These metabolites are then transported into the bloodstream to the kidneys for excretion.

Tubular excretion of weak acids progressively increases with age, reaching adult values at between one and three years of age (Suggs, 2000; Kanneh, 2002b). Glomerular filtration rate (GFR) is low at birth but increases dramatically due to a fall in renal vascular resistance and a subsequent increase in the renal blood flow. GFR reaches adult levels by six months, with tubular secretion maturing slightly later, reaching adult values at about eight months. Because decreased renal function causes decreased renal drug clearance and a prolonged drug plasma **half-life**, lower doses are prescribed or their administration intervals widened in order to avoid drug toxicity in children (Kanneh, 2002b).

Pharmacodynamics

Pharmacodynamics is the study of what the drug does to the body including its biochemical and physiological action and effects of drugs in the body. This includes how drugs operate at their site of action, their mechanism, and their specificity. Medications work through two main mechanisms once they reach their site of action:

1 Alter the cell environment through physical or chemical processes.
2 Alter cell function, mainly through drug-receptor interactions.

Table 7.1 Physical and chemical processes that alter cell function

Physical processes	Example
Alteration of surface tension	Stool softener reducing the surface tension of faeces
Absorption	Activated charcoal given PO to absorb harmful chemicals in the GI tract

Chemical processes	Example
Alterations in pH	Antacids given PO to neutralize gastric acidity
Alterations in body fluid chemistry	Ammonium chloride given IV to reverse metabolic acidosis

Table 7.1 summarizes the physical and chemical processes that alter cell function.

The receptor

Receptors are proteins. They are located on the surface of the cell or inside it and they have two important functions:

1 To bind the body's own chemical messenger chemicals such as hormones and neurotransmitters.
2 To convert the binding event into a signal that the cell can recognize and respond to.

(Greenstein & Gould, 2008)
Receptors have two important characteristics, their specificity and their affinity.

Specificity

Receptors are designed so that they recognize specific chemical configurations, e.g. epinephrine receptors such as β adrenoceptors will bind norepinephrine, but will not bind progesterone. They will also recognize chemicals that are taken into the body, e.g. epinephrine receptors on bronchiolar smooth muscle will bind synthetic epinephrine—e.g. chemicals such as salbutamol.

Affinity

Receptors that are designed to recognize and bind certain chemicals will bind these chemicals tightly. This is called having 'a high affinity' for the chemical and is important as even at very low concentrations of that chemical the receptor will pick up the chemical. Therefore the dose can be kept to a minimum.

Agonists, antagonists, and partial agonists

Agonists

A drug is termed an '**agonist**' when the drug occupies and activates a receptor, thereby producing a cellular response. In other words, an agonist combines with the receptor and produces a response, e.g. terbutaline (bronchodilator).

Antagonist

A drug is termed an '**antagonist**' when it occupies a receptor but does not activate the receptor. The antagonist occupies the space that would normally be occupied by an endogenous **ligand** or an agonist, thereby inhibiting the ability of the endogenous ligand or agonist to cause its effect. Antihistamines are an example of antagonists.

Partial agonist

A **partial agonist** is a drug that is able to both stimulate and block at a receptor. Partial agonists do not have the same maximal effect on a receptor as a full agonist.

The log 10 dose response curve

The dose response curve is a simple x-y graph relating the amount of a drug to the response of the receptor. The x-axis plots the concentration of a drug and the y-axis plots the response. The dose response curve can tell you a significant amount of information about the drug's potency (concentration of a drug required to elicit a biological effect), efficacy (the ability of a drug to elicit an effect—it is the limit of the dose response curve on the response y-axis), and action as an antagonist.

How changes throughout childhood affect the metabolism of medications

Both pharmacokinetics and pharmacodynamics are affected by the age of a child. The term 'child' does not refer to a homogeneous group of children but rather a collection of highly variable subgroups from neonates, infants, and adolescents to young people. Childhood consists of dynamic processes of growth, differentiation, and maturation that set children apart from adults. In addition to growth in physical size, dramatic changes in body proportions, body composition, physiology, neurologic maturation, and psychosocial development take place during infancy and childhood. Age-related differences in pharmacokinetics and pharmacodynamics occur throughout childhood and account for many of the differences between drug doses at various stages of childhood (Summer, 2000). Therefore, children should not be considered as scaled down adults, as the differences in dose are not purely dependent upon body mass.

Growth and development

Growth and development are particularly rapid during the first two years of life. The body weight typically doubles by six months of age and triples by the first birthday. Body length increases by 50% and the body surface area doubles during the first year (Greenstein & Gould, 2008). In pre-school-age children, the ratio of body surface area to body weight, which reflects the relative size of the skin as an organ, is approximately 2.5 times that in adults. The calculation of drug dosage must therefore be based on accurate current body weight of the child.

The gastrointestinal tract undergoes many changes during childhood. The absorptive surface area of the gut is relatively greater in the infant than in the adult and the gastric pH is 7–8 at birth and then falls to less than pH 3 during the first one to two hours of life. However, relative hypochlorhydria (low hydrochloric acid production) persists during the first one to two months of life. Premature infants have impaired gastric acid production until after 32 weeks of gestational age. Gastric emptying and gut transit time may be prolonged in premature and ill newborns. On the other hand, healthy infants may have transit times that are shorter than those for adults. Infants have decreased first-pass metabolism of drugs, with increased levels of uptake until the gut mucosa and liver mature. This may lead to greater bio-availability of drugs that undergo significant first-pass metabolism (Trigg & Mohammed, 2006; Greenstein & Gould, 2008).

Protein binding and infancy

Protein binding of drugs can affect drug pharmacodynamics, toxicity, distribution, and elimination. Maturational differences in protein binding are primarily an issue during infancy. Plasma protein binding of drugs is decreased in the newborn and young infant. This is attributed to decreased levels of circulating protein and also to a decreased affinity for certain **ligands**. Decreased binding may also be attributed to competition for binding sites with other drugs or highly bound endogenous substances.

Body weight proportions

The respective proportions of body weight contributed to by fat, protein, and water change during infancy and childhood. At birth, total body water constitutes approximately 80% of body weight. By five months of age, however, total body water accounts for only 60% of body weight and then remains relatively constant. There is a progressive decrease in extracellular water throughout childhood and into young adulthood. As the proportion of body water decreases, the percentage of body weight contributed by fat doubles by four to five months of age. During this time period the major organ systems grow and mature. Puberty is an important period of childhood when accelerated growth and sexual maturation occur. Physiological changes that occur include large growth spurts, which are caused by surges in human growth hormone and other growth factors. There are also gender-specific changes in body composition, with females acquiring a greater proportion of body fat and males having a larger lean muscle mass (Neill & Knowles, 2004).

Renal function in the first year

Glomerular filtration rates and tubular transport mechanisms are all reduced at birth but increase rapidly during the first month of life and reach maturity before the end of the first year. Maturational changes in renal function have profound implications for drug administration for those medicines primarily eliminated in the kidney.

Care and management of drug administration

The ability to calculate drugs accurately is an essential skill for the children's nurse as poor calculation skills can lead to serious drug errors and patient harm. Watt (2003) suggests that medication administration should be viewed as an essential aspect of nursing care practice, as all drug dosages are calculated on the child's body weight with a set dose of all medication being recommended per kilogram of body weight. Please refer to the current *British National Formulary* (BNF) or the BNF child website for up-to-date recommended drug dosages (**http://bnf.org/bnf/**). Effective drug administration requires essential key steps outlined in Table 7.2.

All nurses should be familiar with and follow their national governing body guidelines as well as local community and/or clinical policy in relation to drug administration. Professional and legal responsibilities in the administration of medications to children are examined in much greater depth in both the An Bord Altranais (ABA, 2007) and the Nursing and Midwifery Council (NMC, 2008) guidelines and these are consistently referenced throughout this chapter. In addition to these guidelines, Table 7.3 provides a helpful summary of the five 'rights' of medication that healthcare professionals must abide by.

Table 7.3 The five rights of medication administration (ABA, 2007; NMC, 2008)

The right **medication**	Check the name of the medication against the prescription
The right **patient**	Check the child's name band against the prescription; verify with parent/guardian
The right **dose**	Check that the dose prescribed is correct for the age of the child
The right **route**	Check that the route prescribed is correct for the child and that the correct medication has been selected
The right **time and frequency**	Check that the time and frequency is correct for the child

7.1 Drug calculations

All student nurses must be proficient in standard unit conversions to accurately calculate drug dosages. Metric unit conversions are outlined in Box 7.1.

Table 7.2 Knowledge and numeracy

Knowledge	Numeracy
■ Knowledge of drug administration guidelines	■ Ability to add
	■ Ability to subtract
■ *Standards for Medicines Management* (NMC, 2008)	■ Ability to multiply
	■ Ability to divide
■ *Guidance to Nurses and Midwives on Medication Management* (ABA, 2007)	■ Ability to convert from one unit to another
■ British National Formulary (**www.bnf.org.uk**)	■ Drug calculation formula
■ Five rights of medication administration	

Box 7.1 Unit conversions

■ 1 kilogram (kg)	= 1000 grams (g)
■ 1 gram (g)	= 1000 milligrams (mg)
■ 1 milligram (mg)	= 1000 micrograms (mcg)
■ 1 microgram (mcg)	= 1000 nanograms (ng)

Nursing Alert

All weights and volumes in any equation must be in the same units prior to drug calculation.

In order to convert a larger unit (e.g. mg) to a smaller unit (e.g. mcg) you must multiply by 1000. The decimal point moves three places to the right:

$$0.125 \text{ mg} = 0.\ 1\ 2\ 5 = 125 \text{ mcg}$$

In order to convert a smaller unit (e.g. mcg) to a larger unit (e.g. mg) you divide by 1000.
The decimal point moves three places to the left:

$$125 \text{ mcg} = 1\ 2\ 5.\ 0 = 0.125 \text{ mg}$$

To avoid confusion with calculations:

- Always place a '0' in front of a decimal point, e.g. 0.4.
- Do not add a decimal point at the end unless necessary, e.g. write 2 mg, not 2.0 mg.
- Avoid working with decimals if possible, e.g. write 250 mg rather than 0.25 g.

Drug calculation formula

Example 1:

A child is prescribed oral paracetamol 80 mg. The drug is available as oral suspension with 120 mg in 5 ml.
You **want** 80 mg.
You **have** 120 mg in 5 ml **volume**.
Therefore: 80 mg divided by 120 mg multiplied by 5 ml = answer.
80 divided by 120 multiplied by 5 = 3.3 ml of the drug.

Example 2:

A child is prescribed oral chloral hydrate 250 mg. The drug is available as an elixir containing 200 mg in 5 ml.

Box 7.2 Drug calculation formula

$$\frac{\text{what you } \textbf{want}}{\text{what you } \textbf{have}} \times \text{volume you have it in}$$

You **want** 250 mg.
You **have** 200 mg in 5 ml **volume**.
Therefore: 250 mg divided by 200 mg multiplied by 5 ml = answer.
250 divided by 200 multiplied by 5 = 6.25 ml of the drug.

Drug administration and the role of the student nurse

The administration of drugs under supervision is an integral part of the student nurse's role. The following website is a useful resource for students in relation to all forms of drug calculations: **http://www.testandcalc.com/quiz/index.asp**. A rare occurrence with drug administration is anaphylaxis or anaphylactic shock. This is a systematic allergic reaction, which if untreated can be fatal. The classic symptoms include hives, swelling around the eyes or mouth, and difficulty breathing or swallowing (Greenstein & Gould, 2008). Management includes control of the airway, breathing, and circulation (ABC). Treatment consists of epinephrine (adrenaline), antihistamines, steroids and ongoing management of the ABC.

Differing routes of drug administration

Drugs can be administered to children via numerous different routes (see Box 7.4), although the most common route of administration is the oral route in liquid or solid form.

7.2 Administering oral medications to children

Oral drugs are the preferred route of drug administration for children. The decision to administer medicines to children orally in liquid or solid form depends on the age at which it is safe to do so without the risk of choking (Trigg & Mohammad, 2006) and the likely compliance of the child. Tablets and capsules are not recommended for children under the age of five years (Royal College of Paediatrics and Child Health & Royal College of Nursing, 2002); however, certain medications may only be available in tablet/capsule form. Maintaining dosage accuracy

Box 7.3 Practise your skills!

Exercise 1

1. Divide the following and write as decimals:

   a) 3.78 ÷ 10 =   b) 3.78 ÷ 100 =   c) 3.78 ÷ 1000 =

2. Change the following to grams:

   a) 2.4 kg =   b) 0.75 kg =   c) 1.625 kg =

3. Change the following to milligrams:

   a) 0.655 g =   b) 0.02 g =   c) 4.28 g =

4. Change the following to grams:

   a) 865 mg =   b) 70 mg =   c) 125 mg =

5. Change the following to micrograms:

   a) 0.08 mg =   b) 0.625 mg =   c) 0.098 mg =

6. Change the following to milligrams:

   a) 825 mcg =   b) 95 mcg =   c) 5 mcg =

7. Change the following to nanograms:

   a) 1 mcg =   b) 500 mcg =   c) 0.635 mcg =

Exercise 2

Do the following calculations:

1. A child is prescribed oral paracetamol 360 mg. The drug is available as an oral suspension with 250 mg in 5 ml (Calpol 6 Plus). How much will you need?

2. A child is prescribed oral phenobarbital (phenobarbitone) 45 mg. The drug is available as 15 mg in 5 ml. How much will you need?

3. A child is prescribed IV metronidazole 75 mg. The drug is available as 100 mg in 20 ml. How much will you need?

4. A baby is prescribed 25 mcg of digoxin IV. The drug is available as 500 mcg in 2 ml. How much will you need?

5. A child is prescribed desmopressin 400 ng by subcutaneous injection. The drug is available as 4 mcg in 1 ml. How much will you need?

Exercise 3

1. Emily is 4 years old and weighs 16 kg. She is prescribed ampicillin (Penbritin) IV 400 mg QDS. There are 500 mg in a vial, which has been made up to 10 ml.

   a) How many ml should Emily receive?

   b) How many mg per kg is Emily prescribed?

2. Fionn is 6 days old and weighs 3.5 kg. He is prescribed ranitidine (Zantac) IV 3.5 mg TDS. Each vial contains 50 mg in 2 ml.

   a) How many ml should Fionn receive?

   b) How many mg per kg is Fionn prescribed?

3. Jade is 18 months old and weighs 12.5 kg. She is prescribed sodium valproate (Epilim) PO 62.5 mg BD. There are 200 mg in 5 ml.

   a) How many ml should Jade receive?

   b) How many mg per kg is Jade prescribed?

4. Libby is 6 months old and weighs 7.8 kg. She is prescribed ibuprofen (Brufen) PO 39 mg TDS.

   a) How many ml should Libby receive?

   b) How many mg per kg is Libby prescribed?

5. A prescription states that 5 mmol of potassium chloride (KCl) is to be added to a 500 ml bag of 0.9% NaCl. Each 10 ml vial of KCl contains 20 mmol.

   How many ml of the drug need to be added to the bag of fluids?

6. Quentin is 1 month old and weighs 4.6 kg. He is prescribed folic acid PO 1150 mcg OD. There are 2.5 mg in 5 ml.

   a) How many ml should Quentin receive?

   b) How many mg per kg is Quentin prescribed?

Box 7.4 Routes of drug administration

- Pills
- Tablets
- Enteric-coated preparations
- Capsules
- Sustained-release preparations
- Topical preparations
- Oral liquid preparations

- Transdermal administration
- Rectal administration
- Vaginal administration
- Parenteral administration
- Subcutaneous administration
- Intramuscular injections
- **Intravenous** injections

- Intra-arterial
- **Intra-thecal** injections
- Epidural injections
- Intra-articular
- Sublingual administration
- Intranasal administration
- Others

can be a major challenge in dispensing childhood medications, for example, certain medications are not available in liquid form and whilst tablets could potentially be crushed or split to achieve dosage requirements, this may also affect the drug's physical and chemical properties (Kanneh, 2002a)—see Nursing Alert below. Chewable tablets tend to improve cooperation as children find them easier to swallow after chewing. Fast-dissolving formulations that melt in the saliva within a few seconds of being put in the mouth are a new approach, for example, a very common paediatric analgesic is now available in this format and may have future significance for children. At present, liquid formulations are preferred to solid dosages in young children (Breithkreutz *et al.*, 1999). Oral medications for children are available in a number of different formats, which are listed in **Box 7.5**.

Medicines can be administered by spoon, measuring cup and spoon, or specifically designed oral plastic syringe (these syringes cannot be attached to intravenous tubing, thus preventing a medication route error). Some medicines have a high sugar content that can damage children's teeth if used for prolonged periods. Good oral hygiene

and rinsing the mouth with water post-administration of the medicine will help to prevent tooth decay.

Nursing Alert

Never crush or split capsules or enteric-coated medications as this will alter the absorption rate and effectiveness of the medication (Watt, 2003). Appropriate advice must always be sought before crushing medicines (ABA, 2007; NMC, 2008).

Procedure: Administration of oral medicines

Preparation

Nursing Alert

- Measure all liquids using a syringe or medicine cup.

- If using a medicine cup, ensure the cup is on a flat surface and measure at eye level.

Safety: Adhere to the five rights of medication administration:
- Right medication.
- Right patient.
- Right dose.
- Right route.
- Right time (ABA, 2007; NMC, 2008).

Equipment

- Correct medicine.
- Non-sterile gloves.
- Oral syringe, medicine cup, spoon.
- Water or juice to drink after administration.
- Drug administration chart and pen.

Box 7.5 Format of oral medications

Liquid
- Syrup
- Suspension
- Elixir
- Solution
- Oil

Solid
- Tablet
- Capsule
- Lozenge
- Granules

Consent and communication

As discussed in Chapter Two, family centred care is a key principle in children's nursing. Hence encouraging and supporting parents to be involved in their child's medication administration will help maintain partnership in care (Watt, 2003). It is very helpful to determine the child's prior experience of taking medicines. Parents know their children best, therefore ask the parent how the child prefers to take medicines, and this information will help you to plan your approach to the procedure. Effective communication and active listening are essential components of medication administration, therefore explain to the child in age-appropriate language why it is necessary to take the medicine and ask the child and parent if they have any questions. Listen to them and allay any fears or anxieties that they may be experiencing. As mentioned in Chapter Two, play is an extremely useful tool for explaining the procedure to the child, eliminating fear, and gaining their cooperation in the administration of all medications. Play is one of the most effective tools used to reduce anxiety, stress, and tension in the hospitalized child (Haiat *et al.*, 2003). Gain consent.

Step-by-step guide to oral drug administration

Procedure

Rationale

	Procedure	Rationale
1	Check prescription and adhere to the five rights of medication administration. All checks must be carried out with another registered nurse or in accordance with local hospital policy. Adhere to your governing body guidelines and local healthcare setting policy.	To prevent medication administration error and ensure the safe administration of medication. Double-checking is common practice in paediatric nursing care for safety reasons.
2	Wash hands and don gloves.	To prevent the spread of micro–organisms.
3	Prepare and carefully measure medicine for administration (see 'Preparation' section above). If a tablet needs to be crushed first, check with the hospital pharmacy department or the *BNF for Children* (British National Formulary, 2008).	To prevent incorrect amount being administered and ensure correct measurement of liquids. Certain tablets are unsuitable for crushing as crushing alters how the medicine is absorbed in the body.
4	Check the child's name band against the prescription chart/ kardex. Ask parent to verify the child's name and date of birth.	To prevent medication administration error. To ensure the correct identity of the child.
5	You must take into consideration the age of the child and their developmental level when preparing them for the procedure.	This will determine the most effective and appropriate way to hold the child during the procedure.
	Infants Ask parent to hold infant firmly in their arms. Ensure that the child's head is in the upright position.	Infants are very attached to their parents and separation from their parent may cause distress and anxiety for them. This position helps to promote swallowing and prevent choking or aspiration.
	Toddlers Ask toddler to sit on their parent's lap or on a chair or bed.	Toddlers are naturally inquisitive and often very independent.

Avoid holding toddlers firmly.	Toddlers should be encouraged to participate
Sit at eye level in front of the toddler and explain with the use of play why they need to take the medicine.	independently in taking their medicine. Incorporating play into the procedure encourages participation and reduces fear for the child (Haiat *et al.*, 2003).
Older children	This position helps to promote swallowing and
Ask child to sit upright on a chair or bed.	prevent choking or aspiration.
Older children must be encouraged to participate fully in medication administration.	Participation promotes independence in the older child. Children with chronic conditions need to gain independence so that they can manage their illness effectively (Horner, 1999).

6 | **Administering of the medication will depend on the age of the child and their developmental level.** | |

Infants	
Encourage the infant to open their mouth; play technique may be helpful.	Administration will be more effective if the infant voluntarily opens their mouth.
Instil the liquid medicine slowly into the infant's mouth using an oral syringe.	Oral syringes prevent damage to the infant's oral mucosa and gums.
Gently press the syringe onto the infant's tongue at the front of their mouth.	This will encourage the swallowing reflex.
Stroke the infant's cheek or chin.	This will encourage the swallowing reflex.
If the infant takes a soother, place their soother into their mouth.	This will encourage the swallowing reflex.
It may be helpful to use a spoon to retrieve any medicine from the chin that may be lost due to natural outward tongue thrust (Watt, 2003).	

Toddlers	
Ask toddler if they are ready for their medicine.	To gain cooperation of the toddler.
Ask toddler to open their mouth. Use play as a therapeutic tool to get toddler to open their mouth.	Administration will be more effective if the toddler voluntarily opens their mouth.
Instil the liquid medicine into the toddler's mouth using an oral syringe or spoon. Some toddlers may prefer to drink their medicine from a medicine cup.	You will have decided with the parent if an oral syringe or spoon or medicine cup is to be used, so that the method is the most suitable for the individual child.
Offer a drink after the medicine has been swallowed.	This will dispel any residual taste in the toddler's mouth.
Praise the toddler after they have taken their medicine.	Praise will have a positive effect on behaviour.

Older children	
Ask child if they are ready for their medicine.	To gain cooperation of the child.
If child is taking medicine in tablet form, give the child the tablets in a medicine cup.	To prevent the spread of micro-organisms.
Also give the child a drink.	To swallow the tablets with.
Tell child to take their time and demonstrate a relaxed and encouraging attitude.	Learning how to take tablets can be difficult for children. It is important not to rush the child and promote success through encouragement.
Praise child after they have swallowed tablets.	Praise will have a positive effect on behaviour.

7 Stay with the child until the medicine is fully taken.

Do not leave medicine on bedside lockers.

Do not leave medicine with parents or children.

It is the responsibility of the children's nurse to ensure the safe administration of medicines to children.

This is unsafe because another child could take the medicine.

This is unsafe because the children's nurse will not know how much of the medicine was actually taken.

8 Dispose of equipment as per local hospital policy.

To prevent the spread of micro-organisms.

9 Remove gloves and wash hands.

To prevent the spread of micro-organisms.

10 Evaluate child for desired effect of medicine or for possible side effects of medication.

Evaluation is an essential component of the nursing process. It is important that the desired effect of medicine is achieved. If the desired effect is not achieved alternative action will be necessary.

11 Document procedure and evaluation in nursing notes.

Documentation necessary to ensure continuity of care.

7.3 Administering eye (optic) and ear (otic) medications to children

Although eye and ear drops are not a painful procedure they can cause a certain level of discomfort for a child and parent. Hence it is important to explain to the child (and parent/s) beforehand how he/she may feel and what the sensations may be like. As mentioned earlier in Chapter Four, children generally cope better with procedures when they know what to expect. Eye drops can cause irritation for the child and blurred vision. Ear drops can also cause a certain level of discomfort on installation. Eye and ear drops are administered by dropper or syringe. Once opened, all eye and ear drops are patient exclusive. Individual containers must be provided for each child (Watkinson & Seewoodhary, 2008; BNF, 2008) to prevent contamination. If separate bottles are being used for each eye, they must be labelled 'left' and 'right'.

Procedure: Administration of eye and ear medicines

Preparation

Safety: Adhere to the five rights of medication administration:

- Right medication.
- Right patient.
- Right dose.
- Right route.
- Right time (ABA, 2007; NMC, 2008).

1 Check prescription. All checks must be carried out with another registered nurse or in accordance with local hospital policy.

2 Wash hands and don gloves.

3 Ensure you have the patient-specific bottle of solution.

4 Check the child's name band against the prescription chart/kardex.

5 Ask parent to verify the child's name and date of birth.

Nursing Alert

Many eye/ear drops expire shortly after opening. The date opened must be documented on each bottle. Check expiry date and date the medication was first opened.

Equipment

- Correct eye/ear drops.
- Non-sterile gloves.
- Eyedropper.
- Drug administration chart and pen.

Consent and communication

As with oral medications, ask the child's parents about their experience with these medicines and any preferences. Encourage the family to be involved to gain cooperation and gain consent. **Box 7.6** outlines some distraction techniques that nurses can ask parents to try during clinical procedures.

Step-by-step guide to eye drug administration

Procedure	Rationale
1 **Adhere to the five rights of medication administration and ensure you have prepared as advised under 'safety' before this box.**	To prevent medication administration error and ensure the safe administration of medication.
2 **You must take into consideration the age of the child and their developmental level when preparing them for the procedure.**	This will determine the most effective and appropriate way to hold the child during the procedure. Nursing strategies are determined by the child's developmental level (Arnold & Underman Boggs, 2007).
Infants and toddlers **Lay the infant supine or across the parent's lap. Alternatively, ask toddler to sit on parent's lap and look up to the ceiling.**	This position allows easy access to the eye area and will also facilitate the drops to go directly into the eye.
Older children **Ask the child if they are ready for their eye drops. Ask the child to lie supine on their bed with their head straight.**	This allows the child to participate in their care and make decisions about their care. This position allows easy access to the eye area and will also facilitate the drops to go directly into the eye.
3 **Cleaning the eye:** **The eye must be clean before eye drops are administered.**	This will ensure maximum effect (Watkinson & Seewodhary, 2008).
Cleanse the eye with cotton wool/gauze and normal saline if the eye appears sticky (Marsden & Shaw, 2003).	This will remove any old residual medication or any crusting around the eye.
Move from the inner canthus of the eye outwards. Use a new cotton wool ball/gauze for each sweep of the eye.	To prevent the spread of micro-organisms. To prevent possible contamination.

Gently rest your dominant hand against the child's forehead. With your other hand gently pull down on the lower eyelid to expose the conjunctival sac.	This will stabilize your hand and the child's head.
Alternatively, with your non-dominant hand gently pull down and out on the lower eyelid to form a cup effect for the medication.	This method is more effective for a child who is sitting upright for the procedure.

 Administration:

Eye drops

Using the dropper instil the prescribed amount of drops into the conjunctival sac of the eye.	This ensures correct placement of the medication.
Be careful not to touch the eye lashes, eye, or eyelid with the dropper.	To prevent contamination (Watkinson & Seewoodhary, 2008; Watt, 2003) and trauma.
Ask the child to close his/her eyes for one minute post-administration.	Facilitates the medication being dispersed over the eye.
If the infant/child refuses to open their eyes, drop the prescribed amount of drops onto the inner canthus of the eye and encourage the child to open their eyes.	When the child opens their eyes the medication will flow into the conjunctiva.

Eye ointment

If eye ointment and eye drops are prescribed at the same time, the eye drops must be administered first.	Ointment 'waterproofs' the eye. For eye drops to be absorbed correctly they must be administered before ointment (Marsden & Shaw, 2003).
Squeeze the ointment tube from the end.	This will prime the nozzle with ointment medication.
Place a thin strip of the ointment along the conjunctival sac going from the inner canthus of the eye to the outer canthus.	Ensures correct coverage of the eye.
Ask the child to close his/her eyes for one minute post-administration.	Facilitates the medication being dispersed over the eye.
Wipe excess medication away with a tissue.	This will prevent weeping of medication around the eye.

5 Dispose of equipment as per local hospital policy.	To prevent the spread of micro-organisms.
6 Remove gloves and wash hands.	To prevent the spread of micro-organisms.
7 Return medication to correct storage area.	To ensure safe storage of medication.
8 Observe child for possible side effects of medication and report. Side effects of ophthalmic medications may include redness or oedema around the eyes.	If the child experiences side effects of the medication alternative action will be necessary.
9 Document procedure and evaluation in nursing notes.	Documentation is necessary to ensure continuity of care.

Administration of ear medicines

Step-by-step guide to ear drug administration

Step	Rationale
1 **Adhere to the five rights of medication administration and ensure you have prepared as advised under 'safety' before this box.**	To prevent medication administration error and ensure the safe administration of medication.
2 **Preparation:** **Infants and toddlers** **Lay the infant across the parent's lap. Use distraction techniques as necessary.**	This will facilitate entry of the drops into the ear canal.
Older children **Ask the child to lie supine with his/her head turned to one side.**	This will facilitate entry of the drops into the ear canal.
Administration: **3** **In children under three years, gently pull the pinna of the ear down and back (Watt, 2003). In children over three years, gently pull the pinna of the ear upwards and back (Watt, 2003).**	This will straighten the external auditory canal for effective drop administration.
4 **Holding the dropper 2 cm above the ear canal, instil the prescribed amount of drops into the ear.**	This will facilitate the entry of the medication into the ear canal and prevent contamination of the dropper.
Be careful not to touch the ear with the dropper.	Prevents contamination of the dropper.
5 **Gently massage the area anterior to the ear canal.**	Facilitates the entry of the medication into the ear canal.
6 **Have the infant/child lie supine with their head turned for 2–3 minutes.**	Allows adequate time for the medication to enter the ear canal.
7 **Repeat on the other ear as prescribed.**	So that both ears are treated as necessary.
8 **Praise the child for holding still during the procedure.**	Praise will have a positive effect on desired behaviour.
Comfort the child post-procedure if they are upset.	Ear drop administration can be invasive and frightening for the child.
9 **Dispose of equipment as per local hospital policy.**	Prevents the spread of micro-organisms.
10 **Remove gloves and wash hands.**	Prevents the spread of micro-organisms.
11 **Return medication to correct storage area.**	Ensures safe storage of medication.
12 **Observe child for possible side effects of medication and report.**	If the child experiences side effects alternative action will be necessary.
13 **Document procedure and evaluation in nursing notes.**	Documentation is necessary to ensure continuity of care.

Box 7.6 Distraction techniques during clinical procedures

The use of distraction or play diverts the infant's attention from the procedure. Asking the parent to distract the infant gives the parent a role and makes them feel included in their infant's care. Suggestions include:

Infants

Ask the parent to sing to the infant or dangle a colourful toy to get the infant's attention.

Toddler

Play some cartoons on a nearby television and ask the parent to talk to their child about the cartoons.

7.4 Administering nebulizers to children

A nebulizer is a device that is designed to atomize drugs into a fine mist for the purpose of inhalation into the lungs (Booker, 2007). Nebulizers are commonly used to deliver bronchodilators, steroids, and antibiotics. This section will discuss the use of jet nebulizers as these are most commonly used in the community and hospital settings. When preparing the child and family, follow the guidelines already discussed and in addition explain the desired effect of the nebulizer to the child and parent/s prior to administration. Differing equipment and techniques are utilized in the administration of nebulizers to children of various age groups.

Nursing Alert

Nebulizer therapy can be a frightening experience for a child who has not received a nebulizer before. The children's nurse should incorporate play into the procedure to encourage participation and reduce fear in the child.

Procedure: Administration of a nebulizer

Preparation

Safety: Adhere to the five rights of medication administration:

- Right medication.
- Right patient.
- Right dose.
- Right route.
- Right time (ABA, 2007; NMC, 2008).

1 Check prescription. All checks must be carried out with another registered nurse or in accordance with local hospital policy.
2 Wash hands and don gloves.

Nursing Alert

Peak flow measurements may need to be recorded pre- and post-administration of the nebulizer.

Equipment

- Correct medication.
- Nebulizer.
- Mask or baby inhaler.
- Tubing.
- Oxygen/air supply.
- Drug administration chart and pen.

7.5 Administering rectal medications to children

Rectal medication administration in the paediatric healthcare setting is not routinely used, due to its invasive nature (Greenstein & Gould, 2008). However, at times it may be necessary for a child who is vomiting and unable to tolerate the oral route or for a child who cannot take medicine orally. Rectal medication is administered in the form of suppositories or enemas. When preparing the child and family, follow the guidelines already discussed.

Procedure: Administration of rectal medications

Preparation

Safety: Adhere to the five rights of medication administration:

Step-by-step guide to nebulizer drug administration

Procedure	Rationale
1	**Adhere to the five rights of medication administration and ensure you have prepared as advised under 'safety' before this box.**	To prevent medication administration error and ensure the safe administration of medication.
2	**Prepare medicine for administration.** **Unscrew the top of the nebulizer chamber. Snap open the top of the solution to be nebulized.**	In paediatric care the dose per plastic 'nebule' of the solution to be nebulized is often greater than the prescribed dose for the infant/child. The prescribed dose must be measured out of the plastic 'nebule'.
3	**Measure the prescribed amount of the drug using a needle and syringe.**	
4	**Safely dispose of the needle.** **Pour the prescribed amount into the chamber of the nebulizer.** **Safely dispose of the syringe.**	Prevents needle stick injury. Ensures only the prescribed amount will be administered. Prevents possible hazard.
5	**Connect tubing to the bottom of the chamber.** **Connect face mask to nebulizer.**	Provides air/oxygen supply to nebulize medication. Face masks are recommended for infants and children (Booker, 2007).
6	**Check the child's name band against the prescription chart/kardex.** **Ask parent to verify the child's name and date of birth.**	Prevents medication administration error. This is to ensure the correct identity of the child.
7	**You must take into consideration the age of the child and their developmental level when preparing them for the procedure:**	Nursing strategies are determined by the child's developmental age (Arnold & Underman Boggs, 2007). This will determine the most effective and appropriate way to hold the child during the procedure.
	Infants **Position infant upright in the cot or in their parent's lap. Ensure infant is positioned safely and securely.**	This position maximizes lung expansion.
	Toddlers **Ask toddler to sit upright on their parent's lap or on a chair or their bed.** **Avoid holding toddlers firmly.**	This position maximizes lung expansion.
	Sit at eye level in front of the toddler and explain with the use of play why they need to take the nebulizer.	Toddlers are naturally inquisitive and should be encouraged to participate independently in taking their nebulizer. Incorporating play into the procedure encourages participation and reduces fear in the child.
	Older children **Ask child to sit upright on a chair or bed.** **Older children must be encouraged to participate fully in their nebulizer therapy.**	This position maximizes lung expansion. This promotes independence in the older child. Children with chronic conditions need to gain independence so that they can manage their illness effectively.

8 Administering the medication:

Infants

Gently place face mask over infant's mouth.
Ask parent to hold face mask to infant's face if it is not possible to place the elastic support around the infant's head.

Face masks must be applied closely to the face to ensure adequate nebulization of the medication (Booker, 2007).

Post-administration of the nebulizer, clean the infant's face.

This ensures that there is no residual medication on the infant's face and promotes comfort for the infant.

Toddlers

Ask toddler if they are ready for their nebulizer.

Gains cooperation of the toddler.

Use play as a therapeutic tool; give teddy his nebulizer first.

This will alleviate possible fear and gain the cooperation of the toddler.

Turn on the air/oxygen supply to 6–8 litres (Booker, 2007; Poter-Jones, 2000).

This vaporizes the medication.

Praise the toddler after they have taken their nebulizer.

Praise will have a positive effect on desired behaviour.

Older children

Ask child if they are ready for their nebulizer.

Gains cooperation of the child.

Ask the child to sit upright in a chair or on their bed.

Maximizes lung expansion and promotes comfort.

Use play as a diversional tool: get the child to choose a book to read; ask the child if they would like to play their Nintendo DS or listen to their iPod.

This will distract the child from the procedure.

9 Stay with the child until the nebulizer is fully taken.

It is the responsibility of the children's nurse to ensure the safe administration of medicines to children.

Do not leave nebulizer on bedside lockers.

This is unsafe because another child could ingest the medication.

Do not leave medicine with parents or children.

This is unsafe because the children's nurse will not know how much of the nebulizer was actually taken.

10 Dispose of equipment as per local hospital policy.

Prevents the spread of micro-organisms.

11 Wash hands.

Prevents the spread of micro-organisms.

12 Evaluate child for desired effect of nebulizer or for possible side effects of medication.
NOTE: Peak flow measurements may need to be recorded pre- and post-administration of the nebulizer.

Evaluation is an essential component of the nursing process. It is important that the desired effect of medicine is achieved.

13 Document procedure and evaluation in nursing notes.

Documentation is necessary to ensure continuity of care.

Step-by-step guide to rectal drug administration

Procedure

Rationale

Procedure	Rationale
1 Adhere to the five rights of medication administration and ensure you have prepared as advised under 'safety' before this box.	To prevent medication administration error and ensure the safe administration of medication.
2 Prepare medicine for administration. Avoid cutting suppositories.	Cutting suppositories prevents the nurse from knowing the exact amount of medication being administered.
3 Check the child's name band against the prescription chart/kardex.	Prevents medication administration error.
Ask parent to verify the child's name and date of birth.	To ensure the correct identity of the child.
4 You must take into consideration the age of the child and their developmental level when preparing the child for the procedure.	This will determine the most effective and appropriate way to hold the child during the procedure.
Infants Ask parent to hold infant in the cot on their left lateral side.	The left lateral position allows for ease of insertion of the medication into the rectum (Dougherty & Lister, 2004).
Toddlers Ask toddler to lie on their bed on their left lateral side. Ask the parent to sit at their child's side and tell them a story. Avoid holding toddlers firmly.	The left lateral position allows for ease of insertion of the medication into the rectum (Dougherty & Lister, 2004). Storytelling is a good method of distraction therapy for toddlers. This would frighten the child and promote resistance to the procedure.
Older children Ask child to lie on their bed on their left lateral side. Ask the child to count to 20. Alternatively ask the child if he/she would like to listen to their iPod, etc.	The left lateral position allows for ease of insertion of the medication into the rectum (Dougherty & Lister, 2004). Counting is a good method of distraction for the older child. Play through modern technology is also a good method of distraction for the older child.
5 Administering of the medication: Don gloves.	Prevents the spread of micro-organisms.
Suppositories Lubricate the tapered end of the suppository. Separate the child's buttocks. Gently insert the suppository into the rectum beyond the anal sphincter, with the lubricated, tapered end first. Hold the buttocks firmly together.	Enables easy application into the rectum. To view the anus. This ensures that the suppository is correctly in place. This will relieve the pressure on the anal sphincter until the urge to expel the suppository has passed (Watt, 2003).

	Enema	
	Place an incontinence pad underneath the child.	In case of possible leakage of the enema.
	Lubricate the funnel of the enema.	Enables easy application into the rectum.
	Separate the child's buttocks.	To view the anus.
	Gently insert the funnel of the enema through the anus following the manufacture's recommendations.	To position the funnel correctly.
	Gently administer the contents of the enema into the rectum.	Excess pressure could cause damage to the child's colon.
	Ask the child to retain the enema for as long as they can.	To avoid premature evacuation of the medication.
	Remind the child of the location of the nearest toilet.	To avoid premature evacuation of the medication.
6	Dispose of equipment and wash hands.	Prevents the spread of micro-organisms.
7	Stay with the child until the procedure is over.	It is the responsibility of the children's nurse to ensure the safe administration of medicines to children.
8	Praise the child for holding still during the procedure.	Praise will have a positive effect on desired behaviour.
9	Evaluate child for desired effect of medicine or for possible side effects of medication.	Evaluation is an essential component of the nursing process. It is important that the desired effect of medicine is achieved. If the desired effect is not achieved alternative action will be necessary.
10	Document procedure and evaluation in nursing notes.	Documentation is necessary to ensure continuity of care.

- Right medication.
- Right patient.
- Right dose.
- Right route.
- Right time (ABA, 2007; NMC, 2008).

1 Check prescription. All checks must be carried out with another registered nurse or in accordance with local hospital policy.

2 Wash hands and don gloves.

Equipment

- Correct medication.
- Water-soluble lubricant.
- Tissues.
- Drug administration chart and pen.

Administering topical medications to children

Certain medications are administered topically via the skin to children. Children have a larger body surface area and less subcutaneous tissue than adults, therefore systematic absorption and medication effects may be greater (Greenstein & Gould, 2008). Topical medications should not be applied to inflamed, red, or broken skin unless specifically ordered. Prior to administration and application of topical medications the children's nurse must assess the child's prior experience of having topical medicines applied. The nurse must also check that the skin is clean and dry before applying topical medicines. When administering topical medicines the children's nurse must follow the guidelines for the application and storage of the medicine as provided by the manufacturer. Please refer to Chapter Fifteen for further detail in relation to the topical administration of medications to children and young people.

7.6 **Administering subcutaneous injections**

A subcutaneous injection (or infusion) is given beneath the epidermis into the subcutaneous tissue underlying the dermis. This type of injection can either be given by a healthcare professional, or can be self-injected by an adult or an older child. Subcutaneous injections are a relatively convenient way to deliver medication that would otherwise be absorbed too slowly or made ineffective if taken by mouth. The subcutaneous route has less blood flow to fatty tissue and the injected medication is generally absorbed more slowly than the intramuscular route. **Box 7.7** outlines medications commonly delivered this way.

Complications of subcutaneous injections

The greatest disadvantage of the subcutaneous route is that it penetrates the body's first line of defence: the skin. Thus it is imperative that aseptic technique is used for the child's safety. Subcutaneous injections often cause pain and bruising (Chan, 2001; Kuzu & Ucar, 2001; Venketasubramanian & Chua, 1998). Kuzu & Ucar (2001) highlight the point that site-pain causes the child physical and psychological discomfort and bruising limits possible sites for subsequent injections.

Box 7.7 Drugs and solutions commonly administered via the subcutaneous route

- Insulin
- Heparin
- Maxalon
- Epinephrene
- Growth hormones
- Hyoscine
- Morphine
- Isotonic fluid

Potential complications include:
- Infection—abscess.
- Bruising and pain.
- Lipodystrophy—due to multiple injections at the same site.
- Sloughing at the site of injection.
- Anaphylaxis.
- Fibrosis.
- Hyperpigmentation.

(Barron & Cocoman, 2008)

Traditionally, nurses administered subcutaneous injections at a 45-degree angle to decrease the depth of insertion of the needle and avoid accidental intramuscular injections. Over recent years, with the introduction of shorter needles, practice has changed from administration at a 45-degree angle to a 90-degree angle. Barron & Cocoman (2008) recommend the use of a 25 to 29 gauge and a shorter needle of 5 or 6 mm long (appropriate to the size and age of the child). Nurses must be aware that the sites they select for the administration of a subcutaneous injection differ in their absorption rates.

Sites for subcutaneous injections

The following parts of the body have subcutaneous layers and are suitable for subcutaneous injections: the lateral aspects of the upper arm and thigh; the buttocks; and the abdomen, except the navel or waistline (**see Figure 7.1**). Rotation of injection sites is recommended to minimize tissue irritation. However, it is important to keep in mind that some drugs may be absorbed at different rates in different areas of the body. For example, insulin is absorbed fastest from the abdominal area, slowest from the leg and buttock, and at an intermediate rate from the arm. Rotation of these sites ensures improved absorption and lessens the risk of irritation.

Procedure: Administering subcutaneous injections
Subcutaneous infusions

Subcutaneous infusions can be given in preference to intravenous treatment, especially if intravenous access is difficult. Subcutaneous infusions can be intermittent or

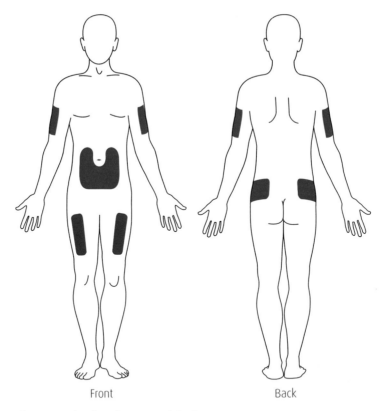

Figure 7.1 Sites for subcutaneous injection

continuous and may also be administered by the older child or parent in the home environment, thus reducing hospital admissions. Fluids that may be administered subcutaneously to children include isotonic fluid replacement (Brown & Worobec, 2000) and immunoglobulin replacement therapy. The abdomen is frequently chosen for infusion of larger volumes (more than 10 ml per hour) as it provides the best absorption of all the subcutaneous sites. However, many children do not like having needles in their abdomen and may prefer you to site the needle in the subcutaneous layer of the upper thigh. Some swelling at the site of infusion may be expected as the fluid may be administered more quickly than it can be absorbed; however, it should reduce rapidly and usually disappears completely 2–4 hours after completion of the infusion. The rate of infusion may vary from greater than 1 ml per hour up to 50 ml per hour (Great Ormond Street Hospital, 2005).

Procedure: Administering subcutaneous infusions

Preparation

Safety: Adhere to the five rights of medication administration:
- Right medication.
- Right patient.
- Right dose.
- Right route.
- Right time (ABA, 2007; NMC, 2008).

1 Check prescription. All checks must be carried out with another registered nurse or in accordance with local hospital policy.
2 Wash hands and don gloves.

Step-by-step guide to subcutaneous injection

Procedure	Rationale
1 A registered nurse or a student nurse in the presence of a registered nurse may administer subcutaneous injections.	To minimize risk of error (ABA, 2007; NMC, 2008).
2 Perform hand hygiene.	To remove transient organisms (Doebbeling *et al.*, 1992) and prevent the spread of micro-organisms (Evans-Smith, 2005).
3 Inspect all equipment and packaging.	To ensure sterility. If damaged or past expiry dates please discard.
4 Identify the patient and discuss the procedure. Evaluate their knowledge.	To ensure that the patient understands the procedure and gives consent (Ellis & Bentz, 2004).
5 Check the child's drug prescription. Administer medication according to the five rights of medication administration: right drug; right dose; right time; right route; right client.	To ensure that the correct child receives the drug as prescribed by physician (ABA, 2007; NMC, 2008).
6 Select the drug in the appropriate volume dilution or dosage. Check expiry date.	To reduce wastage. The expiry date indicates when a particular drug is no longer pharmacologically efficacious (Evans-Smith, 2005).
7 Re-check the drug and dosage against the prescription chart with a registered nurse.	To minimize risk of error (ABA, 2007; Ellis & Bentz, 2004).
8 Ensure you have correctly identified the child and assist them into a position that is comfortable and practical for access to the injection site.	Injection into a tense extremity causes discomfort (Evans-Smith, 2005).
9 Always wear disposable gloves as there is potential for exposure to blood in the administration of SC injections.	Gloves act as a barrier and protect the nurse's hands from accidental exposure to blood (Evans-Smith, 2005).
10 Locate the correct area for injection. The preferred injection site is the abdomen (Ellis & Bentz, 2007). Do not give injections in moles, scarred, inflamed, or oedematous areas (Barron & Cocoman, 2006). Inspect the area prior to injection for bruising from previous injections. Rotation of injection sites is extremely important.	There is unpredictable absorption from these sites. To prevent the formation of lipodystrophy, which is an accumulation of fat in lumps underneath the skin (Barron & Cocoman, 2008).

11	Follow the individual healthcare setting's policy and procedure with regard to cleansing of the injection site.	Cleaning of the injection site is not required in normal circumstances for SC injections.
12	With your non-dominant hand pinch a fold of skin between your fingers and hold it up.	The nurse should always administer the injection with their dominant hand in order to ensure good control of the needle and syringe during administration. Never lift a skin fold with your full hand as this may lead to elevation of muscle and the incorrect administration of an SC injection into muscle.
13	It is not necessary to aspirate prior to administering the medication.	Heparin is an anticoagulant and will cause bruising if aspirated. An insulin needle is so small that aspiration is unreliable in predicting needle placement (Evans-Smith, 2005).
14	Using your dominant hand, pick up the syringe and hold like a dart (Ellis & Bentz, 2007). For the subcutaneous route you can insert the needle at a 90 degree angle, especially for heparin and insulin, or at 45 degrees for a very thin patient.	With the advent of shorter needles a 90 degree insertion is standard practice (Barron & Cocoman, 2008). However, a 45 degree angle may be needed to ensure that the end of the needle does not pierce the muscle with extremely emaciated patients (Ellis & Bentz, 2007).
15	The key to a comfortable injection is swift needle entry followed by slow injection of fluid and finally quick withdrawal of needle.	This is less painful for the patient.
16	Dispose of syringe and needles in the sharps box (never recap a needle).	To prevent needle stick injuries (ABA, 2007; NMC, 2008).
17	Dispose of clinical waste and gloves and wash hands.	To prevent cross infection.
18	Record the medication given in the prescription chart and any other place necessary as indicated by individual hospital policy.	To ensure accurate recording of all medications administered (ABA, 2007; NMC, 2008).

Equipment

- The medication to be administered.
- A luer lock syringe appropriate to the infusion volume.
- Appropriate-sized needles for drawing up the medication.
- Sterile adhesive dressings or clean paper tape.
- Portable syringe pumps, e.g. Graseby.
- Sharps disposal bin.
- Medication chart.
- Non-sterile gloves.

Consent and communication

Prepare the child and family by explaining what you are about to do and asking the parents to be involved.

Step-by-step administration of subcutaneous infusions

Procedure	Rationale
1 Adhere to the five rights of medication administration and ensure you have prepared as advised under 'safety' before this box.	To prevent medication administration error and ensure the safe administration of medication.
2 Check there is no blood in the line; it is not necessary to aspirate.	Re-site the needle if blood is present to ensure the medication/fluids are administered subcutaneously.
3 Secure the needle with suitable tape or occlusive dressing as appropriate.	To prevent the infusion being dislodged (Great Ormond Street Hospital, 2005).
4 Place the child in a position that is comfortable for them.	To gain the child's cooperation and to adhere to your local policy on holding. To ensure safety of the child, family, and nurse.
5 Check the child's name band against the prescription chart/kardex. Ask parent to verify the child's name and date of birth.	Prevents medication administration error. To ensure the correct identity of the child.
6 Lift a skin fold and insert the needle into the subcutaneous tissue. The angle of insertion will depend on the needle length and the amount of subcutaneous tissue the child has.	With the introduction of shorter needles a full depth perpendicular injection of 90 degrees into a raised skin fold is recommended for subcutaneous injections (Barron & Cocoman, 2008).
7 Attach the syringe to the pump and start the infusion, checking the rate. Observe the child throughout the treatment.	To give the infusion at the correct rate. To check the infusion site for pain, excessive redness, or swelling.
8 Record the administration of all medications/fluids in the appropriate drug chart as per your local policy.	To prevent drug errors (ABA, 2007; NMC, 2008).
9 Upon completion of the infusion, remove the tape and/or dressings securing the needle. Remove and dispose of the needle. The frequency with which sites change will depend on the type of infusion device and nature and rate of infusion. It may vary from <1 day–7 days (Ross *et al.*, 2002).	To allow the needle to be removed. For safety reasons. To ensure the medication/fluids are administered subcutaneously.

7.7 **Administering intramuscular injections to children**

Rationale for administering medication via the intramuscular route

Although a common feature in the past, the administration of intramuscular (IM) injections to children in paediatric clinical settings is no longer required as frequently due to the availability of modern alternatives. However, on occasions IM injections are used for the delivery of specific medications that are not recommended for use through other routes of administration. The intramuscular route offers a faster rate of absorption than the subcutaneous route, and muscle tissue can often hold a larger volume of fluid (between 0.5 and 2 ml depending on the child's age and the site) than subcutaneous tissue. However, medication injected into muscle tissues is absorbed less rapidly and takes effect more slowly than medication that is injected intravenously (Rodger & King, 2000). Careful consideration in deciding which injection site is to be used for the prescribed medication is essential. Intramuscular injections should always be avoided if other routes of administration, especially oral, can be used to provide a comparable level of absorption and effect in any given child's situation and condition (Barron & Cocoman, 2008).

Sites for intramuscular injections in children

When considering a site for intramuscular injections with children, the nurse needs to consider the following:

- The size and age of the child: the site recommended may depend on the age/weight of the child. If under two years of age it is currently recommended to use the vastus lateralis site—outer thigh).
- The child's ability to maintain the required position during administration safely.

- The size and accessibility of the muscle: the muscle must be well-developed and capable of tolerating the volume of medication to be administered.
- On the rare occasions of repeated IM injections being required, then rotation of sites into more developed muscles is preferential.
- The type of medication being used and the manufacturer's instructions.

There are two common sites recommended for the administration of intramuscular injections to children: the vastus lateralis (anterior lateral aspect of the thigh) and the deltoid (upper arm) sites. However, the ventrogluteal site is also an option, especially in adolescents.

The vastus lateralis site

The vastus lateralis site has attracted considerable attention in the literature, specifically in relation to the administration of vaccinations to infants, and is recommended by the Royal College of Paediatricians and Child Health & Royal College of Nursing (2002) for use with infants up to two years of age.

The vastus lateralis muscle forms part of the quadriceps muscle group of the upper leg and can be found on the anterior lateral aspect of the thigh. Landmarking of any injection site is vitally important. In young children you will need to remove/open the nappy in order to accurately landmark the site. To locate the site, visually divide the length of the muscle that originates on the greater trochanter of the femur and inserts on the upper border of the patella into thirds. Inject into the middle third of the lateral aspect of the vastus lateralis muscle.

Cook & Murtagh (2005) compared the rates of adverse reactions and parental approval ratings for three different techniques for vastus lateralis thigh vaccination in infants aged two, four, six, and 18 months. They found that the WHO technique (using a 25 gauge, 16 mm long needle inserted at 90 degrees to the long axis of the femur, with the skin compressed between the index finger and thumb) for IM injection into the vastus lateralis site resulted in less irritability in infants and toddlers than the US and Australian techniques, and less bruising at the injection site than the US technique. Cook & Murtagh (2005) therefore recommend the WHO technique as the optimal technique for anterolateral intramuscular injections in children, as it ensures that the injection is intramuscular, results in fewer adverse reactions, and is the easiest technique to perform as it does not require angling of the needle to the long axis of the femur. One of the advantages of the vastus lateralis site is its ease of access; it is also the preferred site for IM injections for infants and young children (Trigg & Mohammad, 2006; Royal College of Paediatrics and Child Health & Royal College of Nursing, 2002) as the muscle mass is adequate to absorb IM medications. Nevertheless, the site has been associated with injuries (Haber *et al.*, 2000) through inaccurate location of the site.

The deltoid site

The deltoid site is located laterally on the upper arm and is the recommended site for intramuscular injections in children over the age of two (Royal College of Paediatrics and Child Health & Royal College of Nursing, 2002) who have acceptable muscle mass development. Unlike the vastus lateralis, the deltoid site has not received a lot of attention in the literature and the evidence-based knowledge is decidedly weaker than that for the vastus lateralis site (Barron & Cocoman, 2008). This is unfortunate as many IM injections to children over the age of two years will be administered via this site. Further research into the use of this site in children over the age of two is needed. Intramuscular injections into the mid-deltoid muscle, like other IM injections, should be given into the densest part of the muscle. Barron & Cocoman (2008) suggest that the injection should be given into an imaginary inverted triangle whose apex is above the level of the axilla/armpit (Kozier *et al.*, 1993). It is essential to expose the arm completely from shoulder to elbow when landmarking the deltoid site.

Insufficient retraction of a shirtsleeve may expose only the inferior portion of the deltoid area. Injury to the brachial artery and/or the radial nerve (if landmarking technique is poor and the injection is given too low) and the limited volume of medication that can be administered (0.5–1 ml maximum) are highlighted as risks associated with the deltoid site. This site is commonly used for small volume IM injections, e.g. vaccines, which are usually administered into the deltoid site for children over two years of age (Mallett & Bailey, 1996). The deltoid site is not recommended for repeated use or large volumes (Rodger & King, 2000).

The ventrogluteal site

The ventrogluteal site is seen by many as the site of choice for IM injections for adults (Beecroft & Redick, 1990; Hahn, 1990; Covington & Trattler, 1997; Greenway, 2004). This site provides the greatest thickness of gluteal muscle (consisting of both the gluteus medius and gluteus minimus), is free of penetrating nerves and blood vessels, and has a narrower layer of fat of consistent thinness than is present in the dorsogluteal site (Zelman, 1961). Evidence-based research endorses the ventrogluteal site as the safer option for the administration of intramuscular injections to adults (Kozier *et al.*, 1993; Beyea & Nicoll, 1995; Dougherty & Lister, 2004). However, the landmarking technique is not suitable or accurate when used with children due to the differences in anatomical size of the child compared to the adult. Further research specifically related to landmarking this site in different sizes and ages of children is required. Despite the evidence supporting the use of the ventrogluteal site, a study by Farley *et al.* (1986) identified that only 12% of the nursing staff in a teaching hospital in the United States used the ventrogluteal site. No current research-based evidence was found to support the use of the ventrogluteal site in children from a UK or Irish perspective.

Z-track technique and intramuscular injections

Z-tracking involves displacing the skin and subcutaneous layer in relation to the underlying muscle to be injected so that the needle track is sealed off when the needle is withdrawn, thus minimizing reflux. This technique can be used in any appropriate muscle group provided that the overlying tissue can be displaced by at least 2 cm. The Z-track technique is endorsed in all literature relating to intramuscular injections (Keen, 1990;

Newtown *et al.*, 1992; Beyea & Nicoll, 1995) with the exception of that on infant vaccination, which advocates compressing the skin between the index finger and thumb (Diggle & Deeks, 2000; Diggle, 2007). In order to make use of the Z-track technique when administering intramuscular injections, the children's nurse should use their non-dominant hand to displace the skin and subcutaneous tissue 0.5 inches or 1 cm laterally to the injection site prior to injecting. The Z-tracking must be kept in place until after the medication is administered and the needle is withdrawn, thus preventing reflux of the medication into the subcutaneous tissue. This manoeuvre seals off the puncture tract and traps the drug in the muscle.

Selection of appropriate syringe and needle

The size of the syringe used should be determined by selecting the smallest possible to accommodate the given volume. Volumes of less than 0.5 ml should be given with low dose 1 ml syringes to ensure accuracy (Zenk, 1993). An administration rate of no faster than 1 ml per ten seconds is recommended to facilitate absorption and minimize pain (Farley *et al.*, 1986; Keen, 1990). To prevent glass contamination, Hahn (1990), McConnell (1993), and Preston & Hegadoren (2004) support the use of a filter needle when drawing medication from a vial or ampoule, in order to prevent shards of glass or rubber particles being injected into the child and reduce or prevent injury. If no filter needle is available nurses are advised to draw up with a 23 gauge needle (Mallett & Bailey, 1996; Dougherty & Lister, 2004) and then replace with the appropriate needle to administer the injection. For all intramuscular injections, the needle should be long enough to reach the muscle mass and prevent the medication from seeping into subcutaneous tissue, but not so long as to involve underlying nerves, blood vessels, or bone (Groswasser *et al.*, 1997; Zuckerman, 2000). The Royal College of Paediatrics and Child Health and Royal College of Nursing (2002) recommend a needle length of 16 mm (five-eighths of an inch) as the minimum for all intramuscular injections, although the Department of Health (DH, 2005) states that a 25 mm (1 inch) needle is considered suitable for

all ages except pre-term or very small infants, when a 16 mm needle is suitable. However, appropriate needle length depends on age and body mass of the individual child, as it would be unreasonable to administer an IM injection with the same gauge and length needle to a two-year-old toddler as you would to a ten-year-old. Different patients need different needle sizes (Zuckerman, 2000).

Cleaning of the injection site

Cleaning of injection sites has been debated for decades with conflicting evidence within the literature. Many authors (McConnell, 1993; Mallett & Bailey, 1996) suggest that antiseptics in current use cannot act in the time that is generally used in practice, about five seconds on average, and cannot possibly provide complete sterility. More current research contends that once the patient's skin is clean, no cleansing is necessary (Royal College of Paediatrics and Child Health & Royal College of Nursing, 2002; Department of Health, 2005). Diggle (2007) declares that a simple wash with soap and water is adequate for a dirty injection site for children.

Aspiration prior to injection

Diggle (2007) argues strongly that aspirating immediately before administering an intramuscular injection for the administration of a vaccine is an outdated and unnecessary procedure. She argues that nurses have traditionally and routinely drawn back on the syringe plunger before an intramuscular injection to ensure the needle is not sited within a blood vessel. However, there is no scientific evidence to support the practice of aspiration before injecting a vaccine and the World Health Organization, the American Academy of Pediatrics (AAP), and the Department of Health have stated that this practice, which serves only to prolong the injection procedure, is unnecessary (AAP, 2003; DH, 2005; WHO, 2006). Absence of proof however does not however mean that the principle is wrong and currently there is insufficient evidence to support the discontinuance of aspiration prior to administering an intramuscular injection to children over the age of two years.

Complications/risks associated with IM injections

Muller-Vahl (1985) and Small (2004) suggest that inadequate training in both the procedure and technique is responsible for many of the complications resulting from intramuscular injections. The most common complications stemming from the procedure are related to local trauma caused by the injection itself or the irritating properties of the drug. Despite knowledge of them, preventable complications still occur. Based on the current evidence base (Barron & Cocoman, 2008) it seems advisable that nurses use the vastus lateralis and deltoid injection sites for intramuscular injections with children, as to date there is minimal evidence available for the correct landmarking for the ventrogluteal site in children. Reported injuries associated with sites other than the ventrogluteal for IM injections include:

- Permanent damage to radial nerves resulting in paralysis.
- Neuropathy.
- Persistent nodules—granulomas.
- Muscle contractures and palsy.
- Peripheral nerve and bone injury.
- Local irritation, pain, local discomfort, and redness at the site.
- Infection, abscess, cellulitis, and tissue necrosis.
- Haematomas, bleeding, arterial punctures, and (in rare cases) gangrene.
- Muscle fibrosis.

(Farley *et al.*, 1986; Hahn, 1990; Beyea & Nicoll, 1995).

Procedure: Intramuscular injections

Preparation

Safety: Adhere to the five rights of medication administration:

- Right medication.
- Right patient.
- Right dose.
- Right route.
- Right time (ABA, 2007; NMC, 2008).

1 Check prescription. All checks must be carried out with another registered nurse or in accordance with local hospital policy.
2 Inspect all equipment and packaging.
3 Wash hands and don gloves to remove transient organisms (Doebbeling *et al.*, 1992).

Equipment

- The medication to be administered.
- Syringe and appropriate-sized needles.
- Dry, sterile gauze swab and bandage.
- Sharps disposal bin.
- Medication chart.
- Non-sterile gloves.

Consent and communication

Prepare the child and family by explaining what you are about to do and asking the parents to be involved. This will ensure that the child and/or family understands the procedure and gives consent (Ellis & Bentz, 2004).

Post-procedural care for intramuscular injections

Discard the used syringe and needle intact as soon as possible in an appropriate sharps box, remembering not to attempt to replace the sheath on the needle, i.e. do not 're-cap' (Greenstein & Gould, 2008). Check the site at least once more, a short time after the injection, to ensure that no **bleeding**, **swelling**, or any other signs of reaction to the medication are present. Monitor the child for side effects, especially if it is the first time the child is receiving the medication; most complications of intramuscular injections are a result of the drug injected and poor injection technique. Minor discomfort and pain is common for a short period following the injection, but usually resolves within a few hours. Document all injections given and any other relevant information. Ask the child and parent to report any localized discomfort or swelling following the injection.

Step-by-step guide to intramuscular injection

Procedure	Rationale
1 A registered nurse or a student nurse in the presence of a registered nurse may administer intramuscular injections.	To minimize risk of error (ABA, 2007; NMC, 2008).
2 Ensure you have prepared by following the guidelines provided before this box.	To prevent medication administration error and ensure the safe administration of medication.
3 Select the drug in the appropriate volume, dilution, or dosage.	To reduce wastage.
Check expiry date.	The expiry date indicates when a particular drug is no longer pharmacologically efficacious (Evans-Smith, 2005).
4 Recheck the drug and dosage against the prescription chart with another registered nurse or student nurse.	To minimize risk of error (An Bord Altranais 2007, Ellis and Bentz, 2004).
5 Select correct syringe and needle size.	Needle size must be sufficiently long to reach the muscle (Greenway, 2004).
6 Ensure privacy and avoid exposing body parts during the procedure.	To maintain patient's privacy and dignity (Barron & Cocoman, 2006).
7 Assist the child into a position that is comfortable and practical for access to the injection site you have chosen.	Injection into a tense extremity causes discomfort (Evans-Smith, 2005).
8 Always wear disposable gloves as there is potential exposure to blood in the administration of IM injections.	Gloves act as a barrier and protect the nurse's hands from accidental exposure to blood (Evans-Smith, 2005).
9 Follow the individual healthcare setting's policy and procedure with regard to cleansing of the injection site.	Some health settings recommend no skin cleansing prior to administration. However, if using an alcohol swab, cleanse the site in a circular motion for 30 seconds and allow to dry for 30 seconds prior to administration (Workman, 1999).
10 When administering an IM injection, insert the needle at a 90-degree angle using the Z-track technique.	The Z-track technique prevents leakage into subcutaneous tissue as the needle is withdrawn, thereby reducing complications.
11 The needle should be inserted into the skin in a dart-like fashion at a 72–90-degree angle.	Katsma & Smith (1997) and *Katsma & Katsma (2000)* demonstrated with the use of trigonometry that an injection given at 72 degrees reaches 95% of the depth of an injection given at 90 degrees. This relation between needle angle and needle depth lends support to the proposal for a new standard of angle administration between 72 degrees and 90 degrees.

12	The plunger should be drawn back, thereby creating a negative pressure in the tissue below it. If a blood vessel has been compromised, blood will appear in the aspirate and the needle should be withdrawn and the whole procedure repeated.	To prevent an intra-artery injection (Rodger & King, 2000).
13	Inject the medication slowly, taking approximately ten seconds per ml. Withdraw the needle quickly and smoothly once all medication has been administered.	This slow, steady rate promotes comfort and allows time for the tissues to expand and begin absorbing the solution (Workman, 1999) and helps to avoid damage to the muscle tissue.
14	Once the needle is out, use a dry, sterile gauze swab to apply gentle pressure at the site. Use a plaster if appropriate and/or requested. Don't massage the site.	Massaging the site could cause tissue irritation (Rodger & King, 2000).

Intravenous infusion

Children may receive fluids and/or medications via the intravenous (IV) route. The student nurse may be asked to prepare the intravenous line for commencing an infusion or change the infusion bag and giving set. There are two main techniques for the administration of intravenous fluids. Infusion pumps are the preferred method of administering IV fluids to children as they accurately deliver a pre-set rate over a specific period of time and they alarm if problems occur with the infusion. In fact, most paediatric nursing units have a policy that children under a certain age with IV fluids/IV medications will be placed on an infusion pump.

Most intravenous solutions come in 500 ml or 1000 ml bags with a separate giving set, which needs to be connected to the IV solution bag using an aseptic technique to prevent cross contamination and sepsis. The giving set is then run through with the IV fluid required to expel any air bubbles from the set. The giving set is then 'fed through' the internal section of an electronic pump. The pressure alarm limit must be set when an infusion is commenced. The tubing is then connected to the IV cannula already sited in the child. It is important that for EACH IV infusion that the signature/initial of the nurse in charge of the infusion is clearly recorded. In addition the pressure of the infusion pump and the volume infused should be recorded on a regular basis (at least hourly).

Minimizing pain associated with injections

Invasive procedures, particularly procedures that involve needles, can cause substantial anxiety and pain to patients (Ellis & Bentz, 2004). In the paediatric clinical setting, many children view injections as one of the most traumatic aspects of being in hospital (Cordoni & Cordoni, 2001). Parents rate needle procedures as the second most distressing event during their child's hospitalization (Sharp, 2004). For some children, a fear of needles may persist into adulthood and can have lifelong negative repercussions, such as preventing them from donating blood or precipitating fainting episodes in response to a needle (Pavlin *et al.*, 1993). Research suggests that if painful procedures such as injections are not properly managed, children may suffer negative psychological effects in both the short and long term, such as nausea, insomnia, and treatment non-adherence (Weisman *et al.*, 1998). Therefore it is important for the nurse to minimize injection-induced pain, thus reducing the child's distress and preventing potential needle phobia.

Topical anaesthetics can help provide pain relief at the insertion point of the needle. Emla, a lidocaine-prilocaine cream, is used predominantly in children beyond neonatal age (Trigg & Mohammad, 2006). The peak action following application of Emla occurs at two hours and lasts for as long as four to five hours (Sharp, 2004). Ametop gel (tetracaine 4%) provides analgesia similar to Emla's but has the advantage of a more rapid onset of action. It works in about 30 to 45 minutes and lasts for four to six hours after a single application (Sharp, 2004). The use of topical anaesthetics gives children a sense of control and they are easy to apply. However, they have a slow onset and may cause further anxiety in children who identify them with needle sticks that are soon to follow. Additional research into the psychological consequences to children of waiting for topical anaesthetics to take effect is required.

Conclusion

Pharmacokinetics is the movement of drugs through the body over time, and addresses the absorption from the site of administration, distribution throughout the body, metabolism of the drug, and its elimination from the body (Kanneh, 2002a). This area was examined as it relates to children. Pharmacodynamics, which is the study of the biochemical and physiological action and effects of drugs in the body, was then introduced and age-related differences that occur throughout childhood were explored, leading to the conclusion that children should not be considered as scaled down adults. Throughout this chapter the importance and method of drug calculations and mental mathematics was discussed in detail, because of their importance in the safe preparation and administration of all medications.

The ability to calculate drug doses accurately is an essential skill for the children's nurse as poor calculation skills can lead to serious drug errors and patient harm. The administration of drugs under supervision is an integral part of the student nurse's role and you must therefore be proficient in standard unit conversions, drug calculation formulas, and mental mathematics. While drugs can and are administered to children via numerous differing routes, the most common route of administration is the oral route in liquid or solid form. The key nursing points to consider when administering medications via differing routes to children were explored based on up-to-date evidence-based practice.

Encouraging and supporting parents to be involved in their child's care is vital to maintain a partnership relationship between the nurse, child, and family (Watt, 2003). Therefore, the student nurse must assess the child's prior experience of taking medicines, as well as asking for the parents' knowledge and experience of their individual child's ability to take medications. Parents know their children best, and this information will help you to plan your approach to the procedure. Effective communication and active listening are essential components of medication administration and all verbal communications with the child must be age appropriate.

Online resource centre

You may find it helpful to work through our online resources including interactive scenarios intended to help you to develop and apply the skills in this chapter. Where material referenced below is available electronically, we're pleased to provide active web links to the source via ⓦ **http://www.oxfordtextbooks.co.uk/orc/coyne/**

References

American Academy of Pediatrics (2003) *Red Book: Report of the Committee on Infectious Diseases, 26th* ed. Elk Grove Village: American Academy of Pediatrics.

An Bord Altranais (2007) *Guidance to Nurses and Midwives on Medication Management*. Dublin: An Bord Altranais.

Arnold, E.C. & Underman Boggs, K. (2007) *Interpersonal Relationships: Professional communication skills for nurses, 5th ed.* St Louis, Missouri: Saunders.

Barron, C. & Cocoman, A. (2006) *Theory and Practice of Intramuscular and Subcutaneous Injections*. Dublin: Campus Print DCU.

Barron, C. & Cocoman, A. (2008) Administering intramuscular injections to children: What does the evidence say? *Journal of Children's and Young Peoples Health* **2** (3), 138–143.

Beecroft, P. & Redick, S. (1990) Intramuscular injection practices of paediatric nurses: Site selection. *Nurse Educator* **15** (4), 23–28.

Beyea, S. & Nicoll, L. (1995) Administration of medications via IM route: An integrative review of literature and research based protocol for the procedure. *Applied Nursing Research* **8**, 23–33.

Bonati, M., Impicciatore, P., & Pandolfini, C. (2001) Medicines for children in Europe at the beginning of the new millennium. *Paediatric and Perinatal Drug Therapy* **4** (3), 82–84.

Booker, R. (2007) Correct use of nebulizers. *Nursing Standard* **22** (8), 39–41.

Breitkreutz, J., Wessel, T., & Boos, J. (1999) Dosage forms for peroral drug administration to children. *Paediatric and Perinatal Drug Therapy* **3**, 25–33.

British National Formulary (2008) *BNF for Children*. UK: BMJ Group and RPS Publishing.

Brown, M. & Worobec, F. (2000) Hypodermoclysis: Another way to replace fluids. *Nursing* **30** (5), 58–59.

Chan, H. (2001) Effects of injection duration on site-pain intensity and bruising associated with subcutaneous heparin. *Journal of Advanced Nursing* **35** (6), 882–892.

Cook, I.F. & Murtagh, J. (2005) Optimal technique for intramuscular injection of infants and toddlers: A randomised trial. *Medical Journal of Australia* **183** (2), 60–63.

Cordoni, A. & Cordoni, L.E. (2001) Eutectic mixture of local anaesthetics reduces pain during intravenous catheter insertion in the paediatrics patient. *Clinical Journal of Pain* **17** (2), 115–118.

Covingston, T. & Trattler, M. (1997) *Fundamentals of Nursing, Human Health and Function, 2nd ed*. New York: Lippincott.

Department of Health (2005) Immunisation procedures. In: *Immunisation against Infectious Diseases*. London: HMSO. Available at: **http://www.dh.gov.uk**

Diggle, L. (2007) Injection technique for immunisation. *Practice Nurse* **33** (1), 34–37.

Diggle, L. & Deeks, J. (2000) Effect of needle length on incidence of local reactions to routine immunisation in infants aged 4 months: Randomised controlled trial. *BMJ* **14** (321), 931–933.

Doebbeling, B.N., Stanley, G.L., & Sheetz, C.T (1992) Comparative efficacy of alternative hand washing agents in reducing nosocomial infections in intensive care units. *New England Journal of Medicine* **327**, 88–93.

Dougherty, L. & Lister, S. (2004) *The Royal Marsden Hospital Manual of Clinical Nursing Procedures, 6th ed*. London: Blackwell Publishing.

Ellis, J. & Bentz, P. (2004) *Modules for Basic Nursing Skills, 7th ed*. Philadelphia: Lippincott Williams.

Evans-Smith, P. (2005) *Taylor's Clinical Nursing Skills: A Nursing Process Approach*. Philadelphia: Lippincott Williams.

Farely, F., Joyce, N., Long, B., & Roberts, R. (1986) Will that IM needle reach the muscle? *American Journal of Nursing* **86**, 1327–1328.

Great Ormond Street Hospital (2005) *Subcutaneous Access (Infusions and Injections) Clinical Guideline*. Available at: **http://www.ich.ucl.ac.uk/ clinical_information/clinical_guidelines/cpg_ guideline_00154**

Greenstein, B. & Gould, D. (2008) *Trounce's Clinical Pharmacology for Nurses, 18th ed*. London: Elsevier.

Greenway, K. (2004) Using the ventral gluteal site for intramuscular injection. *Nursing Standard* **18** (29), 39–42.

Groswasser, J., Kahn, A., Bouche, B., Hanquinet, S., Perlmuter, N., & Hessel, L. (1997) Needle length and injection technique for efficient intramuscular vaccine delivery in infants and children evaluated through an ultrasonographic determination of subcutaneous and muscle layer thickness. *Pediatrics* **100**, 400–403.

Haber, M., Kovan, E., Andary, M., & Honet, J. (2000) Post injection vastus lateralis atrophy: Two case reports. *Archives of Physical Medicine and Rehabilitation* **81** (9), 1229–1233.

Hahn, K. (1990) Brush up on your injection technique. *Nursing* **20**, 54–58.

Haiat, H., Bar-Mor, G., & Shochat, M. (2003) The world of the child: A world of play even in the hospital. *Journal of Pediatric Nursing* **18** (3), 209.

Horner, S.D. (1999) Asthma self-care: Just another piece of school work. *Pediatric Nursing* **25** (6), 597.

Kanneh, A. (1998b) Pharmacological principles applied to children. Part 2. *Paediatric Nursing* **10** (4) 24–27.

Kanneh, A. (2002a) Paediatric pharmacological principles: An update. Part 2. Pharmacokinetics: Absorption and distribution. *Paediatric Nursing* **14** (9), 39–43.

Kanneh, A. (2002b) Paediatric pharmacological principles: An update. Part 3. Pharmacokinetics: Metabolism and excretion. *Paediatric Nursing* **14** (10), 39–43.

Katsma, D. & Katsma, R. (2000) The myth of the 90 degree angle intramuscular injection. *Nurse Educator* **25**(1), 34–37.

Katsma, D. & Smith, G. (1997) Analysis of needle path during intramuscular injection. *Nursing Research* **46**, 288–292.

Kearns, G.L. (1998) Pharmacokinetics in infants and children. *Inflammatory Bowel Diseases* **4** (2), 104–107.

Kearns, G., Alander, S.W., & Leeder, J.S. (2003) Developmental pharmacology—drug disposition, action, and therapy in infants and children. *The New England Journal of Medicine* **349** (12), 1157–1167.

Keen, M. (1990) Get on the right track with Z-track injections. *Nursing* **10**, 59.

Kozier, B., Erb, G., & Blais, K. (1993) *Techniques in Clinical Nursing, 4th ed*. California: Sage.

Kuzu, N. & Ucar, H. (2001) The effect of cold on the occurrence of bruising, haematoma and pain at the injection site in subcutaneous low molecular weight heparin. *International Journal of Nursing Studies* **38**, 51–59.

Mallett, J. & Bailey, C. (1996) *The Royal Marsden NHS Trust Manual of Clinical Procedures, 5th ed*. London: Blackwell Science.

Marsden, J. & Shaw, M. (2003) Correct administration of topical eye treatment. *Nursing Standard* **17** (30), 42.

McConnell, E. (1993) Clinical dos and don'ts: How to administer a Z-track injection. *Nursing* **23**, 18.

Muller-Vahl, H. (1985) Isolated complete paralysis of the tensor fasciae latae muscle. *European Neurology* **24** (5), 289–291.

Neill, S. & Knowles, H. (2004) *The Biology of Child Health: A reader in development and assessment*. London: Palgrave Macmillan.

Newton, M., Newtown, D., & Fudin, J. (1992) Reviewing the big three injection routes. *Nursing* **22**, 34–42.

Nursing and Midwifery Council (2008) *Standards for Medicines Management*. UK: Nursing and Midwifery Council.

Pavlin, D., Links, S., Rapp, S. Nessley, M., & Keyes, H. (1993) Vasovagal reactions in an ambulatory surgical centre. *Anaesthesia & Analgesia* **76**, 931–935.

Poter-Jones, G. (2000) Nebulizers—1: preparation. *Nursing Times* **96** (36), 45–46.

Preston, S. & Hagadonen, K. (2004) Glass contamination in parenterally administered medication. *Journal of Advanced Nursing* **48** (3), 212–215.

Rodger, M. & King, L. (2000) Drawing up and administering intramuscular injections: A review of literature. *Journal of Advanced Nursing* **31** (3), 574–582.

Rose, K. (2005) Better medicines for children—where are we now and where do we want to be? *British Journal of Clinical Pharmacology* **56** (6), 657–659.

Ross, J., Saunders, Y., Cochrane, M. & Zeppetella, G. (2002) A prospective, within-patient comparison between metal butterfly needles and Teflon cannulae in subcutaneous infusion of drugs to terminally ill hospice patients. *Palliative Medicine* **16** (1), 13–16.

Royal College of Paediatrics and Child Health & Royal College of Nursing (2002) *Position statement on injection technique*. London: RCPCH & RCN.

Schmalbach, T.K. & Hoekelman, R.A., (eds.) (1997) *Clinical Pharmacology*. Chapter 30: Primary pediatric care. St Louis: Mosby.

Sharp, D. (2004) Selling comfort: A survey of interventions for needle procedures in a paediatrics hospital. *Pain Management Nursing,* **5** (4), 144–152.

Small, S. (2004) Preventing sciatic nerve injury from intramuscular injections: Literature review. *Journal of Advanced Nursing* **47**, 287–296.

Suggs, D. (2000) Pharmacokinetics in children: History, considerations, and applications. *Journal of the American Academy of Nurse Practitioners.* **12** (6), 236–239.

Summer, Y. (2000) *Ed Rational Therapeutics for Infants and Children. National Academy of Sciences*. USA: National Academy Press.

Trigg, E. & Mohammed, T.A. (2006) *Practices in Children's Nursing: Guidelines for hospital and community, 2nd ed*. China: Churchill Livingstone.

Van den Anker, J.N., & Choonara, I. (1999) ENDIC—European Network for Drug Investigation in Children. *Paediatric and Perinatal Drug Therapy* **3**, 15–16.

Venketasubramanian, N., & Chua, H.C. (1998) Subcutaneous low molecular weight heparin in place of heparin infusion during warfarin dose optimization in cerebral ischaemia. *Clinical Neurology and Neurosurgery* **100**, 193–195.

Watkinson, S. & Seewoodhary, R. (2008) Administering eye medications. *Nursing Standard* **22** (18), 42.

Watt, S. (2003) Safe administration of medicines to children: Part 2. *Paediatric Nursing* **15** (5), 40.

Weisman, S., Bernstein, B., & Schechter, N. (1998) Consequences of inadequate analgesia during painful procedures in children. *Archives of Paediatrics Adolescent Medicine* **152**, 147–149.

Workman, B. (1999) Safe injection techniques. *Nursing Standard* **13**, 47–54.

World Health Organization (2006) *Immunization in Practice. Module 6: Holding an immunization session.* Geneva: WHO.

Zelman, S. (1961) Notes on the techniques of intramuscular injection. *American Journals of Medical Science* **241**, 47–58.

Zenk, K. (1993) Beware of overdose. *Nursing* **23** (3), 28–29.

Zuckerman, J. (2000) The importance of injecting vaccines into muscle: Different patients need different needle sizes. *British Medical Journal* **321**, 1237–1238.

Further reading and URLs

Department of Health (2001) *Seeking Consent: Working with children.* London: The Stationery Office.

European Convention on the Rights of the Child: Consent and Capacity, cited in UN Convention on the Rights of the Child (1989) (20.Xi. 1989; TS 44; Cm 1976).

Glasper, A., & Richardson, J. (eds.) (2006) *A Textbook of Children's and Young People's Nursing.* London: Churchill Livingstone.

Greenstein, B. & Gould, D. (2004) *Trounce's Clinical Pharmacology for Nurses, 17th ed.* London: Churchill Livingstone.

Kanneh, A. (1998a) Pharmacological principles applied to children. Part 1. *Paediatric Nursing* **10** (3), 17–20.

Mallett, J. & Dougherty, L. (2000) *The Royal Marsden Manual of Clinical Nursing Procedures, 5th edition.* London: Blackwell Science.

Royal College of Nursing (2003) *Restraint, Holding Still and Containing Children and Young People. Guidance for Nursing Staff.* London: RCN.

Royal College of Paediatrics and Child Health & Royal College of Nursing (RCN) (2002) *Position Statement on Injection Technique.* London: RCPCH.

Simonsen, T., Aarbakke, J., Kay, I., Sinnott, P., & Coleman, I. (2006) *Illustrated Pharmacology for Nurses.* Oxford: Oxford University Press.

Trigg, E. & Mohammed, T. (eds.) (2006) *Practices in Children's Nursing: Guidelines for Hospital and Community, 2nd ed.* London: Churchill Livingstone.

The BNF child website is useful for up-to-date recommended drug dosages: **http://bnf.org/bnf/**

Nurse Prescribing is the leading UK journal for nurses with prescription rights. It has useful sections on pharmacology, nursing practice, legal and ethical issues, and research and development: **http://www.nurseprescribing.com/**

The following website is a useful resource for students in relation to all forms of drug calculations: **http://www.testandcalc.com/quiz/index.asp**

This website deals with the pharmacokinetics and pharmacodynamics of drugs: **http://www.abdellab.sunderland.ac.uk/Lectures/Nurses/**

Part Three

The respiratory system

8

JAN ORR

Skills

 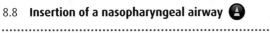
Introduction

The aim of this chapter is to provide an outline of the underpinning theory and relevant information needed to deliver safe and effective, family centred, evidence-based care to the child or young person who presents with breathing difficulties.

Learning outcomes

In is anticipated that at the end of this chapter you will be able to:

- Understand the anatomy and physiology of the respiratory system.
- Discuss the concept of visual assessment of breathing, including monitoring and recording of respiratory rate, oxygen saturation levels, and peak expiratory flow rates.
- Explain oxygen therapy and the use of airway adjuncts.
- Reflect upon methods and equipment used for suctioning.
- Discuss tracheostomy management, care of intrapleural drainage, and endotracheal tubes.
- Apply the concepts and principles outlined relevant to the hospital and community setting.

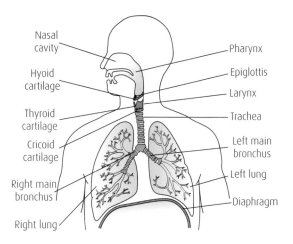

Figure 8.1 The respiratory system

The respiratory system

This is the system through which oxygen is breathed in from the external environment, either by the nose or mouth, and a waste product (carbon dioxide) is excreted. The respiratory system consists of respiratory passages, which carry air via the nose to the lungs, and a network of blood capillaries in the lungs (**see Figure 8.1**). The respiratory passages include the nose, pharynx, larynx (voice box), trachea, two bronchi (one bronchus to each lung), and copious bronchial tubes, which divide and lead to millions of alveoli (tiny air sacs). There are two lungs either side of the heart in the thoracic cavity. They are made up of bronchial tubes, alveoli, blood vessels, and nerves (McCance & Heuther, 2006).

How breathing occurs

Air containing oxygen (O_2) and carbon dioxide (CO_2) is breathed into the lungs. This fills the alveoli. It is separated from the blood in capillaries by two semi-permeable membranes. These make up the walls of the alveoli and capillaries. Oxygen is at a higher concentration in the alveoli. It therefore passes from the alveoli into the blood. Carbon dioxide is higher in concentration in the blood, so it passes from the blood into the alveoli. Oxygen is carried in the blood in haemoglobin (red blood corpuscles). Breathing is the regular inflation and deflation of the lungs, maintaining a steady concentration of atmospheric gases in the alveoli (MacGregor, 2000).

Lung function and effective ventilation

The following are common terminology used in respiratory assessment and support:

- Ventilation: this is the movement of gas between the lungs and atmospheric (ambient) pressure.
- Tidal volume: this refers to the volume of gas that is inspired and expired in one breath. This equates to 6 millilitres (ml) per kilogram (kg) of body weight. For example, a child weighing 20 kg will have a tidal volume of 120 ml.
- Minute volume: this refers to the quantity of gas expired by the lungs in one minute.
- Functional residual capacity: this is the amount of gas that remains in the lungs after normal expiration.
- The anatomical dead space: this is approximately 30% of each tidal volume. It fills the conducting airways and no gas exchange takes place here (Davies & Hassell, 2001).

The descriptions above will help you to understand some of the terminology used in respiratory assessment, support, and care delivery, particularly in the child and young person in respiratory distress. The terminology is commonly used in high dependency and intensive care units for the child requiring respiratory support such as **mechanical ventilation**.

Anatomical differences of the child's respiratory system compared to adults

- A large head and tongue and short neck. This can cause airway obstruction when in the supine position (lying on the back).
- Cartilaginous (pliable) tracheal rings. These can easily collapse causing airway obstruction.
- The face and mandible (lower jaw bone) are small and hyper-plastic (bendy). Care must be taken to ensure the airway is positioned effectively.
- Loose deciduous teeth. These may be inhaled resulting in choking.
- The larynx is high and at the level of the second and third cervical vertebrae in infants, compared to fifth and

sixth vertebrae in adults. Therefore appropriate-sized equipment should be used for airway support.

- The cricoid ring (the ring-shaped cartilage at the lower end of the larynx) is the narrowest part of the airway in children; in adults the larynx is the narrowest. Care should be taken to position the child appropriately for airway support. The child is susceptible to swelling.
- The ribcage is compliant (bendy). This leads to insufficient inspiration causing an increased effort in breathing.

(Davies & Hassell, 2001)

Nursing Alert

The basic principles of paediatric life support are the same as for adults; however, there are specific differences in the techniques required for neonates, infants, and children. Basic life support education is a mandatory requirement for students prior to working in healthcare settings but further reading into this subject is recommended.

Embryology and breathing

Lung growth and development continues through uterine and embryonic stages. In the fourth gestational week on day 22 the lung appears as a bud from the oesophagus below the pharyngeal pouches. Two branches, making up the bronchi, bud out on day 26 to day 28. By the eighth week more branching occurs and the bronchi and hyaline cartilage appear in the walls, together with capillaries and smooth muscles. At 17 weeks' gestation all structures are formed. No gas exchange is possible though, so at this age the foetus is not viable.

From 16 to 25 weeks the bronchioles become highly vascular and some gas exchange occurs. Neonates under 24 weeks gestation can be so fragile that they are at risk of permanent lung damage. However, due to advances in neonatal care, at this age neonates can develop to have healthy lungs. From 24 weeks to birth, the terminal sacs develop. At birth each lung will have 20–70 million of these sacs; adults have 300–400 million. Foetal pulmonary resistance is very high; the lungs are filled with fluid so the alveoli lack oxygen (**hypoxia**). This ensures that pulmonary vasoconstriction and adequate blood flow

nourishes the developing pulmonary tissues. Breathing is not important *in utero* as the foetus receives its oxygen from the maternal circulation. At 26 weeks the muscles of the bronchi and bronchioles are complete (MacGregor, 2000).

Surfactant is a lipid (fatty substance present in body tissues) that is excreted onto the alveoli surface, preventing the sacs from collapsing on expiration. This is achieved by reducing the surface tension on the internal surface. At 22 weeks of gestation surfactant is secreted and this continues to 32–35 weeks' gestation. It flows up the trachea out of the mouth, into the amniotic fluid. Prematurely born babies are at a high risk of respiratory failure due to surfactant deficiency. Surfactant replacement therapy increases their chance of survival. The surfactant is administered through the endotracheal tube (Halliday, 2006).

The lungs at birth

The neonate is hypoxic (low oxygen levels) at birth and breathing responds to the low oxygen. This adjusts to adult requirements by day 7. Oxygen pressures at day 1 are 80 mmHg. Carbon dioxide and blood acidity are normal. In the pre-term birth, the neonate shows reduced sensitivity to oxygen, as it still has the foetal response of elevated breathing movements, reacting to carbon dioxide levels in the circulating blood. After 2–12 weeks of life, the muscles in the pulmonary arteries become thinner, dilate, lengthen, and branch out. This reduces the resistance of the pulmonary circulation in the right side of the heart. After one to two months the pulmonary vessels supplying the bronchi, bronchioles, and alveoli develop. This differs in babies born with cardiac problems (MacGregor, 2000).

Baby breathing

Babies up to the age of four weeks are nose breathers. They are therefore at risk of breathing difficulties if they have a cold or lie with their faces in vomit or bedding. They do not adapt well to mouth breathing. They have small airways, which narrow and block further if they become swollen or blocked with secretions. Young babies who have difficulty breathing will likely have problems feeding. This is because they are unable to swallow and breathe at the same time. They may also lose their appetite as a result of tiredness from any increased respiratory effort (MacGregor, 2000).

> **Nursing Alert**
>
> ■ Babies with breathing problems are likely to lose weight. Consideration of the nutritional requirements of babies is very important (refer to Chapter Twelve).
>
> ■ The patency of the upper airways is maintained by active contractions of muscles in the pharynx and larynx. The muscles are compromised if the neck is flexed or extended, hence the importance of maintaining effective neutral airway positioning in emergency care intervention (Advanced Paediatric Life Support Group (APLS), 2006).
>
> ■ To reduce the risk of cot death, babies should be positioned in their cot on their back, with their feet to the foot of the crib. The covers should reach no higher than the shoulders and should be securely tucked in so they cannot slip over the baby's head. At about five or six months old, it is normal for babies to roll over and they shouldn't be prevented from doing this. The risk of cot death reduces rapidly at this age. Support the baby's family and carers in instigating this practice (Department of Health (DH), 2007). Further reading on reducing the risk of cot death is recommended.

The small child's breathing

The small child has a compliant (easily movable) chest wall. Only the external intercostal muscles stabilize the chest wall. The diaphragm is more horizontal and the lower ribs retract when the child lies supine (flat). The more the ribs retract, the more the diaphragm needs to contract to generate the tidal volume. This is inefficient breathing and takes a lot of effort. Therefore in the child with breathing difficulties, it does not take long for the child to become tired due to increased respiratory effort.

Heat and water are transmitted to inspired air; therefore children lose more body heat and water from body tissues in breathing. Children are therefore more likely to develop mucus plugs when they have respiratory infections. The airway size and length increases after birth. Up until the age of three years the number of immature

alveoli increases. After this it is only the size of the alveoli that increases. This continues until the age of eight years (MacGregor, 2000; McCance & Huether, 2006).

Changes at puberty

From the age of five to puberty the weight of the lungs increases by three times. Total lung volume increases as the lungs grow. This is the same in both boys and girls. Frequency of respiration rate tends to be slightly higher in boys than girls. This is thought to be because of the changing lean body mass as they approach puberty. Lean muscle tissue has a higher metabolic demand than fat (MacGregor, 2000).

By the age of eight, the tissues are mature. From eight to puberty increase in air space occurs through enlargement of the airways. Throughout childhood the lung volume remains constant compared to the body mass. As the child grows and the airways enlarge, resistance to the flow in the airways reduces and the respiration rate increases (McCance & Heuther, 2006).

Sleeping and breathing

During the 'non-rapid eye movement' (NREM) stage of sleep, respiration is regular and ventilation reduces. This is as a result of reduced metabolic demands. This slowing rate occurs in children as they go into their deep sleep state. The parasympathetic nerve supply takes over and the bronchi muscles relax giving a reduction in lumen size. In the 'rapid eye movement' (REM) stage of sleep, respiration becomes irregular. Rhythmic breathing activity is reduced. Arterial oxygen levels are reduced. The tidal volume also reduces. Consideration of the effects of sleep is important when assessing the child or young person's breathing. Small babies have longer REM sleep periods and are often seen to have irregular breathing (MacGregor, 2000).

> **Nursing Alert**
>
> Any swelling of the upper airway will compromise the airway as the soft palate relaxes and the tongue falls back in the pharynx. Take care in positioning babies with respiratory problems; ensure their head is placed in the neutral position and their neck is not extended (APLS, 2006).

Common breathing problems

One common breathing difficulty experienced by children is bronchiolitis. Bronchiolitis is the commonest lower respiratory disease affecting children under one year (APLS, 2006). It is usually caused by respiratory synctial virus (RSV). This virus replicates in the epithelial cells of the bronchioles causing **necrosis** (death of tissues). New epithelial cells are not ciliated (have no hair-like structures). This and increased secretions cause obstruction of the small airways. This impairs gaseous exchange and can result in hypoxia (lack of oxygen).

Nursing Alert

RSV is highly infectious and requires careful protective isolation to avoid cross infection. Refer to the local guidelines of the healthcare setting for information on protective isolation (Fazakerley, 2004).

Asthma is another common respiratory disorder seen in children. It is a chronic inflammatory condition of the airways that results in breathing difficulties and, in severe cases, respiratory distress and arrest (APLS, 2006). The actual cause is not completely understood but it can be precipitated by a specific trigger such as:

- Viral infections.
- Cigarette smoke.
- Allergens, such as animal dander, house mite dust, mould, or pollen.
- Exercise.
- Emotion such as fear, anxiety, or excitement.

Asthma occurs when the muscles around the walls of the airway tighten, in response to the above named triggers or other factors. There may also be swelling of lining of the airways and mucus production. Signs and symptoms of this include coughing, wheezing, breathlessness, and noisy breathing.

The overall aim of asthma management is symptom control, prevention of exacerbations, and enabling the child to lead a full and active life. Treatment includes the use of inhaled drugs called 'relievers' and 'preventers'. The child, family, and other carers (including teachers, childminders, club leaders, and others who spend time with the child) need to be educated in why, how, and when to use these inhalers. Support from asthma care specialists, school nurses, and other community-based care teams is important to help the child to live with this chronic condition (Global Initiative for Asthma (GINA), 2007; McEwing et al., 2003).

Respiratory viral and bacterial infections are spread easily by airborne droplets. Close proximity of children at school, nursery, and other social and communal places results in the spread of infection. In particular, children are not always careful about using disposable handkerchiefs to cough and sneeze into and appropriate hand washing to prevent the spread of infection (Kelsey & McEwing, 2006). Education in community settings such as nurseries and schools is an effective way to promote good 'cough and cold' hygiene. It is important to alert the child and family to the importance of this (DH, 2004). Babies and young children are more vulnerable to respiratory infection as their immune systems have not been exposed to common pathogens. For the most part respiratory infections stay localized and remain in the respiratory tract, without spreading to other organs. However, this is not to say that respiratory conditions are always mild. These conditions can be severe, for example pneumonia, and may require medical intervention (Fazakerley, 2004).

Indeed, respiratory failure is the commonest cause of death in children and conditions can become very severe. Precipitating conditions that lead to death include severe asthmatic attacks, choking, bronchiolitis and other infections, and exacerbation of congenital respiratory problems. Prompt recognition, assessment, and expert multi-professional management of respiratory emergencies are important to ensure good outcomes and prevent such a devastating consequence (APLS, 2006; Rotta & Wiryawan, 2003; Toplis, 2007).

Visual assessment

The visual assessment and early recognition of any breathing problems are very important to ensure effective care outcomes (Aylott, 2006a). When approaching the young child to assess their breathing try and adopt a calm and supportive atmosphere. Further information about clinical observations is outlined in Chapter Five. In keeping with concepts of family centred care discussed in Chapter Two, it is very important to involve the child, their family, and any other carers during this assessment. You should always explain what is happening in words they understand, avoiding medical jargon and abbreviations. This is to ensure they understand what is happening and are not frightened any further (Smith *et al.*, 2002). The use of play and distraction is helpful in such situations (see also Chapter Two and Chapter Five). Involving play specialists at an early stage is useful, to assist with explanations and distraction therapies (Webster, 2000) (see also Chapter Two).

> **Nursing Alert**
>
> Further distress to the child could exacerbate any breathing difficulties (Kelsey & McEwing, 2006).

One approach that is commonly used in practice is consideration of the mnemonic 'ABCD' in relation to visual assessment of the child's respiratory status. This provides a prompt to the nurse, whose assessment may, in conjunction with the use of standard approaches to assessment (Chapter Five) and local evidence-based policies and guidelines, be guided towards a systematic, prioritized, and thorough consideration using each of these letters as an *aide memoire*. The letters relate to the assessment as follows:

- **A**irway
- **B**reathing
- **C**irculation
- **D**isability

This is particularly useful during stressful emergency situations and for healthcare professionals not used to dealing with sick children, to ensure nothing is missed (APLS, 2006). These specifics will now be further discussed.

When giving consideration to the *airway*, it is important to observe the child or young person's mouth to ensure the patency of the airway. Look to see if it is clear and if there is any visible foreign body (APLS, 2006).

> **Nursing Alert**
>
> ■ Only remove foreign bodies from the mouth that can be easily reached. If unable to do so leave it as it is until medical assistance arrives. This is in case it becomes dislodged further into the airway (APLS, 2006).
>
> ■ Do not ask the child to talk too much as they could become more tired and exacerbate breathlessness (Toplis, 2007).
>
> ■ During assessment, if there is no evidence of breathing, the chin lift or jaw thrust should be carried out and basic life support commenced (APLS, 2006; Aylott, 2006a).

When considering *breathing* it is important to bear in mind that under normal circumstances breathing should be effortless, even in the neonate and newborn baby, where breathing is more frequent. During assessment you observe the rate and pattern of breathing (Chapter Five). You look and see if the child is using accessory (supplementary) respiratory muscle groups during breathing, as this is an indicator of respiratory distress. Listen to see if the child has a stridor when breathing. A stridor or wheeze can be heard as a harsh, vibrating, shrill sound but is seen as a child gasping for breath (Kelsey & McEwing, 2006). Other signs to observe that can indicate breathing difficulties as a result of forced air entry include nasal flaring and head bobbing or coughing. If the child is in respiratory distress for long periods of time they become exhausted and the aforementioned signs of increased respiratory effort will decrease (Rotta & Wiryawan, 2003). When the child is at rest, tachypnoea (fast breathing) indicates that increased ventilatory effort is needed to meet the body's demand for oxygen. Reasons for this include lung or airway disease, other lung problems, or metabolic acidosis (abnormal blood gases as a result of hypoxia) (Davies & Hassell, 2001). The clinical signs of respiratory distress that are observed for during examination of respiration are as follows:

- Tachypnoea.
- Altered breathing.
- Use of accessory muscle groups to breathe.
- Nasal flaring.
- **Cyanosis**.
- Wheeze.
- **Dyspnoea**.
- Coughing.
- Stridor.
- Head bobbing.
- Seesaw respirations.
- Decreased chest expansion sounds.
- Silent chest.

> **Nursing Alert**
>
> A stridor is usually caused by a partial obstruction to the larynx or trachea and is a severe medical emergency (APLS, 2006).

When giving consideration to the assessment of *circulation* it is important to look at the colour of the child's skin, particularly the fingers, toes, lips, and ears (known as extremities). In respiratory distress oxygen will be circulated to the major organs, resulting in reduced oxygen distribution to the extremities. Visual signs would include mottling, blue, pale, clammy skin and extremities. This lack of oxygen is known as peripheral shut down and is a result of poor oxygen perfusion (Rotta & Wiryawan, 2003).

Cardiovascular indicators:

- Tachycardia.
- Bradycardia.
- Hyper- and hypotension.
- Cyanosis.
- Cardiac arrest.

Nursing Alert

By the time cyanosis (lack of oxygen, visible by blue or a blue tinge to the skin, lips, and extremities) has occurred, the child is likely to be very near respiratory arrest. It is for this reason that prompt assessment and actions are important (APLS, 2006).

This assessment is also outlined in more detail in Chapter Five and circulation is considered in Chapter Nine.

The final element of the ABCD assessment guide is the consideration of *disability* in a child presenting with a respiratory complaint. This relates to the visual assessment of the child or young person's responsiveness. There are other more general indicators of respiratory distress such as a child that is lethargic or 'floppy', tired, or experiencing pain around the chest and abdomen. The child may also be perspiring. Brain function may also be affected by respiratory insufficiencies and as a result the child may exhibit signs of irritability, headache, confusion, unresponsiveness, pain, altered consciousness levels, or unconsciousness (Kelsey & McEwing, 2006). It is important to ascertain the child's responsiveness by asking questions that are appropriate to the child or young person's age and development. Parents or carers are helpful in this role, as the child or young person is more likely to respond to them (Smith *et al.*, 2002). A more detailed discussion of neurological assessment is provided in Chapter Ten.

Nursing Alert

- Exhaustion is a dangerous sign and can result in respiratory and cardiopulmonary arrest if not treated promptly (APLS, 2006).

- When approaching the child or young person remain calm and friendly to establish a therapeutic relationship and reduce anxiety (Ogden-Burke *et al.*, 2001).

- Consider airway, breathing, and circulation prior to assessing problems with conscious levels to establish a neurological reason for breathing problems. For example, a child with a head injury (Kelsey & McEwing, 2006).

Careful looking and listening to the child is very important in the visual assessment of the child's respiratory status. Monitoring of capillary refill (see Chapter Five), oxygen saturation, and peak expiratory flow compliment in making a holistic, family centred, and individual assessment (McEwing *et al.*, 2003).

Non-invasive assessment of breathing

8.1 Recording respiratory rate

Accurate measurement of breathing is required to determine the child's baseline as a comparison for future measurements. It can indicate any changes in the respiratory rate. It is also an important measurement to assess the effectiveness of respiratory medications and treatments (Aylott, 2006b). Respiratory rate is usually measured when the child is admitted to hospital; however, parents or carers, community nursing staff, and respiratory nurse specialists may also measure respiratory rates in the community. For example, with a child with asthma who is recovering from a chest infection at home, this could be done to ensure that their breathing is responding to antibiotics and asthma inhaler treatments (Kelsey & McEwing, 2006).

Measuring breathing can be difficult, particularly in the younger child or infant who may be distressed and agitated. Ensure that the infant or child is approached in a calm and reassuring way. Involving parents or carers will reduce the infant or child's anxiety. Play specialists are an important part of the multi-professional team involved in the child's care in hospital and in the community. Involving them in the initial assessment and ongoing care of the infant or child and their family reduces anxiety (Webster, 2000).

Procedure: Measuring respiratory rate

Assessment

Before you begin consider the child's age to determine the most appropriate method of measurement to use.

Listening to chests with a stethoscope

Experienced nurses and other healthcare professionals such as physiotherapists, medical staff, paramedics, and community nurse specialists, will assess the child's

Table 8.1 Normal respiratory rates by age at rest (APLS, 2006)

Age (years)	Respiratory rate (breaths per minute)
<1	30–40
1–2	25–35
2–5	25–30
5–12	20–25
>12	15–20

respiratory rate by auscultation. This involves listening for breath sounds and any other added sounds. This includes listening and observing for pitch, intensity, quality, location, and duration of breath sounds. Listening to the child's voice and cry is also helpful in assessing breathing, for example, a hoarse or wheezy voice is a likely indication of respiratory problems. Involving parents or carers in this assessment is valuable in identifying any changes in the child's normal breathing (Kelsey & McEwing, 2006; Thornton, 2007).

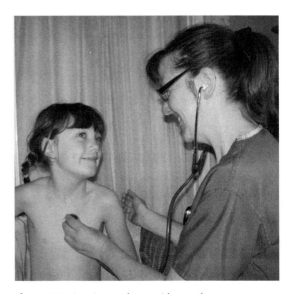

Figure 8.2 Listening to chests with a stethoscope

Step-by-step guide to measuring respiratory rate

Step	Rationale
1 Hand washing.	To prevent cross infection.
2 Pretend to take the pulse or listen to the heart beat at the same time as measuring respirations (Kelsey & McEwing, 2006).	Children may alter their breathing pattern if they are aware they are being counted.
3 Whilst measuring, observe depth of breathing and note symmetry or asymmetry of the chest.	To assess the quality of the breath.
4 In children younger than eight years, assess the presence and equality of the chest rising and falling by counting abdominal movements (Kelsey & McEwing, 2006).	Children this age are predominantly abdominal breathers (Aylott, 2006a; Royal College of Nursing (RCN), 2007).
5 In older children observe the chest wall for inspiration.	To count the respirations.
6 Count respirations for 60 seconds (RCN, 2007).	To ensure accuracy.
7 Whilst counting also note any signs of increased work of breathing (Kelsey & McEwing, 2006).	To indicate breathing difficulties.
8 Record the measurements and observations.	To ensure effective communication.
9 Repeat the measurements and observations as indicated by the child's condition or any interventions. For example, the administration of medication to assist breathing.	To observe and assess for early indicators of exacerbation or improvement of breathing problems.
10 Report any abnormalities to the appropriate healthcare practitioner, e.g. a doctor.	To ensure early medical care intervention.
11 Hand washing.	To prevent cross infection.

8.2 Peak flow monitoring

Peak expiratory flow rate (or peak flow) is a measurement of the highest rate at which air can be expelled from the lungs through an open mouth. Handheld peak expiratory flow rate meters are commonly used to assess lung function and aid the self-management of respiratory and respiratory-related illness, for example, asthma and **cystic fibrosis**. Electronic peak flow meters are also available (Lewis, 2007).

Procedure: Monitoring a peak flow rate

Preparation

Explain the procedure to the child and their parent/carer. This promotes compliance and reduces anxiety. If the child is particularly anxious, it may help to involve a play specialist.

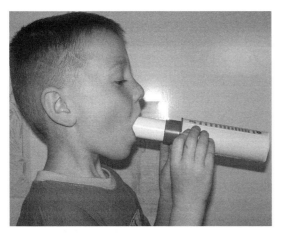

Figure 8.3 Taking a peak expiratory flow rate

Equipment

Ensure the peak flow monitor to be used is the new standard European model, as this will help you to take an accurate reading (Lewis, 2007).

Consent and communication

Explain the procedure, and why you are carrying it out, to the child/family before you begin.

Normal values of peak flow

The reference value for children is best assessed against their baseline peak flow (taken on admission to hospital

---

Step-by-step guide to monitoring a peak flow rate

Step	Rationale
1 Hand washing.	To prevent cross infection.
2 Ensure the child is sitting upright or standing up.	To achieve a larger lung function and more accurate reading.
3 Ask the child to hold the peak flow monitor and ensure the pointer is pushed to the lowest number on the sliding scale. (Lewis, 2007). Ensure the child's fingers are clear of the pointer and gauge (Jevon *et al.*, 2000).	To allow a clear run for the pointer to move.
4 Encourage the child to blow out as much as possible (Lewis, 2007).	To encourage a good deep breath.
5 Encourage the child to take a deep breath (Lewis, 2007).	To fill the lungs to their full capacity.
6 Ensure the child seals their lips around the single-use mouthpiece of the peak flow meter (Lewis, 2007).	To prevent air loss and inaccurate results.
7 Encourage the child to blow out in one breath as hard and fast as they can. This sounds like 'huff' (Lewis, 2007).	A false low reading may be given if maximum effort is not used.
8 Ask the child to repeat the peak flow three times and record the best of the three results (Lewis, 2007).	To allow practice.
9 Record the findings on a peak flow record sheet or diary.	To ensure effective documentation.
10 Hand washing.	To prevent cross infection.
11 Report any abnormalities or improvements to the appropriate healthcare professional, e.g. doctor or respiratory nurse specialist.	To ensure early intervention if there are problems and evaluation of treatments.

or at the first consultation with the child at home). If this is possible, in particular for the child with chronic breathing problems, a record of their best ever value (reference value) should be used as an assessment of deterioration of their respiratory function. In a child with asthma, a peak flow reading below 50% of their reference value indicates a severe asthma attack. Values of less than 33% indicate a life-threatening attack (Booker, 2007).

Although there are other methods of assessing peak flow such as spirometry, the use of handheld peak flow meters is easy and quick to teach children and their parents or carers. It is an easy and accessible method to use at home and is commonly used by children to monitor asthma at home (Miller *et al.*, 2005).

8.3 **Monitoring oxygen saturation and using a pulse oximeter**

Alongside the visual assessment of breathing, pulse oximetry is a commonly used method as part of the respiratory assessment. It is usually performed when a child is admitted to hospital with breathing problems. It is also used in the community setting for children with chronic breathing problems to allow parents or carers to observe for problems in their child's condition and to measure the effectiveness of drugs and treatments. Pulse oximetry is the monitoring of the oxygen saturation (SPO_2) of

haemoglobin in capillary blood. The result is expressed as a percentage (Lewis, 2007).

Procedure: Using a pulse oximeter

Equipment

Check the pulse oximeter is in good working order before beginning the procedure, to ensure safe and accurate monitoring. You will need to ensure that the monitor, sensor probe, and infra-red light are working. Finally check and set the alarm limits so they are appropriate to the child's individual age and development (Syers, 2008).

Consent and communication

Explain the procedure to the child/family to help ensure their cooperation.

Oxygen therapy and airway adjuncts

It is likely that the child with respiratory problems will require oxygen therapy. Oxygen should be prescribed by medical staff or healthcare professionals certified to prescribe, for example, nurse specialist or paramedic. Many clinical and health community settings have care pathways or group directives for the administration of oxygen. This is to prevent any time delay in administering oxygen. When next in a clinical or community placement, it is advised that you refer to local guidelines in regard to this (Langridge, 2004).

The amount of oxygen given to the child is called the fractional inspired oxygen concentration (FiO_2). The lowest possible concentration of oxygen should be delivered to maintain FiO_2. Oxygen should be discontinued as soon as possible (APLS, 2006). In neonates, continuous administration of high levels of oxygen can raise partial pressure of oxygen, known as PO_2. This can result in damage to the retina in the eye (retinopathy of prematurity). Prolonged

Step-by-step guide to using a pulse oximeter

Step		Rationale
1	Hand washing.	To prevent cross infection.
2	Place an appropriate-sized sensor probe around the child's finger, toe, or ear lobe. The chosen site should be warm and well perfused with good capillary refill time (Syers, 2008).	To ensure accuracy of reading.
3	The sensor probe has infra-red diodes on one side of the probe and a detector on the other. They should be directly opposite each other on the selected site.	The processor in the monitor analyses the changes in the light absorption in the peak flow through the capillary bed (Syers, 2008).
4	If there is no reading, re-site the probe.	Too much light may be getting into the sensor because of an incorrectly placed probe (Syers, 2008).
5	Check the wave form on the monitor is regular and has a good volume. Compare the pulse recording to the child's pulse (Syers, 2008).	To ensure accuracy.
6	If continuous oxygen saturation monitoring is required, change the probe site every four hours (Medical Devices Agency, 2001).	To prevent skin damage under the probe. This is particularly relevant in children with fragile skin or infants.
7	Hand washing.	To prevent cross infection.
8	Document the measurements on the appropriate charts. Report any abnormalities or improvements to the relevant healthcare professional, e.g. doctor.	To ensure good documentation and early intervention or change in treatment.

exposure to high oxygen levels, in this group, can lead to permanent lung damage, as the lungs are immature and alveolar tissue is fragile. One example of this type of consequence is the development of broncho-pulmonary dysplasia (Toplis, 2007).

Nursing Alert

Using oxygen concentrations that are too high in children with chronic lung conditions can cause respiratory failure (APLS, 2006).

Methods to deliver oxygen

Oxygen can be provided to children in the clinical environment in several ways.

8.4 **Delivery of oxygen using nasal prongs**

Nasal prongs are a commonly used method of delivering oxygen, as it is tolerated well by most children. With the use of prongs, humidification (which is normally applied when using a mask to deliver oxygen) is not needed as the nasal passages are warm and moisten the oxygen as it enters the airways (Hufton, 2007).

Nursing Alert

Nasal prongs can only be used for the delivery of less than two litres of oxygen, otherwise it dries the mucosa and is uncomfortable (Dougherty & Lister, 2006).

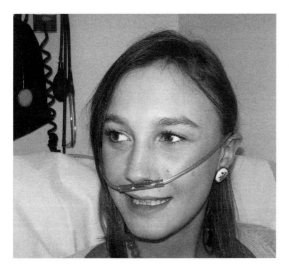

Figure 8.4 Patient with nasal prongs

Procedure: Using nasal prongs to deliver oxygen

Equipment

● Oxygen supply.
● Nasal prongs.

● Monitor.
● Adhesive tape.

Assessment

Before you begin ensure the oxygen is prescribed and assess the need to administer it. Oxygen is toxic and should only be given if needed (Hufton, 2007; Owens, 2008).

Consent and communication

To ensure compliance and reduce anxiety, explain the procedure to the child and their family. Involve a play specialist if required.

8.5 **Delivery of oxygen using a face mask**

There are several types of face mask used in the delivery of oxygen to children. If oxygen over 2 litres is delivered for more than four hours, humidification should be added to prevent drying of the mucosa and to aid loosening of secretions (Kelsey & McEwing, 2006). Humidity is usually

Step-by-step guide to using nasal prongs to deliver oxygen to children

Step		Rationale
1	Hand washing. Wear personal protective equipment (PPE) (e.g. gloves, aprons, visors) as indicated by the local infection control policy.	To reduce cross infection.
2	Apply the nasal prongs in each nostril. In babies ensure the prongs do not block the nasal passages (Hufton, 2007).	Babies are nose breathers.
3	In small children and babies particularly, it is a good idea to secure the nasal prongs in place with adhesive tape.	To keep the prongs in place because the tubing can be easily dislodged.
4	Tighten the tubing around the back of the head, ensuring the child is comfortable.	To promote comfort and ensure the tubing stays in place.
5	Hand washing.	To prevent cross infection.
6	Document and sign the prescription stating amount, timings, and any changes during the delivery of the oxygen.	To ensure effective documentation.

delivered via an electronic and monitored warming system (Hufton, 2007). Inhaled air is normally warmed by the nose and upper respiratory tract. Warming a gas such as oxygen increases its capacity to hold vapour (Hufton, 2007).

Types of mask (APLS, 2006)

- Simple mask without a reservoir bay—commonly used, maximum FiO_2 is 50%.
- Mask without reservoir bay (partial re-breathing)—maximum FiO_2 is 70%.
- Mask with reservoir bay (non-re-breathing)—maximum FiO_2 is 90%.
- Not all children tolerate oxygen masks for long periods of time. Careful planning and preparation, including the child's family, carer, or a play specialist, can help with cooperation (Ogden-Burke *et al.*, 2001).

Procedure: Applying an oxygen face mask

Equipment

- Oxygen mask.
- Oxygen tubing.
- Oxygen supply.
- Flow meter.

Consent and communication

To ensure compliance and reduce anxiety, explain the procedure to the child and their family. Involve a play specialist if required.

Step-by-step guide to applying an oxygen face mask

Step	Rationale
1 Hand washing. Wear PPE.	To prevent cross infection.
2 Have an appropriate size of oxygen mask attached to an adequate length of green tubing.	To ensure comfort and effective administration of oxygen.
3 Place the oxygen mask over the child's face with the elastic securely and comfortably around the back of their head (Owens, 2008).	To ensure comfort.
4 Connect the oxygen tubing to the oxygen flow meter. Assess the need to administer and ensure the oxygen is prescribed (Owens, 2008).	To allow administration of the oxygen from the oxygen supply. Oxygen is toxic and should only be prescribed if needed (Owens, 2008).
5 Turn on the oxygen flow meter to the prescribed amount (in litres). Record amount and duration of oxygen delivery and sign the prescription (Owens, 2008).	For effective documentation and to ensure the correct dose is given.
6 Observe and record the child's pulse, respiratory rate, and oxygen saturations at least hourly.	To observe for improvements or deterioration whilst the oxygen is administered.
7 Report any changes in vital signs to the appropriate healthcare practitioner, e.g. doctor.	To ensure early intervention or changes of treatment.
8 Hand washing.	To prevent cross infection.

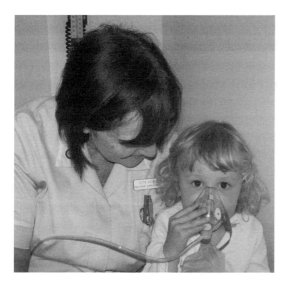

Figure 8.5 Patient using a face mask

8.6 **Delivery of oxygen using a head box**

A head box is only suitable for use in infants under eight months of age. This is because older children would become distressed and anxious, as they could feel trapped in the enclosed space. Younger children are less likely to be aware of this effect, due to their developmental level. Furthermore it can be difficult to use either the nasal prongs or face mask for oxygen delivery to children less than eight months old, so the head box is an effective way of oxygen delivery for this group. The box also allows for FiO_2 monitoring.

Procedure: Delivering oxygen via a head box

Consent and communication

To reduce anxiety and promote family centred care, explain the procedure and why you are using a head box to the parents/carers. Show them ways to comfort the baby whilst in the head box (for example, by stroking the baby's feet).

Using oxygen at home

Many children with chronic breathing problems have oxygen delivery systems at home. This includes portable system

Nursing Alert

Careful monitoring and recording of respiratory rate and oxygen saturation is important to assess the effectiveness and need for oxygen therapy (Aylott, 2006a). However, it is important to remember that babies are unable to be cuddled as once removed from the head box the FiO_2 decreases. Warmed humidification is also required as the cold oxygen cools the baby. Support the parent or carer to touch other areas such as feet to comfort and soothe the baby.

delivery such as portable oxygen in backpacks so that they can attend school, clubs, colleges, etc. Many healthcare settings provide guidelines and equipment loan facilities for this purpose. Careful follow-up by a team of respiratory healthcare professionals is important to ensure the child, their family or carer, and anyone involved in the daily living activities of the child such as teachers, club leaders, other family, or childminders are supported (Henderson, 2005).

Airway adjuncts

Airway adjuncts are used to maintain airway patency and avoid complications related to hypoxia. The two main devices used are an oropharyngeal and nasopharyngeal airway.

Nursing Alert

It is important to select the correct size airway and to insert it safely and correctly to prevent mucosal trauma, or this may worsen airway obstruction. Too large an airway will cause **laryngospasm** (APLS, 2006).

8.7 **Insertion of an oropharyngeal airway**

The oropharyngeal airway is used in the unconscious child to provide a patent airway between the tongue and the posterior pharyngeal wall.

Nursing Alert

The oropharyngeal airway will not be tolerated by an awake child with an intact gag reflex. It will likely induce vomiting and will cause the child distress and discomfort. It may also cause choking and laryngospasm (APLS, 2006).

Step-by-step guide to delivering oxygen via a head box to children

Step	Rationale
1 Hand washing. Wear PPE.	To prevent cross infection.
2 Ensure the oxygen is prescribed and assess the need to administer.	Oxygen is toxic and should only be given if needed (Owens, 2008).
3 Connect green oxygen tubing from the oxygen flow meter to a humidifier (Owens, 2008).	To ensure effective use of the equipment.
4 Check the water level in the humidifier and ensure the water is replaced as required (Hufton, 2007).	To ensure effective humidification.
5 Place the oxygen analyser probe into the head box and set the upper and lower limits of oxygen concentration (Owens, 2008).	To ensure the correct amount of oxygen is given.
6 Position the baby on their side (lateral) or on their back (prone). Place the head box carefully over their head with the shoulders outside the box (Hufton, 2007).	To promote comfort and to prevent a build-up of carbon dioxide as gases can circulate out of the box (Owens, 2008).
Place colourful and washable toys within the baby's visual field. Support the parents/carers to touch and soothe their baby whilst in the head box (Owens, 2008).	To provide visual stimulation. To encourage family centred care.
7 Connect elephant tubing through the port in the head box next to the baby's head. The dial on the humidifier will show the amount of oxygen being delivered. Adjust this to the required oxygen rate (Owens, 2008).	To ensure adequate oxygen is given.
8 Attach the oxygen saturation probe and set it to required limits. Record respirations and pulse at least hourly.	To record vital signs to ensure adequate pulmonary ventilation.
9 Record oxygen saturation and oxygen air mix hourly (Owens, 2008).	To observe for signs of improvement or deterioration.
10 Record skin temperature hourly and feel the baby's skin regularly.	To ensure the baby is not too hot or cold.
11 Sign the prescription chart and record the time and amount of oxygen given.	To ensure effective documentation.
12 Report any abnormalities or improvements to the appropriate health care professional, e.g. doctor.	To allow early intervention in case of problems.
13 Hand washing.	To prevent cross infection.

Step-by-step guide to inserting an oropharyngeal airway

Step		Rationale
1	Hand washing. Wear PPE.	To prevent cross infection.
2	Select the correct size of airway by measuring from the mid-incisor to the angle of the jaw against the face (APLS, 2006; Wilkie, 2007).	To maintain an effective airway.
3	Position the child using the chin lift. Do not hyper-extend the neck (APLS, 2006).	To maintain an effective airway. This will occlude the airway.
4	In infants and small children insert the airway the correct way up.	To prevent trauma to their soft and pliable palate (APLS, 2006).
5	In older children (as with adults) insert the airway upside down until the tip has passed the soft palate, then rotate 180 degrees so that the curve of the airway follows the curve of the tongue and pharynx (Wilkie, 2007).	Allows easier insertion.
6	Once inserted observe and document respiratory rate, pulse, and oxygen saturations.	To observe for signs of improvement or deterioration.
7	Report any changes to the appropriate healthcare professional, e.g. doctor.	To ensure early intervention.
8	Be prepared to change the size of the airway if a patent airway is not achieved (APLS, 2006).	To ensure adequate pulmonary ventilation.
9	Hand washing.	To prevent cross infection.
10	Document the process.	To ensure effective documentation.

Procedure: Inserting an oral pharyngeal airway

Consent and communication

The child's family/carer might be anxious about the procedure, so it is important to explain it to them. As well as easing their concerns, it should also help ensure their cooperation.

8.8 Insertion of a nasopharyngeal airway Ⓐ

This is an advanced skill. You *must* check whether you can assist with or undertake any aspect of this skill, in line with local policy.

Procedure: Inserting a nasopharyngeal airway

Consent and communication

To ensure compliance and reduce anxiety, explain the procedure to the child and their family/carer. Involve a play specialist if required.

The insertion of oral and nasopharyngeal airways is performed by suitably experienced care practitioners. However, experience can be gained through observation, assimilation, and direct supervision.

Suctioning

Children usually clear their airways by sneezing, coughing, or blowing their nose, but there are times when their

Step-by-step guide to inserting a nasopharyngeal airway

This is an advanced skill. You *must* check whether you can assist with or undertake any aspect of this skill, in line with local policy.

Step	Rationale
1 Hand washing and wear PPE.	To prevent cross infection.
2 Select the correct sized nasal airway by measuring from the tip of the nose to the tragus (ear lobe) (APLS, 2006).	To ensure correct size.
3 The airway should fit without blanching to the skin (APLS, 2006).	To ensure the correct size.
4 Lubricate the end of the airway with a water-soluble gel (APLS, 2006).	To aid insertion.
! Insert a large safety pin to the end of the flange (APLS, 2006).	To prevent the airway from slipping in the nose causing airway obstruction and difficulty in its retrieval (APLS, 2006).
5 Insert the tip of the airway into the nostril and direct it backwards along the floor of the nose, where it is gently passed by the turbinates into the pharynx. Continue until the flange and safety pin rest on the nostril (APLS, 2006).	To ensure correct placement.
6 Observe and document respiratory rate, pulse, and oxygen saturations.	To observe for improvements or deterioration.
7 Report any changes or improvements to the appropriate healthcare professional e.g. doctor.	To ensure early intervention.
8 Hand washing.	To prevent cross infection.
9 Document the process.	For effective communication.

Nursing Alert

The nasopharyngeal airway should not be used if there is a confirmed or suspected fracture to the base of the skull, as it could pierce into the meninges and cause cerebral damage and infection. It should also be avoided if there are any nasal problems, bleeding disorders, or nasal trauma, as the insertion could cause further mucosal trauma and bleeding (APLS, 2006).

usual mechanisms are ineffective, for example, immediately after an anaesthetic or when unconscious due to trauma. Suction may be required to remove excess secretions in order to maintain a patent airway and ensure effective breathing (Dougherty & Lister, 2006).

Types of suctioning

- Oral—this is performed to remove secretions from the mouth. It is usually carried out using a larger bore suction catheter. With appropriate explanations and preparation this method is usually well tolerated by the child (Moore, 2003).

- Oropharyngeal—this involves the insertion of a fine catheter through the mouth and pharynx into the trachea. It is used on the child who is unable to maintain their own airway, but is breathing spontaneously (Donaldson & Holliday, 2007).
- Nasopharyngeal—this involves the insertion of a fine catheter through the nasal passage and pharynx into the trachea. This is performed either directly through the nose or with a nasal airway adjunct (Moore, 2003).
- Tracheal—this is done via an artificial opening in the trachea. The presence of an airway adjunct such as a tracheostomy tube, which is a foreign body, increases the production of secretions. Therefore suctioning is required to ensure a patent airway. This will be discussed in more detail in the tracheostomy care section (Wilson, 2005).
- Endotracheal—suctioning is performed through an endotracheal tube. This will be discussed in the endotracheal tube section (Moore, 2003).

The risks involved when performing oropharyngeal and nasopharngeal suctioning include:

- Atelectasis: Failure of part of the lung to expand due to thick secretions in the bronchial tubes.
- Trauma: To the mucosa of the upper and lower airways.

Nursing Alert

- Prior to performing suctioning ensure it is really needed. Could the child sit up and coughing be encouraged? Suctioning can be a frightening experience for the child and their family or carer. Suctioning should only be performed for clinical reasons when needed and not done routinely (Moore, 2003).

- Prepare the child and their family or carer for the procedure through play preparation and explanations, according to the child's age, development, and understanding (Hutchfield, 1999). Ensure permission and full informed consent is obtained from the child (if old enough to understand) and their family or carer (see Chapters Two, Three, and Four for more information on communication, child development, and consent).

- Vasovagal stimulation: Caused by the catheter tip touching the mucosa, or lack of oxygen to the child. This results in bradycardia or tachycardia, cardiac arrhythmias, hypo- or hypertension, and cardiac arrest.
- Laryngospasm: Caused by the larynx being touched.
- Infection: through cross infection.

(Donaldson & Holliday, 2007).

Tracheal and endotracheal suctioning is contraindicated in the child with persistent raised intracranial pressure, as the pressure is likely to be increased further due to the pressure of the suctioning (APLS, 2006).

8.9 **Performing suctioning**

Procedure: Performing suctioning

Preparation

Some children, depending on their medical condition, will require hyper-oxygenation prior to this procedure. This involves the delivery of 100% oxygen given between and after the suction catheter is passed (Woodrow, 2002). Check first with the medical staff or healthcare practitioners if this is required. There is evidence to suggest that hyper-oxygenation prevents a drop in the arterial oxygen level (Hazinski, 1999; Woodrow, 2002).

Consent and communication

Explain the procedure to the child and their parents/carers. They might like to be there when you carry out the procedure, to comfort the child. Involve a play specialist if needed.

After the procedure, ensure the child is comfortable. Ensure the child and parent or carer are fully informed about the whole process and that they are given the opportunity to ask any questions. Allow time to rest before undertaking any other interventions (Hutchfield, 1999). Carefully document the whole process, including consent, whether any supportive holding occurred and by who, and colour, description, and amount of secretions (refer to Chapter Five for more on restraint and control and record keeping).

Step-by-step guide to performing suctioning

Step	Rationale
1 Carefully wash and dry hands. Apply PPE.	To prevent cross infection
2 If possible sit the child upright. If required and appropriate the child could sit on their parent or carer's lap.	To promote pulmonary ventilation and comfort (Moore, 2003). To reassure and reduce the child's anxiety.
3 Remove any oxygen supply. In the ventilated child disconnection of oxygen should not exceed ten seconds (APLS, 2006).	To allow the procedure to take place. To prevent hypoxia (Moore, 2003).
4 Observe respiratory rate including colour and pallor of skin and extremities throughout the process.	To observe for respiratory problems.
5 Introduce the suction catheter gently. Most catheters have holes around the diameter and do not require rotation on insertion, therefore unless indicated direct insertion without rotation is required (Moore, 2003).	To prevent trauma and blockage with thick secretions.
6 Suction should be applied with the withdrawal of the catheter (Wiltshire & Aitken, 2007).	To prevent trauma to the mucosa.
7 Reconnect the oxygen supply as soon as possible after the procedure (APLS, 2006). Assess the child's breathing.	To prevent hypoxia.
8 Withdraw the used catheter gently and discard appropriately (refer to the local policy on waste disposal). A helpful tip is to wrap the used catheter around the gloved hand, pull the glove back over the soiled catheter, and discard safely.	To prevent cross infection.
9 With the suction pressure on, insert the tubing into a receiver of water.	To rinse the tubing.
10 Repeat the process until the airway is clear. Experienced healthcare practitioners or medical staff will auscultate the chest to listen for clear sounds (Moore, 2003).	To ensure effective suctioning.
11 No more than three suction passes are recommended. Seek medical advice if suctioning is not effective after three attempts (Moore, 2003).	Excess suctioning can irritate and cause trauma to the airway. It can be upsetting and uncomfortable for the child (Donaldson & Holliday, 2007).
12 Carefully wash hands and discard PPE.	To prevent cross infection.
13 Use tissues to carefully wipe the child's mouth and nose. The parent or carer may like to do this (Donaldson & Holliday, 2007).	To remove excess secretions and promote comfort. To encourage family centred care.

Table 8.2 Guide to suction catheter size and suction pressure (mmHg) selection (Dougherty & Lister, 2006)

Age	Catheter size	Suction pressure (mmHg)
Neonate	0–6	80–100
Infant	8	80–100
Toddler	10	100–120
School age	12	100–120
Adolescent and adult	14	120–150

Nursing Alert

- Suctioning should only be performed by an experienced and competent healthcare professional. However, confidence and competency can be gained through simulated and supervised practice. Observing the procedure and assisting in supporting the child and their family is a very important part of gaining experience and competence in this skill.

- This is a guide and care should be taken to assess the child according to their individual development and size.

- Anecdotal evidence suggests that inserting sodium chloride into the airway adjunct may assist in the removal of thick secretions. This is not recommended as a safe practice because not all the saline is recovered on suctioning and there is a risk of inhalation. It is also frightening and uncomfortable for the child. Refer to the local guidelines in the clinical area in regards to this (Day, 2002).

8.10 **Obtaining a sputum specimen**

Sputum specimens are often required in a child with respiratory problems, to identify the presence of any infections of the respiratory tract. The specimen is collected using a variety of methods and sent to a microbiology laboratory for analysis (Aylott, 2006a).

Nursing Alert

- When performing suctioning the lowest suction pressure should be used, to prevent mucosal trauma. The suction pressures should be 60–120 mmHg. In infants the pressure should be no higher than 100 mmHg. This is a guide and pressure selection is based on individual clinical need (Donaldson & Holliday, 2007).

- Take care not to insert the suction catheter too far, as this can lead to mucosal trauma. For nasopharyngeal suctioning pre-measure the catheter from the child's nose to the suprasternal notch (top of the ribcage). For oral suctioning, pre-measure from the mouth to the suprasternal notch. The suction tubing should not be inserted any further than this measurement (Buglas, 1999).

- When performing suctioning via the nose or mouth, if any resistance is met withdraw the suction catheter and attempt a second pass. If resistance is still met select a smaller catheter. If resistance is still met, seek medical advice (Donaldson & Holliday, 2007).

Nursing Alert

A visit to a microbiology laboratory is recommended, to observe and understand the processes involved in analysing sputum specimens.

Sputum specimens are frequently requested by medical staff when the child is admitted to hospital with breathing problems. In the community parents or carers of many children with chronic respiratory problems are empowered to seek medical help and obtain sputum specimens when they feel their child has a respiratory tract infection, for example, the child with cystic fibrosis. Children (and their families or carers) with chronic illness should be supported by community health teams to be confident in their ability to recognize early signs and symptoms of changes in their illness, with the aim of reducing hospital admission and preventing or reducing exacerbations of their condition (Elliot *et al.*, 2006).

Respiratory tract infections are initially diagnosed through clinical assessment and symptoms. Refer back to visual assessment and non-invasive assessment in this chapter to revise signs and symptoms of respiratory problems. Chest X-ray is likely to be required to identify the presence of lung infection. Blood samples may be required to assess the blood count and blood cultures for signs of infection (Hazinski, 1999).

Antibiotic medications are usually commenced prior to the analysis and identification (sensitivity) of appropriate antimicrobial medications to use. This is because any delay in treatment of respiratory tract and lung infections can cause deterioration in the child's breathing (Woodrow, 2000).

Before obtaining a sputum specimen, careful assessment is needed to ensure the child understands what they need to do. Involve the play specialist and parent or carer in this, to ensure compliance (Smith *et al.*, 2002). If the child is unable to understand what is required, inform medical staff to determine if another method of specimen can be used, for example, nasopharyngeal aspirate.

> **Nursing Alert**
>
> Ensure the child and their family or carers are fully informed and that consent is gained prior to undertaking the procedure (refer to Chapter Four on consent).

Types of investigations of sputum specimens

Bacterial

The specimen is usually collected in a clean specimen container free from organisms of respiratory origin. Sputum is not sterile as it passes through the nasopharynx and mouth, which contain normal commensals of bacteria. The specimen undergoes microscopic investigation to indicate the causative bacteria. The specimen is usually cultured for 24–48 hours to incubate and grow organisms. This is followed by antibiotic sensitivity testing. This involves the application of paper discs, impregnated with antibiotics, onto agar plates. After overnight incubation the growth of the bacteria may be inhibited by the antibiotic disc. This indicates the degree of the sensitivity of the organism (Dougherty & Lister, 2006).

Viral

The three main laboratory techniques to test for viral infections are: direct microscopy; culture (the isolation of growth in living cell systems); and serology. Specimens of nasopharyngeal aspirate, collected in a clean specimen container, are the usual way that specimens are collected.

Speed of delivery to the laboratory is important as viruses do not survive well outside the body. The specimen should be kept cold at a temperature of 4°C, but not at freezing temperature, to maintain its survival (Dougherty & Lister, 2006).

> **Nursing Alert**
>
> Follow the guidelines of the healthcare setting to ensure specimens are sent at the correct times. If in doubt contact the laboratory for advice. Failure to do this may result in the death of the virus and delay of any treatments (Mandell *et al.*, 2000).

Mycosis and Mycobacterium tuberculosis

This is done to identify pathogenic fungi and bacteria. Sputum specimens are sent in clean specimen containers and the organisms are grown on special mycological media (Mandell *et al.*, 2000).

Protozoa

Most protozoa do not cause disease; however, if there are suspicions of malaria, then sputum is collected in a clean container and sent to the laboratory quickly, as protozoa are mobile. Laboratory investigation involves viewing through a microscope (Mandell *et al.*, 2000).

> **Nursing Alert**
>
> Ensure the correct collection system and accompanying request forms are available as laboratories will be unable to process the specimen if it is in the wrong container or forms are incorrectly filled in. Take care to label containers carefully and in accordance with the local policy of the healthcare setting. Failure to do this will result in stress to the child and family by having to repeat the test. Delay in confirmation or identification of the appropriate antibiotic to use could delay treatment and lead to exacerbation of the problem (Dougherty & Lister, 2006). (Refer to Chapter Five for more on record keeping.)

Procedure: Obtaining a sputum specimen

Preparation

Check you have the correctly completed and signed request form, with the correct details of the child. This is an important safety measure to ensure specimens are not mixed up in the laboratory and are easily identified.

Equipment

- Sputum specimen container (have a spare container nearby in case the procedure needs to be repeated).
- Tissues.

Consent and communication

Inform the child and their parent/carer about the procedure. Involve a play specialist if required.

Nursing Alert

Care should be taken to ensure that the material sent to the laboratory is sputum and not saliva, as this would result in an incorrect analysis.

After the procedure ensure the child and family are comfortable and that they fully understand what has happened.

Document the whole process (refer to Chapter Five for more on record keeping).

8.11 Obtaining a sputum specimen using nasopharyngeal aspirate (NPA)

This method of obtaining a sputum specimen is used in young babies and for the diagnosis of bronchiolitis. This type of specimen is not required routinely as bronchiolitis is usually diagnosed by clinical symptoms (Fazakerley, 2004).

Bronchiolitis, as previously mentioned, is a respiratory condition that occurs in association with viral infections. It is usually diagnosed in babies under 12 months old, and is usually caused by respiratory synctial virus (RSV). It is characterized by breathing difficulties, cough, poor feeding, and irritability. The symptoms usually last 3–7 days. Admission to hospital is usually needed to give oxygen, nasogastric feeding, and suctioning.

Step-by-step guide to taking a sputum specimen

Step		Rationale
1	Careful hand washing. Apply PPE.	To prevent cross infection.
2	If the child is having problems producing sputum, ask them to practise coughing, particularly in the morning. A physiotherapist will be able to assist (Dougherty & Lister, 2006).	To facilitate expectoration.
3	Ask the child to cough and transfer sputum into the specific container.	To provide the specimen.
4	Label the container correctly and send to the laboratory.	To ensure effective patient identification.
5	Wipe the child's mouth with tissues if required.	To ensure comfort.
6	Dispose of PPE appropriately and carry out careful hand washing.	To prevent cross infection.
7	Document the process.	To ensure effective documentation.

> **Nursing Alert**
>
> Specific circumstances requiring an NPA (Wiltshire & Aitken, 2007):
>
> - Infants under six months old.
> - Chronic lung disease.
> - Immunodeficiency.
> - Neuromuscular disease.
> - Very severe bronchiolitis.

The NPA is obtained using a fine suction catheter and a sputum trap. It is sent to the laboratory for microbiological examination. The result can be obtained within an hour, upon request. As mentioned previously the specimen must be sent promptly and stored in cold conditions (Mandell *et al.*, 2000).

Before obtaining the NPA ensure that appropriate and in date equipment are on hand. Oxygen and suction should be easily available in case any emergency interventions are required. Personal protective equipment such as goggles, gloves, and aprons (in accordance with the local healthcare setting guidelines) should be available. The NPA collection device should be connected to the suction device (Wiltshire & Aitken, 2007). A 5 ml ampoule of sterile normal saline is required to assist in the collection of the sample.

> **Nursing Alert**
>
> The specimen should be collected before feeding as vomiting may occur and contaminate the specimen (Wiltshire & Aitken, 2007).

Procedure: Taking a nasopharyngeal aspirate

Equipment

Gather all the equipment you will need before you begin, to ensure that the procedure goes smoothly.

- Suction catheter.
- Container with label for specimen.

Consent and communication

Explain the procedure to the family/carers and involve a play specialist if required. Encourage a family centred approach by involving the family/carers in the procedure. This should also reduce any anxiety.

After the procedure, make sure the infant and the parents or carers are comfortable. Answer any questions. Ensure the whole process is documented appropriately (refer to Chapter Five for more information on record keeping).

> **Nursing Alert**
>
> This method of obtaining an NPA is used when there is a large amount of nasal secretion (coryzal). However, nasopharyngeal lavage or washout is the preferred method of obtaining an NPA. This can be very stressful for infants and is usually performed in older children and adults (Wiltshire & Aitken, 2007).

8.12 Tracheostomy management 🔺

This is an advanced skill. You *must* check whether you can assist with or undertake any aspect of this skill, in line with local policy.

This is a specialist skill only undertaken by qualified nurses and other appropriately trained healthcare practitioners. A tracheostomy is an artificial airway that bypasses the body's natural protective mechanisms of the upper airway (Wilson, 2005). It involves the creation of an opening in the trachea, to facilitate breathing and for the removal of secretions. The tube used is curved to accommodate the anatomy of the trachea (Dougherty & Lister, 2006).

> **Nursing Alert**
>
> The child with a tracheostomy needing basic life support requires breaths to be delivered via the tracheostomy and not the mouth. To do this, cover the child's tracheostomy with the rescuer's mouth. Inflate the lungs by blowing into the tracheostomy tube, until you see the chest rising. As with usual basic life support, give five rescue breaths and continue the cycle as per resuscitation guidelines (APLS, 2006).

Step-by-step guide to taking a nasopharyngeal aspirate

This is an advanced skill. You *must* check whether you can assist with or undertake any aspect of this skill, in line with local policy.

Step / Rationale

Step	Rationale
1. Careful hand washing and apply PPE.	To prevent cross infection.
2. The infant ideally should be held on the parent's or carer's knee, with the head in an extended position. If this is not possible the infant should lie down, with the parent or carer next to them. If parent or carer does not want to be present, a play specialist or another member of the healthcare team should support and reassure the child (McEwing *et al.*, 2003).	For reassurance and to reduce anxiety. To supportively hold the infant safely (refer to Chapter Five for information on restraint and control). To allow ease of passing the suction tube.
3. The suction catheter should be gently passed up the nostril pathway to the pharyngeal space (Wiltshire & Aitken, 2007).	To prevent trauma and reduce discomfort.
4. Suction should be applied with the withdrawal of the catheter.	To prevent trauma to the mucosa.
5. 0.5–1 ml of mucus should be obtained (if possible) and this can be processed in up to 5 ml of sterile normal saline (Dougherty & Lister, 2006).	To ensure an adequate amount of specimen for analysis.
6. Assess the infant's respiratory rate and observe colour and pallor.	For signs of respiratory difficulties.
7. Dispose of PPE safely and carefully wash hands.	To prevent cross infection.
8. Label the specimen correctly and ensure the request form is completed correctly.	To ensure correct patient identification.
9. Ensure the specimen is kept cool. If using melting ice, make sure the specimen doesn't go below freezing.	To ensure survival of the virus.
10. Ensure the specimen is sent promptly to the laboratory (Wilshire & Aitken, 2007).	Viruses do not survive well outside the body.
11. Document that the specimen has been sent and when.	To ensure effective documentation.

The reasons for having a tracheostomy have greatly changed over the past 20 years. Previously and commonly a tracheostomy would be inserted in the child with an airway obstruction secondary to infection. Due to advances in medical care and increased immunization programmes, such incidences are now rare (Wilson, 2005).

Careful ongoing assessment of the child with a tracheostomy is important, as the child is susceptible to infection. Parents/carers of the child at home should be educated in observing for early warning indicators of problems such as infection, to ensure early care interventions (Wilson, 2005).

Multi-professional team working is important to ensure the child and family are supported in the care of a child with a tracheostomy. This includes the paediatric ear, nose, and throat (ENT) team, specialist respiratory teams, and children's community nursing teams (Elliott *et al.*, 2006). It is important that teachers, club leaders, friends, other family members, etc. are supported in providing the health and emotional care needs of the child with a tracheostomy (Wilson, 2005).

Examples of reasons for a tracheostomy

- Congenital abnormalities—laryngeal papilloma, laryngeal haemangioma, vocal cord paralysis, choanal atresia, tracheomalicia, cystic hygroma.
- Trauma—long-term ventilation, road traffic accidents, thermal injuries.
- Infections—epiglottitis, laryngotracheobronchitis (croup), polyneuritis, e.g. Guillain Barré Syndrome.
- Foreign body—inhalation of an object, e.g. a cherry tomato. However, this is more likely to be removed by medical staff or appropriately trained practitioners using a bronchoscope (Wilson, 2005).

Types of tracheostomy

Temporary
This is performed before a surgical procedure, but is rare in children.

Permanent
This is usually performed in the child with congenital abnormalities of the airway, preventing effective breathing. The tracheal cartilages are brought to the surface of the skin and sutured to the neck wall to form a stoma. The end tracheostomy is permanent and the rigid tracheal cartilage keeps the stoma open. The child will breathe through this stoma for the rest of their life. The child with a permanent tracheostomy has no connection between the nasal passages and the trachea.

Emergency
This is carried out when the child has an obstructed airway, for example, due to trauma or infection.

Percutaneous
This technique enables the tissues of the neck to be incised under local anaesthetic. It is usually performed in intensive care units for the purpose of mechanical ventilation due to trauma, swelling, or infection. A sheath is inserted into the trachea between the cricoids and the first tracheal ring. The trachea is dilated with forceps and a guidewire is inserted, ready for the insertion of a tracheostomy tube (Dougherty & Lister, 2006).

Mini tracheostomy
This method is used when frequent suctioning is required, rather than for the purpose of mechanical ventilation. The tube is inserted under local anaesthetic, either via a surgical incision or with the use of a guidewire (Dougherty & Lister, 2006).

Tracheostomy tubes

The type of tube used is based on the child's individual needs, in relation to their clinical condition, anatomy, and body size. Several types of tubes are available. They are made of metal or plastic. They may be cuffed, un-cuffed, or fenestrated (with a hole to allow speech). Un-cuffed tubes are commonly used in children as children have a narrow trachea and a cuffed tube would risk stenosis (narrowing of the trachea). However, cuffed tubes are more commonly used for children on long-term ventilation or with aspiration problems (Wilson, 2005).

Nursing Alert

Parts of tracheostomy tubes (Wilson, 2005)

- Cannula: Curved part of the tube that is inserted into the stoma. This keeps the stoma open and allows for tracheal suctioning.

- Neck flange: This rests against the neck. It has an opening either side for tapes to be tied around the neck, helping secure the tube in place.

- Hub: This is a small connector, to directly attach to a ventilator or bagging circuit.

Tracheostomy care

Humidification
The natural mechanisms of warming and humidifying air do not occur when a tracheostomy is in place. There is a high risk of damage to ciliary function when dry gases are inhaled. Therefore all children with tracheostomies require humidification. This is done by dry humidification using a

connector such as a 'Swedish Nose', or by using nebulized saline. This is done by a connector to an oxygen supply or a compressor that is attached to a chamber containing normal saline. The saline produces a mist, which is delivered to the child via a mask over the tracheostomy (Charlton, 2007).

Humidification assists in reducing the risk of tube blockage by minimizing the production of thick secretions. It is therefore an important aspect of the care of a child with a tracheostomy (Wilson, 2005).

Nursing Alert

The practice of instilling saline during suctioning in the child with a tracheostomy is not recommended, as there is some evidence that it can cause a decrease in oxygen levels. However, in some clinical areas this is still a routine practice. Refer to the policy of the clinical area (Moore, 2003). Any tracheostomy care should take place at least two hours after feeding as touching the stoma may cause retching and vomiting (Woodrow, 2002).

8.13 **Stoma hygiene** 🔺

This is an advanced skill. You *must* check whether you can assist with or undertake any aspect of this skill, in line with local policy.

As a tracheostomy is a surgical wound, the prevention of infection is an important part of the child's daily care. The child and their parents or carers should be supported and taught how to perform stoma site cleaning. The main aim is to keep the area clean and dry, to reduce skin irritation and infection until the stoma is well established. However, this is based on the child's individual needs and more frequent cleaning may be needed (Wilson, 2005).

Nursing Alert

Ensure the child and their parents or carers are fully informed of the procedure and consent is gained. Refer to Chapter Four for more information on consent.

Whilst undertaking the procedure, sitting the child in a chair or on their parent or carer's lap helps to promote comfort and accessibility to the neck. Ensure that the timing of stoma care is conducive to the needs of the child and their parent or carer. Ensure they are involved in this decision to reduce anxiety and promote a family centred approach (Smith *et al.*, 2002).

Nursing Alert

Tracheostomy dressings are not routinely advocated as they can harbour bacteria. The dressing also prevents tracheostomy tapes from being effectively secured and therefore there is a risk of the tracheostomy tube becoming dislodged. The stoma site is usually left uncovered (Wilson, 2005).

Procedure: Cleaning the stoma

Preparation

Help to prevent cross infection by careful hand washing and the application of personal protective equipment.

Equipment

- Sterile non-fluffy gauze or cotton wool applicators (Woodrow, 2002).
- Sterile dressing pack and 0.9% sterile sodium chloride or water.
- Personal protective equipment, e.g. gloves and aprons (check the policy of the clinical area).

Consent and communication

Explain the procedure to the child and their family/carer and involve a play specialist if required. Involve the child and their family/carer and teach them at their own pace. This promotes family centred care, reduces anxiety, and ensures compliance.

After the procedure, check the child and their parents or carers are comfortable. Allow time for asking questions. Document the whole process to ensure effective communication by good record keeping (see Chapter Five).

Changing tapes

The use of tapes to secure the tracheostomy tube is important. Ineffective or no tapes would cause the tracheostomy to become dislodged or removed. The tapes should be changed daily, but more frequent changes

Step-by-step guide to cleaning the stoma

This is an advanced skill. You *must* check whether you can assist with or undertake any aspect of this skill, in line with local policy.

Step	Rationale
1 Open the dressing pack and pour the normal saline or sterile water into a gallipot. Apply sterile gloves.	To maintain asepsis. To prevent cross infection.
2 Visually divide the stoma into four. Work from the centre outwards and use a separate piece of gauze to clean each quarter (Wilson, 2005).	To keep the skin clean and prevent cross infection.
Take care not to let any cleaning solution get under the tracheostomy tube as this is difficult to dry (Wilson, 2005).	To prevent infection risk and discomfort.
3 Use the same technique as above to dry the stoma area.	To maintain comfort and prevent cross infection.
4 Document the process.	To ensure effective documentation.

will be needed if the tapes become contaminated with secretions. Traditional linen tape is used, as this is soft and comfortable for the child. Velcro tapes can be used for children who are less mobile (Dougherty & Lister, 2006).

Nursing Alert

Tapes should be tied on alternate sides each time they are changed, to prevent pressure damage to the skin and discomfort to the child (Wilson, 2005).

A single length of linen tape is inserted into the opening on the flange of the tracheostomy tube. A reef knot is used to secure the tape in place. After tying the tapes at the side of the neck, the tension should be checked (Wilson, 2005).

Nursing Alert

Velcro tape can be used for older children. There is a safety risk as it may become loose. Small children may undo it, therefore risking accidental removal of the tube. You should be able to insert your little finger under the tape, ensuring the tapes are not too loose or tight.

8.14 Suctioning the child with a tracheostomy ⬤

This is an advanced skill. You *must* check whether you can assist with or undertake any aspect of this skill, in line with local policy.

As mentioned previously, the tracheostomy bypasses the usual functions of the upper airways. Secretions can therefore become thick and dry and so may compromise the airway. The child's airway is small and any reduction in the size as a result of thick secretions increases the effort of breathing. Suction is required to prevent airway obstruction, reduce the effort of breathing, increase airway resistance, remove microbial contaminants, and increase oxygenation and ventilation (Ireton, 2007). This procedure should be performed by a competent healthcare practitioner. It is recommended that the student nurse observes or performs the task under supervision. Prior to commencing the procedure, it is important to assess the need for suctioning. This would include the need to remove mucus and secretions to allow for effective and easy breathing.

Care must be taken when suctioning the child with a tracheostomy as there are risks. These include:

- Trauma to the airway.
- Atelectasis.
- Hypoxia.
- Laryngo- and bronchospasms.
- Infection.
- Increased mucus production.

Therefore suctioning should be based on clinical need and not done routinely (Buglas, 1999).

Assess the child's respiratory rate before and during the procedure to detect any complications. Ensure all the equipment is on hand, working effectively, and the correct size for the child. This is to promote safety and to ensure the procedure is prompt and effective to reduce any anxiety and fears of the child and their parent or carer (Wilson, 2005).

Care must be taken to ensure the child and their parents or carers are fully informed of the procedure and consent is obtained (refer to Chapter Four).

Procedure: Performing tracheostomy suctioning

Preparation

Calculate the size of the suction catheter by multiplying the internal diameter of the tracheostomy tube by two. This gives the external diameter of the suction tube. Subtract four to calculate the catheter gauge (FG). For example, if tracheostomy tube is 6 mm: 6 × 2 = 12 mm; 12 − 4 = 8 FG catheter (Moore, 2003).

This is a guide as selection of size is based on individual clinical need.

Ensure that you have a range of catheters in case the estimated size is not effective. A new suction catheter is used each time (Donaldson & Holliday, 2007).

Equipment

- Personal protective equipment, e.g. goggles, gloves, and apron (check the policy of the clinical area).
- A selection of sizes of disposable and sterile suction catheters, including at least five of calculated size.
- Suction machine, portable or wall mounted.
- Clean water and clean receptacle.
- 0.9% saline and nebulizer equipment.
- Oxygen.
- Tissues.

Consent and communication

Find out whether the family/carers wish to be present during the procedure. Explain the procedure to the child and their family/carers, and involve a play specialist if needed.

After the procedure

Support the child and their parent or carer, reassure them, and answer any questions. Allow the child time to rest, as the procedure will likely tire them. Document the whole process, including any supportive holding, amounts and description of secretions, and consent (refer to Chapter Five, particularly in relation to record keeping and restraint and control).

Changing a tracheostomy tube

Regular changing of the tracheostomy tube is recommended to prevent the gradual build-up of mucus, which can block the tracheostomy tube. Refer to the policy of the healthcare setting regarding how frequent this should be. The term 'routinely' differs between healthcare settings. Regular tube changes are not advocated if the child feels unwell or is irritable. Compliance is an important part of tube changing. The prevention of unnecessary stress or anxiety is an integral part

Performing tracheostomy suctioning

Step-by-step guide to performing tracheostomy suctioning

This is an advanced skill. You *must* check whether you can assist with or undertake any aspect of this skill, in line with local policy.

Step	Rationale
1 Hand washing and apply PPE.	To reduce cross infection.
2 Ensure the child and their parent or carer (if they want to be present) are sitting comfortably, preferably in an upright position.	For comfort and to ensure easy access to the neck.
3 Connect suction tubing and check pressure setting. The lowest amount of suction pressure should be used.	To ensure safe and effective suctioning.
4 Pour water into the clean bowl/gallipot.	For cleaning the tubing of debris between suctioning.
5 Administer nebulized 0.9% normal saline if required.	To reduce thick, tenacious secretions (Buglas, 1999).
6 Give oxygen prior to suctioning as indicated. This is known as pre-oxygenation.	Evidence suggests pre-oxygenation reduces hypoxia (Moore, 2003).
7 Pre-measure the suction tubing (refer back to suctioning section). Only suction the length of the tube (Aylott, 2007).	To prevent mucosal trauma.
8 Gently insert the suction catheter into the stoma without using suction, to the pre-measured length (Dougherty & Lister, 2006).	To reduce the risk of hypoxia and prevent trauma to the mucosa.
9 Using a finger tip control, apply continuous pressure while withdrawing the suction catheter (Aylott, 2007).	To remove secretions from the lumen of the tube. To reduce the risk of hypoxia. To maintain comfort.
10 Suction should be quick but effective (refer back to suctioning section for further guidance).	To promote comfort. To reduce anxiety. To prevent hypoxia (Aylott, 2007).
11 If a cuffed tracheostomy tube is used (usually in the older child), the cuff may need to be deflated during suctioning.	To prevent pooling of secretions above the cuff (Buglas, 1999).
12 Assess the child's respiratory rate and the colour and pallor of their skin. Administer oxygen if required (APLS, 2006).	For indications of hypoxia.
13 Dispose of the suction catheter in accordance with the policy of the healthcare setting.	To prevent cross infection.
14 Using the suction catheter, draw up water into the tubing.	To clear away debris.
15 Repeat the suctioning if required.	To ensure suctioning is effective.

of nursing children (Wilson, 2005). Tube changes are undertaken by experienced and competent healthcare practitioners.

Tube changing may need to be done more frequently if the secretions are thick and there are signs of respiratory distress. A larger size of tracheostomy tube may be required if secretions remain thick. Using nebulized 0.9% normal saline may also help. It is recommended in children with new tracheostomies that the tube is not changed for at least two to three days. This is to ensure that the stoma and area around the tracheostomy are healed (Dougherty & Lister, 2006).

Initially when a tracheostomy is formed, the surgeon will use nylon sutures inserted either side of the tracheal opening. If a new tracheostomy tube needs changing within the first two to three days, the suture is used to pull apart the tracheal opening to insert a new tube (Wilson, 2005).

The first tube change will likely be frightening for the child and their parent or carer. It is important that full informed consent, full explanations, play preparation, and diversion are prioritized in the child's plan of care, ensuring the child and family are involved in decision making (refer to Chapter Two, family centred care). To maintain the safety of the child, it is always experienced and competent healthcare professionals who undertake the tube changing procedure in hospital (Woodrow, 2002; Wilson, 2005).

Discharging the child home with a tracheostomy

An individual and supportive care package must be set up prior to the child going home. Parents or carers of the child will be supported and educated to undertake all the required care, including tracheostomy tube changing. They are provided with emergency and spare equipment. It is usually the community nursing services and respiratory care team who support the child and their family at home. This includes ensuring they have the correct and appropriate equipment and being on hand for support and advice. Many children and their families/carers find joining a tracheostomy support group helpful, such as that found at **http://www.tracheostomy.com.**

Consideration

Statement from a parent of a six-month-old baby discharged from hospital following the insertion of a tracheostomy:

'The first night at home, I was terrified; I did not sleep a wink. I was sure he would dislodge the tube and would stop breathing. With support from the community nurses, I gained confidence. He is due to have surgery soon to correct the problem and may not need to have the tracheostomy. Following the surgery I was keen to be discharged home, to try and establish a routine, but was very nervous at the prospect. All the nurses and doctors took the time to listen to my worries. They supported my husband and I when we were learning the tracheostomy care. Without this we would definitely still be in hospital.'

8.15 **Care of intrapleural drainage** ⚠

This is an advanced skill. You *must* check whether you can assist with or undertake any aspect of this skill, in line with local policy.

Intrapleural drainage is a method used to remove a collection of air, fluid, pus, or blood from the pleural space. This is done to restore normal lung functions (Dougherty & Lister, 2006). Intrapleural drainage is done by the insertion of a drain. The drain is inserted into the pleural cavity through the intercostal space by an experienced doctor or healthcare practitioner. The aim is to remove air or fluid safely, preventing their reintroduction, and to promote lung expansion. The drain is usually inserted using sedation or a general anaesthetic in children. Local anaesthetic is used for insertion in an emergency (Allibone, 2003).

An intrapleural drain is a tube made of clear pliable plastic. It often has a radio opaque end, to allow X-ray detection. The drain is inserted into the pleura and has holes to assist drainage. The end of the tube is attached to a drainage system (Dougherty & Lister, 2006). Pre-packed drainage systems are often used for the drainage of a pneumothorax or effusion. The bottle has a screw top with two parts. One part has a length of tube that will sit under the water level in the bottle. The second part has a shorter length of tubing, which acts as a vent. It is exposed to the air or may be attached to a suction unit. This venting prevents the build-up of pressure in the intrapleural drain system, which could prevent the elimination of the fluid or air.

The underwater seal occurs when there is adequate sterile water in the bottle (usually 500 millilitres). The end of the intrapleural drain is attached to the underwater seal part of the bottle and immersed at least 2.5 cm below the level of the water. Air bubbles through the water, preventing the backflow of the air back into the intrapleural space (Hazinski, 1999; Dougherty & Lister, 2006).

Reasons for intrapleural drain requirement

Prior to insertion of the chest drain, medical staff will confirm the site of the pneumothorax or effusion (fluid collection) by a plain X-ray. The drain is usually inserted into the chest at the fifth intercostal space in the mid-auxiliary line, on the side with the pneumothorax or effusion (APLS, 2006).

Nursing Alert

Signs and symptoms of pneumothorax, pleural effusion, haemothorax, and empyema:

- Pallor (due to ineffective pulmonary ventilation).

- Cyanosis (due to ineffective pulmonary ventilation).

- Dyspnoea (due to ineffective pulmonary ventilation).

- Tachypnoea (due to ineffective pulmonary ventilation and compression around the heart).

- Reduced breath sounds on the affected side.

- Decrease in peripheral oxygen saturation (due to compression around the heart).

- Low blood pressure (due to compression around the heart).

- Chest pain (due to increased pressure around the lungs and inflammation of the pleura).

(Hazinski, 1999)

Table 8.3 Reasons an intrapleural drain is needed (Dougherty & Lister, 2006)

Problem	Cause
Pneumothorax	Air in the pleural cavity, usually caused by trauma.
Spontaneous pneumothorax	Caused by a blister on the lung. It can occur in healthy young people due to mechanical stresses on the surface of the lung; air enters the pleural space causing a partial or total lung collapse. Reasons include trauma, surgery, central venous catheter insertion, during positive pressure ventilation, and in lung conditions such as severe asthma, pneumonia, or tuberculosis.
Tension pneumothorax	This occurs when a tear in the visceral pleura remains unsealed and a valve is formed, so air enters the pleural space but is unable to escape during expiration. This can cause complete lung collapse and cardiac arrest.
Pleural effusion	Caused by excessive amount of fluid in the pleural space. This effusion can be caused by trauma, heart failure, and pneumonia.
Haemothorax	Caused by blood in the pleural space, as a result of trauma to the chest, heart, lungs, or major blood vessels.
Haemopneumothorax	Caused by blood and air in the pleural space, for the same reasons as haemothorax.
Empyema	Caused by pus in the pleural space, as a result of the rupture of an abscess in the lung, secondary to pneumonia, pulmonary tuberculosis, or an infection following thoracic surgery.

Procedure: Maintaining a chest drain

Preparation

To help prevent cross infection put on PPE, e.g. gloves and aprons.

Equipment

- Oxygen and suction, to promote safety in case respiratory or cardiac problems occur.
- Two non-toothed clamps.*
- Spare underwater seal chest drain bottle, tubing, and sterile water, to renew the drain should it dislodge.
- Sterile dressing pack.
- Sterile clear occlusive dressing to observe the wound, promote healing, and prevent cross infection.

*In case the chest drain becomes disconnected, to prevent reoccurrence of the pneumothorax or effusion. To prevent the clamp splitting the tube (Dougherty & Lister, 2006).

Consent and communication

Explain the procedure to the parent/carer and involve a play specialist if required, in order to reduce anxiety and ensure compliance.

8.16 Removal of the intrapleural drain Ⓐ

This is an advanced skill. You *must* check whether you can assist with or undertake any aspect of this skill, in line with local policy.

Prior to the procedure ensure that the timing of the procedure is suitable for the child and their parent or carer (if they want to be present). Involve the child and their parent or carer in decisions on timings. Ensure effective pain relief is administered prior to the procedure, as it can be very painful and uncomfortable. If the child is very upset they may require sedation. Discuss this with medical staff (refer to Chapter Six).

Step-by-step guide to maintaining a chest drain

This is an advanced skill. You *must* check whether you can assist with or undertake any aspect of this skill, in line with local policy.

Step	Rationale
1 Careful hand washing and apply PPE.	To prevent cross infection.
2 Monitor and record vital signs. Observe the respiratory rate and colour and pallor of skin and extremities. Initially attach the child to a monitor to record oxygen saturation levels, blood pressure, and pulse for at least 24 hours following the intrapleural drain insertion. The frequency of monitoring the vital signs is dependent on the child's condition (APLS, 2006).	To observe for deterioration in the child's cardiopulmonary function.
3 A large suture is inserted into the child's skin once the drain is in place. This is known as the 'anchor suture'. Another suture is inserted through the skin and the ends left loose. This is called a 'purse string suture'. Ensure the sutures are kept clean and covered by a semi-occlusive dressing.	To keep the tube in place. To seal the skin together when the drain is removed. The purse string suture can also be used in an emergency if the drain falls out, to prevent re-entry of air and fluid (Dougherty & Lister, 2006). To promote wound healing and prevent cross infection.

4	A sterile occlusive dressing should cover the insertion site. Refer to the wound care product instructions and the policy of the healthcare setting for frequency of changing. It is usually every 5–7 days. The dressing should be changed if contaminated exudate is leaking. Any redressing should be done aseptically (Dougherty & Lister, 2006).	To promote healing. To observe the wound for signs of infection. To prevent cross infection.
5	The tubing should be observed visually for holes and kinks (Allibone, 2003). Seek medical help quickly if any holes are present.	Holes and kinks could cause reoccurrence of the pneumothorax or effusion. There is a risk of infection. The tubing will need to be changed quickly.
6	The drainage tubing should be placed in line with the child's ribs. Taping it in place is helpful (Allibone, 2003).	To promote comfort by preventing the tube from moving around.
7	Ensure the water level inside the intrapleural drainage bottle is maintained above the marked minimum level and that the tube inside the bottle is kept beneath the water level (Allibone, 2003).	To maintain the water seal.
8	The intrapleural drainage bottle must remain lower than the insertion site (APLS, 2006). If the tubing disconnects or the bottle breaks, apply non-bolted clamps. A new sterile drainage tube will need to be used to reconnect and re-establish the pleural drainage (Allibone, 2003).	To ensure the correct placement and patency, bubbling air drainage of fluid, and swinging movement in the drainage tubing. To prevent re-entry of air or fluid into the pleural space. To prevent cross infection.
9	The child should be positioned, for the duration of the intrapleural drain being in place, in a semi-upright position towards the chest drain site (if possible) (Allibone, 2003).	To promote drainage and effective pulmonary ventilation. To maintain comfort.
10	Encourage mobility. Liaise with physiotherapy to assist.	To promote optimal drainage and encourage effective pulmonary ventilation.
11	Give regular pain relief and assess pain with a recognized pain tool (refer to Chapter Six, pain assessment and management).	To prevent chest infection and minimize discomfort for the child.
12	It may be necessary to apply suction pressure using a low flow meter or a portable suction unit. This will be requested by medical staff and the required pressure will be indicated (Allibone, 2003).	To assist in the removal of fluid or air from the pleural cavity.

Nursing Alert

Care must be taken to ensure the child and their parent or carer are fully informed and that consent is obtained (refer to Chapter Four).

Ensure oxygen and suction are easily available and working effectively. There is a risk of cardiopulmonary problems, so easy access to full resuscitation equipment is important (APLS, 2006).

Procedure: Removing an intrapleural drain

Equipment

- Sterile dressing pack containing non-fluffy gauze, gallipot, and sterile gloves, to perform the removal of the drain aseptically.
- Sterile cleaning solution, e.g. 0.9% sodium chloride or sterile water, to clean away any debris from around the entry site.
- Sterile stitch cutter to remove the anchor suture.
- Sterile semiocclusive dressing (refer to the policy of the healthcare setting, as the choice of wound care products differs).

- Two chest drain clamps in case the drainage system is accidentally disconnected prior to removal. These can be used to clamp the drain for a trial period, prior to removal, to ensure that it is ready to be removed (Allibone, 2003).
- Protective absorbent pads to collect any exudate or other fluids, to reduce cross infection when the drain is removed. This will also help maintain the patient's comfort.

Consent and communication

Explain the procedure to the child and their family/carers. Ascertain whether or not the parents/carers would like to be there. Answer any questions to ease anxiety and ensure cooperation.

Nursing Alert

- Appropriate preparation and diversion are helpful in ensuring compliance (refer to Chapter Two, preparing the child for procedures).

- Stripping and milking of tubes is still practised in some clinical areas. This practice is not advocated and can result in lung damage. If the tube is occluded it should be changed. Selection of the correct intrapleural drain, should avoid the need to change tubing (refer to the policy of the healthcare setting) (Tang *et al.*, 2002).

Step-by-step guide to removing an intrapleural drain

This is an advanced skill. You *must* check whether you can assist with or undertake any aspect of this skill, in line with local policy.

Step		Rationale
1	Hand washing and apply PPE.	To prevent cross infection.
2	If possible sit the child upright. If the parent or carer wants to be present, ensure they are comfortable and next to the child.	To aid removal of the drain. To ensure effective pulmonary ventilation. To ensure comfort.
	Explain the procedure and involve the play specialist if required.	To ensure compliance and reduce anxiety.

3	Turn off any suction connected to the intrapleural drain system.	To prevent a tension pneumothorax (Dougherty & Lister, 2006).
4	Prepare the aseptic field on a cleaned trolley. Open the dressing pack and place everything in order for use. Open wound care products and any cleaning solutions. Cut off lengths of tape and place on the side of the trolley (refer to Chapter Six, wound assessment and management).	To ensure everything is ready so the procedure takes minimal time. This promotes comfort, reduces infection, and prevents re-entry of air or fluid into the pleural cavity (Allibone, 2003).
5	Position protective absorbent pad underneath the child and the drain.	To prevent exudates soiling the child's clothing and bed linen, thus preventing discomfort and reducing the risks of cross infection.
6	Hand washing should be repeated.	In preparation for the aseptic technique.
7	Remove the dressing from around the drain site. Ensure the anchor and purse string sutures are identified and are easily accessible.	To ensure the anchor suture can be easily removed. To ensure access to the purse string suture, so it can be used to create an airtight seal by bringing the slain edges together on drain removal (Allibone, 2003).
8	Remove the anchor suture with the stitch cutter. Dispose of the sharp safely. Ensure the drain is movable.	In preparation for removal of the drain.
9	Ensure the purse string suture is ready to tie when the drain is removed (Dougherty & Lister, 2006).	To ensure an airtight seal in order to prevent re-entry of air or fluid once the drain is removed.
10	Encourage the child to take a deep breath, while the doctor or healthcare practitioner removes the drain.	To prevent re-entry of air or fluid due to a negative intrathoracic pressure (Allibone, 2003).
11	The second healthcare practitioner ties the purse string suture securely to the skin.	To form an airtight seal and prevent a tension pneumothorax.
12	Clean around the drain site with cleaning solution, dry the area, and apply the occlusive dressing.	To reduce cross infection. To maintain comfort. To reduce the risk of air or fluid re-entry into the pleural space (Dougherty & Lister, 2006).
13	Observe vital signs and record, such as breathing, pulse, conscious level, and blood pressure (refer to Chapter Five, observation of the sick child).	To ensure child's safety.
14	Ensure the child and their parent/carer are comfortable after the procedure. Reassess the child's pain and give further analgesia if required.	To ensure comfort.
15	Document the whole process, including any supportive holding.	To ensure effective documentation.

Nursing Alert

- Clamping of intrapleural drains when mobilizing or transporting patients is not necessary and is discouraged. Clamping can prevent air or fluid leaving the pleural space and can also cause a pneumothorax (refer to the policy of the healthcare setting) (Dougherty & Lister, 2006).

- Full explanations should be given to the child and their parent or carer, particularly if the child is initially awake. It is important that appropriate language is used and that the parent or carer is supported throughout the process. It is at the discretion of medical staff for the parent or carer to remain with the child. However, evidence shows that parents or carers have a reduced anxiety if they are present but need continuous support and explanations of every event (Maxton, 2007).

Nursing Alert

If the child has a suspected cervical spine injury, an experienced healthcare practitioner should stabilize the neck during the cricoid pressure (APLS, 2006).

As a nursing student, direct observation and supervised practice in the care of the child with an ET tube is recommended. It is important to understand the care interventions required during the insertion of the ET tube, to relate it to the physical, social, and psychological family centred needs of the child and their parents or carers (refer to Chapter Two). Places to gain experience of the child with an ET tube include at the scene of an accident with a paramedic Accident and Emergency, anaesthetic rooms, intensive care and high dependency units, children's hospices, and in the community (children with long-term ventilatory support).

8.17 **Care of the child with an endotracheal tube** Ⓐ

This is an advanced skill. You *must* check whether you can assist with or undertake any aspect of this skill, in line with local policy.

An endotracheal tube is used to perform intubation and ventilator support in the child who is unable to maintain a patent airway due to potential or actual respiratory failure (APLS, 2006). This may be due to respiratory infection causing swelling to the airways, trauma, or to maintain effective pulmonary ventilation during prolonged anaesthesia.

Intubation is a frightening, painful, and unpleasant procedure and should not be performed on a conscious or semiconscious child. The child must be totally unconscious or else a doctor, usually an anaesthetist or intensive care doctor, may perform a 'rapid sequence induction'. This involves the administration of muscle relaxant and anaesthetic drugs (Aylott, 2006b). Pressure is applied over the cricoid area, which causes compression of the oesophagus, preventing regurgitation of gastric contents (APLS, 2006). This is done by doctors or appropriately trained healthcare practitioners. The appropriate-sized endotracheal (ET) tube is then inserted and attached to manual or mechanical breathing mechanisms (Aylott, 2007).

Selecting the appropriate size of ET tube (ET)

Nursing Alert

Formula for calculating ET tube requirements:

ET tube size (mm) = age in years ÷ 4 + 4
E.g. 8 years ÷ 4 + 4 = 6 mm

Oral endotracheal tube (cm) = age in years ÷ 2 + 12
E.g. 6 years ÷ 2 + 12 = 15 cm

Nasal endotracheal tube (cm) = age in years ÷ 2 + 15
E.g. 10 years ÷ 2 + 15 = 20 cm

(APLS, 2006)

ET tubes have a cuff along the lumen, which resembles a small balloon. This is inflated using air, given via a syringe, to keep the tube in place. The amount of air required is indicated in the manufacturer's instructions.

Nursing Alert

In the child under eight years of age an uncuffed tube is used, as the larynx at the level of the cricoid cartilage is the narrowest point and will form a natural seal. Using a cuffed tube can cause mucosal damage (Aylott, 2006b).

Table 8.4 ET tube sizes for the child under two (Aylott, 2006b)

Age	Weight in kilograms (kg)	ET tube
Newborn	3.5	3.5
3 months	6.0	3.5
1 year	10.0	4.0
2 years	12.0	4.5

Procedure: Insertion of an ET tube

Preparation

Please note that suctioning will probably be required as mucus accumulation can reduce airway patency and prevent a good view of the vocal cords for intubation (APLS, 2006). Make sure you have a portable or wall mounted suction to hand, set at the appropriate pressure.

Equipment

- Personal protective equipment e.g. mask, gloves, aprons, (refer to the policy of the healthcare setting).

- A working laryngoscope and blade, with a clear light source.
- A straight laryngoscope is used in small children and a curved laryngoscope in older children.*
- For babies a shoulder roll (made with a rolled blanket or towel), to help extend the neck and position the airway in a neutral position to assist intubation.

*Small children have a 'floppy epiglottis'. Older children have a stiff epiglottis (Aylott, 2007).

Consent and communication

Explain the procedure to the child and their parents/carers. This will help ensure cooperation and ease any anxieties.

Once the procedure is completed, ensure the child and their parent or carer are comfortable and understand what has happened. Document the whole process, including sizes of equipment used, to ensure effective record keeping (see Chapter Five).

Nursing Alert

In the child over eight years of age a cuffed tube is required as the cricoid becomes wider. An uncuffed tube would cause air leakage and ineffective pulmonary ventilation (APLS, 2006).

Step-by-step guide to inserting an ET tube

This is an advanced skill. You *must* check whether you can assist with or undertake any aspect of this skill, in line with local policy.

Step	Rationale
1. Hand washing. Apply PPE (refer to policy of the healthcare setting).	To reduce cross infection.
2. Ensure a face mask is giving the child oxygen prior to intubation.	Pre-oxygenation ensures adequate ventilation and oxygenation (APLS, 2006).
3. Apply oral and oral/nasal pharyngeal suctioning (refer to suctioning section).	To remove secretions.

4	In babies, place a rolled towel or blanket under their shoulder.	The baby's large occiput makes extension of the neck difficult (APLS, 2006).
5	Give the anaesthetist, intensive care doctor, or healthcare practitioner the correct bladed laryngoscope. The laryngoscope is placed down the right side of the tongue into the top of the oesophagus.	The blade is used to view the vocal cords as the tube is inserted through the vocal cords. Care is taken to prevent a laryngospasm (APLS, 2006).
6	With the anaesthetist, intensive care doctor, or healthcare practitioner, insert the ET tube.	To insert the tube.
7	The placement is confirmed by listening to breath sounds with a stethoscope and then an X-ray (APLS, 2006).	To ensure appropriate placement.
8	Tapes are attached to the ET tube and tied in place.	To prevent the tube becoming dislodged and maintain comfort.
9	The child is attached to the appropriate ventilator or support. Vital signs including breathing, pulse, blood pressure, and oxygen saturations should be monitored continuously before, throughout, and after the procedure.	To detect deterioration in the child's condition.
10	Once intubation is established, ensure the mouth, nose, and surrounding skin are kept clean and dry. Clean the area with water or normal saline and dry carefully. Frequency of this is dependent on the child's individual needs but should be observed hourly initially.	To prevent skin and pressure damage from the ET tube. To maintain comfort.
11	Perform suctioning as required and not as a routine (refer to the section on suctioning).	To assist pulmonary ventilation.
12	Change the tapes as needed, when they are contaminated with secretions.	To prevent cross infection and promote comfort. To prevent the risk of dislodgement (Aylott, 2007).

Conclusion

The evidence-based, individual family centred care of the child's breathing needs has been discussed. However, further reading around each section is highly recommended. It is hoped that during clinical placements and practice, the theory discussed in this section can be related and make more sense.

General steps of procedures in relation to interventions involved with breathing, particularly in the critically ill child, have been discussed. However, it is important to remember that care interventions may be adapted dependent on the care setting, e.g. hospital or home, due to the individual, physical, social, psychological, cultural, and spiritual family centred needs of the child. It is also important to check the policies and guidelines of the clinical areas as procedures differ.

It is advised that during clinical placements in relation to the child with breathing problems or requiring ventilatory support, under the supervision and support of a relevant competent healthcare practitioner, the student attempts or practises many of the procedures discussed, in order to develop the required skills in the area.

It is important to remember that breathing problems are the commonest type of problem in children and this highlights the importance of careful assessment and monitoring of breathing in the child admitted to hospital and the child with chronic breathing problems and acute respiratory infections in the community setting. It is very important to ensure prompt interventions to try and improve positive care outcomes.

Online resource centre

You may find it helpful to work through our online resources including interactive scenarios intended to help you to develop and apply the skills in this chapter.

🌐 **http://www.oxfordtextbooks.co.uk/orc/coyne/**

References

Advanced Paediatric Life Support Group (2006) *The Practical Approach, 4th ed.* London: Blackwell, BMJ Books.

Allibone, L. (2003) Nursing management of chest drains. *Nursing Standard*, **17** (22), 45–54.

Aylott, M. (2006a) Observing the sick child: Part 2a. Respiratory assessment. *Paediatric Nursing* **18** (9), 38–44.

Aylott, M. (2006b) Caring for children with critical illness. In A. Glasper & J. Richardson (eds.) *A Textbook of Children and Young People's Nursing.* Edinburgh: Churchill Livingstone, Elsevier.

Aylott, M. (2007) Tracheostomy: Suctioning a tracheostomy. In A. Glasper, G. McEwing, & J. Richardson (eds.) *Oxford Handbook of Children and Young Person's Nursing.* Oxford: Oxford University Press.

Booker, R. (2007) Peak expiratory flow measurement. *Nursing Standard*, **21** (39), 42–43.

Buglas, E. (1999) Tracheostomy care: Tracheal suctioning and humidification. *British Journal of Nursing* **8** (8), 500–504.

Bull, P.D. (1996) *Lecture Notes on Diseases of the Ear, Nose and Throat, 8th ed.* Oxford: Blackwell Science.

Chandler, T. (2000) Oxygen saturation monitoring. *Paediatric Nursing* **12** (8), 37–42.

Charlton, C. (2007) Administration of nebulisers. In A. Glasper, G. McEwing, & J. Richardson (eds.) *Oxford Handbook of Children and Young Person's Nursing.* Oxford: Oxford University Press.

Davies, J.H. & Hassell, L.L. (2001) *Children in Intensive Care: A Nurse's Survival Guide.* Edinburgh: Churchill Livingstone.

Day, T. (2002) Suctioning: A review of current research recommendations. *Intensive and Critical Care Nursing* **18** (2), 79–89.

Department of Health (2004) *National Service Framework for Children, Young People and Maternity Services: Asthma.* London: HMSO.

Department of Health (2007) *Reduce the Risk of Cot Death: An Easy Guide.* London: HMSO.

Department of Health (2008) *Dirty Bertie, Catch it, Bin it, Kill it.* National Health Service Publications. Available at: **http://www.dh.gov-uk/en/ publications&statistics/publications/ publicationspolicy&guidance/DH_085121**

Donaldson, P. & Holliday, L. (2007) Oropharyngeal and nasopharyngeal suctioning. In A. Glasper, G. McEwing, & J. Richardson (eds.) *Oxford Handbook of Children and Young Person's Nursing.* Oxford: Oxford University Press.

Dougherty, L. & Lister, S. (2006) *The Royal Marsden Hospital Manual of Clinical Nursing Procedures, 6th ed.* Oxford: Blackwell Science.

Elliott, B., Callery, P., & Mould, J. (2006) Chronic illness and the family. In A. Glasper & J. Richardson (eds.) *A Textbook of Children and Young People's Nursing.* Edinburgh: Churchill Livingstone, Elsevier.

Fazakerley, M. (2004) Clinical effectiveness of an integrated care pathway for infants with bronchiolitis. *Paediatric Nursing*, **16** (1), 30–35.

Gallon, A. (1998) Pneumothorax. *Nursing Standard* **39** (10), 35–39.

Glasper, A. & Haggerty, R.E. (2006) The psychological preparation of children for hospitalisation. In A. Glasper & J. Richardson (eds.) *A Textbook of Children and Young People's Nursing.* Edinburgh: Churchill Livingstone, Elsevier.

Global Initiative for Asthma (2007) *GINA Report, Global Strategy for Asthma Management.* Available at: **http://www.gina.asthma.org**

Halliday, H.L (2006) Recent clinical trials of surfactant therapy for neonates. *Neonatology* **89** (4), 323–329.

Hazinski, M.F. (1999) *Manual of Paediatric Critical Care.* New York: Mosby.

Henderson, Y. (2005) Home oxygen therapy, changes to service delivery. *Primary Health Care* **15** (10), 33–36.

Hufton, R. (2007) Using a humidifier. In A. Glasper, G. McEwing, & J. Richardson (eds.) *Oxford Handbook of Children and Young Person's Nursing*. Oxford: Oxford University Press.

Hutchfield, K. (1999) Family centred care: A concept analysis. *Journal of Advanced Nursing* **29** (5), 1178–1187.

Ireton, J. (2007) Tracheostomy suction: A protocol for practice. *Paediatric Nursing* **19** (10), 14–18.

Jevon, P., Ewens, B., & Maizie, J. (2000) Measuring peak expiratory flow. *Practical Procedures for Nurses* **21** (39), 42–43.

Kelsey, J. & McEwing, G. (2006) Respiratory illness in children. In A. Glasper & J. Richardson (eds.) *A Textbook of Children and Young People's Nursing*. Edinburgh: Churchill Livingstone, Elsevier.

Kelsey, J. & McEwing, G. (2008) *Clinical Skills in Child Health Practices*. Edinburgh: Elsevier.

Langride, P. (2004) Extended independent and supplementary prescribing: An update. *Paediatric Nursing* **14** (11), 32.

Lewis, G. (2007) Peak flow monitoring. In A. Glasper, G. McEwing, & J. Richardson (eds.) *Oxford Handbook of Children and Young Person's Nursing*. Oxford: Oxford University Press.

MacGregor, J. (2000) *Introduction to the Anatomy and Physiology of Children*. London: Routledge.

Mackway-Jones, K., Molyneux, E., Philips, B., & Wieteska, S. (1997) *Advanced Paediatric Life Support: The Practical Approach, 2nd ed*. London: BMJ Publishing.

Mandell, G., Bennett, J., & Dolin, R. (2000) *Principles and Practice of Infectious Diseases*. Philadelphia: Churchill Livingstone.

Maxton, F. (2007) Family and staff support during resuscitation. In A. Glasper, G. McEwing, & J. Richardson (eds.) *Oxford Handbook of Children and Young Person's Nursing*. Oxford: Oxford University Press.

McCance, K.L. & Heuther, S.E. (2006) *Pathophysiology: The Biologic Basis for Diseases in Adults and Children*. St Louis: Elsevier Mosby.

McEwing, G., Kelsey, J., Richardson, J., & Glasper, A. (2003) *Child and Family Health in Foundation Studies for Nursing: Using Enquiry Based Learning*. Basingstoke: Palgrave Macmillan.

McFerran, T. (2003) *Mini Reference Dictionary for Nurses, 5th ed*. Oxford: Oxford University Press.

Medical Devices Agency (2001) *Tissue Necrosis Caused by Pulse Oximeter Probes*. London: Medicines and Health Care Products Regulatory Agency.

Miller, M.R., Hankinson, J., & Brusasco, V. (2005) Standardisation of spirometry. *European Respiratory Journal* **26** (2), 319–338.

Moore, T. (2003) Suctioning techniques for the removal of respiratory secretions. *Nursing Standard* **18** (9), 47–53.

Ogden-Burke, S., Harrison, M.B., Kaufman, E. & Wong, C. (2001) Effects of stress point intervention with families of repeatedly hospitalised children. *Journal of Family Nursing* **7** (2), 128–158.

Owens, K. (2008) Oxygen therapy. In Kelsey, J. & McEwing, G. (eds.) *Clinical Skills in Child Health Practices*. Edinburgh: Elsevier.

Rotta, A.T. & Wiryawan, B. (2003) Respiratory emergencies in children. *Respiratory Care* **48** (3), 248–260.

Royal College Nursing (2007) Vital signs. *Paediatric Nursing* **20** (1), 29.

Smith, L., Colman, V., & Bradshaw, M. (2002) *Family Centred Care: Concept, Theory and Practice*. Basingstoke: Palgrave Macmillan.

Syers, S. (2008) Interpretation of observations. In Kelsey, J. & McEwing, G. (eds.) *Clinical Skills in Child Health Practices*. Edinburgh: Elsevier.

Tang, A., Vellissaris, T., & Weeden, D. (2002) An evidence based approach to drainage of pleural cavity: Evaluation of best practice. *Journal Evaluation Clinical Practice* **8** (3), 333–340.

Thornton, C. (2007) Listening to chests. In A. Glasper, G. McEwing, & J. Richardson (eds.) *Oxford Handbook of Children and Young Person's Nursing*. Oxford: Oxford University Press.

Toplis, D. (2007) Administration of oxygen. In A. Glasper, G. McEwing, & J. Richardson (eds.) *Oxford Handbook of Children and Young Person's Nursing*. Oxford: Oxford University Press.

Webster, A. (2000) The facilitating role of the play specialist. *Paediatric Nursing* **12** (7), 24–27.

Wilkie, L.M. (2007) Airway adjuncts: Uses, sizes and potential hazards. In A. Glasper, G. McEwing, & J. Richardson (eds.) *Oxford Handbook of Children and Young Person's Nursing*. Oxford: Oxford University Press.

Wilson, M. (2005) Tracheostomy management. *Paediatric Nursing* **17** (3), 38–44.

Wiltshire, M. & Aitken, P. (2007) Nasopharyngeal aspirate. In A. Glasper, G. McEwing, & J. Richardson (eds.) *Oxford Handbook of Children and Young Person's Nursing*. Oxford: Oxford University Press.

Woodrow, P. (2002) Managing patients with a tracheostomy in acute care. *Nursing Standard* **16** (44), 39–46.

Cardiovascular system

9

MICHELLE GREEN AND KIRSTEN HUBY

Skills

Introduction

This chapter will outline the anatomy and physiology of the cardiovascular system and the changes that occur during childhood as this body system matures. Signs and symptoms of cardiovascular failure and nursing assessment and monitoring of the child will also be discussed. This knowledge will enable the nurse to recognize cardiovascular failure as early as possible and commence appropriate interventions. A range of interventions and clinical skills required for cardiovascular support are also explained, utilizing evidence-based guidelines. All aspects of care will be discussed using a family centred and child-friendly approach.

The Nursing and Midwifery Council (NMC) introduced the use of essential skills clusters (ESC) to help pre-registration nursing students meet the standards of proficiency required for registration (NMC, 2007b). They are written from the perspective of what the public can expect of a newly qualified nurse and are designed to improve safe and effective practice. The information contained within this chapter covers aspects of most of the skills clusters. In particular, the underpinning principles from: care, compassion, and communication (1); organizational aspects of care (9, 10); infection prevention and control (22, 25, and 26); and nutrition and fluid management (29, 32) which are integrated throughout the discussion.

Learning outcomes

At the end of this chapter you will:
- Understand the anatomy and physiology of the cardiovascular system and the changes that occur during childhood as this body system matures.
- Learn to recognize signs and symptoms of cardiovascular failure.
- Be familiar with nursing assessment and cardiovascular monitoring of the child.
- Understand how the nurse recognizes cardiovascular failure as early as possible and commences appropriate interventions.

- Begin to develop an understanding of the range of interventions and clinical skills required for cardiovascular support.

Anatomy and physiology of the heart

The cardiovascular system is vital for supplying the tissues of the body with blood. This blood supply enables the needs of individual cells for oxygen and nutrients and removal of waste products to be met (metabolic demands). The body is also able to achieve these functions under a variety of circumstances: at rest or sleeping; during exertion through exercise; and during the extra demands placed on the body as a result of illness.

The heart begins to develop during the first month of foetal life and is complete by the end of the second. Whilst in the uterus the foetus relies totally on the placenta to receive oxygen and nutrients from the mother and for removal of waste products. There are a number of adaptations of the foetal circulation that enable this to occur (**see Box 9.1**).

These foetal shunts mean that even if the foetus has a congenital cardiac defect it is usually well tolerated at this stage of development and only becomes a problem when the infant is born. At birth changes in the circulation occur as the infant can no longer utilize the placenta and must rely on its own circulation to meet the tissues' metabolic demands (Horrox, 2002).

The heart is located in the middle of the chest behind the sternum and acts as the pump for the body. The arteries, capillaries, and veins are the transport system delivering oxygenated blood to the tissues and transporting waste products to where they can be excreted. The heart is essentially two pumps. The right side pumps deoxygenated blood to the lungs via the pulmonary arteries. The left side receives oxygenated blood from the lungs via the four pulmonary veins; this blood is pumped around the rest of the body by the left ventricle. The heart is comprised of four chambers: two smaller chambers at the top, the atria, and two larger, more muscular chambers at the bottom, the ventricles (**see Figure 9.1**). The right and left sides of the heart are separated by the septum, and the atrioventricular valves further divide the atria and ventricles. These valves, along with the semi-lunar valves, ensure a one-way flow of blood through the heart (McCance & Heuther, 2006).

The heart receives its own supply of blood from the coronary arteries, which stem from the base of the aorta. Due to its function the heart has a high demand for oxygen and the higher heart rates seen in children increase this demand for oxygen still further (Curley & Maloney-Harmon, 2001).

The heart pumps blood by contracting and relaxing. The cardiac cycle is made up of the heart contracting and relaxing once; the phase of contraction is termed systole and the relaxation phase diastole (McCance & Heuther,

Box 9.1 Foetal shunts

- Ductus venosus: while supplying the liver and abdomen with a small amount of blood, most blood from the placenta is shunted into the inferior vena cava (IVC) and to the heart. This is because the placenta performs the functions of the foetal liver.
- Foramen ovale: shunts blood oxygenated by the placenta from the right to the left atrium, largely bypassing the lungs.
- Ductus arteriosus: shunts oxygenated blood from the pulmonary artery trunk to the aorta, again bypassing the lungs.

These adaptations mean that less than 10% of foetal blood reaches the lungs (Curley & Maloney-Harmon, 2001). Further reading on foetal circulation can be found in Chapter Seven of Neill & Knowles (2004).

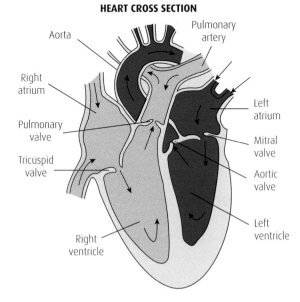

HEART CROSS SECTION

Aorta · Pulmonary artery · Right atrium · Pulmonary valve · Tricuspid valve · Right ventricle · Left atrium · Mitral valve · Aortic valve · Left ventricle

Figure 9.1 The structure of the heart

Diagram © EMIS and PiP 2009, as distributed on http://www.patient.co.uk

2006). How much blood is pumped with each beat is termed stroke volume and the stroke volume multiplied by how many times the heart beats in a minute (heart rate) is termed cardiac output. Factors important in controlling cardiac output are: preload (the amount of blood returning to the heart); heart rate; contractility (force of each heart beat); afterload (the amount of resistance the ventricles have to overcome in order to pump blood); and peripheral vascular resistance (how constricted or dilated the peripheral blood vessels are) (Novak, 2004).

The heart beat itself is stimulated by the sinoatrial node (SA), which lies within the wall of the right atrium (often referred to as the heart's pacemaker). An electrical impulse passes from the SA node through a conduction system throughout the heart (**Figure 9.2** illustrates electrical conduction through the heart). The heart muscle itself is made of specialized fibres that can contract independently of nervous stimulation, but the heart's conduction system ensures this occurs in a coordinated manner (Tortora & Derrickson, 2006). Heart rate and contractility are controlled by the autonomic nervous system and the cardiac centre of the brain located in the medulla oblongata (Horrox, 2002). The sympathetic nervous system and hormones are responsible for increasing heart rate and the parasympathetic nervous system slows the heart rate (Tortora & Derrickson, 2006).

Blood is carried around the body via a system of blood vessels. Oxygenated blood is transported away from the heart via the arterial system comprised of arteries, arterioles, and capillaries. Deoxygenated blood is carried back to the heart via the venous system of venules and veins. Arteries and veins both have three layers: an outer layer of connective tissue (tunica externa); a middle muscular layer (tunica media); and an inner smooth epithelial layer (tunica intima) (McCance & Huether, 2006).

The function of the vessels is reflected in the structure of these layers. As arteries carry blood under high pressures they have thicker walls than veins. The large arteries have outer layers that contain more elastic fibres to allow them to stretch as blood is ejected from the heart, whereas the smaller arteries have more muscle fibres as they are further from the heart and do not need to expand as much (McCance & Huether, 2006). Veins carry blood at low pressure and generally have a wide enough diameter to cope with any fluctuations in blood volume. In order to assist venous return many veins contain valves that prevent the blood travelling at low pressure from backing up, particularly in the limbs (Tortora & Derrickson, 2006). Capillaries connect the arterial and venous circulation. The function of capillaries is to carry nutrient-rich blood to the tissues and enable removal of waste products. Their cell walls are only one cell thick to allow for the exchange of nutrients and waste products between the blood supply and the tissues (Tortora & Derrickson, 2006).

During childhood the heart and circulation undergo a number of developmental changes starting in the first few hours and days after birth, when the ductus arteriosus and foramen ovale close. At birth the ventricles are of a similar size with the right ventricle slightly thicker than the left. As the workload of the left ventricle increases it grows in size and becomes the dominant ventricle during childhood (Novak, 2004). Heart rate is faster in children to compensate for a smaller stroke volume; as the child develops, the heart grows and stroke volume increases, resulting in a decrease in heart rate (Novak, 2004).

Shock

A number of clinical conditions affect a child's cardiovascular status but in order to be able to recognize an abnormality it is important to have an understanding of normal parameters and how these vary according to the child's age (see Tables 9.1 and 9.2). The circulatory system is said to be failing when blood flow fails to meet the metabolic demands of cells; this condition is termed shock. It can occur for a range of reasons and unless it is

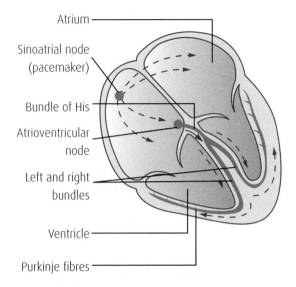

Atrium
Sinoatrial node (pacemaker)
Bundle of His
Atrioventricular node
Left and right bundles
Ventricle
Purkinje fibres

Figure 9.2 Electrical conduction through the heart

recognized and treated it may eventually result in injury to the cells and cell death, which in turn can lead to cardiorespiratory arrest (Resuscitation Council UK, 2006).

A range of conditions may result in failure of the circulatory system, for example, if the respiratory system fails; hypoxia (lack of oxygen), unless treated, may eventually lead to failure of the circulation. One of the commonest causes of shock in children is failure of the cardiovascular system due to hypovolaemia. This is when loss of fluid (severe dehydration) or loss of blood (haemorrhage) means the circulation cannot be maintained effectively (Resuscitation Council UK, 2006). Other causes of shock include severe infection (sepsis) and heart failure. In children heart failure is most likely to be the result of a congenital cardiac condition.

The body has a range of mechanisms to ensure the metabolic needs of the tissues are met despite a failing circulation, including increasing heart rate and contractility, constriction of veins supplying blood to less essential parts of the body such as the skin, and the kidneys excreting less water resulting in reduced urine output. However, when these mechanisms eventually become exhausted, the body decompensates and shock may progress rapidly (Resuscitation Council UK, 2006).

Normal ranges of heart rates for children

A key part of cardiovascular assessment in children is observing heart rate. In order to assess if a heart rate is

Table 9.1 Normal heart rates in children

Age	Heart rate
Premature	100–180
0–1 month	100–180
1–3 months	100–160
6–12 months	80–140
1–5 years	75–120
6–10 years	70–110
11–16 years	60–100

abnormal it is important that nurses are able to recognize normal heart rates in children of a range of ages. This information is contained in **Table 9.1** and also discussed in Chapter Five.

Assessment and monitoring of the child

9.1 **Visual assessment of cardiovascular status**

Observation of the child's physical appearance and behaviour can provide important information in regard to cardiovascular status, therefore the nurse's skill in carrying out a thorough assessment of the child and obtaining a history from the child and parents is extremely important. The assessment needs to include past medical history as well as that concerning the current illness. More details about admission procedures and clinical observation, including vital sign monitoring, are outlined in Chapter Five.

The clinical observation and physical assessment of the patient needs to be undertaken and recorded regularly so that any changes in the child's condition can be detected and the effectiveness of interventions can be evaluated. It should be remembered that a single assessment or assessment of a single parameter is not as useful as performing a structured, comprehensive assessment. This should be repeated regularly and the information obtained correctly interpreted and documented. The timing of repeat assessments is determined on an individual basis, guided by both the child's condition and local policies and guidelines.

In order to help the nurse perform a thorough assessment, a conceptual model or framework is often used. There is a large amount of information available in the published literature on these models and further discussion is outlined in Chapter Five. These models will underpin all nursing care, if used. Of course if the child is acutely ill or their condition is deteriorating rapidly, the assessment and planning process may need to be carried out very quickly and focused on the area of concern (Casey, 2006). One such emergency situation is shock. The Resuscitation Council (UK) provides guidance on recognition of shock in children that is summarized on the following page.

Procedure: Undertaking observations for recognition of shock (see following page)

Recording pulse/heart rate

This information can be found in Chapter Five in the section on assessing and recording vital signs.

9.2 **Recording blood pressure using all devices**

As the name suggests blood pressure (BP) is how much pressure is exerted on the walls of vessels as blood is pumped around the body (Tortora & Derrickson, 2006). The systolic blood pressure is the highest pressure in the arteries during contraction of the ventricles and the diastolic blood pressure is the lowest pressure in the arteries during the relaxation phase of the cardiac cycle. The mean arterial pressure (MAP) is the average pressure during the cardiac cycle (Tortora & Derrickson, 2006). Blood pressure is dependent on a range of factors including rate and force of the heart beat, volume of blood, and vascular resistance, which is affected by blood vessel length and diameter and blood viscosity (Tortora & Derrickson, 2006). An abnormality in any of these parameters can affect blood pressure with the result that it may be abnormally high or low.

Blood pressure is measured in millimetres of mercury (mmHg) as when this parameter was first measured mercury sphygmomanometers were routinely used. Due to health and safety concerns regarding mercury, their use these days is becoming increasingly rare with manual blood pressure measurement more commonly being undertaken using aneroid manometers (Medicines and Healthcare products Regulatory Agency (MHRA), 2006). Although these do not have the risks associated

with mercury they have the disadvantage that they are likely to become less accurate with wear and tear (O'Brien *et al.*, 2003). Other methods of blood pressure measurement include oscillometric and using an arterial catheter (the latter is mostly used in intensive care or the operating theatre). Errors can be made by healthcare professionals when assessing blood pressure; therefore appropriate training must be undertaken whichever method of measurement is used (O'Brien *et al.*, 2003). It is also important that equipment is in good working order. Normal blood pressure ranges for children of different ages are shown in **Table 9.2**.

Manual blood pressure measurement

This section applies to manual blood pressure measurement using either a mercury sphygmomanometer or aneroid gauge. When manually measuring blood pressure the age of the child must be taken into consideration; it is not possible to accurately hear **Korotkoff sounds** in children younger than one year and it may be difficult in children younger than five years. In these circumstances other more sensitive methods should be used (O'Brien *et al.*, 2003). Korotkoff sounds are the noises heard when auscultating (listening) using a stethoscope to the brachial pulse. Children's nurses working in the community may use a sphygmomanometer and not an automated oscillometric monitor.

Table 9.2 Normal blood pressure ranges in children

Age (years)	Systolic blood pressure (mmHg)
<1	70–90
1–2	80–95
2–5	80–100
5–12	90–110
>12	100–120

Step-by-step guide to undertaking observations for recognition of shock

Step	Rationale
1 Check skin colour. When well a child's skin is pink (remember this may be difficult to assess in more darkly pigmented skin; look at nail beds and mucous membranes). If the child appears pale or has mottled skin this is an abnormal sign.	Change in skin colour may be an early sign of the body compensating for shock. Blood vessels near the skin constrict ensuring blood is conserved for vital organs such as the heart and brain.
2 Check capillary refill time (CRT). Apply pressure sufficient to blanch the skin to an area such as the sternum or forehead for five seconds, then release. Count how long it takes for normal colour to return. This should be within two seconds (three seconds for neonates) (Royal College of Nursing (RCN), 2007).	Increased CRT indicates that peripheral vessels are constricted and is one of the signs of shock.
3 Check skin temperature. Feel child's hands and feet in relation to their head and trunk; if cold feel up the arms and legs for the demarcation line (where the coldness begins).	Normally child's hands and feet will feel warm, unless they have been in a cold environment. Cold hands and feet indicate shock. The more this progresses towards the trunk, the worse the degree of shock.
4 Check heart rate. Palpate pulse and assess rate. If difficult to palpate (or child is under two years) listen over the heart's apex with a stethoscope and assess for one minute.	A fast heart rate is a sign of shock as the body is trying to deliver adequate oxygen to the tissues despite a failing circulation (but remember that shock is only one of many causes of increased heart rate in children). A very slow heart rate is a dangerous sign and means circulation is failing and the child may progress to cardiopulmonary arrest.
5 Check respiratory rate. Child's respiratory rate should be observed for a full minute, observing not only rate but effort and efficacy of breathing.	Child presenting with tachypnoea (fast breathing) but minimal signs of respiratory distress may have a cardiovascular problem for which the respiratory system is attempting to compensate.
6 Urine output should be measured or a history of urine output in the last 12 hours obtained.	Conserving water is one of the body's compensatory mechanisms when dehydrated or in shock. Decreased urine output can also indicate an inadequate supply of blood to the kidneys as a result of cardiovascular failure.
7 Check child's mental status. Observe if the child appears lethargic/drowsy or agitated/irritable. The acronym AVPU may be used for quickly assessing mental status: A for alert; V for responds to voice; P for responds to pain; U for unresponsive even to painful stimulus.	Deteriorating mental status is a sign of a gradual decrease in blood supply to the brain. However, remember a young child is likely to be frightened by the hospital environment and this may influence their responses. Ask the parents how the child's behaviour compares to their normal behaviour.

| 8 | **Check blood pressure. While it is important to recognize normal and abnormal blood pressure in children and blood pressure monitoring may be used to assess the effectiveness of treatment, it cannot be relied upon as an early indicator of cardiovascular failure.** | Low blood pressure is a very late sign of shock in a child and indicates the body's compensatory mechanisms have failed. The signs discussed above allow shock to be recognized more quickly and treated earlier. |
| 9 | **Consider how frequently assessment needs to be repeated and ensure all observations are documented.** | Frequency of observations will depend on seriousness of child's condition. Documentation will provide important information on improvement or deterioration. |

Procedure: Manual blood pressure measurement

Preparation

Wash hands.

Equipment

- Monitoring device.
- Correctly sized cuff.
- Stethoscope.

Ensure that this is clean (particularly the earpieces and diaphragm of the stethoscope) and in good working order.

Consent and communication

Introduce yourself and explain the procedure to the child and/or parent, including that the cuff when inflated will cause a tightening sensation, but this will only be for a short period of time. The child and family need to understand why the procedure is being carried out and what will happen during it. If the child is distressed this will affect the accuracy of the reading. Gain consent.

Blood pressure using automated oscillometric monitor

This method for measuring blood pressure is widely used in the hospital setting. The monitor contains a sensor, which measures blood flow and calculates blood pressure from the data it collects. Before use it is important to ensure that the equipment is in good working order and is used according to the manufacturer's instructions. Choose an appropriately sized cuff (see the procedure for manual recording of blood pressure). The cuff should ideally be placed on the upper arm but can be placed on the child's lower leg if the arms cannot be used for any reason; however, it must be recognized that this will give a higher systolic reading (RCN, 2007).

The advantage of this method of monitoring is that it allows serial observation of blood pressure as an automated monitor can be set to take readings at regular intervals. This will clearly demonstrate improvement, maintenance, or deterioration in the child's condition. However, if blood pressure is consistently high or low for the child's age or is unobtainable using an automated monitor, it should be rechecked manually (RCN, 2007).

Blood pressure monitoring via arterial catheter

Arterial blood pressure is a more invasive method of assessing blood pressure as it is measured via a catheter placed in an artery, such as the radial or femoral artery or one of the umbilical arteries in a neonate. This method of blood pressure monitoring is not without risk and nurses need additional training in caring for a patient who is undergoing this type of monitoring. The catheter is attached to a fluid-filled system that in turn is attached to a monitor and this provides a waveform with beat to beat monitoring of the patient's systolic, diastolic, and mean blood pressure.

Care of the child during arterial blood pressure measurement includes monitoring of the catheter site and

Step-by-step guide to manual blood pressure measurement

Step	Rationale
1 Ensure BP device has been regularly calibrated and that it reads 0 prior to use.	Equipment must be functioning correctly in order to obtain an accurate result. It should be checked and calibrated regularly according to local policy.
2 Wash hands/apply alcohol gel.	Hand washing reduces the cross transmission of infection from patient to patient, which reduces the incidence of hospital acquired infection (Pratt *et al.*, 2007).
3 Ensure patient has been at rest for three minutes prior to measurement.	Activity (including eating or crying) prior to taking reading will affect accuracy (British Hypertension Society, 1999).
4 BP should be measured in the middle of the upper arm; remove any tight clothing.	Measuring BP in the arm gives a more accurate reading.
5 Ensure patient is comfortable and that the arm is supported and is at heart level.	If the arm is below heart level gravity may cause a falsely high systolic BP. If it is above the level of the heart it can give a false low reading (British Hypertension Society, 1999).
6 Use a correctly sized cuff. The bladder should cover 100% of the arm (RCN, 2007) and the width should cover two thirds of the elbow to shoulder distance (Novak, 2004).	Incorrectly sized cuffs lead to inaccurate results. A cuff that is too small will give a falsely high reading and one that is too large will give a falsely low reading.
7 Feel for the brachial artery running down the inner aspect of the elbow.	To aid accurate placement of the stethoscope once the cuff is inflated.
8 Whilst palpating the brachial pulse the cuff is inflated by squeezing the attached rubber bulb, until the pulse disappears. Note at what point this happens and deflate the cuff by releasing the screw on the inflation bulb.	Allows estimation of the systolic blood pressure. Young children may not tolerate the tightening sensation of the cuff. If extremely distressed abandon procedure and seek further advice.
9 Inflate the cuff 20–30 mmHg above the point where previously the pulse disappeared.	Allows the nurse to accurately monitor reading when Korotkoff sounds are first heard.
10 Place the stethoscope over the brachial artery and deflate the cuff at 2–3 mmHg/second until Korotkoff sounds can be heard. Note when this happens (British Hypertension Society, 1999).	This is the systolic blood pressure and should be recorded to the nearest 2 mmHg. Deflation of the cuff that is too rapid can lead to inaccurate measurement.
11 Listen until the Korotkoff sounds disappear and note this number. Remove cuff and leave patient comfortable.	This is the diastolic blood pressure and should be recorded to the nearest 2 mmHg.
12 Clean stethoscope, clean hands.	Reduces risk of cross infection.

13 Consider the significance of the findings. Was the blood pressure higher or lower than expected? Document findings.

Accurate documentation is required so that any abnormality or abnormal trend in blood pressure readings may be recognized and appropriate action taken.

14 Blood pressure status should only be decided after it has been measured on a number of occasions (O'Brien *et al.*, 2003).

Single measurements may give an inaccurate reading for a range of reasons.

ensuring perfusion (adequate blood supply) of the limb in which the catheter is inserted. The monitoring system and line infusion (usually heparinized saline to maintain patency of the line) will need to be replaced every few days (in accordance with local policy). The nurse needs to ensure that the monitoring system is at the correct level (heart level) and that the quality of the waveform is observed, otherwise accuracy of monitoring can be affected. Alarm parameters for acceptable blood pressure limits for the child's age and condition must be set. Potential complications associated with arterial lines include: disconnection of the system resulting in serious haemorrhage; introduction of infection; and blood clot or air embolus in the system, which may lead to inadequate blood supply to the limb in which the line is inserted. Careful monitoring and use of aseptic technique when accessing the line should be used (Horrox, 2002).

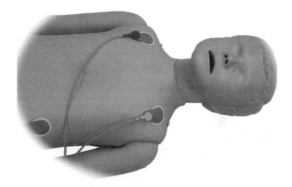

Figure 9.3 Normal placement of ECG leads and ECG complex

toring is useful to provide a continuous reading of the patient's heart rate and rhythm. Should an **arrhythmia** be suspected a more detailed 12 lead ECG should be performed. **Figure 9.3** shows correct placement of monitoring leads and includes a diagram of a normal ECG complex. **Table 9.3** explains the ECG complex in relation to heart function.

Electrocardiogram (ECG)

If using continuous electrocardiogram (ECG) monitoring the practitioner should be trained in the correct use of equipment and the limitations and risks associated with its use (RCN, 2007). This is particularly important due to the wide range of monitors available on the market, which incorporate a variety of functions.

An ECG measures the electrical activity in the heart associated with contraction of the muscle, and transmits and records it on a monitor (Horrox, 2002). ECG monitoring will provide information about heart rate and rhythm, which the operator needs to interpret in order to recognize both normal and abnormal variation and to work out why it exists and what it means. Three lead ECG moni-

9.3 **ECG monitoring**

This is an advanced skill. You *must* check whether you can assist with or undertake any aspect of this skill, in line with local policy.

It must be remembered that arrhythmias are relatively rare in children. A normal heart rhythm is termed sinus rhythm (**see Figure 9.3**); this is fairly regular but there may be some variation between beats and the rhythm is also affected by respirations (Curley & Maloney-Harmon, 2001). The most common

Table 9.3 ECG complex in relation to heart function

ECG representation	Physiological event in the heart
P wave	Atrial depolarization is stimulated by the sinoatrial (SA) node, which is located in the right atrium. This leads to contraction of the atria (atrial systole). The muscle mass of the atria is smaller than the ventricles and this is reflected in the smaller wave on the ECG.
P–Q interval	Electrical conduction continues to the atrioventricular (AV) node and down through the ventricles via the AV bundle and the Purkinje system.
QRS complex	Ventricular depolarization occurs, the ventricles begin to contract and the atria relax. The ventricles are more muscular and therefore the size of this part of the complex is much bigger.
S–T segment and T wave	This represents repolarization of the ventricles and occurs as the ventricles relax (diastole).
Relaxation period	Following the T wave and ventricular repolarization the atria and ventricles are relaxed. The faster the heart beats the shorter this period of relaxation.

abnormalities are sinus tachycardia (normal rhythm but a fast rate for the child's age) and sinus bradycardia (normal rhythm but a slow rate for the child's age). Severe sinus bradycardia is often linked to hypoxia in children and may progress to asystole (no electrical activity and absence of heart beat).

Procedure: ECG monitoring (see following page)

Preparation

Consider how you will place the monitoring leads on the child as indicated in **Figure 9.3**. This will include where to set up the machine, the length of the leads, and the needs of the child.

Equipment

- ECG monitor.
- ECG leads.
- ECG electrodes.

Consent and communication

Before placing the leads explain the procedure to the family and child and gain consent.

Cardiac catheterization

This is an advanced skill. You *must* check whether you can assist with or undertake any aspect of this skill, in line with local policy.

Cardiac catheterization is a specialist skill and is beyond the remit of this book; however, student nurses and nurses may be asked by patients to explain what it is and what is involved. Cardiac catheterization is a procedure used for the diagnosis of a number of cardiac conditions; it can provide detailed information about heart anatomy, blood flow, and pressures within the heart (Curley & Maloney-Harmon, 2001). Catheterization is achieved by inserting a radio-opaque (visible on X-ray) catheter into one of the large arteries or veins, threading the catheter up into the heart, injecting contrast medium (radio-opaque dye), and taking X-rays (angiography) (Horrox, 2002).

Catheterization is used to diagnose and treat abnormal electrical conduction through the heart. It is also used to relieve symptoms or treat a number of cardiac defects (Curley & Maloney-Harmon, 2001). Catheter procedures can delay surgical intervention and in some cases replace it. While less invasive than surgery, the procedure is not without risk of complications; these include cardiac arrhythmias, vascular complications such as haemorrhage from the catheter site or thrombosis (blood clot),

ECG monitoring

Step-by-step guide to ECG monitoring

This is an advanced skill. You *must* check whether you can assist with or undertake any aspect of this skill, in line with local policy.

Step	Rationale
1 The leads for the ECG monitor are connected to the child through use of electrodes. There are a range of sizes and types on the market and the nurse must be familiar with the type used locally.	To ensure they can carry out the procedure correctly.
The electrodes have a metal stud on one side (or an integrated lead) and conductive adhesive on the other.	This adhesive allows the electrode to stick to the chest and conduct the electrical impulses from the heart.
2 Ensure the skin is clean and dry.	If the skin is wet or oily the electrodes will not adhere and may give a poor or inaccurate trace on the monitor.
3 Peel the backing off and place the electrodes at the left and right shoulders of the patient with the third electrode on the left side of the abdomen or on the leg (see Figure 9.3).	Correct placement of the electrodes and leads is important; if misplaced the ECG recording will be affected.
4 The leads are often colour coded. Commonly this is red on the right, yellow on the left, and green (or black) on the abdomen or left leg. Three individual leads connect to a single lead that is plugged into the monitor.	Incorrect lead placement can result in inaccurate monitoring. Lead colours for individual monitors may vary.
5 Electrodes may require replacement from time to time.	The conductive adhesive dries out, giving a poor signal and trace on the monitor, and the electrodes may no longer adhere to the child's skin.
6 Switch the monitor on and check which lead is being used for monitoring. Lead II is used most commonly.	The monitor reads through lead I, II, or III. The leads give a view of the heart from different angles across the body. Lead II gives a clear picture of the PQRS.
7 Set alarm parameters according to the age of the child, their clinical condition, and the baseline heart rate.	Alarm parameters need to be wide enough to allow for normal fluctuations in rate, but still enable recognition of any condition that is likely to require further assessment and intervention.
8 Careful cleaning of the monitor and especially the leads (unless disposable) is required between patients. Manufacturer's instructions or hospital policy should be followed.	To ensure effective cleaning and prevent cross infection or damage to the equipment.

9	All electrical equipment should be regularly maintained according to local policy and manufacturer's instructions.	Defective equipment may result in inaccurate monitoring.
10	Nurses must be able to recognize sinus rhythm and common abnormalities and when to seek further assistance regarding significance and interventions.	Abnormal heart rhythms may be life-threatening and rapid intervention may be required.
11	Patients on continuous ECG monitoring must have their heart rate documented regularly; any abnormalities must also be documented in the nursing notes.	To ensure effective documentation.

and allergic reactions to the contrast medium (Horrox, 2002). In order to minimize these risks the child needs careful preoperative assessment and preparation and close monitoring postoperatively of heart rate, rhythm, and blood pressure. Horrox (2002, p 398) includes a detailed care pathway for children undergoing cardiac catheterization.

Blood transfusion

9.4 Administering a blood transfusion ▲

This is an advanced skill. You *must* check whether you can assist with or undertake any aspect of this skill, in line with local policy.

Transfusions of red cells or blood products are often life-saving therapies for children with a range of acute and chronic conditions. However, there are also a number of risks associated with this procedure and these must be weighed against the potential benefits before transfusion is requested. Nurses are closely involved in all aspects of the transfusion process and practice must ensure that the risks of transfusion are minimized. The traceability of all transfusions is now a legal requirement in the UK and the

final fate of every blood component issued by transfusion services must be documented and a record of this kept for 30 years (RCN, 2005b).

A further legal requirement is that any serious adverse event or reaction is reported on the serious adverse blood reactions and events (SABRE) system. This can be accessed via the Serious Hazards of Transfusion (SHOT) website at **http://www.shotuk.org**. A range of adverse reactions to transfusions can occur but unfortunately the most common adverse event in children is that the incorrect blood component is transfused to the patient. Such errors can increase morbidity and even result in the patient's death, and furthermore they are entirely preventable (SHOT, 2006).

The guidance provided here is for the administration of a transfusion required for clinical reasons in the non-emergency situation. Additional guidance should be sought if a transfusion is required in an emergency as a result of a major haemorrhage and for specialist neonatal transfusions. McClelland's (2007) handbook of transfusion was utilized to develop the following procedure and is a good reference point for detailed guidance on all aspects of transfusion.

Nursing Alert

Transfusing an incorrect blood component is the most common error of transfusion.

Procedure: Administration of a blood transfusion

Preparation

Preparing the blood

The transfusion must have been prescribed by a doctor and the prescription should contain patient identification details, the blood component, the quantity to be transfused, and the duration of the transfusion. Incomplete or unclear prescriptions or acceptance of verbal orders has led to a number of serious untoward events (SHOT, 2005; 2007).

Correctly fill in the blood request form documenting patient details, the product required, the reason for transfusion, any special requests, and the requesting doctor's details. Ensure the sample for compatibility testing is correctly labelled after the sample has been collected (RCN, 2005b). Check the patient's ID bracelet and ask the patient or parent to confirm their identity. Prior to blood product administration a sample of the patient's blood must be sent to transfusion services to find the child's blood type and test for antibodies. Transfusing an incorrect blood component is the most common error of transfusion. This includes sending a sample from the wrong patient for compatibility testing. In infants younger than four months a sample of maternal blood must also be sent in a correctly labelled tube to test for maternal as well as the infant's antibodies.

The blood is dispensed by transfusion services and the nurse must record when the blood pack has been removed from the fridge (and if it is returned to the fridge for any reason). Take a form with the patient's identification (ID) details and match them to the blood pack, as part of the traceability of the blood and to ensure that the correct blood component is withdrawn from the fridge.

When the blood is removed from the fridge a few minutes should be allowed for it to warm to room temperature. With infants and/or large transfusions use of a blood warmer should be considered. A large transfusion of cold blood may lead to hypothermia, which in turn will have an adverse effect on the patient's condition. Never warm blood in an uncontrolled manner such as with a microwave or hot water.

Observation

Observations of temperature, pulse, and blood pressure are performed before transfusion commences and when the transfusion is completed. These should be recorded on the observation chart (RCN, 2005a; 2005b). This will provide a baseline of what is normal for that patient, for monitoring of any adverse reaction.

> **Nursing Alert**
>
> Signs of adverse or allergic reactions during a transfusion include: fever, flushing, itching and rash, hypotension, restlessness and anxiety, pain at the site of transfusion, loin pain, or respiratory distress.

Equipment

- Blood pack.
- Administration set including filter with a 170–200 µm pore size.
- Cannula.
- Saline.
- Apron, gloves, and disposal unit.
- Equipment to monitor temperature and other vital signs.

Consent and communication

Ensure written and verbal information has been provided for the child (appropriate to their level of understanding) and parents regarding the advantages and risks associated with transfusions and any alternatives available. This will provide an opportunity to discuss any concerns and enables the child and family to make an informed choice.

Although not a legal requirement, it is good practice that the doctor gains consent for the transfusion and a record of this is made in the patient's notes. Clear documentation of reasons for the transfusion, type of transfusion, and the information given to the family is necessary to minimize risk of errors.

Step-by-step guide to administration of a blood transfusion

This is an advanced skill. You *must* check whether you can assist with or undertake any aspect of this skill, in line with local policy.

Step	Rationale
1 Ensure you have undertaken the preparation outlined above.	To ensure the nurse and patient are ready for the procedure.
2 The blood pack label should be checked against the ID bracelet for the patient's minimum identification data. This data constitutes first and last name, gender, date of birth, and hospital identity number (address is also required in some areas). These checks must be performed at the patient's bedside by a qualified nurse.	Minimum identification data is a standardized method for correctly identifying patients and so reducing errors.
3 Check that the donation number on the compatibility label (tie on tag) and label on the blood pack match.	Ensures correct component for the patient has been dispensed by transfusion services.
4 Positively identify the patient by asking them their name and date of birth. Ask a parent if the child is unable to provide this information (RCN, 2005b).	The child's age or condition may prevent them from giving positive identification.
5 Local policy should be followed for the number of staff required to check a transfusion.	Careful checks are required to ensure patient safety and minimize risk of errors.
6 Wear personal protective equipment and adhere to local infection control guidance including the use of hand washing, gloves, and aprons, and correct disposal of hazardous waste (RCN, 2005a).	To limit exposure to blood-borne pathogens and the potential for injury (RCN, 2005a).
7 Refer to the transfusion prescription to check patient identification details, the blood component, the quantity to be transfused, and the duration of the transfusion.	Incomplete or unclear prescriptions or acceptance of verbal orders has lead to a number of serious untoward events (SHOT, 2005; 2007).
8 Check the expiry date on the pack and inspect for any discolouration, clots, or leaks.	Ensures the blood is in optimum condition for transfusion.
9 Check any special requirements, e.g. cyto-megalovirus (CMV) negative blood, have been met.	Failure to meet special requirements may result in an incorrect blood component being transfused (SHOT, 2005).
10 A qualified IV competent nurse should flush the cannula with 0.9% saline.	Ensures cannula is patent and has been cleared of fluid that may not be compatible with the blood transfusion.

11	Administration sets must contain a filter with a 170–200 µm pore size (British Committee for Standards in Haematology Blood Transfusion Task Force, 1999).	Reduces transfusion of particulate matter and microscopic clots (RCN, 2005a).
12	Ensure infusion device is suitable for administration of blood and use an appropriate administration set.	Some pumps may cause blood **haemolysis** (RCN, 2005a).
13	Check the set is intact and the packet sealed before use. The set is primed with the blood to be transfused using aseptic technique according to local policy.	Minimizes risk of transfusion-induced infection.
14	Drugs should not be added to the blood pack and compatibility of IV fluids through the same line should be checked.	Certain medications and IV fluids are not compatible with blood and may cause haemolysis or the blood to clot.
15	The patient's temperature and pulse should be monitored 15 minutes after the start of the transfusion and at the start of each subsequent blood pack. These should be recorded on the observation chart.	Adverse reactions to transfusions result in pyrexia and tachycardia and are more likely to occur at the beginning of a transfusion.
16	The patient requires close monitoring during the transfusion.	This is especially important in young children as they may not be able to report early symptoms.
17	Frequency of further observations is dependent on the patient's condition and local policy.	More frequent observations may be required if a reaction is suspected or for some patient groups.
18	If an adverse reaction is suspected (see Nursing Alert box) stop the transfusion immediately and call for medical help. Stay with the patient and reassure them; monitor vital signs including blood pressure and urine output. Ensure the cannula remains patent by infusing 0.9% saline. Also check the patient's identity against the blood compatibility label.	Medical assistance will be required to stabilize the patient. Observing vital signs allows monitoring of improvement or deterioration in the patient's condition. It is important to establish if the reaction is allergic in origin or due to an incorrect blood component being transfused.
19	With minor reactions it may be decided to restart the transfusion following medication.	Minor reactions are not uncommon and may be managed with medication to relieve symptoms, and by infusing the blood at a slower rate.
20	The transfusion should be completed within four hours of removing the pack from the fridge (RCN, 2005b). If the blood is out of the fridge for more than 30 minutes but not transfused, it should not be returned to the fridge. Seek advice from the transfusion department.	The blood warms once removed from the fridge and this is associated with increasing risk of infection (RCN, 2005b).

21 Following completion of the transfusion, document the start and finish times and the volume of blood transfused on the fluid balance chart. The donation number, component type, and date of transfusion should be documented in the patient's notes.	To ensure accurate documentation and traceability of all aspects of the transfusion.
22 Administration sets should be discarded after 12 hours for continuing transfusion or on completion of a transfusion. Ensure safe disposal of the set; the empty transfusion bag should be discarded according to local policy.	For infection control and to prevent contamination of blood giving sets with incompatible drugs or fluids.
23 A qualified IV competent nurse should flush cannula with 0.9% saline.	Ensures the cannula is patent and is clear of blood ready for further use.
24 Errors or adverse reactions must be documented in the patient notes and should be reported according to local policy and national reporting procedures (RCN, 2005a).	This is a legal requirement and is important for managing risk and learning from errors.

Intravenous (IV) access and fluid management

Recording fluid balance

When children are receiving IV fluids it is important to monitor their overall fluid status. Fluid balance charts (see Figure 9.4) are one way of monitoring this but in order for this to be an accurate record all types of input and output need to be recorded. This could also include information from parents (see Table 9.4). Weighing the child will also give an indication of their level of hydration.

9.5 **Administering IV fluids**

The intravenous (IV) route can be used to administer many different types of fluids including maintenance fluids (meeting normal daily requirements), resuscitation fluids, and blood products. Total parenteral nutrition

(TPN) is usually given via central venous lines rather than peripheral venous lines due to risk of tissue damage from extravasation. These need to be prescribed by a

Table 9.4 Types of input and output

Input	Output
Oral food and drink including breast milk	Urine
Enteral feeds, e.g. gastrostomy, nasogastric, or jejunostomy	Stool/stoma
IV fluids	Vomit
Total parenteral nutrition (TPN)	Output from drains or wounds
Blood products, e.g. packed cells, platelets, human albumin solution (HAS)	Gastric aspirate (if discarded)
Drug infusions	Secretions

Working Weight 12 Kg Mls/kg/24 hours 1100 mls Total mls/hr 46 mls/hr	Surname JONES First Name JOHN Unit No AB1234 Date 10 JUNE	24 Hour Fluid Balance Chart

TIME	Type & Amount Taken: ORAL	NG	Total	Type Packed Cells: Hourly	Total	Type: Hourly	Total	IV Site Check Sign.	URINE: Amount	Total	STOOL TYPE	VOMIT / ASPIRATE: Amount	Descriptior
0700	Cows Milk		150										
0800				42	42			[illegible]				small	Milky
0900				42	84			[illegible]	100	100	BNO		
1000				42	126			[illegible]					
1100				42	168			[illegible]					
1200													
1300													
1400													

Figure 9.4 Fluid balance chart

doctor, nurse prescriber, or delivered under a patient group direction (RCN, 2005a). The nurse administering the fluid should have a clear understanding of why the infusion is necessary, the nature of the fluid being infused, and any potential side effects.

Ensuring the correct volume of fluid is administered is an extremely important aspect of IV fluid administration in order to prevent a range of adverse side effects such as dehydration and fluid overload. There are a number of methods of calculating maintenance fluids; examples from Mackway-Jones *et al.* (2005, p 285) are contained in Table 9.5.

For example, a child weighing 23 kg would require 1000 + 500 + 60 = 1560 ml/day. This figure is then divided by 24 to provide an hourly rate (65 ml/hour).

Table 9.5 Calculation of maintenance fluids

Body weight	Fluid requirement per day (ml/kg)	Fluid requirement per hour (ml/kg)
First 10 kg	100	4
Second 10 kg	50	2
Subsequent kg	20	1

The use of an infusion device to deliver intravenous fluids allows the fluid to be delivered at a set rate over a specific period of time. Where infusion devices are used to deliver intravenous fluids all staff should have been given appropriate training and be competent in the safe use of the device (Department of Health (DH), 2004). Intravenous administration sets can be left *in situ* for 72 hours without causing an increased risk of infection to the patient (O'Grady *et al.*, 2002). Administration sets used for fluids that promote microbial growth such as TPN should be changed more frequently. Pratt *et al.* (2007) advise parenteral nutrition sets are changed at the end of the infusion or at least every 24 hours. Some manufacturers may suggest that their administration sets are changed more frequently than these recommendations. Clear documentation is required to ensure that administration sets are changed at appropriate times. The procedure for administering IV fluids is outlined below.

Procedure: IV fluid administration

Preparation

Ensure the prescription is accurately written and fluids are prescribed on the correct chart. Ensure patient details are correct. The calculation of fluid type and volume and fluid

Step-by-step guide to IV fluid administration

Step	Rationale
1 Ensure you have undertaken the preparation as outlined above.	To ensure the prescription has been correctly written and the nurse and patient have been prepared.
2 Check the patient's name and date of birth verbally and against their ID band.	Ensures that the correct fluid is administered to the correct patient.
3 Open administration sets and if more than one is needed connect together using an aseptic or non-touch technique in line with local policy. Ensure all lines are clamped. The number of lines and additional connections should be kept to a minimum. If more than one type of fluid is to be administered through one vascular access device at the same time then both fluids must be compatible.	Aseptic or non-touch technique should be used to prevent contamination of the fluid. Lines and connection should be kept to a minimum to reduce the risk of infection (DH, 2003).
4 Expose port on fluid bag by removing the protective covering. Remove the protective cap from the spike of the administration set.	Administration sets need to be primed to remove air from the system.
Spike the bag of fluid with the bag held below eye level. Hang the bag on the IV stand.	Holding the bag below eye level prevents splashes into eyes.
5 Squeeze the drip chamber of the administration set until this is half full. Open the roller clamp and prime the administration set following manufacturer's guidelines.	Prevents air from the drip chamber being drawn down the administration set.
6 Correctly insert administration set into appropriate pump. Set pump according to prescription and following manufacturer's instructions.	To reduce risk of error the administration set must be loaded correctly and the rate and volume to be infused must be accurately entered (DH, 2004).
7 Collect equipment required for connecting administration set to venous access device. This will depend on the type of vascular access, the cap that is in place, and whether it needs to be removed.	To ensure the correct equipment is ready for use.
When needleless connectors are in use the catheter hub may be decontaminated prior to and after use with single patient alcohol wipes (Pratt *et al.,* 2007).	To prevent cross infection.

8	A qualified IV competent nurse should flush the venous access device with 0.9% saline.	This checks for patency of the device and prevents precipitation of incompatible fluids.
9	Connect administration set to vascular access device. All connectors should be leur lock devices. Commence IV infusion according to prescription.	Leur lock devices reduce the risk of administration sets becoming disconnected.
10	Remove and dispose of gloves. Wash hands/use alcohol gel.	To prevent cross infection.
11	Document time and date of start of infusion in line with organizational guidelines. If replacing a previous infusion, document the stop time and date.	To ensure effective documentation.

administration rates should be checked and documented prior to commencing an infusion in order to reduce the risk of error (DH, 2004).

Select the correct bag of fluid to be administered. Two qualified practitioners must check the fluid to be administered against the prescription and sign the chart (NMC, 2007a). Some calculations may be complex and should be independently calculated by two practitioners. The use of a calculator should aid not replace arithmetical skills (NMC, 2007a).

Wash hands or use alcohol gel and put on gloves to reduce the cross-transmission of infection from patient to patient and the incidence of hospital acquired infection (Pratt *et al.*, 2007).

Equipment

Collect equipment required, selecting appropriate administration sets for the fluid to be infused. Some intravenous giving sets contain filters to remove particulate matter from the solution. Local policy and manufacturer's guidance should be used. Wear gloves.

Consent and communication

Explain the procedure to the child and family and gain consent. This provides an opportunity to discuss any concerns in order that the child and family can make an informed choice.

IV cannulation

A cannula is a tube that is inserted into a body cavity or duct (Scales, 2005). An intravenous cannula is inserted into a peripheral vein in order to provide access to the circulation to give drugs, fluids, blood products, or nutrition. Common veins that may be cannulated are those in the antecubital fossa (inner aspect of the elbow) where the basilic, cephalic, and median cubital veins are found close to the skin's surface. Other veins that can be used are those on the dorsum of the hand and foot; scalp veins may also be cannulated if necessary. The vein that is chosen should ideally not have been previously cannulated and should be easily accessible. If possible the non-dominant side of the body should be used to cause least disruption to the child's mobility and functioning.

Whilst the use of intravenous cannulae is commonplace in the management of children, their in-hospital use carries associated risks including: infection, phlebitis, infiltration, and extravasation (Callaghan *et al.*, 2002). In order to reduce the risks associated with intravenous cannula use, care must be taken during insertion and monitoring must occur frequently whilst the cannula is *in situ*.

9.6 **Preparing the child for venepuncture and cannulation**

This is an advanced skill. You *must* check whether you can assist with or undertake any aspect of this skill, in line with local policy.

Procedure: Preparing for venepuncture and cannulation

The nurse's role in relation to **venepuncture** and **cannulation** is explained here.

Preparation

Venepuncture and cannulation can be traumatic for the child and their family. Preparation and careful planning of the procedure are essential for reducing fear and future psychological problems (**see Box 9.2**). Preparation of the child and family must involve:

- Explanation.
- Consent.
- Distraction.
- Pain relief.

Box 9.2 Preparation of the child and family for venepuncture or cannulation

> Explaining the procedure to the child and family is the first step in preparing the child. Both verbal and non-verbal communication needs to be age and developmentally appropriate and take into consideration past experience. Lavery & Ingram (2005) suggest that particular attention needs to be paid when a child has had a previous traumatic experience of venepuncture or cannulation so that action can be taken to avoid the same outcome. It is also beneficial to ascertain what has previously worked well so that similar interventions can be utilized.
>
> Venepuncture is invasive and the necessity of carrying out the procedure must be explained. Consideration should be given to the likelihood of needing venous access for multiple interventions. If this is the case a cannula will be more appropriate and the child and family should be prepared that this will be left *in situ*.

Consent and communication

Introduce yourself and explain the procedure to the child and family using effective age-appropriate verbal and non-verbal communication. Play can be a useful strategy to help children prepare for procedures. Ideally children should be given the opportunity to play with safe equipment prior to the procedure (Willock *et al.*, 2004); this can help assess any misconceptions that the child and family may have.

Consent must be obtained before any procedure is undertaken (NMC, 2004). Children may be competent to consent even if they haven't reached the legal age limit and therefore should be included in the explanations and discussions to allow their views to be heard. The legal age limit for consent varies between countries.

9.7 **Care of an intravenous cannula**

This is an advanced skill. You *must* check whether you can assist with or undertake any aspect of this skill, in line with local policy.

Whilst the risk of infection and phlebitis can be reduced by using an aseptic technique when the cannula is inserted (Ingram & Lavery, 2007) there is still an associated risk as long as the cannula is *in situ*. Localized infection can occur at the exit site as well as systemic infection occurring due to bacteria entering the bloodstream through the cannula. Observation of the cannula site and removal if any complications are noted can help to prevent severe complications occurring. The cannula site should be observed frequently when in use (Lavery & Smith, 2007; Callaghan *et al.*, 2002). However, there is little consensus as to whether this constitutes daily or hourly observation; local policy and guidelines should dictate the frequency of observations.

Nursing Alert

Observation of the cannula site and removal if any complications are noted can help to prevent severe complications occurring.

Step-by-step guide to preparing for venepuncture and cannulation

This is an advanced skill. You *must* check whether you can assist with or undertake any aspect of this skill, in line with local policy.

Step	Rationale
1 Select appropriate method of pain relief.	The most appropriate form of pain relief depends on the child and availability of drugs, equipment, and appropriately trained staff. Local anaesthetic creams if used (Ametop, Emla) need to be applied in advance following manufacturer's guidelines. Ethyl chloride spray rapidly cools the skin and has rapid onset but short-term effects so the procedure must be accurately timed (Willock *et al.*, 2004). Nitrous oxide and oxygen mixture (Entonox) is an inhaled, rapid onset, short-acting analgesic (Harrop, 2007). Cooperation is required from the child and practitioners must be appropriately trained so it may not be suitable in all cases. Local anaesthetic or inhaled analgesia are more effective than other forms of analgesia that have slower onset of action.
2 Utilize distraction techniques or diversional play to reduce anxieties and fears.	Such techniques can refocus the child's attention away from the procedure and onto some other, non-threatening stimuli (Cavender *et al.*, 2004). The child needs to have been involved in choosing the distracter and distraction needs to begin prior to the procedure starting.
3 Ensure that the child is positioned comfortably with the area to be cannulated accessible. If possible they should sit next to a parent or on a parent's lap. As a last resort when all alternatives have been tried it may be necessary to immobilize the child by holding them still. Minimum force should be used (RCN, 2003).	The child needs to be still but able to engage with any distraction techniques being used. Sitting next to a parent or on a parent's lap has been found to be less distressing than lying flat (Cavender *et al.*, 2004). Immobilizing the child should be a last resort as it can make the procedure more frightening for the child.

Procedure: Care of an IV cannula (see following page)

Preparation

Wash hands.

Equipment

- You may need to apply new bandages and dressings.
- Saline.

Consent and communication

Explain the procedure to the child and parents and gain consent.

9.8 **Removal of an IV cannula** 🅰

A cannula should be removed if there are signs of infection, phlebitis, or infiltration, or if the cannula has become blocked or is no longer being used (Ingram & Lavery, 2007). The length of time the cannula has been indwelling is considered a risk factor for developing phlebitis and infection. Elective replacement of a cannula at specific time periods has been suggested (Idvall & Gunningberg, 2006) although this is not always possible within the paediatric population due to difficulty in accessing veins and distress caused by cannulation (Oishi, 2001).

Procedure: Removal of an IV cannula (see page 250)

Preparation

Wash hands, wear gloves.

Equipment

- Gauze and dressing.
- Sharps bin.

Consent and communication

Explain the procedure to the child and parents and gain consent.

Care of a central line

Central venous access devices (CVAD) provide access to the central circulation, with their tips terminating in the superior vena cava (**see Figure 9.5**). They are used for several reasons, including: the delivery of high volumes of fluids; multiple blood sampling; delivery of multiple intravenous therapies; and central venous pressure monitoring. They reduce the need for repeated venepuncture and cannulation and therefore reduce the trauma caused to children and their families.

The type of central line inserted will depend on the length of time that therapies need to continue. Peripherally inserted central catheters (PICCs) and non-tunnelled catheters are used for short-term access and may be seen in children in the intensive care unit. Tunnelled lines

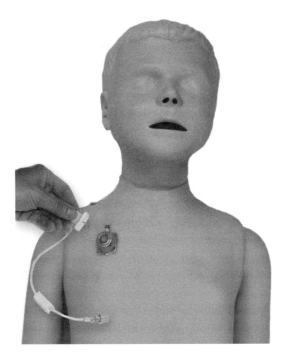

Figure 9.5 Position of central line and Huber needle

Step-by-step guide to care of an IV cannula

This is an advanced skill. You *must* check whether you can assist with or undertake any aspect of this skill, in line with local policy.

Step	Rationale
1 **Wash hands/apply alcohol gel.**	Hand washing reduces the cross-transmission of infection from patient to patient, which reduces the incidence of hospital acquired infection (Pratt *et al.*, 2007).
2 **If *in situ* the bandage must be removed fully. Any splint also needs to be removed.**	The cannula exit site needs to be observed for signs of infection, phlebitis, and infiltration. The limb needs to be checked for adequate circulation. It is not possible to recognize problems early if the site is not observed fully by removing the bandage.
3 **Observe cannula exit site for signs of phlebitis, infection, or infiltration. It is recommended that a phlebitis scale is used when observing the cannula site (RCN, 2005a).**	Such scales enable assessment for signs of erythema (redness), pain, swelling, induration (hardness), and pyrexia. The use of a validated scale can help with consistent scoring when more than one practitioner is undertaking the task.
4 **If phlebitis, infection, or infiltration is suspected then the cannula should be removed.**	To prevent further complications.
5 **Ensure cannula remains secured with an appropriate dressing. Transparent, gauze-based, and combined dressings are often used. The dressing will need to be changed if it has become wet or soiled.**	Securing the cannula is essential to reduce the risk of accidental dislodgement and mechanical phlebitis. No difference in infection rates has been observed between the types of dressing (O'Grady *et al.*, 2002). Transparent dressings have the advantage of allowing the exit site to be observed without removing the dressing. The dressing should be changed if wet or soiled to prevent infection (RCN, 2005a).
6 **A qualified IV competent nurse should flush the cannula with 0.9% saline.**	The cannula should be flushed at least once every 24 hours in order to maintain patency (RCN, 2005a). It should also be flushed before and after the delivery of any medication to ensure the drug is delivered and the line is clear of incompatible fluids.
7 **Reapply bandage if needed and ensure any splint is appropriately positioned.**	Splinting may be necessary if the cannula is situated near to a joint or the child is young (Workman, 1999) to prevent excessive movement of the limb and occlusion of the line. A bandage can reduce the anxiety felt at seeing the cannula and prevent children from attempting to remove the device (Callaghan *et al.*, 2002). However, bandages should be used with caution as they restrict the view of the exit site.
8 **Wash hands/apply alcohol gel.**	To reduce cross-transmission of infection and the incidence of hospital acquired infection.
9 **Record observations on appropriate documentation.**	To ensure effective documentation.

Step-by-step guide to removal of an IV cannula

This is an advanced skill. You *must* check whether you can assist with or undertake any aspect of this skill, in line with local policy.

Step	Rationale
1 Wash hands/apply alcohol gel.	Hand washing reduces the cross-transmission of infection from patient to patient, which reduces the incidence of hospital acquired infection (Pratt *et al.*, 2007).
2 Put on gloves.	To protect the healthcare worker as there is the potential for exposure to blood and other bodily fluids (Pratt *et al.*, 2007).
3 Remove the dressing leaving the cannula *in situ*.	Allows the cannula to be removed freely.
4 Place gauze across the cannula exit site and apply pressure as the cannula is removed. The cannula must be observed to ensure that it is intact.	Applying pressure prevents bleeding and formation of a haematoma (bruise). The cannula must be checked to ensure that no part remains within the patient (Ingram & Lavery, 2007).
5 Dispose of used cannula into a sharps bin (Ingram & Lavery, 2007).	For safety reasons.
6 Apply pressure until bleeding stops.	This prevents formation of a haematoma.
7 Apply a dressing/plaster to the site.	Prevents any leakage of blood before clot is completely formed.
8 Dispose of all equipment and waste in line with organizational guidelines. Clinical waste needs to be disposed of separately to normal household waste.	For safety reasons and to prevent cross infection.
9 Remove and dispose of gloves. Wash hands.	Gloves are for single use only and should be disposed of after each patient contact. They may allow leakage of bacteria even when they appear intact so hands must be decontaminated after their removal (Pratt *et al.*, 2007).
10 Document the time and date of cannula removal in an appropriate place (DH, 2003).	To ensure effective documentation.

(Hickman, Broviac) and implanted ports (portacaths) are for longer term use (months to years) and are often used in children with complex problems, for example, those requiring chemotherapy, long-term parenteral nutrition, or multiple courses of antibiotics (McIntosh, 2003).

Implanted ports are accessed using a specialist Huber needle (these needles are designed to minimize damage to the port hub) (see Figure 9.5). All CVADs should be accessed aseptically to reduce the risk of infection being transmitted into the catheter. Whilst allowing complex treatment to be delivered, CVADs are not used without risk, the greatest risk being that of infection. The use of aseptic or non-touch techniques must be strictly adhered to when handling them.

9.9 **Central line dressing change** Ⓐ

This is an advanced skill. You *must* check whether you can assist with or undertake any aspect of this skill, in line with local policy.

Differences may occur in the way a CVAD is dressed depending on the type of catheter in use; however, the principles are the same. Dressings should be changed weekly or earlier if soiled. Ports that are not accessed do not require a dressing. For children who have an implanted port or a tunnelled CVAD, their families can be taught basic line care in order to reduce the number of hospital or healthcare provider visits.

Procedure: Central line dressing change (see following page)

Preparation

Wash hands/apply alcohol gel to reduce the cross-transmission of infection from patient to patient, which reduces the incidence of hospital acquired infection (Pratt *et al.*, 2007)

Equipment

Collect the equipment for the procedure. As a minimum you will require a container for your antiseptic solution, antiseptic solution, swabs, and dressing.

Consent and communication

Explain the procedure to the child and family, and discuss any concerns. Seek consent.

For children who have a long-term CVAD *in situ*, effective teaching and support needs to be given to the family in order that the devices are safely managed at home (see Box 9.3).

Flushing a central line

It is the role of the registered practitioner who has undergone additional intravenous administration training to

Box 9.3 Supporting children with a long-term CVAD

Teaching and support for the family includes how to reduce the risks of infection, how to recognize signs of infection, and what to do if the catheter becomes dislodged or damaged. With support, families can also be taught how to flush the devices and remove Huber needles from implanted ports. This can have positive benefits for both child and family in that it can reduce the number of visits to hospital, and it has been shown that it may reduce the frequency of the line occluding (Gordon & Dearmun, 2003). In order to be able to safely and effectively manage the CVAD the family must be given all the necessary equipment to take home and be informed where they can obtain further supplies.

flush a CVAD. Parents who have had specific training may also undertake this role when the child is at home. Central lines need to be flushed to ensure patency is maintained. The frequency of flushing will depend on the type of line *in situ* and unit policy. In general implanted ports need flushing once a month (McInally, 2005) when not in use, whilst external catheters need flushing at least once a week. They need to be flushed with both saline and heparin solutions to ensure that blood deposits do not collect within or around the line causing the catheter to become occluded. If the line has multiple lumens each lumen will need to be flushed separately.

9.10 **Cardiopulmonary resuscitation (basic life support)**

Cardiopulmonary arrest in children is predominantly due to hypoxia, with the most likely cardiac rhythm being bradycardia progressing to asystole, unlike the cardiac origin of most adult arrests (Bingham *et al.*, 2005). This means that there are differences in guidance between resuscitation of infants and children and resuscitation of adults. The same principles are followed whether the child has a cardiopulmonary arrest in the community or in hospital.

Step-by-step guide to changing a central line dressing

This is an advanced skill. You *must* check whether you can assist with or undertake any aspect of this skill, in line with local policy.

Step	Rationale
1 Clean a suitable surface area with antiseptic solution. Open equipment onto prepared surface. Fill container with antiseptic solution.	A clean surface is essential to ensure that the dressing change is carried out safely.
2 Remove and dispose of soiled dressing. The soiled dressing and the clean equipment must be kept apart.	To prevent contamination.
3 Wash hands and apply new gloves	To prevent contamination.
4 Observe exit site for signs of infection (including redness, swelling and oozing) or dislodgement (are any sutures still in place, is the catheter secure, is the Huber needle secure in an implanted port?). If infection is suspected take a swab for microscopy, sensitivity, and culture (MC&S).	So that any problems can be addressed.
5 Clean exit site and line according to local policy. There is some evidence to suggest that 2% chlorhexidine is the most effective method of skin decontamination (O'Grady *et al.*, 2002; Pratt *et al.*, 2007).	You must adhere to local policy as there may be some groups of patients where this is not an appropriate solution.
6 Apply sterile dressing and secure the line to prevent it from being pulled or hanging in the nappy area. A specialist skin fix or piece of tape can be used to secure the catheter to the abdomen. Transparent semi-permeable polyurethane (TSP) dressings, such as Tegaderm or Opsite, are preferred to gauze dressings.	Transparent dressings allow the exit site to be observed (O'Grady *et al.*, 2002). If the catheter site is oozing then a gauze dressing will be more appropriate to absorb the fluid.
7 Dispose of equipment according to local policy, remove gloves, and wash hands. Clinical waste needs to be disposed of separately to normal household waste.	To prevent cross infection.
8 Document dressing change in appropriate place.	To ensure effective documentation.

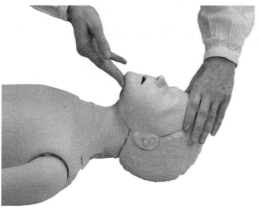
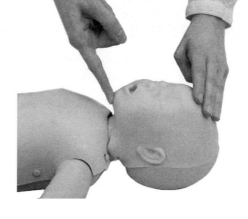

Figure 9.6 Airway position in infant and child

An infant is defined as being less than one year of age and a child between one year and puberty (Bingham *et al.*, 2005). The following guidance is for two rescuers with a duty to respond (including children's

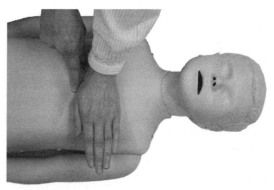

Figure 9.8 Hand position for compressions in a child

Box 9.4 Guidelines for lone rescuer

If you are a lone rescuer then there are some variations from the above guidance.
- If there is no response to the initial shout for help perform one minute's basic life support before going to get help (ILCOR, 2005).
- Single rescuers may choose to follow the adult guidelines (with a ratio of 30 compressions to two breaths) in order to improve the number of compressions. This is especially important if the rescuer is having difficulty moving between ventilation and compressions (Biarent *et al.*, 2005).
- When performing compressions on an infant as a single rescuer it is more effective for moving between breaths and compressions to use two fingers on the sternum instead of the two thumb technique (ILCOR, 2005).

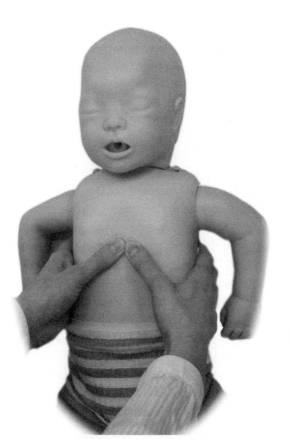

Figure 9.7 Hand position for compressions in an infant

Step-by-step guide to resuscitation of a child

▶ Step	Rationale
1 Ensure safety of rescuer and child.	So the child or rescuer is not exposed to further danger.
2 Gently stimulate and speak loudly to the infant or child: 'Are you alright?' Do not shake.	The aim of stimulating the child is to elicit a response but if this is too vigorous it may result in injury.
3 If the child responds, leave in the position found. Reassess regularly and obtain further help if needed.	If the child is conscious they do not require basic life support.
4 If there is no response shout for help or send a second rescuer to get help. Out of hospital telephone emergency services; in hospital put out a cardiac arrest call.	Emergency services or further help will be required to assist the child wherever the child has collapsed.
5 Airway: open the airway by tilting the head back with one hand on the forehead and the other on the bony point of the chin (head tilt, chin lift).	Placing the fingers on the soft tissues under the chin can obstruct the airway.
6 The head should be in a neutral position for an infant and a 'sniffing' position for a child (see Figure 9.6).	Over-extension of the head or allowing the chin to flop on the chest can obstruct the airway.
7 The jaw thrust is an alternative manoeuvre for opening the airway: place your hands on either side of the child's head. Two or three fingers are placed under the angle of the lower jaw and the jaw is lifted upwards.	This manoeuvre is useful if you have difficulty opening the airway. It also allows opening of the airway with minimal head movement if neck injury is suspected.
8 Look in the mouth for foreign body airway obstruction. Only put your finger in the child's mouth if a foreign body is clearly visible.	'Blind' finger sweeps may cause a foreign body in the mouth to further obstruct the airway.
9 Breathing: assess for breathing by positioning your cheek just above the child's mouth and nose. *Look* for rise and fall of the chest and/or abdomen, *listen* for breath sounds, and *feel* for air movement on your cheek for no longer than ten seconds.	This enables the rescuer to establish if the child is unconscious or is not breathing.
10 If the child is breathing effectively, get help and if there is no suspicion of neck injury place the child in the recovery position.	Although breathing the child is unconscious and requires medical assessment. Placing the child in the recovery position helps keep the airway open and reduces the risk of choking should the child vomit.
11 If the child is not breathing or only breathing infrequently give five rescue breaths.	Most cardiopulmonary arrests in children originate from lack of oxygen, so it is important to breathe for the child.

12 For the infant place your mouth over the infant's nose and mouth. In the child pinch the nose and place your mouth over the child's mouth.

To create a good seal and ensure inflation of the lungs.

13 Each breath should be delivered slowly over 1–1.5 seconds and provide enough volume of air to make the child's chest rise and fall.

Ensures the lungs are inflated and minimizes risk of gastric distension and vomiting.

14 The rescuer should take a breath between each of the five breaths delivered to the child.

Maximizes the amount of oxygen and minimizes the amount of carbon dioxide delivered to the child.

15 Circulation: the healthcare professional should check for a pulse. Feel for the brachial pulse (on the upper inner arm) in an infant and a carotid pulse (on the neck) for a child. Feel for no longer than ten seconds.

This is an important aspect of assessing circulatory status. However, finding a pulse in a collapsed child can be difficult, even for trained healthcare professionals.

16 As well as feeling for a pulse assess for other signs of a circulation, looking for any movement, coughing, or regular breathing.

Results in a more thorough assessment of the child's circulatory status.

17 If you can feel a pulse greater than 60 beats/minute, continue rescue breathing at a rate of 12–20 breaths/minute.

The child has had a respiratory arrest but still has an adequate circulation.

18 If the pulse is fewer than 60 beats/minute (fewer than ten beats in ten seconds) or is absent with no signs of a circulation or you are unsure, start chest compressions.

A heart rate less than 60 is inadequate to support the circulation. It is safer to start compressions in a child that is not breathing even if you are unsure if you can feel a pulse.

19 Landmarks for chest compressions: feel for the point where the ribs join in the middle (**xiphisternum**) and compress the sternum one finger's breadth above this.

To avoid compressions over the stomach or on the xiphisternum.

20 The recommended ratio for infants and children is 15 compressions followed by two breaths. The sternum should be compressed to one third the depth of the chest at a rate of approx. 100/minute, ensuring pressure on the chest is released between each compression.

This method results in more ventilations than the adult guidelines, which is important due to the likely hypoxic cause of the arrest in children.

21 To deliver compressions in an infant the thumbs are used side by side with the hands partially encircling the infant's chest (see Figure 9.7). The second rescuer delivers rescue breaths.

This technique is likely to provide more consistent compressions of the correct depth.

22 In the child the heel of one hand or two hands one on top of the other may be used (see Figure 9.8). Lift the fingers to ensure pressure is not applied over the ribs.

The number of hands used should depend on the size of the child and the rescuer and how much pressure is required to deliver effective compressions.

23 Continue resuscitation until the child shows signs of life, help arrives, or the rescuers become exhausted.

To give the best chance of recovery.

nurses); the guidelines are reviewed every five years and were most recently updated in 2005 by the International Liaison Committee on Resuscitation (ILCOR), European Resuscitation Council (ERC), and Resuscitation Council (UK). Their recommendations have been used as a basis for the procedure that follows. It follows the ABC format useful for the recognition and management of the seriously ill child.

There are slight but important variations in the guidance if there is only a lone rescuer or if the patient being resuscitated is a newborn infant; please see Boxes 9.4 and 9.5.

Box 9.5 Newborn resuscitation

The guidance on resuscitation of a newborn infant is different to that given for older infants and children. Most infants do not require any help to start breathing at delivery; they simply need drying (which also provides stimulation to breathe), keeping warm by wrapping in a towel or blanket, and handing to the mother (Resuscitation Council UK, 2006). However, if following assessment the baby is not breathing, has a slow heart rate (less than 60), and is blue centrally, resuscitation should be commenced.

The Resuscitation Council UK (2006) offer the following guidance on how to achieve this and more detailed information can be obtained from their website or the Neonatal Life Support manual (Richmond, 2006). This guidance applies to both full term and premature neonates.

- Ensure the baby's airway is open and deliver inflation breaths, which need to be at a higher pressure and last for longer (2–3 seconds) than rescue breaths delivered in other circumstances. This is because until the baby has taken its first breath the lungs are filled with fluid and longer breaths delivered at higher pressure are required to clear the fluid.
- Breaths are delivered for 30 seconds, if the chest is moving when the breaths are delivered, but if the baby still does not breathe and the heart rate remains below 60, cardiac compressions should be commenced.
- The landmarks for thumb placement and depth of compression are the same as for an older infant; however, the ratio of compressions to breaths is different. Three compressions to one breath should be performed.
- Check the heart rate after 30 seconds of compressions and if it is above 60 stop compressions and continue ventilating the infant until adequate breathing is achieved or assistance arrives.

A very important aspect of nursing care during resuscitation of an infant or child is care of the family. This is summarized in **Box 9.6**.

Box 9.6 Care of the family

Cardiopulmonary resuscitation of the child is an extremely traumatic experience for the family to witness. Until the last few years parents would have been excluded or strongly discouraged from witnessing attempts to resuscitate their child, but more recently families have been provided with the choice to stay at the bedside (Fulbrook et al., 2007). Such is the change in attitude that the European Resuscitation Council now recommends encouraging parental presence during resuscitation. This allows them to see that everything possible has been done for the child and provides the opportunity to say goodbye should the resuscitation be unsuccessful (Biarent et al., 2005). Therefore parents should be offered the choice to stay during resuscitation, respecting individual preferences.

However, this remains a controversial subject with some nurses and medical staff concerned that performance during resuscitation may be affected by parental presence. Concerns include the possibility that distressed relatives may interrupt the resuscitation, that there may not be enough staff to adequately support the parents, or that they may suffer adverse psychological effects (Fulbrook et al., 2007). However, there is little research evidence to support these concerns and it is an aspect of care where further research and guidance is required.

Conclusion

After reading this chapter you should have an understanding of the complexity of the anatomy and physiology of the cardiovascular system and the vital role it plays in meeting the demands of the body for oxygen and nutrients and removal of waste products. The system matures and develops during foetal life and this continues throughout childhood. Therefore as a nurse caring for children it is essential that you have knowledge of this developmental process and how it influences cardiovascular parameters both in health and illness. Such knowledge will enable you to effectively assess a child's cardiovascular status and allow you to respond appropriately to an identified need ranging from the minor, such as a child requiring venepuncture, to life-threatening, for example imminent circulatory failure.

There are a range of skills required to effectively manage irregularities of cardiovascular function. This chapter has drawn on an evidence base to discuss a number of these skills. These take into consideration a child's age and condition and are examined from a child friendly and family centred perspective. The information contained within this chapter should be utilized in conjunction with other relevant chapters within the book, wider reading, and local policy.

Online resource centre

You may find it helpful to work through our online resources including interactive scenarios intended to help you to develop and apply the skills in this chapter. Where material referenced below is available electronically, we're pleased to provide active web links to the source via **http://www.oxfordtextbooks.co.uk/orc/coyne/**

With thanks to Bruce Holiday for his contribution to the artwork within this chapter.

References

Biarent, D., Bingham, R., Richmond, S., *et al.* (2005) European Resuscitation Council guidelines for resuscitation 2005. Section 6: Paediatric life support. *Resuscitation,* **67S1**, S97–S133.

Bingham, R., Zideman, D., & Simpson, S. (2005) Paediatric basic life support. In A. Handley, (ed.) *Resuscitation Guidelines*. London: Resuscitation Council UK.

British Committee for Standards in Haematology Blood Transfusion Task Force (1999) Guidelines on the administration of blood and blood components and the management of transfused patients. *Transfusion Medicine* **9**, 227–238.

British Hypertension Society (1999) *Blood Pressure Measurement: Recommendations of the British Hypertension Society, 3rd ed.* Available at: **http://www.abdn.ac.uk/medical/bhs/**

Callaghan, S., Copnell, B., & Johnston, L. (2002) Comparison of two methods of peripheral intravenous cannula securement in the pediatric setting. *Journal of Infusion Nursing* **25** (4), 256–264.

Casey, A. (2006) Assessing and planning care in partnership. In A. Glasper & J. Richardson (eds.) *A Textbook of Children's and Young People's Nursing.* London: Elsevier Ltd.

Cavender, K., Goff, M.D., Hollon, E.C., & Guzzetta, C.E. (2004) Parents positioning and distracting children during venepuncture: Effects on children's pain, fear and distress. *Journal of Holistic Nursing* **22** (32), 32–56.

Curley, M. & Maloney-Harmon, P. (2001) *Critical Care Nursing of Infants and Children, 2nd ed.* Philadelphia: W.B. Saunders Company.

Department of Health (2003) Winning ways: Working together to reduce healthcare associated infection in England. London: DH.

Department of Health (2004) *Building a Safer NHS for Patients: Improving medication safety*. London: DH.

Fulbrook, P., Latour, J., & Albarran, J. (2007) Paediatric critical care nurses' attitudes and experiences of parental presence during cardiopulmonary resuscitation: A European survey. *International Journal of Nursing Studies* **44**, 1238–1249.

Gordon, K. & Dearmun, A.K. (2003) Occlusion problems in central venous catheters: The child and family perspective. *Journal of Child Health Care* **7**, 55–69.

Harrop, J.E. (2007) Management of pain in childhood. *Archives of Disease in Childhood, Education and Practice* **92**, 101–108.

Horrox, F. (2002) *Manual of Neonatal and Paediatric Heart Disease*. London: Whurr Publishers.

Idvall, E., & Gunningberg, L. (2006) Evidence for elective replacement of peripheral intravenous catheter to prevent thrombophlebitis: A systematic review. *Journal of Advanced Nursing* **55** (6), 715–722.

Ingram, P., & Lavery, I. (2007) Peripheral intravenous cannulation: Safe insertion and removal technique. *Nursing Standard* **22** (1), 44–48.

International Liaison Committee on Resuscitation (2005) Part 6: Paediatric basic and advanced life support. *Resuscitation* **67**, 271–291.

Lavery, I. & Ingram, P. (2005) Venepuncture: Best practice. *Nursing Standard* **19** (49), 55–65.

Lavery, I. & Smith, E. (2007) Peripheral vascular access devices: Risk prevention and management. *British Journal of Nursing* **16** (22), 1378–1383.

Mackway-Jones, K., Molyneux, E., Phillips, B., & Wieteska, S. (2005) *Advanced Paediatric Life Support, 4th ed.* Oxford: Blackwell Publishing Ltd.

McCance, K. & Heuther, S. (2006) *Pathophysiology: The Biologic Basis for Disease in Adults and Children, 5th ed.* London: Elsevier Mosby.

McClelland, D.B.L. (ed.) (2007) *Handbook of Transfusion Medicine, 4th ed.* London: The Stationery Office.

McInally, W. (2005) Whose line is it anyway? Management of central venous catheters in children. *Paediatric Nursing* **17** (5), 14–18.

McIntosh, N. (2003) Central venous catheters: Reasons for insertion and removal. *Paediatric Nursing* **15** (1), 14–18.

Medicines and Healthcare products Regulatory Agency (2006) *Device Bulletin: Blood Pressure Measurement Devices.* Available at: **http://www.mhra.gov.uk**

Neill, S. & Knowles, H. (eds.) (2004) *The Biology of Child Health.* Hampshire: Palgrave Macmillan.

Novak, B. (2004) Internal transport: Heart and circulation. In S. Neill & H. Knowles (eds.) *The Biology of Child Health.* Hampshire: Palgrave Macmillan.

Nursing and Midwifery Council (2004) *The NMC Code of Professional Conduct: Standards for conduct, performance and ethics.* London: NMC.

Nursing and Midwifery Council (2007a) *Standards for Medicines Management.* London: Nursing and Midwifery Council.

Nursing and Midwifery Council (2007b) *Guidance for the Introduction of the Essential Skills Clusters for Pre-registration Nursing Programmes (Annexe 1 to NMC circular 07/2007).* London: Nursing and Midwifery Council.

O'Brien, E., Asmar, R.. Beilin, L., *et al.* (2003) European Society of Hypertension recommendations for conventional, ambulatory and home blood pressure measurement. *Journal of Hypertension* **21**, 821–848.

O'Grady, N.P., Alexander, M., Dellinger, E.P., *et al.* (2002) Guidelines for the prevention of intravascular catheter-related infections. *Morbidity and Mortality Weekly Report* **51** (RR-10), 1–26.

Oishi, L. (2001) The necessity of routinely replacing peripheral intravenous catheters in hospitalized children. *Journal of Intravenous Nursing* **24** (3), 174–179.

Pratt, R.J., Pellowe, C.M., Wilson, J.A., *et al.* (2007) Epic2: National evidence-based guidelines for preventing healthcare-associated infections in NHS hospitals in England. *Journal of Hospital Infection* **65S**, S1–S64.

Resuscitation Council UK (2006) *European Paediatric Life Support, 2nd ed.* London: Resuscitation Council UK.

Richmond, S. (ed.) (2006) *Newborn Life Support. Resuscitation at Birth, 2nd ed.* London: Resuscitation Council UK.

Royal College of Nursing (2003) *Restraining, holding still and containing children and young people.* London: Royal College of Nursing.

Royal College of Nursing (2005a) *Standards for Infusion Therapy.* London: Royal College of Nursing.

Royal College of Nursing (2005b) *Right Blood, Right Patient, Right Time: RCN guidance for improving transfusion practice.* London: Royal College of Nursing.

Royal College of Nursing (2007) *Standards for Assessing, Measuring and Monitoring Vital Signs in Infants, Children and Young People.* London: Royal College of Nursing.

Scales, K. (2005) Vascular access: A guide to peripheral venous cannulation. *Nursing Standard* **19** (49), 48–52.

Serious Hazards of Transfusion (2005) *Serious Hazards of Transfusion for Children.* Manchester: SHOT.

Serious Hazards of Transfusion (2006) *Annual Report 2006 Summary.* Available at: **http://www.shotuk.org**

Serious Hazards of Transfusion (2007) *Annual Report 2007 Summary.* Available at: **http://www.shotuk.org**

Tortora, G. & Derrickson, B. (2006) *Principles of Anatomy and Physiology, 11th ed.* New Jersey: John Wiley and Sons Inc.

Willock, J., Richardson, J., Brazier, A., Powell, C., & Mitchell, E. (2004) Peripheral venepuncture in infants and children. *Nursing Standard* **18** (27), 43–50.

Workman, B. (1999) Peripheral intravenous therapy management. *Nursing Standard* **14** (4), 53–60.

Further reading and URLs

British Committee for Standards in Haematology Blood Transfusion Task Force (2004) Transfusion guidelines for neonates and older children. *British Journal of Haematology,* **124**, 433–453.

10 Neurological system

COLLEEN O'NEILL AND THERESE NESTOR

Skills

Introduction

This chapter aims to give you knowledge and understanding of the skills required to provide safe and effective care to a child presenting with a neurological disorder. The chapter will focus mainly on the more frequently encountered neurological conditions and procedures both in a hospital and community setting. In addition the importance of family centred care (Chapter Two) and a culturally sensitive approach to care will be discussed.

Learning outcomes

- The rationale for undertaking a neurological assessment and how to carry out a neurological assessment on a child.

- The important elements of care of the child with a **head injury** based on the best practice.
- Key responsibilities of the nurse before, during, and after a **lumbar puncture** procedure.
- Various approaches to neurological imaging and the main principles involved in preparing a child for these.
- The main causes of **seizures** in childhood.
- The main principles involved in caring for a child with a convulsive seizure.
- The nurse's role in caring for an unconscious child.

Background

Good knowledge of national and local polices and guidelines in relation to this area are recommended to compliment learning in this chapter. Furthermore it is essential for students to have a good understanding of the anatomy and physiology of the neurological system when caring for a child with a neurological disorder. A thorough understanding and knowledge of the key structures and functions of the brain will assist in understanding neurological conditions and will help in appreciating the significance and relevance of monitoring neurological status (this section will concentrate mainly on the structure and function of the brain). Nevertheless, it is advisable to revise in more depth the nervous system in your core anatomy and physiology book. Knowledge from other chapters is also advisable in order to understand the interdependence between body systems and the brain.

Anatomy and physiology

The nervous system comprises of three intimately connected parts: the central nervous system; the peripheral nervous system; and the autonomic nervous system.

1 *The central nervous system:* this is composed of the two cerebral hemispheres, the brain stem, the cerebellum, and the spinal cord. The brain and the spinal cord together make up the central nervous system, which communicates with the rest of the body through the peripheral nervous system.

2 *The peripheral nervous system:* this consists of 12 pairs of cranial nerves extending from the cerebrum and brain stem.

3 *The autonomic nervous system:* this regulates the life support systems of the body, without conscious direction. It automatically controls the muscles of the heart, digestive system, and lungs, certain glands, and homeostasis. The autonomic nervous system itself is controlled by nerve centres in the spinal cord and brain stem and is fine-tuned in higher areas in the brain, such as the midbrain and cortex.

Brain development

In contrast to other body tissues, which mostly grow rapidly after birth, the nervous system grows proportionally more rapidly *before* birth. Rapid brain cell growth occurs at weeks 15 to 20 and again at 30 weeks gestation and extends until one year of age (Hockenberry *et al.*, 2003). Cerebral blood flow and oxygen consumption in childhood (up to six years of age) is almost twice that of adults, which reflects an increased metabolic rate consistent with growth and development. This rapid growth during infancy continues during early childhood and then slows down during late childhood and adolescence. In children less than three years of age, rapid brain growth is assisted by the fact that the skull (**cranium**) is not yet fully developed. Normal brain growth can occur quite freely, without being restricted by the skull, as it has flexibility towards expansion. This is because the sections of the skull, which will ultimately merge together to form a solid and complete skull, consist at this point of *unfused sutures*. The **anterior fontanelle**, for example, stays open until around 18 months of age (Trengrove, 2008).

The brain

The brain is the control centre for body movement, sleep, hunger, thirst, and virtually every other vital activity necessary for survival. All human emotions are controlled by the brain. It also receives and interprets the countless signals that are sent to it from other parts of the body and from the external environment. Each section of the brain plays a pivotal role in the regulation and control of body function.

The brain consists of three separate but connected parts: the cerebrum; the cerebellum; and the brain stem (see Figure 10.1).

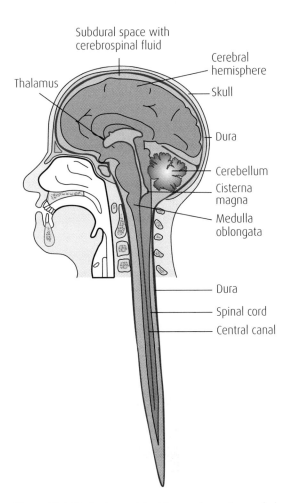

Figure 10.1 The brain consists of the cerebrum, the cerebellum, and the brain stem

- The cerebrum is made up of two distinct hemispheres and is responsible for higher brain functions including thinking and emotions.
- The cerebellum is responsible for control of balance and muscular coordination.
- The brain stem is a central core that gradually becomes the spinal cord and is responsible for basic body functions such as heart beat regulation.

These will now be considered individually.

Cerebrum

Most high-level brain functions take place in the cerebrum. The cerebrum receives information from all the sense organs and sends motor commands (signals that result in activity in the muscles or glands) to other parts of the brain and the rest of the body. The cerebrum is divided into two hemispheres (left and right). The two cerebral hemispheres are partially separated from each other by a deep fold known as the longitudinal fissure. The cerebrum consists of four main regions or lobes: the frontal; parietal; occipital; and temporal lobes (see Figure 10.2).

- *The frontal lobe* is important for the 'higher cognitive functions' and the determination of the personality. Damage to the frontal lobe may cause personality changes, altered intellectual function, and memory and language deficits.
- *The parietal lobe* contains the primary sensory cortex, which controls sensation. Damage to this area may cause language dysfunction, **aphasia**, and **apraxia**.

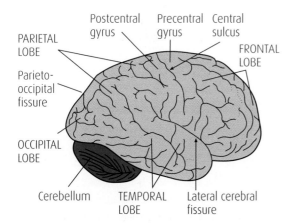

Figure 10.2 The four lobes of the cerebrum

- *The occipital lobe* has responsibility for visual reception; it also contains association areas that help in the visual recognition of shapes and colours. Damage to this lobe can cause visual deficits.
- *The temporal lobe* has responsibility for receiving and interpreting stimuli for taste, vision, sound, and smell. Damage to this lobe may cause inability to interpret meanings of sensory experiences.

Cerebellum

The cerebellum is located at base of the brain, beneath the occipital lobes, and divides into two lateral lobes connected by white fibres known as vermis (see Figure 10.2). Through receipt of instruction from the motor cortex (located in the cerebrum), the cerebellum coordinates voluntary movements. Therefore it has responsibility for the overall coordination of body movements and all motor activity is dependent upon its function. It also has an important role in the maintenance of posture and balance, through sensing the position of the limbs.

Brain stem

The brain stem is a lower extension of the brain and connects the brain to the spinal cord (see Figure 10.1). It is responsible for sustaining the basic functions of life, such as breathing and maintenance of normal blood pressure. It comprises three main structures that lie between and below the two cerebral hemispheres: the medulla oblongata; the midbrain; and the pons.

The medulla oblongata acts principally as a communication centre for the crossing of motor tracts between the spinal cord and the brain. It also contains the respiratory, vasomotor, and cardiac centres, as well as many mechanisms for controlling reflex activities such as coughing, gagging, swallowing, and vomiting.

The topmost structure of the brain stem is the midbrain. It contains major relay stations for neurons transmitting signals to the cerebral cortex, as well as many reflex centres—pathways carrying sensory (input) information and motor (output) commands. Relay and reflex centres for visual and auditory (hearing) functions, as well as relay centres relating to pain, temperature, and touch, are located in the midbrain.

The pons is a bridge-like structure that links different parts of the brain and serves as a relay station from the medulla to the higher cortical structures of the brain. It contains the respiratory centre.

Brain membranes

The brain (beneath the cranium) is covered by three membranes, known as meninges, which afford protection to the brain. The outermost membrane is called the dura mater. Below this lies the middle membrane, known as the arachnoid layer. The innermost membrane, the pia mater, consists mostly of tiny blood vessels and carefully follows the contours of the surface of the brain.

Cerebrospinal fluid

A clear liquid, the cerebrospinal fluid (CSF), bathes the entire brain and fills a series of four cavities, called ventricles, near the centre of the brain. The cerebrospinal fluid protects the internal portion of the brain from varying pressures and transports chemical substances within the nervous system.

From this outline you will see that the brain performs a highly specialized function that determines many essential components of human life. When faced with a child who presents with a potential injury to the brain, nurses in practice perform a range of clinical observations aimed at contributing to the overall assessment, diagnosis, and prevention of brain injury. While the usual physical assessment and clinical observations that are performed on a child receiving healthcare are outlined in Chapter Five, specific observations are also performed that are aimed at determining the child's level of consciousness.

10.1 **Assessment of level of consciousness**

Assessment of level of consciousness (LOC) is the most significant indicator of a patient's brain function. It can assist in determining improvement or deterioration in a patient's neurological status (Fergusson, 2008). Impaired level of consciousness may be due to a specific disease, for example **encephalitis**, or injury to the brain such as a head injury. Neurological observations assist in the assessment of brain function through the use of a structured neurological assessment tool or coma scale.

Coma scales

A coma scale is a standard means by which neurological observations can be assessed and recorded. These scales were initially developed to help to standardize health professionals' assessment of patients with altered levels of consciousness, within and across institutions. The Glasgow Coma Scale (GSC) is one of the most commonly used coma scales and its use is recommended by the National Institute for Health and Clinical Excellence (NICE, 2007), particularly for head injury patients.

The scale was published in 1974 by Graham Teasdale and Bryan Jennett from the neurosurgery department at the University of Glasgow (Teasdale & Jennett, 1974). This scale permits assessment of a patient (child or adult) against predetermined criteria. The resulting responses, from observation by the nurse, give rise to a numerical score that identifies the person's Glasgow Coma Score (or GCS). However, while the GCS works well for children over the age of five years, it has been found to be less responsive to those less than five. It is therefore not suitable for younger children and infants as they are unable to respond to directions or to fully verbalize. As a result of this the scale was further modified, to increase its sensitivity. The version thus used for children is known as the Paediatric Glasgow Coma Scale (PGCS).

The layout and appearance of the PGCS will vary depending on the healthcare institute in which you work. However, regardless of the layout the scale will comprise of three basic assessments or tests: that of eye, verbal, and motor responses. The three values separately, as well as their sum, are considered. The score is taken as an indicator of the child's neurological state. The maximum score is 15, indicating that the child is responsive and alert, i.e. fully awake or easy to wake if asleep. The lowest possible PGCS (the sum) is three, indicating a deep coma (Waterhouse, 2005). Thus lower PGCS scores are reflective of increased condition severity. Whilst 15 is the maximum score, the sensitivity of the scale warrants that once the score drops below 12, the child needs to be very closely monitored, in terms of frequent PGCS calculations and other clinical observation (NICE, 2007). This will alert staff in a timely fashion to either recovery or worsening of the condition, and ensure timely intervention. Once this score drops below 8, vital functions are severely compromised and would most likely require mechanical support with respiration, such as intubation and ventilation (NICE, 2007). A range of different staff may be involved in monitoring the PGCS, but for consistency of observation and recording it is advisable, where possible, for one single nurse to take responsibility for this. At change of shift, this nurse may then pass information about techniques and observations to the next nurse, perhaps performing the PGCS assessment together. This way subtle observations, for example of pupil size, may be discussed, to gain consensus on approach, ensure accuracy of assessment, and reduce the potential for discrepancy among staff (Warren, 2006).

Eye opening

Eye opening contained within the assessment is designed to assess level of arousal within the brain stem. Eye opening response is appraised within the scale in accordance with four criteria. It is ascertained whether or not a child opens their eyes spontaneously, to voice, to pain, or not at all. If spontaneous eye opening does not occur as you approach the child, then proceed by assessing the child's reaction to speech. It is good practice to involve the parents with this assessment, if appropriate, as the child may respond quicker to a parent's voice. A painful stimulus may be necessary to determine the child's ability to open their eyes. **Table 10.1** outlines methods of applying painful stimulus in children.

> **Nursing Alert**
>
> It must be noted that swollen eyes may not open and this does not necessarily indicate a fall in consciousness. Eyes closed due to swelling should be documented in the Glasgow coma scale by using the letter C (Waterhouse, 2005).

Verbal response

Verbal response evaluates the child's orientation as well their ability to communicate and recall. Verbal response may be evaluated by asking questions. An adult or older child who is awake should be able to state their name, the current year, and the month (Waterhouse, 2005). However, younger children may not have the ability to respond in this way; therefore the PGCS adapted its assessment to meet the needs of preverbal children. A grimace response, for example, may also be used to assess verbal response (NICE, 2007). Verbal response is further categorized according to its presentation, as follows.

In children under the age of five years, their verbal response may be described as any of the following:

- Babbles, coos, words, or sentences to usual ability.
- Less than usual ability, irritable cry.
- Cries to pain.
- Moans to pain.
- No response to pain.

In those aged five years or over it is described as follows:

- Orientated, alert.
- Confused.
- Inappropriate words.
- Incomprehensible sounds.
- No response to pain.

When assessing verbal response it must be remembered that simply because a child does not speak does not always indicate an alteration in consciousness. Developmentally the child may not speak and their responses may be described as outlined above. The child who is verbal may also choose not to speak, or may perhaps be traumatized or frightened. A full assessment of the ability to speak needs to be carried out, in consultation with the family, and indeed the parents/guardians can assist in assessing the child's ability to respond to questions asked (the response may be assessed in relation to the child's response to parents' verbalizations rather than the nurse's in this case). This is in keeping with contemporary approaches to family centred care, about which a more complete discussion takes place in Chapter Two.

Other situations that may prove challenging for assessment are where the child's first language may not be English. Similarly, if the parents do not speak English, the child's lack of understanding is further compounded. In these cases the services of an interpreter may be required, to ensure evaluation of the child's verbal response is correct. However, interpreters may not always be available in the service where you are working, and it may be useful to have a range of simple phrases available for use, in commonly presenting languages. Extended family may also be useful in this regard.

The presence of interpreters within the healthcare situation will depend on a variety of factors including need. In the United States, for example, it is common for interpreters to be employed to translate for Spanish-speaking patients whose first language is not English. Even where facilities are in place, it may not always be possible to match the specific language required in each case, although many interpreters will have a range of languages. Emergency situations also prove difficult, particularly out of normal office hours, when increased time will be required to avail of such services. In any case, if an interpreter is available to the team, it is important to work closely with them to establish child and family needs in this regard (do not assume you know the language requirement simply because of country of origin, as several countries have various languages and language dialects). You also need to assist the interpreter to build up relationships with the family and child, by introducing them, and accompanying them in their task. This will assist in ascertaining the maximum response from the child.

There are other special situations where verbal response assessment of a child's neurological status may be inhibited. For example, a child's treatment may require the insertion of an endotracheal or tracheostomy tube, thus rendering verbal response difficult to measure. In these cases specific guidelines for assessment may be developed within the multidisciplinary team.

Motor response

The brain is capable of converting sensory information input into a proper motor response. However, if there is damage to the area of the brain responsible for motor activity then this may be reflected in a child's ability to respond to a motor command or to pain. To properly assess motor response it is advisable to ask the child to obey at least two different commands. Results from the assessment of motor responses within the PGCS may be categorized in children as follows.

For those children less than five years old, their motor response may be described as any of the following:
- Normal, spontaneous movements.
- Localizes to pain or withdraws from touch.
- Withdraws from pain.
- Abnormal flexion to pain (decorticate).

- Abnormal extension to pain (decerebrate).
- No response to pain.

For those children more than five years old, their motor response may be described as any of the following:
- Obeys commands.
- Localizes to pain.
- Withdraws from pain.
- Abnormal flexion to pain (decorticate).
- Abnormal extension to pain (decerebrate).
- No response to pain.

Pupillary activity

Assessing the reaction of the pupils to light is another significant element of neurological assessment. In this part of the neurological observation, the nurse notes the size, shape, equality, and reaction of pupils to light in both eyes. Under normal circumstances both pupils should constrict quickly and equally to light. However, if there is damage to the brain through disease or injury then pupils may not react as normal, and may be dilated. An alteration in pupil size and response to light could indicate a raise in **intracranial pressure** and compression of the cranial nerve that controls pupil constriction (Waterhouse, 2005). It is vital that any change is documented and reported immediately to the doctor.

Painful stimuli

Applying a painful stimulus and observing the response is used to assess a patient's ability to respond to pain. The reaction permits indirect assessment of the brain's ability to recognize pain and deal with pain (Waterhouse, 2005). Traditionally small amounts of painful stimulus have been applied to patients during neurological assessment, to elicit the body's response. **Table 10.1** outlines the various methods of painful stimulus application in children and provides a brief outline of the usual techniques used.

Nursing Alert

It must be noted, however, that the trapezius squeeze (**Table 10.1**) should not be used as a method of applying a painful stimulus in children under the age of five, because the trapezius muscle is not fully developed (Waterhouse, 2005).

Table 10.1 Main methods of applying a painful stimulus in children

Method	Technique
Supraorbital ridge pressure	Place pressure on the notch or groove in the bony ridge along the top of the eye. This approach is reserved for children who are in a deep coma and should only be practised by highly skilled trained practitioners (Waterhouse, 2005).
Trapezius squeeze	Pinch the muscle at the side of the neck (trapezius muscle).
Sternal rub/pressure	Apply pressure with the knuckles of a clenched fist over the sternum.
Side finger pressure	Place a pencil to the side of a finger near the tip and apply gentle pressure. However, this technique may achieve a spinal rather than a central response (Fergusson, 2008).

Of course painful stimuli should be used judiciously, using minimal pressure to elicit a response in the first instance. This can be slowly increased in intensity, to last a maximum of 30 seconds (Trengrove, 2008) after which time the stimulus should be stopped (Edwards, 2001). It is very important that care is taken not to mark or bruise the child's skin when applying a painful stimulus, and this should be prevented if the recommended sites are utilized (**Table 10.1**) using the minimal pressure, for a short period of time. It is also important that local hospital and community guidelines on this issue are used in the first instance. As with restraint (Chapter Five), there is controversy surrounding the use of painful stimuli in children. Therefore in some cases, rather than utilizing the full GCS, the child's response to pain is not assessed if the verbal responses are within acceptable limits. You need to seek advice from your local policies to guide you in this area. As a student, you first need to seek advice from your mentor or preceptor before attempting painful stimulus or other neurological assessments. If response to painful stimulus is used as an assessment method, and the child does not appear to have any response, this may be a sign of severe neurological damage and the medical team needs to be informed immediately.

Nursing Alert

If response to painful stimulus is used as an assessment method, and the child does not appear to have any response, this may be a sign of severe neurological damage and the medical team needs to be informed immediately.

Limb movement

Assessment of limb movement is a component of the neurological assessment aimed at determining the patient's mobility. Damage to the motor nervous system will affect movement, and thus assessment of limb movement is an indirect way of measuring brain, and in particular motor, function. Brain lesion or raised intracranial pressure can cause weakening of the limbs. Each limb is assessed separately to determine muscle strength, tone, coordination, and reflexes.

Posturing

The presence of body movements known as *posturing*, particularly decerebrate and decorticate posturing, is considered abnormal and indicates severe cerebral dysfunction (Advanced Life Support Group, 2005). Decerebrate posturing is characterized by rigid extension of the arms and legs (**see Figure 10.3**), while decorticate posturing involves flexion of the arms on the chest with wrists and hands also flexed and the lower extremities extended (**see Figure 10.4**).

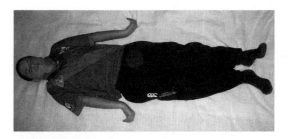

Figure 10.3 Decerebrate posturing

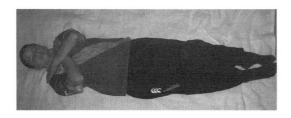

Figure 10.4 Decorticate posturing

Vital signs

Measurement of vital signs is an important element of neurological assessment. Clinical assessments and observations that are commonly referred to as vital signs include the monitoring and recording of respirations, temperature, pulse, blood pressure, and oxygen saturations. These are outlined in more detail in Chapter Five. Of particular concern in relation to neurological status are the rate, character, and pattern of a child's respirations, as respiratory function is controlled by the brain, and brain damage may result in altered respiratory patterns or indeed cessation of respiration. The measurement of both blood pressure and pulse also provides important evidence of a potential rise in intracranial pressure (observed by a reducing pulse and rising blood pressure). Body temperature is also a crucial observation to record and monitor, as children with brain injury may suffer fluctuating temperatures, indicating damage to the hypothalamus. Any such patterns need to be reported to senior staff (Fergusson, 2008).

Procedure: Neurological assessment

Equipment

Gather the necessary equipment prior to undertaking a neurological assessment:

- Pen torch.
- Thermometer.
- Blood pressure monitor.
- Oxygen saturation monitor.
- Neurological observation chart.

Assessment

Undertake a through assessment of the child including a detailed history of the child's health and developmental history. This will determine the child's normal abilities and any underlying condition that may affect the child's response. This can be achieved by consulting with the child (if capable) and parents.

Consent and communication

Explain to the parents, in clear terms, what is involved in a neurological assessment to ensure they understand the assessment and its importance. Encourage the parents to take an active part in the assessment, as a child is more likely to respond to or obey a command given by a parent than by a healthcare professional, and this also promotes family involvement. Explain the assessment to the child in a manner appropriate to the child's age and developmental level to reduce the child's anxiety and gain their cooperation. Essential skills clusters (Nursing and Midwifery Council (NMC), 2007) recommend that information provided to patients is clear, accurate, and meaningful at a level the patient can understand.

Other factors: Community perspective

In the community, during emergency situations, rapid assessment of neurological status may be necessary to determine the seriousness of a child's condition or injury. The AVPU responsiveness scale may be more appropriate to use in urgent situations as an alternative to the PGCS, as it allows for an immediate and rapid assessment of a child's neurological state. The AVPU scale consists of four basic categories that aid rapid assessment. The child is assigned to a category, depending on the child's response (Trengove, 2008). The four categories are **A**: Alert; **V**: Responds only to voice; **P**: Responds only to pain; or **U**: Unresponsive to all stimuli. These latter classifications have a relationship to GCS scores, although the direct correspondence between the AVPU scale (i.e. A, P, V, or U) and the GCS (0–15) has not been clearly determined (Kelly *et al.*, 2004). Kelly *et al.* (2004) identified the relationship between the AVPU scale and the median scores of the GCS as follows: A = GCS 15; V = GCS 13; P = GCS 8; and U = GCS 3. There is a suggestion that a classification of U indicates a GCS of less than eight and requires immediate medical attention, as intubation may be required to maintain an open airway (Advanced Life Support Group, 2005).

Step-by-step guide to neurological assessment

Step	Rationale
1 *Eye opening*: Assess child's eye opening ability. If child's eyes do not open spontaneously on approaching the child, ask the parent to call the child's name gently initially, and if no response increase tone and volume of voice.	To assess the child's level of arousal.
2 *Verbal response*: Talk to the child and ask child specific questions in relation to time/place/person appropriate to his/her age and developmental level.	To establish whether the child's level of consciousness is deteriorating. If the child is becoming disorientated, changes may occur in orientation to time/place/person.
3 In the preverbal child, score against his/her normal vocal ability or grimace response.	To determine any change in child's normal verbal response.
4 *Motor response*: Ask the child to perform two activities, for example, ask the child to squeeze and release your fingers and then to stick out their tongue.	To evaluate motor responses.
5 In younger children who may not be able to follow commands, observe spontaneous movements.	To allow for assessment of motor responses in younger children.
6 If the patient does not respond, apply painful stimuli.	Reponses grow less purposeful as the child's level of consciousness deteriorates.
7 Explain what is involved in applying a painful stimulus and why it is necessary to both child and parents/guardians.	To prepare child and parents for the procedure as well as to gain consent from the parents/guardians.
8 Before applying a painful stimulus, try to arouse child by softly shaking the child.	To verify child is in a deeper level of unconsciousness so as to avoid unnecessary pain and distress to the child.
9 Apply chosen painful stimulus once parental consent is given and document child's response to painful stimulus. Choose the most appropriate stimulus for the individual child depending on the condition of the child.	To allow early detection of deterioration in child's condition.
10 *Pupil reaction*: Darken the room and reduce overhead lightening before assessing pupil reaction.	To ensure optimal environment for assessment of pupils.
11 Wash hands prior to assessing pupil reactions as you will need to make contact with the child's eyes.	To prevent cross infection.
12 Hold the eyelids open and note the size, shape, and equality of the pupils.	To assess the size, shape, and equality of the pupils, as changes may be an indication of brain damage.

13	Hold each eyelid open in turn. Move torch from the outer aspect towards the centre of the eye. Shine light directly into the eye. This should constrict the pupil immediately.	To assess the reaction of the pupils to light. A slow reaction may indicate damage to the area of the brain stem that regulates pupil constriction.
14	*Limb movement*: Assess each of the four limbs separately.	To identify level of strength in each limb.
15	Flex and extend all the child's limbs. Note how well the movements are resisted.	To test muscle tone.
16	Ask the child to lift his or her arms straight out in front, with palms upwards, for 20 to 30 seconds with their eyes closed.	The weaker limb will fall away; this demonstrates weakness in that limb.
17	Stand in front of the child and extend your hands. Ask the child to push and pull against your hands.	To test arm strength.
18	Ask the child to raise each leg off the bed and push or pull their feet towards your hand.	To test flexion and extension strength in child's leg by having the child push and pull against your resistance.
19	*Physiological signs*: Monitor the rate and pattern of child's respirations and oxygen saturation levels.	Respirations are controlled by different areas of the brain. When disease or injury occurs in these areas it may cause respiratory changes.
20	Record child's temperature.	Changes in child's temperature may indicate damage to hypothalamus, the temperature-regulating centre in the brain.
21	Monitor child's blood pressure and pulse rate and note any irregularities in pulse.	Physiological changes may indicate increased intracranial pressure.
22	*Frequency of assessment*: Neurological assessment should be continued until a GCS score of 15 is achieved and the child's condition improves. GCS scores below 15 should be assessed on a half-hourly basis until the score is 15. Once this score is achieved, neurological observations should continue every half-hour for two hours, then hourly for four hours and then two-hourly thereafter. Any decline in the score indicates a need to revert to half-hourly observations and should be reported to the medical team immediately (NICE, 2007).	So that changes in the child's condition are appropriately monitored. Allows for quick intervention if necessary.
23	Document precisely what is being observed on the neurological assessment chart. Ensure the assessment chart used is the correct chart for the age of the child.	It is important that nursing staff record and document precisely what is being observed. They should avoid comparing and being influenced by a previous set of observations as changes to the patient's condition can be rapid and may require an immediate response (Dawes *et al.*, 2007).
24	Report any changes in child's neurological assessment immediately to a senior medical doctor.	Allows for prompt medical assessment and intervention if required.

Both the AVPU and the PGCS are used to assess neurological status. There are many causes of neurological dysfunction. A common cause, head injury, is one that you may see in practice.

10.2 **Head injury**

Head injury is defined as any trauma to the head and may involve the scalp, the cranium, the brain, or its protective membranes. Head injury is the most common of childhood injuries and a major cause of death and disability, with 5% being fatal and 20% having long-term disabilities related to the injury (Hogan *et al.*, 2007). As the head of an infant or toddler is significantly larger and more weighty in relation to other body parts, it is particularly vulnerable to injuries (Hockenberry *et al.*, 2003). A head injury is something that you may come across in the community setting, and the immediate care of this condition is now considered.

Community perspective: Emergency care of a head injury patient

It is important, in the presence of a suspected head injury in a child, that the child's airway, breathing, and circulation (if possible) are attended to before attention is given to other injuries. Adequate function of these is vital to life, as reduced air supply and circulatory difficulty may have serious consequences (as outlined in Chapters Eight and Nine). It is important to assess and stabilize circulatory and respiratory function in the first instance. If a child has suffered a severe head injury, spinal damage must be suspected. In such cases, the child should be kept firmly in a position that fully immobilizes the spine until full assessment and imaging can rule out spinal damage (NICE, 2007). Manual immobilization must be maintained by placing the child's head in alignment with the spine.

Failure to immobilize the spine in this way could lead to severe secondary injuries such as permanent paralysis or even death. It is important to maintain constant manual immobilization in this way until emergency services arrive with appropriate equipment such as a spinal board. During this time the child's level of consciousness is assessed regularly using the AVUP (alert, verbal, painful,

unresponsive) system, as it can provide a rapid evaluation to determine the need for airway protection. However, a full regular assessment using the Glasgow coma scale will still be required (Scottish Intercollegiate Guidelines Network (SIGN), 2000). You will need to assess for any signs of nausea, vomiting, or presence of headache or pain. Health professionals who are providing initial care for these patients in the community should refer any child who has sustained a head injury to the local Accident and Emergency department immediately for a thorough assessment (NICE, 2007). They should also alert the hospital facility in advance of the child's condition and volunteer all necessary information prior to the child's arrival. This ensures that appropriately experienced professionals are available to treat the patient, and that care required may be anticipated in advance (NICE, 2007).

In these situations the child is not permitted to eat or drink, at least until arrival and assessment at the emergency department. It is also suggested that analgesia (Chapter Six) is not given at this time as it can mask signs of deterioration in the child (Hockenberry *et al.*, 2003).

Nursing care

Once a child arrives in a hospital setting it is important that a detailed health history and events surrounding the head injury are obtained. For children with head injuries it is important to make a holistic and systematic assessment of the child's core nursing care issues and develop a comprehensive plan of care that is in the best interests of the child and that promotes their health and well-being (NMC, 2007). Information relating to any symptoms following a head injury, such as any loss of consciousness, length of **unconsciousness**, any vomiting or nausea, blurring of vision, or headache, must be established. Accurate neurological assessment, including the use of the PGCS, and understanding the significance of the findings is an important aspect of caring for a child with a head injury. The SIGN (2000) recommend that all medical and nursing staff involved in the care of head injured patients should be trained in the use and recording of the Glasgow Coma Scale. Regular nursing and neurological assessment can provide information needed to establish an accurate diagnosis, detect signs and symptoms of increased intracranial pressure, assist in determining treatment options, and prevent complications (Hockenberry *et al.*, 2003).

The other key responsibilities of the nurse involve: maintaining adequate respiratory function and circulation; monitoring for signs of increased intracranial pressure; and supporting the child and family during the recovery phase. The child's nutritional needs need to be addressed within the hospital setting, and enteral feeding may need to be commenced, depending on the severity of the condition (see Chapter Twelve). If the child is not able to eat in the normal way, enteral feeding should be initiated as soon as possible to ensure nutritional requirements are met. Commencement of early enteral nutrition is associated with better patient survival and outcome (Härtl *et al.*, 2008). In any patient with a head injury a nasogastric tube should be avoided to prevent accidental passage of the tube into the brain via a base of skull fracture. An orogastric tube is used as an alternative (Greaves *et al.*, 2001). It is also an important nursing activity to observe for potential complications for a head injury.

Procedure: Nursing assessment of a child with a head injury

Preparation

This often presents as an emergency so there can be little or no time to prepare. The equipment needed to assess vital signs should be within reach.

Other factors to consider

Complications

Head injury can often lead to complications, which the nurse must carefully monitor for. Box 10.1 outlines these.

Box 10.1 Potential complications of a head injury

- Haemorrhage:
  - sub-dural haemorrhage
  - extra-dural haemorrhage
  - intra-cerebral haemorrhage.
- **Cerebral oedema**, which may cause an increase in intracranial pressure.
- Seizures.
- Risk of infection.

Nursing Alert

- Any child who complains of headache, nausea, or vomiting and demonstrates a decrease in conscious level should be reviewed by a doctor immediately, as this child may be developing raised intracranial pressure.

- Decreased heart rate and high blood pressure accompanied by respiratory depression (also referred to as Cushing's triad) is a late sign of brain damage and should be reported to the medical team without delay.

Discharge advice

Recovering from a head injury can be a long process. Ensure the child and parents are aware of the possibility of delayed complications and disabilities. It is important that advice is given well in advance of the date of discharge, to allow child and parents time to ask questions and for information to be absorbed. For patients and families who do not speak English, utilize an interpreter to assist in the communication process (NICE, 2007). All patients should receive verbal advice and a written head injury advice leaflet before discharge; leaflets should be available in a number of different languages. Discharge information and leaflets should include details of services parents could contact should their child experience any long-term problems.

10.3 **Lumbar puncture**

This is an advanced skill. You *must* check whether you can assist with or undertake any aspect of this skill, in line with local policy.

Definition

The term lumbar puncture (LP) refers to a clinical procedure in which a needle is introduced into the subarachnoid space in the spinal canal. It is performed for the purpose of aspirating cerebrospinal fluid (CSF) or to measure CSF pressure. Lumbar puncture is primarily indicated for the evaluation and diagnosis of patients who present with symptoms consistent with **meningitis**, **meningoencephalitis**, and

Step-by-step guide to assessment of a head injury

Step

Rationale

Step	Rationale
1 Assess child's airway, breathing, circulation.	In emergency situations airway, breathing, and circulation need to be assessed to establish priority of care.
2 Assess for altered levels of consciousness. Assess for any loss of consciousness and determine length of time child was unconscious for.	Neurological assessment using a neurological assessment chart such as Glasgow Coma Scale must be carried out on all head injury patients. Neurological assessment assists in evaluating the seriousness of a head injury.
3 Assess for signs of shock such as irritability, increase in heart rate, pallor, and decrease in urinary output.	Shock is a likely complication following a head injury and early detection and treatment is vital, as shock can be life-threatening if left untreated.
4 Perform a general assessment of the child. Observe for obvious physical signs of head injury and for other related injuries.	Head injuries are often accompanied by other injuries such as spinal injuries and injuries to the skin and extremities. It is important that such injuries are identified so that they can be treated accordingly.
5 Assess vital signs such as patient's heart rate, blood pressure, temperature, respiratory rate and rhythm, and oxygen saturation.	This provides a baseline for future observations, ensures early detection of deterioration in patient's condition, and allows for early identification of complications.
6 Temperature should be recorded every four hours or more frequently if condition indicates.	To assist in the detection of infection and possible hypothermia. Changes in child's temperature may indicate damage to hypothalamus.
7 Assess for signs of raised intracranial pressure (ICP), for example hypertension, bradycardia, and changes in respiratory rate.	Raised ICP is a complication of head injury and early detection is vital so that prompt treatment can be initiated.
8 Assess for any episodes of nausea and vomiting.	One or more episodes of vomiting may be an early indication of deterioration after a head injury.
9 Observe and assess for unusual behaviour. Interpret unusual behaviour with parental assistance and in relation to the child's normal behaviour.	A change in a child's normal manner may indicate damage to the area of the brain that controls personality and behaviour.
10 Observe and assess for seizure activity. Assess for type of seizure, duration of seizure, limbs affected.	Seizures are a potential complication of head injury.
11 Assess for drainage from nose or ears. Note the amount and characteristics of any drainage.	Bleeding from the nose or ears may indicate a possible basal skull fracture.
12 Assess child's level of pain using a pain assessment tool and assess for signs of a headache.	A child may complain of headache or pain following a head injury. Using a pain assessment tool will assist in determining the severity of pain.

13	Assess child's position and movement.	Any abnormal posturing may indicate severe cerebral damage and an interruption of nerve pathways from the brain's cortex to the spine.
14	Document all findings following assessment of the patient.	To ensure accurate records of assessment are maintained.

subarachnoid haemorrhage. It may also be used to administer intra-thecal chemotherapy (Farley & McLafferty, 2008). Lumbar puncture should only be performed if there are no contraindications. If a child or infant is too acutely ill, or has an increase in intracranial pressure, then the procedure should be delayed until they are in a stable condition as there is a risk of cerebral herniation (Hough & Gekas, 2008).

Procedure: Lumbar puncture

Preparation

The older child should empty his/her bladder to avoid accidental incontinence during the procedure. At one hour before the procedure, apply topical local anaesthetic cream to the child's back around the area of L4–L5 where LP is normally performed (in the interspaces between the lumbar vertebrae). This local anaesthetic helps to numb the area prior to procedure. Prepare the sterile field using aseptic technique to maintain effective standard infection control precautions as recommended in essential skills clusters (NMC, 2007).

> **Nursing Alert**
>
> Apply prescribed topical anaesthetic cream (usually Emla or Ametop cream) *at least an hour* prior to the procedure and remove after one hour. Emla needs to be applied at least one hour before the procedure and Ametop requires at least 45 minutes to be effective (British National Formulary, 2008).

Equipment

- Pre-packaged LP pack.
- Three sterile specimen bottles.
- Betadine solution.
- Sterile gloves.
- Spinal needle—a 22 gauge needle is typically used for children.
- Opsite spray.
- Sterile dry dressing, for example Mepore Dressing.

Assessment

Perform a thorough assessment of the child/infant, particularly their vital signs and neurological status, prior to the procedure to provide a baseline for future observations. Assess degree of cooperation of the child to remain in position without excessive movement. Cooperation is necessary if possible as movement can cause injury from the spinal needle.

Consent and communication

Assess parents' and child's knowledge of the procedure and reinforce explanation as appropriate. The child and parents should be fully informed of the nature of the procedure, including the risks and benefits; this will help to reduce fear of the unknown and promote cooperation (Farley & McLafferty, 2008). Informed consent should be obtained from the child's parent/guardian prior to the procedure by the person performing the procedure (Department of Health, 2001).

> **Nursing Alert**
>
> Where there are three failed attempts at the lumbar puncture procedure, the nurse has a professional responsibility to ensure that the performing doctor ceases and seeks assistance from another doctor before making another attempt.

Step-by-step guide to lumbar puncture

This is an advanced skill. You *must* check whether you can assist with or undertake any aspect of this skill, in line with local policy.

Step	Rationale
1 **Double check vital signs and neurological status have been assessed.**	Provides baseline data for comparison with post-procedural measurements.
2 **Ensure that the prescribed topical anaesthetic cream has been applied to the child's back around the area of L4–L5 an hour before the procedure.**	LP is performed in the interspaces between the lumbar vertebrae, usually at the L4–L5 level. The application of a local anaesthetic helps to numb the area prior to procedure—Elma needs to be applied at least one hour before the procedure and Ametop requires at least 45 minutes to be effective (British National Formulary, 2008).
3 **Ensure the sterile field has been prepared.**	To prevent infection and maintain effective standard infection control precautions.
4 **Assist child into required position exposing the lumbar region (see Figure 10.5). Maintain child in the lateral position (foetal) with their back arched to the edge of examination table. A pillow may be placed under the head and between the knees of an older child.**	Complete control of the child is imperative for the safety and success of this procedure.
5 **Clean the skin covering the lower region of the back with an antibacterial solution and alcohol. Drape the child beneath their flank and over the back with the spine accessible to view.**	To prevent spread of infection.
6 **Observe the child throughout the procedure.**	Respiratory and circulatory impairment can occur through over-flexion of the neck.
7 **Have specimen tubes ready and clearly numbered 1, 2, and 3. Collect 8 to 10 drops of CSF in each tube.**	The first sample is collected for glucose and protein, the second sample for Gram stain and culture and sensitivity (C&S), and the third sample is for cell count and differential.
8 **After the sample is collected, the needle is withdrawn and a bandage is placed on the site. Observe for any leakage of fluid or blood from wound site.**	May indicate CSF leakage post-lumbar puncture.

9 Monitor and record patient's neurological status, level of consciousness, temperature, blood pressure, pulse, and respirations post-lumbar puncture.	Frequent observation ensures early detection of deterioration in patient's condition and allows for early identification of complications.
10 Encourage the patient, if able, to lie prone for 3–4 hours.	To prevent leakage and headache. Prophylactic bed rest is common practice post-lumbar puncture, despite some evidence that bed rest is of no benefit and prolonged bed rest is ineffective in preventing headache (Ebinger *et al.*, 2004; Thoennissen *et al.*, 2001). Nevertheless it continues to be widespread practice in most healthcare institutes; therefore it is important to refer to local hospital guidelines in relation to this practice.
11 Encourage child to drink as much fluid as possible for the first 24 hours after the procedure.	This can help decrease the likelihood of a headache afterwards.
12 Documentation should be carried out as soon as possible after providing care. Document the procedure appropriately including details of: a. Specimens sent to laboratory. b. Condition and reaction of child.	To ensure accurate record of procedure has been maintained. Documentation of any procedure is vital to ensure an accurate record of what has occurred (NMC, 2005; An Bord Altranais, 2002).

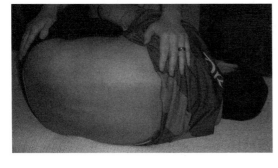

Figure 10.5 Position for lumbar puncture

After the procedure

Nursing Alert

A minimum of one set of neurological observations should be carried out post-procedure. Thereafter neurological observations should be carried out as the child's condition indicates.

Consideration

List some of the nursing priorities that need to be considered before, during, and after a lumbar puncture.

10.4 **Preparing the child for neuro-imaging (X-ray, CT, MRI)**

Diagnostic tests are a valuable adjunct to the treatment regimen in children with neurological conditions and provide essential information about the child's neurological state. Neuro-imaging can vary from a simple X-ray to more complex detailed imaging such as a CT (computed tomography) scan and MRI (magnetic resonance imaging). **Figure 10.6** illustrates an MRI scanning machine.

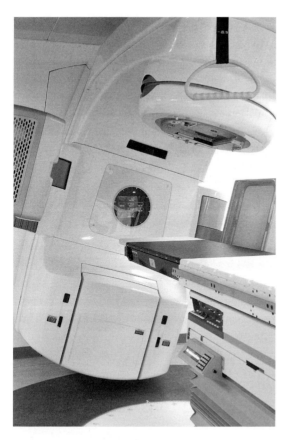

Figure 10.6 MRI machine
© Elgaard-Fotolia.com

Box 10.2 Types of neuro-imaging performed in children

X-ray

An X-ray is a high-energy electromagnetic wave capable of penetrating solid matter and acting on photographic film. X-ray films are commonly ordered in a child with a neurological condition to determine the size, shape, and functioning of the brain.

Computed tomography

A computed tomography or CT scan is a non-invasive X-ray procedure. It is a method by which a body part such as the brain can be scanned from different angles with an X-ray beam and a computer that calculates varying tissue densities and records a cross-sectional image on paper.

Magnetic resonance imaging

Magnetic resonance imaging (MRI) is an advanced scanning technique that uses magnetism and radiofrequency waves to produce cross-sectional images of body tissues on a computer screen. This diagnostic tool can provide unique information about the chemical makeup of tissues *without* the risks associated with radiation.

Cranial ultrasound

This is a non-invasive test that is primarily performed to detect intraventricular haemorrhage (IVH) in infants.

The nurse assumes a variety of roles and responsibilities when a child requires neuro-imaging. Assessing each child's particular needs as well as his or her response to the testing procedure requires individualized nursing care. The following section discusses the nurse's main responsibilities in relation to issues such preparing the child, obtaining consent, and sedation. Box 10.2 outlines the main types of neuro-imaging procedures and diagnostic tests performed in children.

Preparing the child

Preparing the child for neuro-imaging incorporates both physical and psychological preparation. Physical preparation may be simple or extensive depending on the type of neuro-imaging to be carried out. Some tests require a simple explanation whereas more involved measures such as sedation may be necessary before other procedures. Anxiety, fear of the unknown, and misgivings

about pain are often associated with diagnostic procedures. Lack of information about treatments and procedures can intensify anxiety levels and leave the child unprepared (Coyne & Conlon, 2007). These issues are further discussed in Chapter Two.

Explanations by the nurse need to take into account the child's level of understanding and previous experience of hospital procedures. In addition to providing explanation, techniques such as guided imagery and therapeutic play can assist in preparing children and increase understanding of diagnostic procedures. A child who is adequately prepared is more likely to cooperate during the procedure and be less anxious. As well as preparing the child, it is also important to prepare the parents and family. In stressful situations, such as undergoing diagnostic procedures, parents often become anxious for the well-being of their child. The anxiety experienced by parents is concerning because of the potential transmission of that anxiety to the child. Consequently, minimizing parental anxiety is crucial to the success of child preparation. Play has an important role in hospital in reducing the child's anxiety and this is discussed in more detail in Chapter Two.

Obtaining consent

The physician is responsible for obtaining a signed consent form before any diagnostic test. The general consent a parent/guardian signs on admission to the healthcare facility may be sufficient to indicate consent for diagnostic testing, whereas some more invasive procedures may require an additional consent form before the test. For a parent/guardian to make an informed decision about any neuro-imaging test, it is important that they are equipped with adequate information regarding the test. Further information about consent may be found in Chapter Four.

Sedation

Diagnostic imaging can be achieved without the need for sedation; however, this depends largely on the age and cooperation of the child and the type of imaging being performed, as well as good preparation of the child and parents. A CT scan and an MRI are considered non-invasive procedures; however, these procedures require the child to remain still while the images are taken (SIGN, 2004). Oral sedation such as chloral hydrate is often used for children undergoing diagnostic procedures. It is important that informed consent for sedation is obtained and documented before administration. To facilitate this, venous access should be established prior to the procedure (see Chapter Nine). The child is not recommended to eat or drink prior to the procedure as sedation can cause vomiting, regurgitation, and possible aspiration (SIGN, 2004). You will need to follow local policy and guidelines in relation to the relevant fasting procedure; however, it is recommended that a child should not eat solid food for up to four hours before the procedure (this includes bottle and breast milk) and must abstain from clear fluids for two hours prior (Woodthorpe *et al.*, 2007). It is considered good practice to have emergency equipment readily available prior to administration of sedation. This includes

oxygen, suction, resuscitation bag, mask and airways of correct size, and an emergency trolley.

Oral sedation can be administered by an oral syringe or a spoon; however, there is more success if a syringe is used. As oral sedatives can have a sour taste, the use of a small amount of juice may be used to mask the taste (SIGN, 2004). Observation of the child is important and should commence from the time sedation is administered. This includes monitoring vital signs, particularly respiratory rate and pattern and oxygen saturation levels. Document any reaction to the sedation and inform medical staff if there is any change in the child's condition.

> **Nursing Alert**
>
> Sedation for neuro-imaging is contraindicated for children with decreased level of consciousness and for children with evidence of increased intracranial pressure.

Different types of imaging and nursing considerations

Electromyogram (EMG)

An EMG is a procedure that measures electrical potentials of individual muscles (Hogan *et al.*, 2007). The main role of EMG is to help to differentiate neuropathies and myopathies. To perform an EMG, a sterile needle electrode is inserted through the skin into the muscle tissue and the electrical activity is detected by this needle. The activity is displayed visually on a monitor and may also be displayed audibly through a microphone. Normal muscles at rest make certain normal electrical sounds when the needle is inserted. The electrical activity is studied while the muscle is at rest. Abnormal spontaneous activity might indicate some nerve and/or muscle damage. The patient is asked to contract the muscle (e.g. bend the leg) and the activity is studied and recorded.

Nerve conduction velocity (NCV)

An NCV measures the speed and intensity of electrical signals travelling along the nerves and the time it takes to respond to these signals. It is used to detect neuromuscular disorders. For the NCV two electrodes will be placed in a specific location. These electrodes will pick up the electrical signal as it travels along the nerve in that area. A stimulating electrode sends a tiny electrical charge (shock) along the nerve. The patient may feel a tingle or the muscle may twitch.

Nursing considerations for EMG and NCV

In addition to psychological preparation, the main nursing consideration for a child undergoing an EMG or NCV is the administration of analgesia, as the procedures may cause some degree of patient discomfort. Analgesics such as paracetamol or ibuprofen should be sufficient to reduce any pain or discomfort a child may experience (see Chapter Six).

Electroencephalogram (EEG)

An electroencephalogram (EEG) is a procedure using multiple electrodes placed on the head to record changes in electric impulses in the brain (Hogan *et al.*, 2007). It is a valuable tool that aids in the diagnosis of **epilepsy** and cerebrovascular diseases. During the test 21 surface electrodes are positioned on the head using the international 10–20 measuring system (**see Figure 10.7**). Two electrocardiogram electrodes are used to monitor the heart rate. The electrodes are connected to an EEG computer system where the electrical activity of the brain is amplified and displayed on a screen. As part of the test, the child may

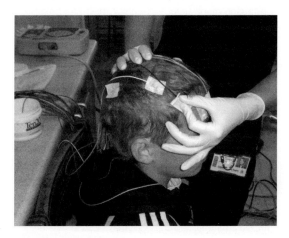

Figure 10.7 Positioning of electrodes for EEG

be asked to breathe deeply and rapidly for a short period of time or view a series of flashing lights. These activities may activate a seizure pattern, which is recorded on the EEG tracing.

Nursing considerations

The child undergoing an EEG needs a thorough explanation of the procedure and reassurance that no electricity will be transferred to the body. It is important that the child's hair is cleaned thoroughly prior to the procedure and again after the test to remove the paste residue from the scalp. There are no restrictions on food and fluid intake.

10.5 Care of the child with convulsive seizure

Seizures

A seizure is the manifestation of an abnormal and excessive synchronized discharge of a set of cerebral neurons (Hogan *et al.*, 2007). The most common cause of convulsive seizures in children is epilepsy. Epilepsy is characterized by unprovoked recurrent seizures (defined as two or more episodes) (Hockenberry *et al.*, 2003). When a child has a seizure, it is important to distinguish whether the episode was an epileptic or non-epileptic event. Box 10.3 highlights the main causes of seizures in children and **Box 10.4** outlines the main types of seizure activity.

Box 10.3 Common causes of convulsive seizures in children

- Epilepsy.
- Infections, e.g. meningitis, encephalitis.
- Fever.
- Cerebral abscess.
- Head injury.
- Brain tumours.
- Cerebral stroke.
- Hypoxia.
- Acidosis.
- Metabolic disorders.
- Toxic ingestion.
- Brain malformations, e.g. cortical dysphasia.

Box 10. 4 Classification of seizures

Partial seizures

- Simple partial seizures.
- Complex partial seizures.
- Secondary generalized seizures.

Generalized seizures

- Tonic-clonic seizures.
- Absence seizures.
- Akinetic seizures.
- Myoclonic seizures.
- Atonic seizures.
- Status epilepticus.

Psychogenic seizures

- Events that look like seizures but are not due to epilepsy are called 'non-epileptic seizures'. Also known as NEAD (non-epileptic attack disorder).

Procedure: Nursing assessment of a seizure

Assessment

Care of a child with a convulsive seizure requires astute assessment on the part of the nurse. The procedure below outlines the main nursing assessment of a child with a convulsive seizure. When a child has a seizure, the main priority is to keep the child safe. During seizure activity, it is important to position the child in the recovery position. You will need to ensure that the environment is safe, e.g. check cot sides are in place and remove any unnecessary objects. Positioning a blanket, soft object, or padding may help prevent injury occurring. Call for assistance but never leave any child unattended who is having a seizure. Ensure the seizure is timed. Anticonvulsant medication may need to be administered according to local clinical guidelines. It is important to monitor the child's vital signs (Chapter Five) and support respiratory and circulatory function (Chapters Eight and Nine). Oxygen may be required depending on these latter assessments and the child's mouth may need suctioning if it becomes overly moist or if sputum is present (Chapter Eight). Record keeping (Chapter Five) is important including clear

documentation of the nature, type, and length of seizures on the seizure events chart.

Nursing Alert

Restraint is discussed in Chapter Five; however, it is important not to restrain a child who is experiencing a seizure. If used this could result in injury to either the nurse or child.

Other factors to consider

Anticonvulsant therapy

Seizures of a recurrent nature are treated primarily with anticonvulsant medication. If seizures are a manifestation of infection, trauma, or a metabolic problem the treatment is aimed at the underlying cause. Eighty-five per cent of children who have seizures, especially those with epilepsy, are usually well controlled through the use of a single type of anticonvulsant medication (Hogan *et al.*, 2007). If the drug does not sufficiently control seizures a second drug is added, in gradually increasing doses. The type of medication prescribed will depend upon the type of seizure. Once seizures are controlled the drug or drugs are continued for a prolonged time, and reviewed by the physician as appropriate. It is important that the nurse educates the child and family about the use of anticonvulsant medication. It is vital to explain to the child and family the importance of taking the medication, even if the child feels very well or is perhaps not having fits. Some families may see this as a sign to stop medication, therefore it must be emphasized that the drug is preventative. Concordance with treatment can be improved through good explanation and advice to the child and family, ensuring a good understanding of the drugs effects and side effects. Sudden withdrawal can cause an increase in the number and severity of seizures; this must be emphasized to both the child and parents. You also need to give advice to the parents on what to do in the event of another seizure (**see Box 10.5**). The timing and amount of drug to take also needs to be carefully explained, perhaps backed up by written instructions. In cases where there are literacy or language barriers, the education material and approach may need to be modified.

Step-by-step guide to assessment of seizures

Step	Rationale
The following information must be gathered and documented:	
1 A description of the seizures should be obtained from the eyewitnesses, e.g. nurse, doctor, parent, carer, teacher, etc.	To assist in diagnosing a seizure and the type of seizure.
2 Any warning/aura before the event.	To assist in determining if partial onset or generalized seizure.
3 Any impairment or loss of consciousness.	To assist in determining if simple partial or complex seizure.
4 Any stiffening or shaking of the body—if so what side or if whole body affected.	To assist medical team in determining what side of the brain is affected.
5 Eye movements.	To assist medical team in determining what side of the brain is affected.
6 Note the presence of cyanosis, frothing at the mouth, incontinence, and post-ictal state.	To assist in diagnosis of type of seizure.
7 Duration of seizure.	Seizures need to be treated after a specific time.
8 Child's history and any relevant clinical findings should be evaluated.	To assist in identifying any underlying cause or predisposing factors.
If child has a previous history of seizures or epilepsy, the nurse must also determine and document the following:	
9 If rescue medication was administered, and if so what time.	To ensure continuity of care and so team is aware of drugs already given.
10 Any known triggers or precipitating factors to seizures, e.g. lack of sleep and fatigue, activity, noise, bright flashing lights, menstruation, non-compliance, stress.	May indicate why seizure occurred—appropriate advice can then be given.
11 Clarify what anticonvulsant medication and dosage the child is taking.	To ensure compliance in taking medication.

Box 10.5 Care of a child during a seizure: Advice for parents

- Ensure safe environment.
- Do not attempt to restrain child or use force.
- Place small cushion/blanket under child's head.
- Remove hazards such as furniture.
- Do not put anything into child's mouth.
- Loosen any clothing as it may restrict breathing.
- Time the seizure and note limb involvement.
- Call ambulance.
- Stay with child until help arrives.

Discharge advice

Witnessing a convulsive seizure can cause huge distress to a family. A sensitive approach by the nurse can assist parents to come to terms with the child's condition. After the immediate treatment and management of the child, it is essential the nursing staff educate and support the family regarding how to deal with the occurrence of a seizure. It is important that the nurse educates the child and family about anticonvulsant medication, including the possible side effects, duration, right times to give the medication, and the right doses. Discharge advice may also include information about follow-up appointments, and who to consult if difficulties arise.

10.6 **Care of the unconscious child** Ⓐ

This is an advanced skill. You *must* check whether you can assist with or undertake any aspect of this skill, in line with local policy.

Definition

Consciousness is a state of awareness of self, the environment, and one's response to that environment (Dougherty & Lister, 2008). Unconsciousness is defined as the inability to respond to sensory stimuli and have subjective experiences due to depressed cerebral function. In an unconscious patient the normal reflexes are lost making the patient totally dependent.

Box 10.6 Causes of unconsciousness in children

- Increase in brain volume, e.g. brain tumours.
- Increase in cerebral blood flood, e.g. cerebral haematoma.
- Increase in CSF volume, e.g. hydrocephalus.
- Metabolic causes, e.g. electrolyte imbalance.
- Poisons and drugs, e.g. alcohol, gases.
- Infections, e.g. septicaemia.

There are numerous causes of unconsciousness and the length of time a child remains unconscious varies and may depend on the initial cause of the coma. **Box 10.6** highlights the main origins of unconsciousness in children.

Nursing care of the unconscious child

There are physical and psychological issues to consider when caring for an unconscious child. As all systems in the body may be affected by loss of consciousness, physical care involves caring for and maintaining all normal bodily functions from respiratory and cardiac functions to care of skin integrity. The procedure box outlines the main nursing activities for an unconscious child.

Procedure: Care of the unconscious child

Equipment

Gather all necessary equipment and leave at the bedside. Including the following:

- Two airways.
- Oxygen.
- Suction.
- Intravenous infusion equipment.
- Feeding equipment (as indicated), e.g. NG tube.
- Eye care pack.
- Mouth care pack.
- Catheter care pack.
- Documentation charts, e.g. neurological chart, intake and output charts.

Step-by-step guide to care of the unconscious child

This is an advanced skill. You *must* check whether you can assist with or undertake any aspect of this skill, in line with local policy.

Step	Rationale
1 Assess child's airway. Check the patency and maintenance of the airway. Insert oral airway/nasopharyngeal or orotracheal tube if indicated.	To ensure child maintains an open airway.
2 Assess child's breathing. Assess respiratory rate, rhythm, and use of accessory muscles.	To ensure breathing is stable.
3 Evaluate circulatory status by measuring child's heart rate, peripheral and central pulses, skin perfusion, and blood pressure (Resuscitation Council UK, 2004).	To ensure circulatory status is stable.
4 Nurse child in a highly visible area near the nurse's station.	To facilitate rapid assessment of the child's condition.
5 Nurse the child in a bed/cot with a firm base and detachable bed head.	To facilitate emergency situations such as cardiac or respiratory arrest or intubation.
6 Position child's body in alignment with spine.	This position helps maintain musculo-skeletal function and prevent contractures (Geraghty, 2005).
7 Elevate head of bed 15 to 30 degrees.	This will minimize ICP elevation (Hogan *et al.*, 2007).
8 Support the child's arms and wrists on pillows and place a pillow between the child's knees.	This will help to prevent skin breakdown and prevent wrist and foot drop (Geraghty, 2005).
9 Using the Glasgow Coma Scale, perform neurological assessment as frequently as child's condition indicates.	To detect changes in child's neurological condition.
10 Assess and monitor for signs of raised ICP.	Early detection enables prompt intervention.
11 Avoid activities that may increase ICP such as head rotation, flexion of the neck, Valsalva manoeuvre, painful stimuli.	To minimize the risk of raising ICP.

12 Assess pain: observe for signs of pain such as increase in heart rate, respiratory rate, and blood pressure. Agitation may also indicate pain.

To detect presence of pain in the unconscious child.

13 Prevent and relieve pain using pharmacological and non-pharmacological methods of pain relief. Administer pain relief medication as prescribed; however, avoid narcotics.

Pain must be controlled as unrelieved pain can cause an increase in ICP. Narcotics must be avoided as elevated intracranial pressure may become masked by narcotic analgesics (Hogan *et al.*, 2007).

14 Assess for seizure activity and employ measures to prevent and treat seizures.

To allow for early detection and treatment of seizures.

15 Pass nasogastric tube as indicated.

To empty gastric contents regularly. Paralytic ileus may occur in the unconscious patient and this may lead to aspiration of stomach contents (Hockenberry *et al.*, 2003).

16 Maintain feeding regime as indicated via prescribed route, e.g. nasogastric tube/central venous catheter.

To prevent weight loss and maintain optimal nutritional status.

17 Administer intravenous fluids as prescribed.

To maintain fluid and electrolyte balance.

18 Maintain strict intake and output chart.

To avoid over-hydration, which contributes to cerebral oedema.

19 Employ universal precautions while caring for the unconscious child.

To prevent transmission of infection.

20 Assess pressure areas at least two hourly and reposition child frequently or as per doctor's instructions.

To prevent development of pressure sores.

21 Daily bed baths as condition indicates.

To maintain hygiene needs.

22 Perform eye care.

During a state of unconsciousness a patient's blink reflex is absent and this may cause corneal drying, irritation, and ulceration (Dougherty & Lister, 2008).

23 Perform mouth care.

To maintain a clean, moist mouth and to prevent mouth infections.

24 Insert catheter as indicated and maintain regular catheter care.

Insertion of catheter enables adequate monitoring of urinary output and proper, frequent catheter care prevents infection.

25	Administer stool softener as prescribed.	To prevent constipation and to avoid straining, as the Valsalva manoeuvre can increase ICP.
26	Keep child's family informed of any changes in child's condition and involve them in caring for the child.	Keeping parents and family informed will help them adjust to the situation and promotes family centred care.
27	Document all care given and report any changes in condition to medical team.	To ensure a written record of nursing practice is maintained to assist in continuity of care.

Consent and communication

Caring for an unconscious child involves not only physical care but psychological care for the child and family. It is suggested that an unconscious patient is aware of what is occurring around them and can hear conversation (Jacobson, 2000). It is therefore important that the nurse communicates to the child on every point of contact and explains each procedure before starting. Call the child by their name and encourage the family to talk to the child about familiar things such as school, their hobbies, or friends (see Chapter Two). This may help to keep the child orientated. The psychological effect on the patient's family also requires special attention. Having a child in an unconscious state can be a traumatic event for the family and time is needed for the family to adjust. Care of the unconscious child involves numerous medical interventions and procedures, which can be frightening for parents and families. Nurses should provide adequate preparation and explanation prior to and during all procedures and interventions.

Conclusion

This chapter highlights the complexity of caring for children with neurological disorders. It is of fundamental importance that nurses who are caring for a child with a brain injury are able to recognize and depict a change in a child's level of consciousness (Kirkham *et al.*, 2008). Early detection of a change in neurological status facilitates prompt intervention and treatment. By developing an understanding of the impact of a neurological disorder and by acquiring the knowledge and skills necessary to care for children with neurological conditions, the nurse can enhance and improve the experience of hospitalization for these children and their families.

Online resource centre

You may find it helpful to work through our online interactive scenarios intended to help you to develop and apply the skills in this chapter. Where material referenced below is available electronically, we're pleased to provide active web links to the source via **http://www.oxfordtextbooks.co.uk/orc/coyne/**

References

Advanced Life Support Group (2005) *Advanced Paediatric Life Support: The practical approach, 4th ed.* London: Blackwell Publishing.

An Bord Altranais (2002) *Recording Clinical Practice: Guidelines to nurses and midwives.* Dublin: An Bord Altranais.

British National Formulary (2008) *British National Formulary for Children, 2008.* London: BMJ Publishing Group.

Coyne, I. & Conlon., J (2007) Children's and young people's views of hospitalization: 'It's a scary place'. *Journal of Children's and Young People's Nursing* **1** (1), 16–21.

Dawes, E., Lloyd, H., & Durham, L. (2007) Monitoring and recording patients' neurological observations. *Nursing Standard* **22** (10), 40–45.

Department of Health (2001) *12 Key Points on Consent: The law in England.* London: Department of Health.

Dougherty, L. & Lister, S. (2008) *The Royal Marsden Hospital Manual of Clinical Nursing Procedures, 7th ed.* Oxford: Wiley-Blackwell.

Ebinger, F., Kosel, C., Pietz, J., & Rating, D. (2004) Strict bed rest following lumbar puncture in children and adolescents is of no benefit. *Neurology* **62** (6), 1003–1005.

Edwards, S.L. (2001) Using the Glasgow Coma Scale: Analysis and limitations. *British Journal of Nursing* **10** (2), 92–101.

Farley, A. & McLafferty, E. (2008) Lumbar puncture. *Nursing Standard* **22** (22), 46–48.

Fergusson, D. (2008) *Clinical Assessment and Monitoring in Children*. Oxford: Blackwell Publishing.

Geraghty, M. (2005) Nursing the unconscious patient. *Nursing Standard* **20** (1), 54–64.

Greaves, I., Porter, K., & Ryan, J. (2001) *Trauma Care Manual*. London: Arnold.

Härtl, R., Gerber, L.M., Ni, Q., & Ghajar, J. (2008) Effect of early nutrition on deaths due to severe traumatic brain injury. *Journal Neurosurgy* **109**, 50–56.

Hockenberry, M.J., Wilson, D., Winkelstein, M.L., & Kline, N.E. (2003) *Wong's Nursing Care of Infants and Children, 7th ed.* Philadelphia: Mosby.

Hogan, M.A., White, J.E., Falkenstein, K., & Brancato, V. (2007) *Child Health Nursing Reviews and Rationales, 2nd ed.* London: Pearson Hall.

Hough, A. & Gekas, J. (2008) Caring for the child requiring a lumbar puncture. In J. Kelsey & G. McEwing (eds.) *Clinical Skills in Child Health Practice*. London: Churchill Livingstone.

Jacobson, A.F. (2000) Caring for unconscious patients. *American Journal of Nursing* **100** (1), 69.

Kelly, C.A., Upex, A., & Bateman, D. (2004) Comparison of consciousness level assessment in the poisoned patient using the alert/verbal/painful/unresponsive scale and the Glasgow coma scale *1, *2, *3, *4. *Annals of Emergency Medicine* **44** (2), 108–113.

Kirkham, F.J., Newton, C.R., & Whitehouse, W. (2008) Paediatric coma scales. *Developmental Medicine and Child Neurology* **50**, 267–274.

National Institute for Health and Clinical Excellence (2007) *Head Injury: Triage, assessment, investigation and early management of head injury in infants, children and adults. Clinical guideline 56.* London: NICE.

Nursing and Midwifery Council (2005) *Guidelines for Records and Record Keeping.* London: NMC.

Nursing and Midwifery Council (2007) *Introduction of Essential Skills Clusters for Pre-registration Nursing Programme, Circular 07/2007.* Available at: **www.nmc-uk.org**

Resuscitation Council (UK) (2004) *European Paediatric Life Support Course, Provider Manual.* London: Resuscitation Council UK.

Scottish Intercollegiate Guidelines Network (2000) *Early Management of Patients with a Head Injury: Clinical Guideline 46* Edinburgh: Scottish Intercollegiate Guidelines Network.

Scottish Intercollegiate Guidelines Network (2004) *Safe Sedation of Children Undergoing Diagnostic Procedures and Therapeutic Procedures: A national clinical guideline.* Edinburgh: Scottish Intercollegiate Guidelines Network.

Teasdale, G. & Jennett, B. (1974) Assessment of coma and impaired consciousness. *The Lancet* **2**, 81–84.

Thoennissen, J., Herkner, H., Lang, W., Domanovits, H., Laggner, A.N., & Müllner, M. (2001) Does bed rest after cervical or lumbar puncture prevent headache? A systematic review and meta-analysis. *CMAJ*, **165** (10), 1311–1316.

Trengove, R. (2008) Neurological assessment. In J. Kelsey & G. McEwing (eds.) *Clinical Skills in Child Health Practice.* London: Churchill Livingstone, 96–103.

Warren (2006) Neurological observations and coma scales. In E. Trigg & T.A. Mohammed. *Practices in Children's Nursing. Guidelines for Hospital and Community, 2nd ed.* London: Churchill Livingstone.

Waterhouse, C. (2005) The Glasgow Coma Scale and other neurological observations. *Nursing Standard* **19** (33), 56–64.

Woodthorpe, C., Trigg, A., Ailson, G., & Sury, M. (2007) Nurse led sedation for paediatric MRI: Progress and issues. *Paediatric Nurisng* **19** (2), 14–18.

Further reading and URLs

Gough, L. (2006) Lumbar puncture. In E. Trigg & T.A. Mohammed (eds.) *Practices in Children's Nursing. Guidelines for Hospital and Community, 2nd ed.* London: Churchill Livingstone.

Helpful addresses

HEADWAY
The National Head Injuries Association
7 King Edward Court
King Edward Street
Nottingham NG1 1EW
Tel: 0115 924 0800
Website: **http://www.headway.org.uk**

The British Institution for Brain-Injured Children (BIBIC)
Knowle Hall
Bridgwater
Somerset TA7 8PJ
Tel: 01278 684060
Website: **http://www.bibic.org.uk**

11 The renal system

ELEANOR HOLLYWOOD, PAUL COSTELLO, MARGARET CHAMBERS, AND AOIFE MORAN

Skills

Introduction

The focus of this chapter is the renal system and the clinical skills that are associated with renal dysfunction. By the end of this chapter you will be knowledgeable in relation to these skills and your new knowledge will be underpinned by up-to-date evidence-based best practice.

Learning outcomes

It is anticipated that you will be able to do the following once you have read and studied this chapter:

- Understand urine sampling techniques and urine testing methods and their significance in clinical practice.
- Understand the various procedures and investigations that the infant, child, or young person may have to endure for renal system evaluation.

Anatomy and physiology

The urinary system is important in maintaining the correct water and electrolyte concentrations in the body. Waste products and excess water and ions are eliminated from the body in the urine.

The kidneys are situated on either side of the vertebral column in the abdomen. The ureter, renal blood vessels, nerves, and lymphatics enter the kidney at a cleft on the medial side called the hilum. The adrenal gland lies on top of the kidney.

The outside of each kidney is lined by:

- The renal capsule—a layer of collagen fibres.
- The adipose capsule—a layer of fat.
- The renal fascia—a layer of dense connective tissue.

These three layers of tissue protect and support the kidney.

The inside of each kidney contains an outer area (the cortex) and an inner area (the medulla). The cortex is lighter in colour compared to the dark reddish-brown medulla. The medulla contains cone-shaped areas of tissue called the medullary pyramids, which point towards the hilum. The cortex extends in between the medullary pyramids forming the renal columns. Urine forms at the tip of the pyramids (papillae) and drains into the minor calyx, then into a larger major calyx. Two or three major calyces join together to form the renal pelvis, a funnel-shaped chamber that leads into the ureter (**see Figure 11.1**).

Nephrons are the functional units of the kidney, the structures where urine is formed. Each kidney contains over one million nephrons. Each nephron is divided into a glomerulus and a tubule (**see Figure 11.2**). The glomerulus is a ball of intertwined capillaries that lies inside the Bowman's capsule. The glomerulus and Bowman's capsule combined are called the renal corpuscle. The lining of the glomerular capillaries contains many small pores that allow fluid to filter out of the blood and into the capsular

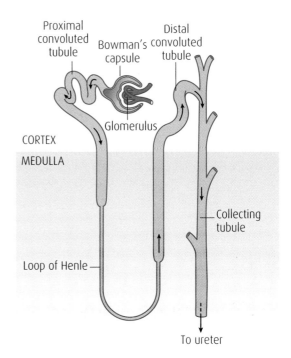

Figure 11.2 A nephron

space. The volume of filtrate formed each minute by the kidneys is called the glomerular filtration rate. Nearly all the fluid in the filtrate is later reabsorbed by the tubules. Only about 1% of the original filtrate is excreted as urine. Red blood cells and proteins are too large to pass through the filter and so remain in the capillaries.

The renal tubules receive the filtrate from the renal corpuscle. They alter the filtrate by absorption (removing substances from it) and secretion (adding substances to it). Any substances left in the filtrate after it has passed through the tubules will be excreted in the urine. The first part of the tubule is the proximal convoluted tubule. Its function is to absorb important substances that the body needs (ions, organic molecules, nutrients, water) and to secrete toxins, drugs, and acids into the filtrate. More than 90% of water in the filtrate is absorbed here. The next part of the tubule is the loop of Henle, which contains a thin descending part and a thicker ascending part. The thin part absorbs more water from the filtrate. The thick part absorbs ions and helps create a concentration gradient, which is necessary for water absorption. The distal convoluted tubule is sensitive to the hormone aldosterone, which stimulates the absorption of sodium from the filtrate and the secretion of potassium into the filtrate. Finally the collecting duct absorbs water under the influence of antidiuretic hormone.

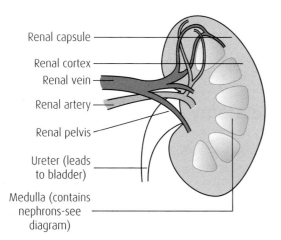

Figure 11.1 The kidney

Blood supply

The kidneys receive 25% of the total cardiac output. The renal arteries arise from the abdominal aorta and supply each kidney. The arteries enter the kidney at the hilum and divide into successively smaller branches, supplying the kidney tissue. The afferent arterioles are very small vessels that lead into the network of glomerular capillaries. After the blood leaves the glomerular capillaries it enters the efferent arterioles and from there enters the venous system. The blood leaves the kidney at the hilum through the renal vein.

Functions of the kidney

The kidney has several important functions in the body, which are listed in **Box 11.1**. The first of these is the regulation of blood volume and blood pressure. The kidney controls the amount of fluid excreted in the urine. Urinary volume can change according to the fluid needs of the body. In cases of dehydration, the blood becomes more concentrated, which is detected by the posterior lobe of the pituitary gland in the brain. It secretes antidiuretic hormone into the blood and this circulates to the kidney, causing the distal convoluted tubule and collecting ducts to reabsorb more water. So if blood concentration increases above normal levels, the kidneys reabsorb more water and produce a smaller volume of concentrated urine. In a situation where blood volume is increased, antidiuretic hormone secretion is inhibited, and the kidneys produce a larger volume of dilute urine. Since blood volume is a factor in blood pressure, the kidney also controls blood pressure by changes in body fluid volume.

Blood volume and blood pressure are also controlled by the renin-angiotensin-aldosterone system. Renin is secreted by the kidney in response to low blood volume and low blood pressure. It converts the plasma protein angiotensinogen into angiotensin I, which in turn is converted into angiotensin II. Angiotensin II causes increased secretion of aldosterone from the adrenal glands. Aldosterone circulates to the kidneys and stimulates the reabsorption of sodium and water, which increases blood volume and blood pressure.

The kidney is also involved in the removal of waste products from the body. The body produces waste products through metabolism that are excreted in the urine. These include urea, uric acid, and creatinine. The kidney also has an important function in the control of the blood acid-base balance. The pH (acid-base balance) of the blood is kept at a normal level by controlling the concentration of hydrogen ions in the blood. The proximal convoluted tubules of the kidney help control the pH by secreting hydrogen ions into the filtrate. Some hydrogen ions secreted combine with bicarbonate to form carbon dioxide and water, whilst others combine with ammonium and hydrogen phosphate and are excreted in the urine.

Other functions include the regulation of sodium and other ion levels, secretion of the hormone erythropoietin, and vitamin D synthesis. Excess sodium is excreted in the urine. Its concentration in the blood is controlled by the hormone aldosterone, which increases sodium reabsorption from the filtrate at the distal convoluted tubule. The kidney also regulates the levels of other ions such as potassium and calcium. Secretion of the hormone erythropoietin stimulates red blood cell production in the bone marrow. The kidney is also important for the activation of Vitamin D, which is required for bone development.

Micturition

Urine leaving the kidney flows through the two ureters to the bladder. Urine is stored in the bladder before it passes into the urethra for elimination (**see Figure 11.3**).

The wall of the bladder is composed of the detrusor muscle, which expels urine by contracting. The trigone is a triangular-shaped area on the inner surface, which lies between the entry of the ureters and the urethra. It is sensitive to increased pressure as the bladder fills. The urethra contains an internal sphincter, which is involuntary, and an external sphincter, which is under voluntary control. The process of urination (**micturition**) is under the control of the nervous system. As urine accumulates in the bladder, the trigone is stimulated and impulses are sent to the brain, which creates the urge to micturate.

Box 11.1 Functions of the kidney

- Regulation of blood volume and blood pressure.
- Removal of waste products.
- Control of the blood acid-base balance.
- Vitamin D synthesis.
- Regulating levels of sodium and other ions.
- Secretion of the hormone erythropoietin.

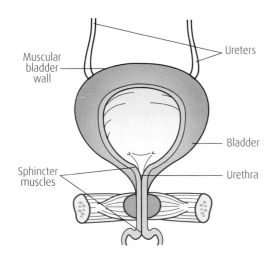

Figure 11.3 The bladder

Children who are toilet trained can resist the urge to micturate by constricting the external urethral sphincter. Micturition occurs in toilet trained children when the detrusor muscle contracts and the internal and external sphincters relax.

In children who are not toilet trained, the neural connections between the brain and the bladder have not fully developed. They cannot voluntarily constrict the external sphincter and so micturition occurs as urine accumulates in the bladder.

For further reading on the anatomy and physiology of the urinary system you may go to the following link: **http://www.le.ac.uk/pa/teach/va/anatomy/case4/4_1.html**

Changes in bladder and kidney function

Bladder capacity changes as the child grows and research has shown that an increase in a child's age strongly predicts the capacity of their bladder (Kaefer *et al.*, 1997). A child's bladder capacity can be calculated by using the following formula:

- age in years + 2 = bladder capacity in ounces (oz)
- NOTE: 1 ounce = 30 ml

Therefore the bladder capacity of a five-year-old would be 7 oz or 210 ml. The increase in bladder capacity allows the growing child to have longer periods between

voiding urine. The bladder also changes shape as the child grows. The infant's bladder is round but it becomes oval/square in shape transversely in older children. In the kidney, the glomerular filtration rate, tubular secretion, and reabsorption are reduced in a child compared to an adult. This can increase the risk of dehydration and the risk of raised blood levels of potassium. The renal system does not fully mature until about 18–24 months after birth.

Toilet training

Toilet training is the process whereby the young child learns how to use the toilet for the purpose of urination and defecation. Toilet training is often referred to as 'potty training' or 'achieving dryness' and it is one of the greatest tasks that the toddler will face in early childhood. Toilet training is a process that most commonly takes place in the home and it is a process that is usually parent led (Jansson *et al.*, 2008). Although there is no consensus regarding the age at which a child should commence toilet training, in general children tend to become toilet trained between the ages of two-and-a-half and four years (Zickler & Richardson, 2004). Girls also generally achieve dryness before boys do (Bray & Sanders, 2006). The most important aspect of toilet training for any child is determining 'readiness' of that child to commence toilet training. The children's nurse plays a significant role in helping parents identify when their child is ready to toilet train, and the three key aspects that determine a child's readiness are explained in **Box 11.2**.

Achieving bladder and bowel control is a complex process that takes time and patience for a child and their family (Jansson *et al.*, 2008). Children with learning difficulties may experience delayed toilet training skills; however, this should not be a barrier to acquiring such skills (Harris, 2004). For more information on continence issues for children please go to the following link: **http://www.eric.org.uk/**

Urinary tract infection

Urinary tract infection (UTI) is a common bacterial infection in children, found in 5% of all febrile children under

Box 11.2 Determining a child's readiness to toilet train

Physical readiness

- Voluntary control of urethral sphincters.
- Ability to stay dry for two hours; decreased number of wet nappies in a 24-hour period.
- Gross motor skills: walking, sitting, squatting.
- Fine motor skills: can open clothing, e.g. buttons, zips.

Psychological readiness

- Expresses interest and curiosity about toilet habits of parents or siblings.
- Willingness to please.
- Desire to be changed once nappy is wet.
- Cognitive ability to follow directions.
- May express the urge to micturate through verbal and non-verbal communication.

Parental readiness

- Recognition that their child is ready to toilet train.
- Can identify the specific aspects of readiness in this child.
- Willingness to invest time in process.
- Absence of familial stressors, e.g. moving house.

the age of two presenting to emergency rooms (Van der Voort *et al.*, 1997). Symptoms and signs in younger children include fever, vomiting, irritability, and poor feeding. Older children may complain of abdominal pain and of passing urine more frequently (National Institute for Health and Clinical Excellence (NICE), 2007). In a suspected urinary tract infection, a **urine sample** is collected to identify the bacteria causing the infection and to choose the correct antibiotic treatment. *Escherichia coli* accounts for most UTIs. Other bacteria include *Klebsiella*, *Proteus*, *Staphylococcus*, and *Pseudomonas*. *Proteus* infection is more common in older boys and *Staphylococcus* infection is more common in adolescence, especially in girls. The incidence of *Klebsiella* infection decreases in older children. *Escherichia coli* is found in the anal and perineal region, close to the urethral opening, which allows the bacteria to travel up the urethra (ascending infection). To prevent UTI in a child, the parents and child can be taught the importance of perineal and toileting hygiene. The child should empty the bladder completely to prevent the risk of bacteria infecting any residual urine. Adequate fluid intake prevents dehydration, which can

lead to increased concentration of any bacteria present in the urine. Although ascending infection is the most common route of infection, spread of bacteria in the blood to the urinary tract may also occur. UTIs are also associated with constipation, infrequent voiding of urine, and structural abnormalities of the urinary tract such as renal scarring.

Log on to the following website for NICE clinical guidelines in relation to managing a child with a urinary tract infection: **http://www.nice.org.uk/nicemedia/pdf/ CG54fullguideline.pdf**

Collecting a urine sample

Urine samples can be used to determine infection and the levels of other substances in the urine such as glucose, protein, and blood. Raised or decreased levels of these substances may indicate disease. A number of methods can be used to obtain a urine sample. The method of collecting a urine sample depends on whether the child is toilet trained; that is whether the child has bladder control and can use the toilet for urination and defecation. A clean catch is a urine sample caught cleanly during voiding and is the recommended method for urine collection (NICE, 2007). Toilet trained children can void urine when requested into a container (although this is not always successful). Non-toilet trained children cannot cooperate with this process and the parent or nurse must wait until the child voids spontaneously.

Since collecting a clean catch urine sample may be time-consuming in this situation, other methods such as urine collection bags and urine collection pads placed inside the nappy may be used. However, contamination of the sample with bacteria outside the urinary tract can lead to inaccurate diagnosis and unnecessary tests and treatments (Lewis, 1998). It is a problem with all methods but clean catch specimens show less contamination when compared to collections using pads or bags (Alam *et al.*, 2005; MacFarlane *et al.*, 1999). Since urine collection pads and bags are in prolonged contact with the skin, they naturally have a greater risk of contamination. There are insufficient data to determine if urine collection pads or urine collection bags are more accurate in detecting urinary tract infection (NICE, 2007), but use of pads for collection is more comfortable for the child and a sufficient amount of urine can be extracted without difficulty (Farrell *et al.*, 2002). Rao *et al.* (2004) recommend that the pad is changed every 30–45 minutes to reduce the risk of contamination. Clean catch, bag collection, and pad collection can be performed outside the hospital environment.

When it is not possible to collect a urine sample by clean catch, pad, or bag collection (for example, if the child is very ill) an internal catheter (into the urethra) or suprapubic aspiration (directly through the skin to the bladder) may need to be used (NICE, 2007). Catheterization and suprapubic aspiration are usually only suitable for a child who is in hospital, due to the potential risk of infection. Catheterization is a method of collecting urine by inserting a catheter (purposeful small narrow tube) into the urethral orifice. When the tip of the catheter enters the bladder, urine flows into a container.

Suprapubic aspiration is the collection of a urine sample by inserting a needle directly into the bladder through the anterior abdominal wall. Suprapubic aspiration is indicated if a child is seriously ill, and a urine sample is needed before treatment is started. Lack of urine in the bladder and infection of the anterior abdominal wall are contraindications (Austin *et al.*, 1999). It is an invasive procedure and a minimum number of attempts should be made to avoid complications such as bleeding and infection (Chu *et al.*, 2002). Suprapubic aspiration is not performed by the nurse; however, the nurse often assists the doctor with the procedure. It is unpleasant for the child and can cause anxiety for parents (Ross, 2000), but it is the most accurate method of detecting urinary tract infection since the risk of contamination is extremely low (Jodal, 2002). Before performing suprapubic aspiration, the child should be adequately hydrated to ensure that there is urine in the bladder. The presence of a dry nappy and no voiding in the previous 30 minutes has been used to predict urine in the bladder (Gochman *et al.*, 1991), although Chu *et al.* (2002) did not substantiate these findings. Before suprapubic aspiration is performed, Jodal (2002) recommends routine administration of fluid and demonstration of urine in the bladder using percussion over the suprapubic area or verification using ultrasound. For further information on urine testing in children please go to: **http://www.patient.co.uk/show-doc/23068848/**

Urine collection at home

With increasing moves towards community care, it is possible that parents are required to collect urine specimens in the home. In these cases they should be helped to make decisions about their child's care. Healthcare professionals should give parents and guardians appropriate information on prompt recognition of symptoms and urine collection (NICE, 2007). Non-invasive urine collection procedures (clean catch, bag collection, and pad collection) can be performed by parents at home and the skills needed can be demonstrated to parents or guardians by healthcare professionals and supplemented by leaflets on urine collection (Liaw *et al.*, 2000).

Parents' views differ on the best method of collecting a urine sample (Liaw *et al.*, 2000). They note that bag collection can leak urine and leave red marks on the skin. Some parents find emptying urine from the bag to be awkward. Parents consider the pad comfortable but some also find it difficult extracting urine from the pad. Overall, Liaw *et al.* (2000) found that most parents dislike the clean catch method, but in contrast Owen *et al.* (2003) noted that parents found obtaining a clean catch was the easiest method. If parents are educated and shown the technique, they will support clean catch sampling (Owen, 2003). A clean catch is a urine sample caught cleanly during voiding and is the recommended method for urine collection (NICE, 2007).

Child and family preparation

It is important to ask the parents or guardians about the child's toilet training history and find out if the child experienced any difficulties during toilet training. You may also assess whether or not the child and family understands the need for the urine collection procedure. The ability of the child to understand the procedure depends on their age and cognitive level. Stress and anxiety may also affect the child's and parents' ability to understand the procedure. For a young child, ask the parents what word the child uses for urine. Use that word when talking to the child. Explain the procedure to the child and family and why it is necessary. Provide the opportunity to ask questions and demonstrate the equipment used in the procedure. Provide privacy for the child during the procedure.

The various methods of collecting urine specimens will now be further explained. For each of the methods listed below, it is important to explain to the child and their family why you are taking the urine specimen, and the procedure you will be using. Gather all the equipment you will need before you begin to ensure the procedure goes smoothly.

11.1 **Clean catch**

A clean catch urine specimen is the preferred method of urine collection. The child should be able to urinate when required and so this procedure is not suitable for non-toilet trained children. Proper cleaning of the genitalia is needed to reduce the risk of contamination of the urine sample (Vaillancourt *et al.*, 2007).

Procedure: Obtaining a clean catch urine specimen (see following page)

Equipment

- Examination gloves.
- Sterile gloves.
- Sterile specimen container.
- Washcloth, towel.
- Antimicrobial swabs.
- Marker/adhesive label.

11.2 **Bag collection of urine**

This method is suitable for a child who is not toilet trained. A urine collection bag is inserted around the genitalia inside the nappy.

Procedure: Obtaining a bag collection urine specimen (see page 295)

Equipment

- Examination gloves.
- Urine collection bag.
- Sterile specimen container.
- Washcloth, towel.
- Marker/adhesive label.

11.3 **Pad collection of urine**

This method is also suitable for a child who is not toilet trained. A pad is inserted inside the nappy and urine is collected from the pad using a syringe.

Procedure: Obtaining a pad collection urine specimen (see page 296)

Equipment

- Examination gloves.
- Urine collection pad.
- Sterile syringe, 5 ml/10 ml.
- Sterile specimen container.
- Washcloth, towel.
- Marker/adhesive label.

11.4 **Collection during catheter insertion**

A urine sample may be collected during the insertion of a urinary catheter. The catheter is inserted into the urethra until urine begins to flow. You may let about 10 ml of urine flow into a specimen container. Put the lid on the container, avoiding contact with the inside of the container or the inside of the lid. Label the specimen and send to the laboratory for analysis.

11.5 **Suprapubic aspiration**

When it is not possible to collect urine by non-invasive methods, suprapubic aspiration may be used. This method is performed by a doctor and assisted by a nurse. It is an invasive procedure and is not suitable as a method of urine collection in primary care. Local anaesthetic is applied at the skin over the bladder. A needle is inserted through the skin into the bladder under ultrasound guidance and urine is drawn into the syringe.

Step-by-step guide to obtaining a clean catch urine specimen

Step	Rationale
1 Put on the examination gloves and wash the child's genital area with warm water and soap. The child may be able to do this themselves.	Removes potential sources of contamination.
2 Remove the lid of the container and place on a clean surface with the inside of the lid facing upwards.	Prevents contamination.
3 Remove the examination gloves, wash hands, and put on the sterile gloves. The child should also wear sterile gloves if assisting.	Prevents contamination of specimen by skin bacteria.
4 For a young child who is not toilet-trained, remove the nappy. Clean around the child's urethral opening using the antimicrobial swabs. Discard the used swabs.	Removes contaminating bacteria from the urethral opening.
5 Have the nurse or parent place a waterproof pad across their lap and place the child on the pad. Hold a sterile bowl underneath the child's genitalia and wait for the child to urinate.	To obtain the sample.
6 After the specimen is collected, put on gloves and replace the nappy on the child.	Prevents contamination of the sterile field.
7 For an older child, clean around the child's urethral opening using the antimicrobial swabs. Ask the child to void a small amount of urine into the toilet first.	Removes contaminating bacteria from the urethral opening.
8 Ask the child to urinate into the container, collecting about 10–20 ml of urine. The child can finish urinating into the toilet after the collection.	To obtain the sample.
9 Put the lid on the container, avoiding contact with the inside of the container or the inside of the lid.	Prevents contamination of specimen.
10 Label the specimen and send to laboratory for analysis.	So that the sample is correctly identified for analysis.
11 Dispose of used equipment and waste appropriately.	Decreases risk of transmission of micro-organisms.

Step-by-step guide to obtaining a bag collection urine specimen

Step	Rationale
1 Wash hands and put on gloves.	Prevents contamination of specimen.
2 Place the child on their back with legs apart and remove the nappy.	Facilitates cleaning of genital area and allows placement of collection bag.
3 Clean the genital area. Avoid oils/lotions/soaps that might interfere with adhesive on the bag. Clean the anus region last.	Prevents contamination of specimen.
4 Attach urine collection bag according to manufacturer's instructions. For males, insert the penis and scrotum into bag opening and press adhesive against the skin. For females, position bag against perineum region first and then press adhesive against skin in an upwards direction. Ensure the bag does not cover the anus.	Correct placement avoids leakage.
5 Remove gloves and wash hands.	Prevents contamination of specimen.
6 After the child has voided urine into the bag, put on gloves and remove the bag.	Prevents contamination of specimen. To obtain the sample.
7 Hold the bag over the specimen container, remove the tab on the lower corner, and direct the urine into the container.	To obtain the sample.
8 Put the lid on the container, avoiding contact with the inside of the container or the inside of the lid.	Prevents contamination of specimen.
9 Label the specimen and send to laboratory for analysis.	So that the sample is correctly identified for analysis.
10 Dispose of used equipment and waste appropriately.	Decreases risk of transmission of micro-organisms.

Step-by-step guide to obtaining a pad collection urine specimen

Step	Rationale
1 Wash hands and put on gloves.	Prevents contamination of specimen.
2 Remove the nappy and clean the genital area.	Prevents contamination of specimen.
3 Attach the pad according to manufacturer's instructions. Position the urine collection pad over the urethra (female) or penis (male).	Correct placement avoids leakage.
4 Fix the pad to the inside of the nappy using the adhesive strips. Replace the nappy.	So that the pad is secured in the correct position to absorb the sample.
5 After the infant has voided urine, put on gloves and remove the nappy with the pad.	To prevent contamination of specimen. To collect the sample.
6 Press the tip of a sterile syringe into the pad and withdraw the plunger to remove a sample of urine.	Sterile syringe prevents contamination of specimen.
7 Hold the syringe over the sterile container and press the plunger to transfer the urine sample into the container.	To obtain the sample.
8 Put the lid on the container, avoiding contact with the inside of the container or the inside of the lid.	Prevents contamination of specimen.
9 Label the specimen and send to laboratory for analysis.	So that the sample is correctly identified for analysis.
10 Dispose of used equipment and waste appropriately.	Decreases risk of transmission of micro-organisms.

Procedure: Assisting with a suprapubic aspiration (see following page)

Preparation

Prepare the equipment before the procedure begins, to decrease the time the child will be away from their bed. Transport the child to the procedure room.

Equipment

- Sterile gloves.
- Sterile drapes.
- Skin antiseptic solution.
- Sterile gauze.
- Local anaesthetic with syringe and needle.
- Sterile syringe, 5 ml/10 ml.
- Needle, 22 gauge.

Step-by-step guide to assisting with a suprapubic aspiration

Step	Rationale
1 Prepare equipment.	Decreases time child will be away from their bed.
2 Transport child to treatment area.	So the procedure can begin.
3 Wash hands and put on gloves.	Decreases transmission of micro-organisms.
4 Position child on back and stand at head of child. Hold child's legs flexed.	Prevents movement of child during procedure.
5 Assist practitioner as required during procedure.	To ensure a successful procedure.
6 After procedure apply pressure with gauze at insertion site as required.	Reduces bleeding.
7 Apply bandage to site.	Protects site.

Consent and communication

Before you begin, carefully explain why you are taking the urine sample and the procedure you are using to the child and their family.

11.6 24-hour urine specimen collection

A 24-hour urine collection is used to determine the levels of certain proteins and chemicals excreted in the urine over that time period. An increase or decrease in those levels may indicate a particular disease. The test is typically used to compare the level of creatinine in the urine with that in the blood (creatinine clearance). Creatinine is a naturally occurring substance in the blood that is filtered by the kidneys and excreted in the urine. The creatinine clearance gives an estimate of the glomerular filtration rate. Low glomerular filtration rate may indicate kidney diseases such as glomerulonephritis and acute nephritic syndrome. If the child is not toilet trained, a urine collection bag may be used to collect urine over 24 hours. An indwelling catheter may also be used to collect the sample.

Procedure: 24-hour urine sample collection (see following page)

Preparation

Place collection container at bedside, as the child's urine must be collected in the same container over 24 hours.

Equipment

- Collection bottle.
- Bedpan or toilet specimen container.
- Marker/adhesive label.

Consent and communication

Explain the procedure and why you are collecting the urine to the child/family.

Nursing Alert

Record and document the urine collection procedure. Record the volume, colour, and any particular odour of the urine. In the case of a 24-hour collection, note the time the collection began and finished.

Step-by-step guide to 24-hour urine specimen collection

Step	Rationale
1 Put on gloves.	Prevents contamination of specimen.
2 Ask child to void bladder. Discard the voided urine. If a catheter or collection bag is present, discard any urine. Note the time the urine was discarded.	The test must commence with an empty bladder and be timed over 24 hours.
3 Pour urine from each void into collection bottle. If an indwelling catheter or collection bag is used, empty into collection bottle every two hours.	To collect the specimen.
4 In some instances the collection bottle may need to be kept on ice.	Ice preserves the urine sample.
5 Soon before the end of the 24-hour time period, ask the child to urinate into the container. Add this final urine sample to the collection bottle.	To complete the specimen.
6 Label the collection bottle and send to laboratory immediately for analysis.	So that the sample is correctly identified for analysis.
7 Record the time the collection began and finished.	So that the timing of the collection is correctly documented for future reference.

Urine testing

Urinalysis (testing urine) using **reagent strips** (chemical analysis strips) is a straightforward, reliable, and cost-effective way of identifying a number of disorders in their early stages (Nursing Standard Quick Reference Guide, 1999).

Urinalysis is used to screen specimens for substances that are not normally present in the urine and is a fundamental aspect of the initial clinical assessment of the child (Wilson, 2005). Examples of substances screened for in urinalysis are **haematuria** (blood in the urine), **glycosuria** (glucose in the urine), nitrites, and leucocytes (white blood cells) (see **Table 11.1**).

Urinalysis

There are a number of issues to take into account when undertaking routine urinalysis. Firstly, contact with bodily fluids can lead to the transmission of infection. Within the healthcare setting this risk is commonly referred to as a biohazard, and **universal precautions** (precautions to be undertaken when handling body fluids) must be observed in order to protect others, including yourself, from infection (Torrance & Elley, 1992). Measures for this are agreed locally within your hospital and you should familiarize yourself with these procedures. In general they refer to the wearing of appropriate gloves when managing situations where bodily fluids are involved, and correct and safe storage and labelling of specimens. Other considerations that need to be taken into account are as follows:

Table 11.1 Substances screened for in urinalysis

Substance	Indication
Blood	May indicate: ■ Infection ■ **Renal calculi** (kidney stones) ■ Injury to kidneys or other part of renal tract ■ Some drugs (e.g. sulphonamides) ■ Glomerulonephritis (inflammation of the glomeruli of the kidney) ■ Malignancy, e.g. **Wilm's tumour** (cancer of the kidney) ■ Bleeding disorders
Protein	May indicate: ■ Infection ■ Glomerulonephritis ■ Nephrotic syndrome
Glucose	May indicate: ■ Diabetes mellitus ■ Physiological stress, e.g. following a grand mal seizure ■ Some drug therapies e.g. corticosteroids and salicylates
Ketones	May indicate: ■ Uncontrolled diabetes mellitus ■ Starvation, e.g. before or after surgery ■ Anorexia ■ Vomiting ■ Fasting ■ Pyrexia
Bilirubin	May indicate: ■ Liver or biliary disease
Urobilinogen	May indicate: ■ Liver disease ■ Haemolytic disorders (abnormal destruction of red blood cells), e.g. haemolytic anaemia
Nitrites	May indicate: ■ Urinary tract infection
Leucocytes	May indicate: ■ Urinary tract infection (especially when found together with nitrites)
pH values: normal range 5.0–8.0 (Higgins, 2007)	pH measures the acidity of the urine: ■ A pH greater than 7 may indicate urinary tract infection
Specific gravity (SG): normal range in urine 1.001–1.035 (Marieb, 2008)	SG measures the total solute concentration in a fluid: ■ A high SG indicates concentrated urine, e.g. in dehydration or when the urine contains glucose or other solutes ■ A low SG indicates diluted urine, e.g. diabetes insipidus (Steggall, 2007)

- As urine is more concentrated first thing in the morning, specimens taken at this time are believed to be optimal for routine urinalysis as they are increasingly likely to be accurate (Wilson, 2005).
- When undertaking urinalysis using reagent strips the urine should be tested immediately for the most reliable results (Wilson, 2005).
- Specimens of urine should be stored in a refrigerator unless tested within one hour of voiding, and then warmed to room temperature before testing.

Bayer Diagnostics Europe (2004) highlight a number of important factors that also need to be taken into account when performing urinalysis. These are as follows:

- When testing for bilirubin and urobilinogen it is important to use a fresh specimen as both are unstable compounds that may be affected by light and room temperature.
- Unpreserved urine stored at room temperature may show increased micro-organisms and change in pH.
- A positive blood reaction could be caused by bacterial growth of contaminating organisms.
- False positive results for protein may be caused by highly alkaline urine.

11.7 **Observations of urine: Amount, colour, and odour**

The amount of urine passed by a child with a urinary tract infection is often noted by the nurse. There may be a specific instruction to measure the urine and record the amount in the child's records to establish whether this is a satisfactory amount. Reduced amounts of urine may be passed in urinary tract infection (McFarlane, 2006) and dehydration (Kanneh, 2006), whilst urinary output may be increased in certain conditions, for example, in diabetes insipidus (Steggall, 2007; Wilson, 2005).

Another common observation of urine during analysis is the colour. Urine is normally a clear straw colour. Urine should be observed for the following abnormalities:

- *Cloudy urine* is usually caused by the presence of particles suspended in the urine. Particles normally settle if the urine is left to stand but may be a sign of infection.

- *Pink or red urine* may indicate the presence of red blood cells but beware—it may also mean that the patient has been eating beetroot!
- *Yellow or orange urine* may indicate the presence of conjugated (yellow) and unconjugated (brown) bilirubin.
- *Blue/green urine* may also indicate the presence of bilirubin but could also be the result of pseudomonas infection.
- *Orange urine* may be caused by urobilinogen or some drugs, e.g. rifampicin.

The odour of urine is also considered by the nurse. Fresh urine should have little or no smell but if urine is left standing it may develop a slight smell of ammonia (Nursing Standard Quick Reference Guide, 1999). However, urine that is infected may have a fish-like odour. In children with diabetes, the presence of **ketones** (due to keto-acidosis, the by-product of fat metabolism) may lead to a characteristic sweet smell. Ketones may also be detected where a child or young person is starving due to neglect or anorexia nervosa, is fasting, e.g. before and after surgery, or has pyrexia. It is of interest to note during your observations that eating strongly flavoured foods may also affect the odour of urine (Cook, 1996). Thus establishing the child's particular history, through speaking with the child and family, is an important component of urine observation, the findings of which are not considered in isolation of this context. To further augment and supplement visual and auditory findings, simple urine testing systems (a reagent strip) are usually available within hospital and community settings and provide some basic diagnostic indicators in relation to a range of conditions (**Table 11.1**). These preliminary urinalysis findings prompt the healthcare team towards a particular possible underlying condition that may well be followed up by more extensive tests. Thus urinalysis is used as a diagnostic indicator to guide assessment and further management. The mechanism for urinalysis will now be explained.

Nursing Alert

Whenever urine must be stored for any length of time prior to being sent to the laboratory it must be stored in a refrigerator.

▶ 11.8 **Urinalysis: Testing with a reagent strip**

Urinalysis is normally undertaken using reagent strips. It is important that these strips are stored and used correctly to ensure reliable and accurate results.

Strips should be:

- Stored in the bottle supplied by the manufacturer, and the desiccant should never be removed from the bottle. The bottle lid should be replaced as soon as possible after removal of the strip.
- Used before the expiry date on the bottle or discarded when that date is reached.
- Dipped into fresh urine ensuring that all the reagent areas are immersed and immediately removed, with excess urine being removed by running the strip against the rim of the container.
- Compared against the colour chart on the bottle label using a watch with a second hand to ensure accurate timing.

Accurate timing in accordance with the manufacturer's instructions is essential because the reagent pads all follow a colour reaction curve that has three phases (**see Table 11.2**).

Following the correct procedure is important. Once the urinalysis has been completed, the strip should be discarded in the appropriate clinical waste bag and the urine disposed of in the sluice or toilet (Cook, 1996). The results of the urinalysis should be accurately recorded as soon as possible in the patient's notes.

For further reading about urinalysis please follow the links below:

http://en.wikipedia.org/wiki/Urinalysis
http://library.med.utah.edu/WebPath/TUTORIAL/URINE/URINE.html

Further, more extensive examinations are available that may be used to support a more comprehensive diagnosis in children with urinary problems. There are a range of diagnostic imaging tests available such as ultrasound, micturating cystogram, and dimercaptosuccinic acid (DMSA) scanning, which will now be further explained.

Preparing the child for diagnostic imaging

Imaging of the renal tract may be necessary either during an acute illness episode or following recovery in order to ascertain any damage that may have occurred to the bladder or kidneys (McFarlane, 2006). Screening may also take place in order to identify abnormalities of the urinary tract in babies and young children. There are three important imaging methods: ultrasound scan; micturating cystogram; and DMSA.

Table 11.2 Colour reaction curve of reagent pads

Phase	Reaction
Kinetic phase	Colours developing in intensity—reading the strip too soon will give inaccurate results.
Stable phase	The time at which the pads should be compared with the chart according to the manufacturer's instructions.
Decline phase	Colours begin to fade—reading the strip during this phase will also result in inaccurate results.

11.9 **Preparing the child for ultrasound**

A kidney ultrasound is a non-invasive investigation used to assess the size, shape, and location of the kidneys and the blood flow through them. This is a painless investigation that involves exposing the appropriate parts of the child's body to high frequency sound waves in order to produce pictures of the child's renal tract. The images are produced when the sound waves are directed into the body by a transducer and then reflected back to a scanner that measures them. The images are captured in real time and so are able to show the structure of the renal kidneys, ureters, and bladder, as well as the blood flowing through the blood vessels.

The ultrasound transducer looks like a small paint roller that is swept back and forth over the area of the body being scanned. When the kidneys are scanned, the child is asked to lie on their back or side on an examination table and gel is applied to the skin allowing the transducer to define the organs as clearly as possible. The gel allows for smooth movement of the transducer over the skin and eliminates air between the skin and the transducer that may interfere with the imaging.

Ultrasound scanning of the kidneys is performed on a full bladder so the child must be requested to drink plenty of water before the scan and not to pass urine until instructed to do so by the sonographer during the investigation. This can be very difficult in young children. Enlisting the help of the parents as well as the cooperation of the sonographer regarding timing of the examination is crucial. The investigation is non-invasive and the child does not need to be fasted or sedated for it.

11.10 **Preparing the child for a micturating cystogram**

A micturating cystogram is an X-ray examination that allows observation of the bladder, ureters, and the urethra during micturition (when passing urine out), thus providing information about the flow of urine through the renal tract. The procedure involves passing a catheter into the bladder and then filling the bladder with contrast media. Prior to passing the catheter, a small amount of anaesthetic gel may be introduced into the urethra. (Some children may find the introduction of a catheter unpleasant or slightly uncomfortable but it should not hurt. However, they may be given a sedative in order to keep them calm during the procedure.) An X-ray camera is used to observe the bladder and kidneys whilst the contrast media is being poured into the bladder, and more X-ray pictures are taken once the bladder is full. The child is then asked to pass urine so that pictures can be taken of how the bladder empties. (Some children find this difficult to do on demand and on an X-ray table so it is important to have the encouragement of their parents or carers at this time.)

The physical preparation for this examination needs consideration. As there is a small risk of introducing infection via the catheter, the child may be prescribed a short course of antibiotics prior to the procedure. The test is not painful but may be frightening for the child, so clear explanations before the procedure of what to expect are helpful. The child may be permitted to eat, as there is no particular requirement for an empty stomach (fasting). For further reading on micturating cystogram please see the following link: **http://www.e-radiography.net/technique/mucg/mcug.htm**

11.11 **Preparing the child for DMSA**

Dimercaptosuccinic acid (DMSA) scanning is another diagnostic imaging examination available that can be used when an acute infection of the upper renal tract is suspected. It allows acute changes in the kidney associated with inflammation of the kidney tissue to be identified. It can also be used to establish the presence of kidney scarring following infection. The scan is performed by injecting a small amount of radiopharmaceutical into one of the child's veins. This involves the insertion of a cannula into an appropriate vein. After 3–4 hours (this allows time for the kidneys to absorb the radiopharmaceutical) the child is asked to pass urine and then the imaging is undertaken. The imaging procedure takes about 30 to 40 minutes and it is important that child lies still during this time in order to ensure the best possible images. Again the support of parents or carers is vital. Once complete the images are viewed for quality. If there has been too much motion the imaging may need to be repeated.

No physical preparation is required for this investigation. However, it is important that psychological preparation is undertaken, and since an intravenous cannula needs to be introduced into the child's vein prior to imaging, preparation for cannulation is essential. This particular element of care is more fully addressed in Chapter Nine.

Psychological preparation for all procedures

The importance of the psychological preparation of children for invasive and non-invasive procedures is an essential aspect of the nursing care of children, as seen earlier in Chapter Two. The child and family should be prepared verbally for the procedure and play can also be a part of preparation, using established therapeutic play techniques as discussed in Chapter Two. Methods of preparation should be age specific and should take into account the child's prior knowledge of the procedure and other medical experiences. They include approaches such as therapeutic play, photographs and filmed modelling, and medical play modalities, which will now be briefly outlined.

Therapeutic play is a useful tool for preparing children and their parents/guardians for invasive procedures. Effective therapeutic play techniques can help to alleviate the effects of hospitalization and create a more positive experience for the child and family.

Photographs and filmed modelling can be used and still photographs depicting the process of the procedure are a regular feature of most pre-admission clinics and prior to emergency surgery and medical procedures. With the help of the play specialist this is a simple tool to develop. All the stages of the procedure should be identified and photographed, usually using a cooperative child and a parent. The child is then able to model his or her behaviour on that of the child in the photographs. It is important that the photographs depict the actual environment that the child will find themselves in, including the ward or outpatient unit and the scan machine and transducer or X-ray camera itself. Filmed modelling (Melamed & Siegel, 1975) is a preparation method in which children watch a short film of a child and parent undergoing the procedure for which the child is being prepared. In contrast to still photographs, the film appears real to the child, who is then more able to model his or her behaviour on that of the child in the film (Chambers, 2008).

Medical play modalities include both directed medical play and non-directed medical play. Non-directed medical play (free play with medical equipment) can be used to allow the child to become familiar with medical equipment and the hospital environment. Directed medical play (medical play with specific therapeutic objectives, e.g. preparation for procedures) can be used to prepare the child specifically for a renal scan. The use of the Zaadi doll (anatomically correct male or female soft doll) can demonstrate the position of the bladder and kidneys and can be catheterized. A body outline doll—a small stuffed doll shaped like a gingerbread man (Chambers, 2008)—can be used with a model of a scan machine and transducer to demonstrate the child within the scanner. Both of the above dolls can also be used to demonstrate intravenous cannula insertion and urinary catheterization. The procedure of urinary catheterization will now be further explored.

11.12 Urinary catheterization

Urinary catheterization is the insertion of a drainage device into the urinary bladder using an aseptic technique, for the purpose of emptying the bladder or instilling fluid into the bladder. Children in hospital and at home in the community require urinary catheterization for many reasons (see Box 11.3).

Urinary catheterization may be performed intermittently or an indwelling catheter may be left in position for a period of days or weeks. Short-term catheterization refers to a catheterization period of up to 14 days and long-term catheterization refers to a catheterization period of up to 12 weeks (Robinson, 2001). Intermittent catheterization is often referred to as CISC: clean intermittent self-catheterization (Senior, 2001) or IC: intermittent catheterization (Collins Pellatt, 2007). Intermittent catheterization is often performed by parents at home for children with neurogenic bladders, e.g. spina bifida.

Nursing Alert

Currently in Ireland nurses are not trained to catheterize male patients, therefore nurses who trained in Ireland do not commonly perform catheterizations on male patients. For further information follow the link below:

http://www.nursingboard.ie/Scope/scope4/try1.asp

Box 11.3 Reasons for urinary catheterization

- Urinary retention: to relieve pressure on the urinary sphincter and provide comfort.
- Postoperative urine monitoring.
- Investigations, e.g. micturating cystourethrogram (MCUG) in order to fill the bladder with fluid and visualize on X-ray.
- Bladder neuropathy: to empty bladder completely and prevent stasis and infection (may be carried out intermittently).
- Critically ill child: may be preferable to using continence pads, especially if accurate urine output is required.
- Obtaining a sterile urine specimen for culture.

Catheterization is a common procedure in paediatric healthcare and has psychological, physical, and social implications beyond the drainage of urine (Bray & Sanders, 2006). Catheterization can be frightening for the child and cause considerable stress for the parent, so promoting best practice in catheter care is essential to enhancing good patient care (Robinson, 2001) and will help to alleviate the fear and stress of the child and their family.

> **Nursing Alert**
>
> Cultural awareness: The children's nurse must be aware that some cultures may be extremely upset and worried about the procedure of urinary catheterization in girls. This is because they may think that the procedure will affect the girl's virginity. Concerns of this nature must be identified prior to the procedure and dealt with through education. This can be achieved by using a manikin to explain that although the urethral opening is situated near the vagina, the openings are completely separate.

Preparation

- Assess the child's prior experience of having a urinary catheter inserted. Parents know their children best, therefore ask the parents how the child coped before with the procedure. A child who has experienced a traumatic catheterization in the past will almost never cooperate in the future (Robson *et al.*, 2006).
- Effective communication is essential if an effective catheterization is to be achieved. Explain to the child in age appropriate language and to the parent why it is necessary to have the urinary catheter inserted.
- Active listening is an intrinsic element of effective communication. Ask the child and parent if they have any questions. Listen to their questions and any possible fears or anxieties that they may be experiencing.
- Incorporate play as a therapeutic tool to explain the procedure to the child, eliminate fear, and gain the cooperation of the child. Acting out the procedure on dolls or playing with materials that will be used for the procedure is often effective for preparing the child and family (Bray & Sanders, 2006).

- Diversional play can be useful during the procedure. Alternative techniques are also useful: counting, deep breathing, or guided imagery.
- All patients have a right to be catheterized by someone of their own sex (Robinson, 2004).

> **Nursing Alert**
>
> Parental presence: A parent or guardian should always be present with their child during the procedure (Robson *et al.*, 2006). Parental presence during invasive procedures has been shown to reduce a child's anxiety (Messeri *et al.*, 2004).

Selecting a catheter

When selecting a urinary catheter two aspects must be considered: firstly the type of catheter required and secondly the size of the catheter required. The type of catheter required will depend on the reason for the catheter insertion. The most common type of indwelling catheter is the Foley catheter. The Foley catheter is retained in the bladder by means of a balloon system. The balloon is located at the tip of the catheter and is inflated with sterile water, thus preventing it from falling out of the bladder. The balloons typically come in two different sizes: 5 cc and 30 cc. Foley catheters are most commonly made of silicone rubber or natural rubber.

Urinary catheters are made from various materials, the most common of which are rubber, silicone, PVC plastic, or Teflon. Rubber catheters or latex-coated catheters should be avoided for children who have latex allergies. Children with chronic illnesses are more susceptible to latex allergy (Sapan *et al.*, 2002). Latex allergy or sensitivity can cause uriticaria, contact dermatitis, asthma, and in severe cases anaphylaxis. Research has shown that there is no consensus in relation to the size and type of catheter to use in the paediatric population (Bray & Sanders, 2006; Smith, 2003; Smith & Adams, 1998).

Charrière (Ch) is the measurement used to express catheter diameter. The smallest diameter catheter that will effectively empty the bladder should be used (Pellowe *et al.*, 2001). Cost should be the least consideration when selecting a catheter (Smith, 2003). Feeding tubes are

Table 11.3 Recommended catheter sizes for paediatric patients

Age in years	Charrière (Ch) size
0–2	6
2–5	6–8
5–10	8–10
10–16	10–12

not recommended for urinary catheterization (Bowden & Smith Greenberg, 2008; Smith, 2003; Carlson & Mowery, 1997) as they have a tendency to knot easily and can cause patient harm. **Table 11.3** indicates the recommended catheter size for paediatric patients (Bowden & Smith Greenberg, 2008; Bray & Sanders, 2006).

Important aspects of care

- Due to the invasive nature of catheterization you will want to carry out the procedure as swiftly as possible. It is useful to have a second nurse to assist you with the procedure. Parents must not be used as helpers (Henderson & Leitch, 2006) because their only role is to comfort their child.
- If catheterizing a girl and no urine is obtained, it is likely that the vagina was accessed. In this instance you should leave the catheter in place and ask for a second catheter to be opened for you. This will ensure that the vagina is not accessed a second time.
- Ensure that you have a selection of catheters available at hand in case of contamination during the procedure.
- All catheters should be inserted gently to decrease pain and discomfort for the child.
- When inserting any catheter, if you experience difficulty stop and seek medical help.
- Ensure that there are no kinks in the tubing before securing the drainage bag to prevent complications.
- Before emptying a catheter bag, wash your hands with antibacterial soap and don a pair of non-sterile gloves (Bray & Sanders, 2006).
- It is recommended that the catheter tap is cleaned with an alcohol swab before and after emptying (Mallett & Dougherty, 2000).

- Drainage bags should be changed every five to seven days (Bray & Sanders, 2006).
- The longer a urinary catheter is in place, the greater the risk of the child developing a urinary tract infection (Curran, 2001). Observe for signs and symptoms of infection in the catheterized child.
- A child with an indwelling urinary catheter may experience bladder spasms. These are caused when the trigone of the bladder is irritated by the presence of the urinary catheter balloon. Bladder spasms cause significant distress for the child and their family and must be identified and treated. Antimuscarinic drugs can reduce the incidence of bladder spasms; however, these medications have significant side effects such as dry mouth, constipation, dry skin, flushed face, and sleep disturbances (British National Formulary (BNF), 2008).

Procedure: Insertion of a urinary catheter

Equipment

- Trolley.
- Sterile catheterization pack.
- Sterile gloves.
- Disposable pad.
- Selection of appropriate catheters.
- Anaesthetic lubricating gel.
- Sterile water.
- Syringe and needle.
- Drainage bag and stand.
- Disposable apron.

Documentation

Documentation after the insertion of a urinary catheter is essential to maintain continuity of care for the child and family. **Box 11.4** outlines the details that should be documented post-catheter insertion. It would also be advisable to document how the child tolerated the procedure in case they require the procedure again in the future.

Step-by-step guide to inserting a urinary catheter

Step	Rationale
1 Wash hands.	Prevents the spread of micro-organisms.
2 Prepare sterile trolley and wash hands again.	Preparation is the key to success and ensures an organized approach to the procedure of catheterization.
3 Draw curtains around the child's bed or close the door into the child's room.	Ensures privacy and dignity of the child.
4 Raise the bed to a comfortable height.	Prevents back injury.
5 Put on an apron and apply sterile gloves.	Reduces spread of micro-organisms.
6 Ensure that the child is positioned comfortably. Girls: ask them to lie supine with their legs in a 'frog leg' position (Robson et al., 2006). Boys: ask them to lie supine. Place a rolled towel under their knees and ensure that the penis and scrotum are raised up onto the thighs.	If the child is comfortable there will be a greater chance of a successful catheterization. The 'frog leg' position permits the nurse to visualize the labia. Permits the nurse to visualize the glans penis and promotes comfort for the child.
7 Place the drape over the genital area. Place disposable pad under the child's bottom.	The drape will obscure the child's view of the procedure and this may be helpful (Robson et al., 2006). Prevents possible soiling of the child's bed.
8 Apply topical anaesthetic lubricating gel: • Girls: gently separate the labia. Apply gel around the perimeatal area or place some gel onto a cotton gauze and place on the perineal area (Robson et al., 2006). • Boys over three years: gently introduce tip of the applicator onto urethra. Squeeze applicator to instil gel into the penis as per manufacturer's instructions. Gently squeeze the dorsal penis for 2–3 minutes to hold gel in place (Algren & Arnow, 2007; Robson et al., 2006). • Boys under three: place several drops of anaesthetic gel at the urethral meatus and leave for 3 minutes.	Algren & Arnow (2007) and Bardsley (2005) advocate the use of topical anaesthetic lubricating gel because research has proven that it reduces the procedural pain experienced by children who undergo urethral catheterization. Lubricant gel needs 3–5 minutes to become effective (Bray & Sanders, 2006).

9 Cleanse the urethral meatus with sterile saline on sterile gauze (Bray & Sanders, 2006; Smith, 2003).
- Girls: gently separate the labia majora with the finger and thumb of the non-dominant hand. Cleanse both sides of the labia from front to back using a separate cotton ball or gauze piece.
- Boys: with the non-dominant hand gently retract the foreskin and clean around the entire surface of the glans penis. Dry the area and replace the foreskin.

Research has shown that there is no advantage of using an antiseptic preparation for cleansing the urethral meatus before catheterization (Department of Health, 2001).

10 Remove soiled gloves, wash hands, and re-glove.

Prevents contamination.

11 Smear lubrication gel onto the appropriate size of catheter and gently insert the catheter into the urethra. See Figure 11.4.
Have the connecting end of the catheter placed in a sterile container and wait for urine to flow out.

Facilitates ease of insertion.

This will allow for specimen collection for culture.

12 Once urine flows out insert the catheter a further 2 cm into the urethra.
Inflate balloon with sterile water (Bray & Sanders, 2006; Bardsley, 2005) as per the manufacturer's instructions.

Gently tug on the catheter.

To allow room for the balloon to be inflated. Sterile NaCl is not used because it can cause crystallization in the inflation channel and difficulty in deflating the balloon (Bardsley, 2005).
This will ensure that the catheter is securely in place in the bladder.

13 Once the catheter is in place the sterile drainage bag should be connected.

Maintaining a closed system prevents contamination and possible infection (Tew *et al.*, 2005; Department of Health, 2001). Nurses have a key role to play in maintaining a closed urinary drainage system (Win, 1996).

14 Attach the drainage bag to the stand and hang at the bedside below the level of the bladder.

Once positioned below the level of the bladder, gravity will aid urine drainage.

15 Return child's bed to appropriate level.

Reduces possible risk of injury.

16 Dispose of equipment as per local hospital policy.

Prevents spread of micro-organisms.

17 Remove the gloves and apron. Dispose of as per local hospital policy.

Prevents spread of micro-organisms.

18 Praise and reassure the child and family.

This promotes a positive feeling of well-being.

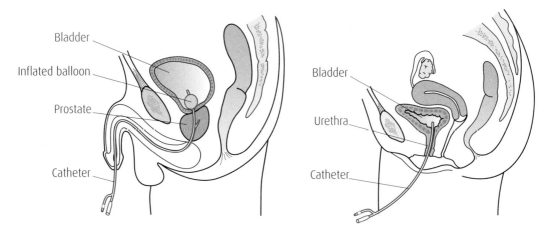

Figure 11.4 Insertion of a urinary catheter

Box 11.4 Recommended documentation post-insertion of urinary catheter

- Catheter size.
- Batch number.
- Catheter type.
- Amount of water inserted into balloon.
- Date and time of insertion.
- Consent gained.
- Analgesia administered.

(Simpson, 2001)

Removal of urinary catheter

Removal of the urinary catheter should occur as soon as the child's condition permits.

- Explain to the child in age-appropriate language, and to the parent/s, that the catheter must be removed.
- Position child as per catheter insertion.
- Place a disposable pad under the child's buttocks to prevent soiling of the bed.
- Remove the correct amount of water from the balloon with a syringe. Check the documentation and the catheter itself to see how much water was inserted into the balloon.
- Gently pull on the catheter to remove.
- If you experience resistance, stop and seek medical help.

- Reassure child and parent/s.
- Dispose of catheter as per hospital policy for clinical waste management.
- Document the child's first void post-catheter removal.

Percutaneous renal biopsy

A percutaneous renal biopsy is a procedure performed to determine the underlying cause and extent of renal disease. It is performed when the person develops unexplained acute renal failure, persistent protein or blood in the urine, or kidney transplant rejection/failure (Richard, 2001; Roebuck, 2001). A biopsy needle is inserted through the skin and kidney tissue is removed for study by microscopy.

A renal biopsy in children is either performed using local anaesthesia with sedation, or short-acting general anaesthesia (Hicklin & DeSousa, 1997; Nammalwar *et al.*, 2006). According to Hicklin & DeSousa (1997), general anaesthesia is more commonly used in younger children, while local anaesthesia and sedation is used in older children. Renal biopsy may also be performed on an inpatient or day case basis (Mahon & Hattersley, 2002; Hussain *et al.*, 2003).

11.13 Preparation for percutaneous renal biopsy Ⓐ

This is an advanced skill. You _must_ check whether you can assist with or undertake any aspect of this skill, in line with local policy.

Prior to providing consent for renal biopsy, the child and family should receive information about the procedure and have all their questions and concerns addressed by healthcare providers. Percutaneous renal biopsy is usually successful but there are potential risks, which need to be discussed with the family. Since the biopsy needle is passed into a highly vascular organ, there is the possibility of bleeding (Nammalwar _et al._, 2006). The extent of the bleeding can range from mild haematuria to prolonged and severe bleeding requiring blood transfusion and possible surgery. Other serious complications include injury to other internal organs and damage to the biopsied kidney (Nammalwar _et al._, 2006).

On the day of admission, the nurse should introduce him/herself to the child and family and orientate them to the ward environment and the child's allocated bed space. The nursing admission should be completed and the child's baseline observations and weight should be recorded. Percutaneous renal biopsy is considered unsafe if a bleeding disorder is present, or if the child is hypertensive. These complications significantly increase the risk of haemorrhage in the biopsied kidney (Mukhtar _et al._, 2005). Therefore, any abnormalities in vital signs should be reported to the medical team responsible for the child's care. In addition, various blood tests should be taken including a coagulation screen, full blood count, group and save, and full biochemical and immunology profile.

The nurse should assess whether the child has been fasting for the specified amount of time. It is now accepted that children should not be fasted overnight prior to procedures and that a minimum fasting period of two hours may be sufficient (Meurling, 2004). However, it is important to be aware of hospital policy on fasting before informing parents of the fasting period for their child. If the biopsy is performed using local anaesthesia, it is beneficial to teach the child to practise deep breathing and breath-holding prior to the procedure. If the patient can cooperate with breath-holding on demand, the risk

of misplacement of the sharp biopsy needle is reduced (Mahon & Hattersley, 2002).

Immediately prior to the procedure, encourage the child to empty his/her bladder. Ensure that the child's name and hospital number are correct and legible on the wrist band. Ensure premedication is administered correctly as prescribed. Ensure that the child's case notes, X-rays (if applicable), and nursing documentation are present. Confirm that the consent form has been completed and signed. If there is a delay with the procedure, it is important to keep the parents informed to reduce stress and anxiety.

The child and family should also be informed of the care interventions that will be provided following the renal biopsy. For instance, the child will be maintained on bed rest for up to 24 hours (Mahon & Hattersley, 2002; Nammalwar _et al._, 2006). However, this duration may vary depending on the length of the child's stay in hospital, and whether the child receives local or general anaesthesia during the procedure. It is necessary to refer to the hospital policy to get specific information related to these issues. The nurse will frequently monitor the child's vital signs and check the biopsy wound site for bleeding. Analgesics will be administered for the relief of pain. If fluid restrictions are not required, the child will be encouraged to drink liberal amounts of water to dilute the urine and prevent clots forming in the kidney (Richard, 2001). Urinalysis will be carried out to monitor for blood in the urine.

The parents should be prepared for what to expect when they take the child home after the biopsy. They must monitor the child for signs and symptoms of infection, persistent blood in the urine, and/or persistent pain (Richard, 2001; Mahon & Hattersley, 2002). The parents must be advised to contact the ward in the event that these complications occur. The child must not be allowed to participate in strenuous activity for two weeks following renal biopsy.

Sometimes percutaneous renal biopsy is considered unsafe and open laparascopic kidney biopsy is performed (Mukhtar _et al._, 2005). In this procedure, surgery is performed, the kidney is exposed, and the biopsy needle is inserted into the kidney. The preparation of the patient for an open/laparoscopic renal biopsy is similar to any major abdominal surgery and also incorporates the preparation for a percutaneous renal biopsy (Richard, 2001).

Renal replacement therapy

11.14 **Renal replacement therapy** 🔺

This is an advanced skill. You *must* check whether you can assist with or undertake any aspect of this skill, in line with local policy.

The care of children with end stage renal disease (ESRD) has improved dramatically as a result of the technological advances in renal replacement therapies. The primary modalities of renal replacement therapy are dialysis and kidney transplantation. Within this section, the two modalities of renal replacement therapy will be discussed, beginning with dialysis therapy.

Dialysis therapy

The excretion of metabolic waste products and body fluids decreases as a result of renal disease. The accumulation of fluid and other harmful substances in the child's blood can lead to serious and sometimes life-threatening consequences, including pulmonary oedema, convulsions, coma, and cardiac arrhythmia (Gruskin *et al.*, 1992). Dialysis is a process where the excess fluid and toxic substances in the child's blood are removed, thus maintaining excretory function and prolonging life. There are two types of dialysis therapy: peritoneal dialysis therapy and haemodialysis therapy.

Peritoneal dialysis therapy

During peritoneal dialysis, the peritoneal membrane is used as a natural filter to remove toxic substances and fluid from the child's blood. The peritoneum is a membrane lining the abdominal wall, the liver, stomach, and intestines. The peritoneal cavity, which exists within this membrane, can hold large volumes of fluid making it suitable for dialysis.

There are two main types of peritoneal dialysis: continuous ambulatory peritoneal dialysis (CAPD) and automated peritoneal dialysis (APD). Both forms of peritoneal dialysis are managed independently by the child and

family at home. CAPD is a manual procedure, which involves the instillation of a dialysis solution into the peritoneal cavity via a peritoneal catheter.

A peritoneal catheter is surgically created through the child's abdomen to allow the instillation of the dialysis solution. A proportion of the catheter tubing lies outside the child's abdomen allowing for connection/disconnection of the dialysis solution to the catheter. Therefore, the catheter must always be securely fixed to the child's abdomen to avoid pulling and trauma on the exit site. The dialysis solution is left to dwell in the peritoneum, allowing dialysis to take place. The dialysis fluid is then drained away with the excess toxins and fluid from the child's blood. The CAPD process is usually repeated four times a day (Rees *et al.*, 2007).

Automated peritoneal dialysis (APD) requires a machine, which repeatedly inserts and drains the dialysis solution to and from the peritoneal cavity. APD is the preferred method of peritoneal dialysis for children because the therapy is undertaken at night while the child sleeps.

Complications of peritoneal dialysis

The most common complication associated with peritoneal dialysis is peritonitis (infection of the peritoneum) (Rees *et al.*, 2007; Li *et al.*, 2008). Peritonitis can occur during connection/disconnection of the dialysis bag or dialysis cycler machine, or by damage to the dialysis line. It may also occur if the tunnel of the dialysis catheter or exit site is infected (Rees *et al.*, 2007). The child and family should inspect the exit site and catheter each day. They must also be advised to contact the hospital immediately if the child complains of stomach pain, fever, or diarrhoea.

For more information on the treatment of children with kidney disease please follow the link below:
http://www.aakp.org/aakp-library/Dialysis-Centers-Accommodate-Children/
For information on treatment methods for kidney failure in children, please follow the link below:
http://kidney.niddk.nih.gov/kudiseases/pubs/childkidneydiseases/treatment_methods/

Haemodialysis therapy

During haemodialysis therapy, the child's blood is circulated outside the body through a dialyser (artificial kidney). The dialyser acts as a semi-permeable membrane, which allows the passage of water and toxic substances out of the child's bloodstream during dialysis. Once the water and solutes are removed, the blood is returned to the patient via the venous blood system. There are two types of dialyser: parallel flow (plate), and hollow fibre. Hollow fibre dialysers are preferable for children because they are developed to hold relatively small volumes of blood (Montagnino & Hockenberry, 2007). In order for haemodialysis therapy to be performed, access to the child's circulatory system is required. This allows the passage of the child's blood through the dialyser or artificial kidney during treatment.

Vascular access

An arterio-venous fistula is the preferred mode of vascular access for children with ESRD because it provides a more long-term form of vascular access. A fistula involves the surgical anastomosis (joining) of an artery to a vein. This allows arterial blood to flow through the vein, causing it to enlarge and expand. If the child's vessels are inadequate for an arterio-venous fistula, a synthetic graft may be formed. A graft involves the implantation of a small piece of synthetic tubing between an artery and a vein. Once the fistula or graft is given time to 'mature' or develop, two needles can be inserted to allow access to the child's circulation during haemodialysis therapy. The size of some children's blood vessels makes it difficult to create a fistula or graft. Therefore, a catheter is inserted into a central vein to allow immediate access to the bloodstream.

Complications of haemodialysis therapy

There may be various complications associated with haemodialysis therapy in children. For instance, complications such as infection and thrombosis (clotting) can occur in the child's vascular access. Therefore, the child and family must be taught to keep the access clean and to recognize the signs and symptoms of infection, such as fever and/or pain, heat, redness, and swelling in the access.

The child and family must be advised to avoid venepunctures and blood pressure measurements in the fistula/graft arm. They must also be taught to check the 'thrill' or pulsating sensation that can be felt when the fistula/graft is palpated. This pulsation of blood through the access is always present in a functioning fistula and

graft. The child must avoid sleeping on the access arm and also avoid wearing anything tight or restrictive on the arm, e.g. jewellery, watch, or bandages.

The exit site of a central venous catheter should be covered with a non-occlusive dressing and should be inspected regularly by the child and family. The catheter should be taped to the skin to prevent pulling. The end ports and clamps should also be taped to prevent accidental disconnection. When taking a bath or shower, the catheter should be protected from water and not immersed (Wright, 2004). Some activities, such as sport, must be avoided to prevent accidental dislodgement of the catheter. In the event that complications occur in the child's access, the family should be told to contact the hospital immediately for advice.

There are acute complications that occur during the haemodialysis procedure itself, which include hypotension, cramps, nausea, and vomiting (Challinor, 1998; Turner, 1998; Kotanko & Levin, 2008). It is important that the child's vital signs, such as blood pressure, pulse, and respiratory rate, are monitored frequently throughout the treatment to prevent and manage these complications.

The insertion of needles into an arterio-venous fistula or graft can be very distressing for children. Furthermore, the need to regularly attend the hospital makes haemodialysis therapy a particularly restrictive treatment. Some children may find it difficult to spend long hours attached to the haemodialysis machine. Therefore, to prevent boredom and ensure the child's cooperation, diversionary activities must be provided during the treatment. For further information about the support available to children who suffer from kidney disease please follow the links below:

http://www.ika.ie/
http://www.thechildrenskidneyfoundation.org/
http://www.kidskidneyresearch.org/
http://www.kidney.org.uk/links.html

Kidney transplantation

Kidney transplantation is the most effective treatment for children with ESRD (Rees *et al.*, 2007). Children may be referred for transplantation at different stages in the illness trajectory. It is more suitable for children to receive a kidney transplant within the six-month period prior to commencing dialysis therapy (Rees *et al.*, 2007). This is known as pre-emptive transplantation. However, it may not be possible to perform pre-emptive transplantation on all children as this procedure depends on the availability of donor organs, severity of renal disease at the time of presentation, underlying cause of renal disease, and the suitability of the child for transplantation (Ward, 2002). Therefore, the child who is unable to receive a pre-emptive kidney transplant must commence either haemodialysis or peritoneal dialysis therapy prior to receiving a kidney transplant.

11.15 **Preparing a child for kidney transplantation** Ⓐ

This is an advanced skill. You *must* check whether you can assist with or undertake any aspect of this skill, in line with local policy.

There are several issues that need to be discussed with the child and family prior to kidney transplantation. It is important that the nurse communicates effectively to ensure their questions and concerns about the process of transplantation are addressed. Repeating information about transplantation to the child and family on a regular basis is also essential to ensure that information is reinforced and misunderstandings are rectified.

The various types of donation must be discussed in detail with the family to allow them to decide which is most appropriate to their circumstances. For instance, the majority of kidney transplants are obtained from cadaveric donation (Franklin, 2002). These donors are patients who have suffered irreversible brain stem damage and cannot survive without a ventilator. Living-related donation involves a relative donating one of their kidneys to the child with ESRD (Montagnino & Hockenberry, 2007). Living non-related donation involves a person who is not biologically related to the patient donating one of their kidneys, e.g. spouse or close friend. There are ethical issues that may arise in the case of live donation. While it is beneficial for the recipient to receive a kidney transplant, the potential complications that may occur to the donor have to be considered and discussed in detail. Thus,

the physical and psychological health of the donor and the motivation behind their decision to donate must be rigorously assessed before proceeding with transplantation.

The potential benefits of kidney transplantation should be discussed with the family. According to Rees *et al.* (2007), the disruptions in lifestyle, schooling, and social activities created by dialysis are alleviated by a kidney transplant. The dietary and fluid restrictions associated with the treatment are avoided. The child's health status, growth, and development are improved. In addition, mortality is lower for children after transplantation than on dialysis (Rees *et al.*, 2007).

The child and family should also be fully informed about the potential risks and disadvantages of kidney transplantation. For instance, the survival rates for kidney transplantation should be highlighted. According to Kidney Research UK (2006), the survival rate for cadaveric kidney transplants is 85–90% at one year, 70% at five years, and 50% at 15 years, while the survival rate for live donor kidney transplants is 90–95% at one year, 80% at five years, and 60% at 15 years.

The child and family should be made aware of the general complications associated with any major surgery, such as bleeding, infection, and wounds. The immunosuppressive drugs required for transplantation and their side effects must be discussed in detail with the child and family. While immunosuppressive medication is necessary to avoid rejection of the kidney transplant, these drugs create unpleasant side effects, such as growth failure, obesity, acne, and changes in facial features. Non-adherence with drug therapy is a major cause of illness and transplant failure, especially in adolescents (Rees *et al.*, 2007). The most common reason for non-compliance is the distressing side effects of the immunosuppressive medication (Montagnino & Hockenberry, 2007). Therefore, it is essential that the child and family are well prepared for these side effects to ensure effective outcomes in the post-transplant stage. The possibility of kidney transplant rejection must be discussed with the child and family. They must also be informed of the potential risk of malignancy and infections (bacterial, viral, and fungal) following transplantation (Rees *et al.*, 2007).

Once the family decide to proceed with transplantation, blood tests are taken for blood group and tissue typing. The child's routine immunization schedule is completed. The child's immunity status to viruses associated with significant complications post-transplantation, e.g. cytomegalovirus, Epstein-Barr virus, and varicella (chicken pox), is assessed (DeSousa & Ward, 1998). A dental check including advice about dental hygiene is arranged for the child. During this transplant 'work-up' period, the nurse will have time to reiterate information about kidney transplantation, and address the concerns and anxieties of the child and family. A tour of the transplant unit should be organized to allow them to meet with healthcare professionals who will be involved in the child's care.

When the pre-transplant preparation is complete, the child will be 'on call' for a cadaver kidney or a date will be arranged for a live donor transplant (DeSousa & Ward, 1998). Waiting times for cadaver transplants are impossible to predict. Therefore, Franklin (2002) emphasizes the need to inform the child and family that the transplant waiting list is different to other hospital waiting lists. The waiting list for a transplant is not merely based on their name reaching the top of the list, but on finding a suitable donor match.

The final surgical preparation and checklist of the child for kidney transplantation is essentially the same as that used for any child prior to surgery. In addition, a final cross match is performed to ensure the suitability of the donor kidney. To exclude infection, most units take swabs of skin, nose, throat, exit sites of peritoneal catheters, and central venous catheters (Terrill, 2002). Preoperative dialysis may also be required if the child has excess fluid or has elevated potassium levels (hyperkalaemia).

The process of kidney transplantation may have a significant impact on the psychosocial functioning of the child, which subsequently impacts on the entire family. Therefore, continual psychosocial support for the child and family is central to the overall success of this treatment for ESRD.

Conclusion

Altered renal function can be extremely problematic for the child and their family. Nurses working with children need to have evidence-based knowledge and skills in order to be able to care effectively for the child or young person with renal dysfunction. This chapter has comprehensively covered several aspects of this particular care,

and provides you as a student with an insight into the requirements of a children's nurse who is knowledgeable and skilled in relation to all aspects of renal dysfunction. Through using this information, together with local policy guidelines, adequate child and family preparation, and a family centred approach, it is anticipated that the family will be fully supported through what could be quite a traumatic experience for both child and family, and that good nursing care will have a positive and lasting effect on the child and their family.

Online resource centre

You may find it helpful to work through our online resources including interactive scenarios intended to help you to develop and apply the skills in this chapter. Where material referenced below is available electronically, we're pleased to provide active web links to the source via 🌐 **http:// www.oxfordtextbooks.co.uk/orc/coyne/**

References

Alam, M.T., Coulter, J.B., Pacheco, J., *et al.* (2005) Comparison of urine contamination rates using three different methods of collection: clean-catch, cotton wool pad and urine bag. *Ann Trop Paediatr* **25**, 29–34.

Algren, C.L. & Arnow, D. (2007) Pediatric variations of nursing interventions. In M.J. Hockenberry & D. Wilson (eds.) *Wong's Nursing Care of Infants and Children.* Missouri: Mosby.

Austin, B.J., Bollard, C. & Gunn, T.R. (1999) Is urethral catheterization a successful alternative to suprapubic aspiration in neonates? *Journal of Paediatrics and Child Health* **35**, 34–36.

Bardsley, A. (2005) Use of lubricant gels in urinary catheterisation. *Nursing Standard* **20** (8), 41–46.

Bayer Diagnostics Europe (2004) *Practical guide to urine analysis.* Newbury, Berkshire: Bayer Healthcare.

Bowden, V.R. & Smith Greenberg, C. (2008) *Pediatric Nursing Procedures, 2nd ed.* Philadelphia: Lippincott Williams & Wilkins.

Bray, L. & Sanders, C. (2006) Nursing management of paediatric urethral catheterisation. *Nursing Standard* **20** (24), 51–60.

British National Formulary (2008) *British National Formulary No. 53*. London: BMJ Publishing Group LTD & Royal Pharmaceutical Society of Great Britain.

Carlson, D. & Mowery, B.D. (1997) Standards to prevent complications of urinary catheterization in children: Should and should nots. *JSPN* **2** (1), 37–41.

Challinor, P. (1998) Complications of haemodialysis. In P. Challinor & J. Sedgewick (eds.) *Principles and Practice of Renal Nursing*. Cheltenham: Stanley Thornes.

Chambers, M. (2008) Therapeutic play in hospital. In J. Kelsey & G. McEwing (eds.) *Clinical Skills in Child Health Practice*. Edinburgh: Elsevier.

Chu, R.W., Wong, Y.C., Luk, S.H., & Wong, S.N. (2002) Comparing suprapubic urine aspiration under real-time ultrasound guidance with conventional blind aspiration. *Acta Paediatr* **91**, 512–516.

Collins Pellatt, G. (2007) Urinary elimination: Part 2—retention, incontinence and catheterization. *British Journal of Nursing* **16** (8), 480–485.

Cook, R. (1996) Urinalysis: Ensuring accurate urine testing. RCN Continuing Education. *Nursing Standard* **10** (46), 49–52.

Curran, E. (2001) Reducing the risk of health care acquired infection. *Nursing Standard* **16** (1), 45–52.

Department of Health (2001) Guidelines for preventing infections associated with the insertion and maintenance of short-term indwelling urethral catheters in acute care. *Journal of Hospital Infection* **47**, Suppl, S39–S46.

DeSousa, M. & Ward, G. (1998) Renal failure in childhood and adolescence. In P. Challinor & J. Sedgewick (eds.) *Principles and Practice of Renal Nursing*. Cheltenham: Stanley Thornes.

Farrell, M., Devine, K., Lancaster, G., & Judd, B. (2002) A method comparison study to assess the reliability of urine collection pads as a means of obtaining urine specimens from non-toilet-trained children for microbiological examination. *Journal of Advanced Nursing* **37**, 387–393.

Franklin, P.M. (2002) Renal transplantation. In N. Thomas (ed.) *Renal Nursing, 2nd ed*. London: Bailliere Tindall.

Gochman, R.F., Karasic, R.B., & Heller, M.B. (1991) Use of portable ultrasound to assist urine collection by suprapubic aspiration. *Ann Emerg Med* **20**, 631–635.

Gruskin, A., Baluarte, H., & Dabbagh, S. (1992) Haemodialysis and peritoneal dialysis. In C. Edelmann (ed.) *Paediatric Kidney Disease, 2nd ed*. Boston: Little Brown & Co.

Harris, A. (2004) Toilet training children with learning difficulties: What the literature tells us. *British Journal of Nursing*. **13** (13), 773–777.

Henderson, M. & Leitch, K. (2006) Urine testing and urinary catheterisation. In E. Trigg, S. Huband, & T.A. Mohammed (eds.) *Practices in Children's Nursing: Guidelines for Hospital and Community*. Churchill Livingstone, London.

Hicklin, M. & De Sousa, M. (1997) Children with renal problems. In T. Smith (ed.) *Renal Nursing*. London: Bailliere Tindall.

Higgins, C. (2007) *Understanding laboratory investigations: For nurses and health professionals, 2nd ed*. Oxford: Blackwell Publishing.

Hussain, F., Watson, A.R., Hayes, J., & Evans, J. (2003) Standards for renal biopsies: Comparison of inpatient and day care procedures. *Pediatric Nephrology* **18**, 53.

Jansson, U.B., Danielson, E., & Hellstrom, A.L. (2008) Parents' experiences of their children achieving bladder control. *Journal of Pediatric Nursing* **23** (6), 471–478.

Jodal, U. (2002) Suprapubic aspiration of urine in the diagnosis of urinary tract infection in infants. *Acta Paediatr* **91**, 497–498.

Kaefer, M., Zurakowski, D., Bauer, S.B., *et al*. (1997) Estimating normal bladder capacity in children. *The Journal of Urology* **158** (6), 2261–2264.

Kanneh, A.B. (2006) Caring for children with body fluid and electrolyte imbalance. In A. Glasper & J. Richardson (eds.) *A Textbook of Children's and Young People's Nursing*. Edinburgh: Elsevier.

Kidney Research UK (2006) *Kidney Health Information: Kidney Transplantation*. Available at: **http://kidneyresearchuk.org/content/view/256/321/**

Kotanko, P. & Levin, N.W. (2008) Common clinical problems during haemodialysis. In A.R. Nissenson & R.N. Fine (eds.) *Handbook of Dialysis Therapy, 4th ed*. Philadelphia: Saunders Elsevier.

Lewis, J. (1998) Clean-catch versus urine collection pads: A prospective trial. *Paediatrics Nursing* **10**, 15–16.

Li, P.K.T., Leung, C.B. & Szeto, C.C. (2008) Peritonitis in peritoneal dialysis patients. In A.R. Nissenson & R.N. Fine (eds.) *Handbook of Dialysis Therapy, 4th ed.* Philadelphia: Saunders Elsevier.

Liaw, L.C., Nayar, D.M., Pedler, S.J., & Coulthard, M.G. (2000) Home collection of urine for culture from infants by three methods: Survey of parents' preferences and bacterial contamination rates. *BMJ* **320**, 1312–1313.

Mahon, A. & Hattersley, J. (2002) Investigations in renal failure. In N. Thomas (ed.) *Renal Nursing, 2nd ed.* London: Bailliere Tindall.

Mallett, J. & Dougherty, L. (2000) *The Royal Marsden Hospital Manual of Clinical Nursing Procedures, 5th ed.* Oxford: Blackwell Science.

Marieb, E., & Hoehn, K. (2008) *Anatomy and Physiology.* USA: Pearson Benjamin Cummings.

Melamed, B.G. & Seigal, L.A. (1975) Reduction of anxiety in children facing hospitalisation and surgery by use of filmed modeling. *Journal of Consulting and Clinical Psychology* **42** (940), 511–521.

Messeri, A., Caprilli, S., & Busoni, P. (2004) Anaesthesia induction in children: A psychological evaluation of the efficiency of parents' presence. *Paediatric Anaesthesia* **14** (7), 551–556.

Meurling, S. (2004) Paediatric aspects: No fasting in children? *Scandinavian Journal of Nutrition* **48**, 83.

McFarlane, K. (2006) Caring for children with genito-urinary problems. In A. Glasper & J. Richardson (eds.) *A Textbook of Children's and Young People's Nursing.* Edinburgh: Elsevier.

McFarlane, P. I., Houghton, C., & Hughes, C. (1999) Pad urine collection for early childhood urinary-tract infection. *The Lancet* **354**, 571.

Montagnino, B.A. & Hockenberry, M.J. (2007) The child with renal dysfunction. In M.J. Hockenberry & D. Wilson (eds.) *Wong's Nursing Care of Infants and Children, 8th ed.* Missouri: Mosby Elsevier.

Mukhtar, Z., Steinbrecher, H., Gilbert, R.D., & Deshpande, P.V. (2005) Laparoscopic renal biopsy in obese children. *Pediatric Nephrology* **20**, 495–498.

Nammalwar, B., Vijayakumar, M., & Prahlad, N. (2006) Experience of renal biopsy in children with nephrotic syndrome. *Pediatric Nephrology* **21**, 286–288.

National Institute for Health and Clinical Excellence (2007) *Urinary Tract Infections in Children: Diagnosis, Treatment and Long-term Management.* Available at: **http://guidance.nice.org.uk/CG054** (last accessed August 2009).

Nursing Standard Quick Reference Guide (1999) Urine testing. *Nursing Standard* **13** (50).

Owen, D., Vidal-Alaball, J., Mansour, M., Bordeaux, K., Jones, K.V., & Edwards, A. (2003) Parents' opinions on the diagnosis of children under 2 years of age with urinary tract infection. *Fam Pract* **20**, 531–537.

Pellowe, C., Loveday, H., Harper, P., Robinson, N., & Pratt, R. (2001) Preventing infections from short-term indwelling catheters. *Nursing Times* **97** (14), 34–35.

Rao, S., Bhatt, J., Houghton, C., & MacFarlane, P. (2004) An improved urine collection pad method: A randomised clinical trial. *Arch Dis Child* **89**, 773–775.

Rees, L., Webb, N.J.A., & Brogan, P.A. (2007) *Paediatric Nephrology.* Oxford: Oxford University Press.

Richard, C.J. (2001) Assessment of renal structure and function. In L.E. Lancaster (ed.) *American Nephrology Nurses' Association: Core curriculum for nephrology nursing, 4th ed.* New Jersey: Anthony J Jannetti.

Robinson, J. (2001) Urethral catheter selection. *Nursing Standard* **15** (25), 39–42.

Robinson, J. (2004) A practical approach to catheter associated problems. *Nursing Standard* **18** (31), 38–42.

Robson, W.L.M., Leung, A.K.C., & Thomason, M.A. (2006) Catheterization of the bladder in infants and children. *Clinical Pediatrics* **45**, 795.

Roebuck, D. (2001) Paediatric interventional radiology. *Imaging* **13**, 302–320.

Ross, J.H. (2000) Urinary tract infections: 2000 update. *Am Fam Physician* **62**, 1777–1780.

Sapan, N., Nacarkucuk, E, Canitez, Y., & Saglam, H. (2002) Evaluation of the need for routine pre-operative latex allergy tests in children. *Pediatrics International* **44** (2), 157–162.

Senior, J. (2001) Clean intermittent self-catheterisation and children. *British Journal of Community Nursing* **6** (8), 381–386.

Simpson, L. (2001) Indwelling urethral catheters. *Nursing Standard* **15** (46), 47–53.

Smith, A.B. & Adams, L.L. (1998) Insertion of indwelling urinary catheters in infants and children: A survey of current practice. *Paediatric Nursing* **24** (3), 229–234.

Smith, L. (2003) Which catheter? Criteria for selection of urinary catheters for children. *Paediatric Nursing* **15** (30), 14–18.

Steggall, M.J. (2007) Urine samples and urinalysis. *Nursing Standard* **22** (14), 14–16.

Terrill, B. (2002) *Renal Nursing—A practical approach.* Melbourne: Ausmed Publications.

Tew, L., Pomfret, I., & King, D. (2005) Infection risks associated with urinary catheters. *Nursing Standard* **20** (7), 55–61.

Torrance, C. & Elley, K. (1992) Urine testing—1. Observation. *Nursing Times* **88** (5) Continence Supplement, 64.

Turner, K. (1998) Complications and nursing interventions associated with peritoneal dialysis. In P. Challinor & J. Sedgewick (eds.) *Principles and Practice of Renal Nursing.* Cheltenham: Stanley Thornes.

Vaillancourt, S., McGillivray, D., Zhang, X., & Kramer, M.S. (2007) To clean or not to clean: Effect on contamination rates in midstream urine collections in toilet-trained children. *Pediatrics* **119**, 1288–1293.

Van der Voort, J., Edwards, A., Roberts, R., & Verrier Jones, K. (1997) The struggle to diagnose UTI in children under two in primary care. *Fam Pract* **14**, 44–48.

Ward, G. (2002) Renal care in childhood and adolescence. In N. Thomas (ed.) *Renal Nursing, 2nd ed.* London: Bailliere Tindall.

Wilson, L.A. (2005) Urinalysis. *Nursing Standard* **19** (35), 51–54.

Win, C. (1996) Basing catheter care on research principles. *Nursing Standard* **10** (18), 38–40.

Wright, E. (2004) Assessment and management of the child requiring chronic haemodialysis. *Paediatric Nursing* **16**, 37–41.

Zickler, C.F. & Richardson, V. (2004) Achieving continence in children with neurogenic bowel and bladder. *Journal of Pediatric Health Care* **18**, 276–283.

Further reading and URLs

Trigg, E. & Mohammed, T.A. (eds.) *Practices in Children's Nursing: Guidelines for hospital and community.* China: Churchill Livingstone.

http://www.le.ac.uk/pa/teach/va/anatomy/case4/4_1.html

http://www.patient.co.uk/showdoc/23068848/

http://en.wikipedia.org/wiki/Urinalysis

http://library.med.utah.edu/WebPath/TUTORIAL/URINE/URINE.html

http://www.e-radiography.net/technique/mucg/mcug.htm

http://www.nursingboard.ie/Scope/scope4/try1.asp

http://www.aakp.org/aakp-library/Dialysis-Centers-Accommodate-Children/

http://kidney.niddk.nih.gov/kudiseases/pubs/childkidneydiseases/treatment_methods/

http://www.ika.ie/

http://www.thechildrenskidneyfoundation.org/

http://www.kidskidneyresearch.org/

http://www.kidney.org.uk/links.html

Gastrointestinal system

MARY CLYNES AND CAROLINE O'CONNOR

Skills

 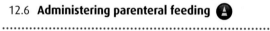
Introduction

The aim of this chapter is to provide you with knowledge and understanding of the skills required in providing care to the child with a gastrointestinal disorder. This chapter will focus primarily on the most frequently encountered procedures both in the hospital and in the community setting. In addition, the importance of family centred care and a multicultural approach to care will be discussed. Some of the skills outlined in this chapter may be classified as advanced skills, for example, caring for a child on parenteral nutrition, and therefore you should seek appropriate guidance/supervision when undertaking these practices. Moreover, it is essential that the student follows appropriate care plans, works within his/her scope of professional practice, and adheres to local policy in relation to carrying out nursing care (Nursing and Midwifery Council (NMC), 2007).

Learning outcomes

This chapter will enable you to:

- Briefly describe the anatomy and physiology of the gastrointestinal system.
- Understand the procedures outlined in the chapter.
- Explain the rationale for the care you provide.
- Understand the importance of the holistic needs of the child when carrying out procedures.
- Understand the importance of family centred care and a multicultural approach to care.

Prior knowledge

Knowledge of national and local policies and guidelines are recommended to enhance learning, e.g. National Institute of Health and Clinical Excellence (NICE) guidelines. Where reference is made to national guidelines, students are advised to refer to them for more detailed information. It is important that the student has a comprehensive knowledge of the anatomy and physiology of the gastrointestinal system to support understanding of many of the clinical skills described in this chapter. The following section will briefly outline the structure and function of the gastrointestinal tract. Knowledge of the changes that occur in the gastrointestinal tract as the child grows and develops is paramount to providing appropriate care and these will be signposted as they relate to skills throughout this chapter. For more detailed information refer to an anatomy and physiology textbook.

It is beyond the scope of this chapter to comprehensively incorporate all aspects of holistic care, so this chapter should be read in association with other chapters in this book in order to gain a comprehensive picture of how is holistic care is delivered. In particular you will need to examine Chapters Two, Three, Four, Five, Six, and Seven.

Overview of the anatomy and physiology of the gastrointestinal system

Anatomy of the gastrointestinal tract

The gastrointestinal tract (GIT) is a long tube that extends from the mouth to the anus. It consists of the mouth, pharynx, oesophagus, stomach, small intestine (duodenum, jejunum, and ileum), and large intestine (caecum, colon, rectum, and anal canal) (see Figure 12.1). Four accessory organs, the salivary glands, the liver, the gall bladder, and the pancreas, secrete digestive juices into the tract. The primary functions of the GIT are the

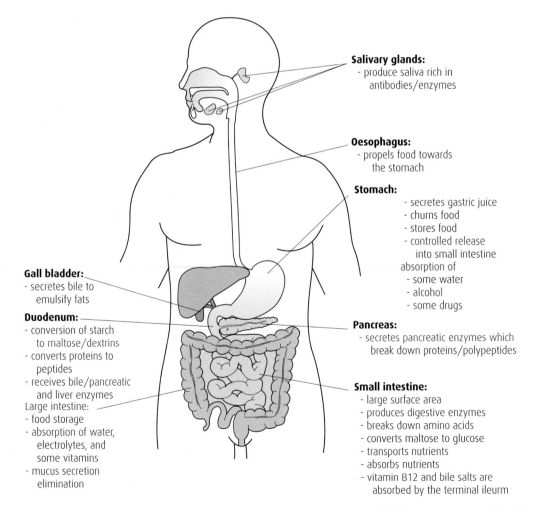

Figure 12.1 The digestive system (with permission from Elsevier. This figure was published in *Anatomy and Physiology in Health and Illness*, Anne Waugh and Alison Grant, *The Digestive System*, page 282, Elsevier, 2006).

ingestion, digestion, and absorption of nutrients and the elimination of undigested and unabsorbed food from the body.

The pharynx is a muscular tube that extends from the back of the mouth to the oesophagus and serves both the respiratory and digestive system. During swallowing, the epiglottis, a small flap of tissue that sits at the base of the tongue, closes the airway. The oesophagus continues from the pharynx and descends through the thoracic cavity, passes through the diaphragm, and empties into the stomach. Entry to the stomach is guarded by the lower oesophageal sphincter (LES) or cardiac sphincter. The outlet of the stomach into the duodenum is guarded by the pyloric sphincter. The small intestine extends from the pyloric sphincter to the ileocaecal valve where it joins the large intestine. The duodenum is the short, curved portion of the small intestine, which circles around the head of the pancreas. Ducts from the pancreas, liver, and gall bladder enter the duodenum through the hepatopancreatic ampulla (ampulla of Vater). The jejunum is the middle portion of the small intestine and is continuous with the third section, the ileum. Millions of tiny finger-like projections called villi line the small intestine, thus providing a greater surface area for the digestion and absorption of food.

The large intestine extends from the end of the ileum to the anus. It is divided into four sections: the caecum, colon, rectum, and anus. The caecum is a sac-like structure that makes up the first part of the large intestine. It is continuous with the colon above and the vermiform appendix is attached to the end of the caecum. The colon consists of four parts:

- The ascending colon continues upwards from the caecum to the under-surface of the liver where it curves to the left at the right colic flexure to become the transverse colon.
- The transverse colon extends across the abdomen to the under-surface of the spleen and bends downwards at the left colic flexure.
- The descending colon passes down the left side of the abdomen, curves towards the midline, and enters the pelvis where it becomes the sigmoid colon.
- The sigmoid colon forms a loop and lies within the pelvis, and continues down to become the rectum. The rectum continues down to become the anal canal.

The anal canal goes downwards and backwards and ends at the anus. Two sphincters control the anus: the internal sphincter, which is under the control of the autonomic system, and the external sphincter, which is under voluntary control to keep the anus closed.

The digestive process

The digestion of food consists of a mechanical and chemical process. The mechanical digestion of food begins in the mouth where the teeth cut and crush the food. Chemical digestion of **carbohydrates** begins when food is mixed with saliva, which contains an enzyme called salivary amylase. In the stomach the mechanical and chemical digestion of food continues. The gastric mucosa secretes gastric juice, which aids the digestion of food and protects the gut from micro-organisms. Peristaltic contractions of the stomach mash and churn food and it mixes with gastric juices to form chyme. When the pyloric sphincter relaxes the chyme passes into the small intestine.

Most of the digestion and absorption of food takes place in the small intestine. When partially digested food reaches the duodenum, hormones are released that stimulate the release of intestinal juices, bile from the gall bladder, and pancreatic juice from the pancreas. The absorption of nutrients takes places almost entirely in the villi of the small intestine. Amino acids and simple sugars pass into blood capillaries in the villi and are transported by the hepatic portal vein to the liver. Fatty acids are absorbed into lymph vessels called lacteals in the villi and circulate through the lymph system before entering the blood.

As unabsorbed material passes through the large intestine, water and salt are absorbed. Undigested and unabsorbed foods as well as bile pigments are eliminated in the form of faeces from the body. Strong waves of peristalsis move material along the pelvic colon. Mass movements propel the faeces into the rectum, which becomes distended and the urge to defecate occurs. The internal sphincter relaxes and the external sphincter remains contracted until it is relaxed voluntarily. In infancy and early childhood, the external sphincter relaxes following rectal distension and defecation occurs as in an involuntary act. Voluntary control is achieved during early childhood, usually between 18 months and two years old.

The structures of the GIT system are well developed at birth; however, many of its functions are immature. These will be referred to throughout the chapter as they apply to specific sections. As one of the primary functions of the gastrointestinal tract is to digest and absorb nutrients to maintain metabolic activities and ensure adequate growth and development, it is vital that the child's nutritional intake is adequate. The following section will examine methods of assessing a child's nutritional status. It is recognised that the nurse has a significant role to play in carrying out nutritional assessment in order to identify potential or actual nutritional problems and to monitor response to treatment (Holden & MacDonald, 2000).

Nutritional assessment

Nutritional assessment is used to establish a child's nutritional status, in order to identify children likely to need nutritional support (Bowling, 2004). The assessment provides valuable baseline data against which the effectiveness of nutritional support can be monitored. There are a number of elements to consider when conducting an assessment. These include physical assessment, dietary assessment, and measurement of weight, height/length, and head circumference (Holden & MacDonald, 2000).

Physical assessment

Considerable information regarding a child's nutritional status can be obtained from a physical assessment. Physical assessment involves observing the child's general appearance, noting whether the child appears under- or overweight. The condition of the child's skin, hair, mouth, teeth, lips, gums, tongue, and eyes is also a good indicator of nutritional status. These areas are particularly susceptible to alternation from normal appearance because of the rapid turnover of the epithelial and mucosal tissue (Hockenberry & Barrera, 2007). It is important to establish whether the child has any medical condition that may result in loss of nutrients or failure to absorb nutrients, e.g. fistula, vomiting, or diarrhoea (Fergusson, 2008). **Box 12.1** outlines the key observations to be made during the physical assessment.

Box 12.1 Physical assessment

General appearance

- Does the child have a healthy complexion or is s/he pale? Is the skin thin and shiny?
- Is his/her hair dull, lacklustre, or thinning?
- Are her/his lips red, inflamed, or fissured at the corners?
- Are the gums swollen, bleed easily, or inflamed?
- Are the teeth discoloured, with/without dental caries?
- Is the tongue smooth, swollen, pale, red, or painful?
- Are the nails brittle?
- Are there any abnormalities of the abdomen, e.g. distension, flabby, larger, poor musculature? In younger children, the normal abdomen is cylindrical and prominent because the pelvis is narrow and more abdominal contents are therefore suprapubic (Neill & Knowles, 2004). The abdomen is normally flat in older children.
- Are the buttocks wasted? A healthy child has firm, rounded buttocks.
- Is there muscle wasting, short stature, thin arms and legs, or prominent bones?
- Weight loss, loose subcutaneous skin folds, and apathy are signs of acute malnutrition in infancy. Chronic malnutrition manifests by pallor, thinness, prominent bones, protuberant abdomen, hypotonia, flat buttocks, and apathy (Gill & O'Brien, 2007).

Measurements of weight, height, and head circumference are key parameters used to monitor growth and overall nutritional status. Growth is predominantly dependent on nutrition in the first 2–3 years of life (Hussain & Preece, 2006). However, growth patterns may vary depending on whether the child is breast or bottle fed and ethnic variation in growth patterns may exist. New UK-WHO growth measurement charts have been devised for children from birth to four years, which take into consideration these variables (Royal College of Paediatrics and Child Health, 2009). The existing UK90 Growth Charts can continue to be used for children born before the new charts came into existence and for children over four years. It is important that measurements of weight, height, and head circumference are recorded accurately and consistently using appropriate equipment and carried out by trained staff. Refer to Chapter Three for procedural steps for taking weight, height/length, and head circumference measurements.

Dietary assessment

Vital information can be obtained by asking the child and his/her parent/carer about their eating habits. In order to carry out a complete assessment of dietary intake it may be necessary to ask the child and family to keep a food diary and record total intake over a number of days. Alternatively they may be asked to recall food intake over the previous few days. The following are key questions to ask the parent/carer and child in order to ascertain the child's dietary intake (**Box 12.2**). It is important to remember to pose these questions in an open manner, e.g. 'Tell me what you take to school for lunch' (RCN, 2007a).

Box 12.2 Assessing infants' and young children's dietary intake

- Ascertain infant's birth weight. Was the infant preterm?
- Is the infant breast or formula fed? Is breastfeeding being supplemented by other types of feed?

If breastfed

- For how long?
- How often?

If formula fed

- What formula?
- How often, how much, and total in 24 hours?
- Who feeds the baby?
- Who prepares the feeds?
- Does the baby have any feeding problems such as difficulty sucking and swallowing or spitting up?
- Is there any history of regurgitation/vomiting?

Weaning

- When were solids introduced?
- What types of solids were introduced?
- Do you make your own baby food or do you use commercially produced foods?
- Is the child taking food of different textures and age-appropriate food?
- Does the infant feed himself/herself, or use a bottle, cup, or beaker?
- Is the infant taking a bottle or being breastfed as well?
- Does the infant take cow's milk and when was it introduced?
- Does the infant take other fluids other than formula, breast milk, or cow's milk? It is important

to establish if the child is taking whole milk or semi-skimmed milk. Semi-skimmed milk is not recommended for children under two years of age (Bowling, 2004).
- How much milk or other fluids does the infant take?

Other information

- Does the infant take vitamin or mineral supplements? If so what type?
- Has the child got food allergies or is there a history of food allergies in the family?
- What is the child's bowel pattern? Enquire about stool frequency and consistency.
- Is the child in childcare? This may influence the dietary intake and parents may not be fully aware of the child's intake.

Additional questions that may be used with an older child are outlined in **Box 12.3**.

Box 12.3 Assessing dietary intake: Additional questions for older children

- Tell me what you usually eat for breakfast, lunch, and dinner. The parent may add additional information as the child may forget what s/he eats. Enquire about portion size.
- What are your favourite foods, drinks, and snacks? How much do you eat of each? How often do you snack and eat sweets? What type of drinks do you usually have? How often do you eat fruit and vegetables?
- What do you take to school for lunch or do you get school lunches?
- What type of food and drinks do you dislike?
- Do you eat meals while watching television?
- Do you clean your teeth after meals?
- Do you take regular exercise?

Questions that can be addressed to the carer

- Does the family eat meals together?
- Does the family eat at the table?
- How is most food prepared, e.g. boiled, baked, fried, or grilled?
- Does the family eat out in restaurants or eat 'takeaway' food?
- Does the child need assistance with feeding?
- Describe your child's appetite, e.g. good, fussy eater, etc.
- Has your child lost or gained weight recently?

When carrying out the assessment it is necessary to be aware that cultural practices may influence dietary intake and that some ethnic food may be consumed by the child and family (Hockenberry & Barrera, 2007). Food choices may be influenced by people's religion and eating patterns may be based on this. Nevertheless it is imperative not to make assumptions as to what people eat because some families may adhere more strictly to religious guidance than others (Albon & Mukherji, 2008). Therefore the nurse must practise in a non-discriminatory manner and acknowledge the differences in beliefs and cultural practices of individuals and families (NMC, 2007). It is important to remember when assessing dietary intake that young children require proportionately more energy than older children and adults because they are growing at a fast pace. Additionally at this time their brains are developing rapidly and require an adequate supply of essential fatty acids. Therefore, their diet should contain a higher fat proportion than older children and adults (Albon & Mukherji, 2008).

The impact of budgetary constraints on the food that a child eats should not be underestimated. Although it is possible to maintain a healthy diet on a low budget, parents may simply feel this is impossible and may rely on less healthy convenience foods through their own beliefs or lack of skills. Financial issues may indeed cause the child to be undernourished and it is important, through questioning, to carefully assess the diet that a child is receiving.

The nurse should demonstrate sound clinical judgement and recognize when it is necessary to refer the child to another member of the healthcare team, e.g. dietician (NMC, 2007). If the assessment highlights any areas of concern, these need to be documented, discussed with parents/carers, and the information passed on to the appropriate specialist (RCN, 2007a).

Infant nutrition

Appropriate early childhood nutrition is essential to ensure proper growth and development and to establish healthy eating habits. Breastfeeding is the ideal way of providing young infants with the nutrients necessary for normal growth and development and exclusive breast-feeding is recommended for the first six months of life (WHO, 2003). For mothers who cannot or choose not to breastfeed, infant formula milks should be used. The nurse should not be judgemental about the method of feeding the mother chooses or allow personal beliefs about formula or breastfeeding to influence the care, support, or information provided for a mother (NMC, 2004). Breastfeeding is not an instinctive behaviour, but a learned skill (Spencer & Jones, 2002) and therefore support and advice should be available to the mother. Written information should be supported with face-to-face advice and women whose first language is not English should have access to interpreting services and information in a format and language they can understand (NICE, 2008).

12.1 Helping a mother to breastfeed

Sometimes it is not possible to breastfeed a baby (for example, when an infant is too sick and unable to do so, perhaps due to respiratory difficulty—see Chapter Eight). At these times mothers should be offered information and advice on how to express and store breast milk. Breast milk can be stored for up to five days in a fridge at 4°C or lower and for longer in a domestic freezer (NICE, 2008). Expressed breast milk may be given to babies using a bottle, or through nasogastric feeding if the child's condition requires it. The principles of providing support to breastfeeding mothers are outlined below.

Procedure: Helping a mother to breastfeed (see following page)

Preparation

Where possible any medical or nursing care should be scheduled to take place between feeds to prevent disruption to feeding patterns.

Pull curtains as appropriate to ensure privacy and dignity, as recommended in the essential skills clusters (NMC, 2007).

Breastfeeding should be a pleasant experience for both mother and baby. Make sure you discuss with the mother the most comfortable position for breastfeeding. She may choose to sit with her back well supported or lie down. The cradle hold, whereby the mother holds the baby with his/her head on her forearm and the baby's entire body facing the mother, is the most commonly used and comfortable position for mothers (Torgus *et al.*, 2006).

Equipment

Offer a footstool to support the mother's feet. This can help prevent backache.

Assessment

Assess the mother's knowledge and confidence regarding breastfeeding and provide practical advice as required.

Step-by-step guide to helping a mother to breastfeed

Step	Rationale
1 **The baby should be positioned so that s/he is lying close to mother with baby's head in line with body.**	To ensure correct positioning and that the baby latches on. Incorrect position can cause sore and cracked nipples and inadequate milk supply.
Bring baby to breast rather than breast to baby. **Line up baby's nose and mouth to nipple.** **Allow baby's tongue and lips to touch nipple.**	This encourages the baby to open his/her mouth. Triggers the 'rooting' reflex.
2 **Mother may need to tilt the baby's head back slightly so that his/her mouth opens and then bring baby back to the breast gently.**	This will help the baby take areola, nipple, and as much breast tissue as possible into his/her mouth, so that enough milk can be squeezed out of the ducts.
3 **Inform mother to observe baby's jaw moving back and forth during feeding. She should be able to hear the baby swallowing.**	To observe sucking action. Indicates that the baby is feeding.
Remind mother that breastfeeding should not hurt. If it is painful she should stop feeding by inserting a finger in corner of baby's mouth. This will make baby open his/her mouth (latch off) and the mother may begin the latching on process again.	The baby has not latched on properly.
4 **Explain to mother that baby will normally release the breast when s/he has fed enough from that breast. Mother should avoid removing baby prematurely from breast and allow sufficient time for baby to receive rich hind milk.**	To ensure that both fore and hind milk is released and the baby gets enough calories. The fore milk is released when baby initially feeds and is lower in fat than the hind milk, which is released later (Mitchell, 2002).
5 **Explain to mother how she will know if her baby is getting enough milk: baby appears content after the feed; her breasts feel empty and softer after feeds; after a few days the baby should have 5–6 wet nappies; after about two weeks the baby begins to gain weight.**	The mother may have concerns about whether the baby is getting enough milk.

Discharge support

Mothers may be more likely to continue feeding at home if they feel confident about feeding before leaving the hospital. A drop-off in breastfeeding after the mother and baby return home is not uncommon. Exclusive breast-feeding at birth in the UK is 75% but this falls to 21% after six weeks (Infant Feeding Survey, 2005).

Before the mother and baby leave the hospital, ensure that the mother:

- Can demonstrate how to position and attach the baby to the breast.
- Can identify signs that the baby is feeding (see above).
- Has contact details for local voluntary organizations providing ongoing support to complement NHS breastfeeding services (NICE, 2008).

12.2 **Formula feeding**

Infant formulas are derived from cow's milk that has been modified to meet the nutritional needs of the growing infant (Rudolf & Levane, 2006). Standard formulas fall into two groups: whey-based milks and casein-based milks. Whey-based formula is easy to digest and has a protein profile resembling breast milk. Casein-based milks are closer in composition to cow's milk and are marketed for hungrier babies as it is believed that curds formed by higher casein levels may stay in the stomach for longer. Follow-on formulas have a higher iron content, which is intended to meet the nutritional needs of infants aged 6–12 months while they are weaned and before they are obtaining adequate iron supplies from a solid diet. Other more specialized types of formula are recommended for infants depending on their health status and these include preterm formulas and soya-based formulas. Nurses should be aware of the different types of formula available and give advice as appropriate to parents (RCN, 2007b). In addition the nurse should be able to provide advice on the amount of feed the infant is expected to take on a daily basis.

Due to the small size of the newborn stomach and the speed at which it empties (2.5 to 3 hours), an infant tends to ingest small, frequent feeds. As the infant grows and the stomach enlarges the frequency of the feeds decreases and the volume consumed at each feed

increases. During the first week of life a newborn infant will take on average up to 120 ml/kg per day and may feed as frequently as every 2–3 hours. This increases to 150 ml/kg per day thereafter and the frequency of feeding is reduced (Holden & MacDonald, 2000). There may be occasions when these calculations are not adhered to for medical reasons, e.g. if a child has cystic fibrosis and additional calories are required. The equipment and procedure required for formula feeding are outlined below.

Procedure: Formula feeding (see following page)

Preparation

Prior to commencing feeding check the baby's nose is clean and that the baby has a clean, dry nappy. This is because babies do not feed as well if their nose is blocked with mucus or if the nappy is wet or soiled.

Equipment

- Plastic apron.
- Sterile bottle of correct milk in appropriate quantity.
- Sterile teat.
- Bottle warmer or jug of hot water.
- Comfortable chair with support for arm.
- Wash hands before removing bottles and teats from the sterilizer.

After the procedure

It is important to maintain a record of intake and output. Document the type of feed offered, quantity taken, and if there was any vomiting.

Clear away the equipment, disposing of any single use items. Wash bottles with warm, soapy water and rinse carefully, as the presence of milk will render sterilizing solution incapable of sterilizing the equipment. The bottle and teat may be sterilized by steeping in a chemical solution, steaming, or microwaving. If using a chemical solution submerge the bottle and teat completely in sterilizing solution and leave it for at least 30 minutes. Discard sterilizing solution every 24 hours or sooner if there is evidence of contamination.

Step-by-step guide to helping parents with formula feeding

Step	Rationale
1 Wash hands thoroughly and put on apron.	To prevent cross infection.
2 Warm bottle of feed (if preferred by baby) under warm running water or place in a jug of warm water. Ensure that the water does not cover the cap of the bottle.	Warming feeds for term babies is not necessary but most infants prefer warmed feed.
Do not microwave the feed.	A microwave heats liquids unevenly and may result in hot spots.
3 Ensure the feed has not expired and in the case of Ready to Feed formula that the button in the middle of the cap has not been popped.	To ensure feed has not expired.
4 When opening a bottle of special feed prepared in the formula room ensure that the feed is labelled with the name of the patient and is within date.	To ensure feed is given to the correct patient.
5 Place teat on bottle and test temperature by squirting a small amount onto the inside of the wrist. The milk should feel warm not hot.	To ensure feed is not too hot as it may result in burning of the baby's mouth.
6 Ensure that teat is appropriate size. Use baby's own bottle and teat if required.	It is important that the teats are an appropriate size. Teats with small openings require the baby to suck strongly to get the milk and may lead to frustration or a tired baby to give up. Large openings may lead to gagging or choking as the milk will come too fast.
7 Hold the baby in a comfortable position with the head supported in an upright position.	Reduces risk of accidental aspiration. The positioning of the infant is influenced by high position of stomach in the abdomen and its horizontal lie (Chamley *et al.*, 2005).
8 Bring bottle gently to baby's lips. If baby is reluctant to take the bottle stroke the side of the baby's mouth or under his/her chin.	To promote feeding.
9 Hold bottle in a position that ensures that the teat is always full of milk.	This prevents the infant swallowing air thus resulting in wind.
10 Make eye contact with baby, talk to baby, and observe development of baby.	To promote comfort and make experience a more pleasurable one for the baby. To assess if the baby is meeting developmental milestones.

11	Observe child for signs of discomfort, e.g. wind. The baby may cry or stop feeding due to wind. Most babies may be able to drink up to half the quantity of the feed before requiring winding (Trigg & Mohammed, 2006).	To allow infant to continue feed in comfort.
12	Wind by removing bottle, sitting the baby in upright position, and supporting the head and neck.	Brings up any air swallowed during feeding. In this position the stomach is positioned with the cardiac sphincter of the stomach upright so that air will rise up the straight oesophagus into the mouth (MacGregor, 2008).
	Patting the baby's back may help to release the trapped air. Alternatively, the baby may be placed onto one shoulder.	This may be comforting for carer but may not be as effective as holding the baby in the upright position (MacGregor, 2008).
	Ensure back and shoulder is protected.	Baby may posset.
13	Do not prolong feeding beyond 30 minutes.	Infants feed at different rates, and some may be slow feeders. Most infants will have completed feed by 20 minutes and feeding beyond 30 minutes will result in infant becoming tired and bored.
14	Wind again after the feed is completed.	To ensure that the baby is comfortable.

Regardless of the method of sterilization used, mothers should be made aware of the need to clean and sterilize the bottles and teats after every feed to protect the baby from getting gastrointestinal infections.

Community perspective

It is essential that parents and carers know how to prepare a formula feed prior to discharge from hospital. Particular attention should be paid to ensuring that bottles and teats are sterilized prior to use. Freshly boiled water cooled to a temperature of about 70°C should be used to make up feeds (RCN, 2007b). It will take about 20 to 30 minutes from the time of boiling for the water to cool to this temperature. One level scoop of powder should be added to each 30 ml of water and any excess powder can be removed with the straight edge of the blade of a knife. A heaped scoop of powder would make the feed too concentrated and may lead to hypernatraemic dehydration (Rudolf & Levane, 2006). The bottle should be cooled under running water before feeding. It is best practice to make up infant formula for each feed. However, where it is not possible or practical

a day's supply of feeds may be made up provided the milk can be stored in a refrigerator at a temperature below 5°C (RCN, 2007b).

Enteral feeding

Oral feeding is the preferred method of feeding for children with an effectively functioning gastrointestinal tract. However, if oral intake is inadequate, or if the infant is too ill and unable to feed from the breast or bottle, then **enteral feeding** may be necessary.

Enteral feeding is an artificial method of supplying the child with nutrients via a tube into the gastrointestinal tract. Feed may be administered via a nasogastric/ orogastric tube, a gastrostomy tube, or a jejunostomy tube. The need for enteral feed may be short term but for many children it may be a long-term requirement. Artificial nutritional support is required when oral intake is absent or likely to be absent for a period >5–7 days. Earlier instigation of enteral feeding may be needed for those who are malnourished. Although nutrition may be administered intravenously (parenteral nutrition) it is more beneficial physiologically to administer nutrition via the gastrointestinal route even if the mouth and oesophagus must be bypassed (Hanks & McEwing, 2009).

Feeds are available in different forms such as **ready to use**, non-sterile, or modular. **A modular feed** is formulated from separate ingredients. It allows adjustment of protein, carbohydrates, and fats to meet the needs of the individual patient. Ready to use feeds, which are commercially prepared and only require attaching to the administration set or feeding tube, should be used in preference to feeds requiring decanting, reconstitution, or dilution whenever possible (NICE, 2003; Food Safety Authority of Ireland (FSAI), 2007; Paediatric Group of the British Dietetic Association, 2007). This reduces the risk of cross contamination. Decisions on route, content, and management of nutritional support are best made by the multidisciplinary team.

Oral feeding is a normal activity and part of the parenting role and consequently the decision to commence enteral feeding can be difficult for both parent and child. Furthermore the passing of a nasogastric (NG) tube can be very distressing for the child and parent. Preparation of the child and family is therefore essential before enteral feeding is commenced. The play therapist may be involved in preparing the child and parent by using dolls and puppets to enact nasogastric or gastrostomy feeding. Colouring and story books are also useful aids (further information on distraction may be found in Chapter Five). The nurse can augment this teaching by reinforcing the information and answering questions as required, or s/he may lead on the information giving. The child's level of understanding and previous experience of hospital must be taken into consideration when giving information. Reducing parental anxiety through information giving can have a positive impact on the child, as parental anxiety may be transmitted to the child. During the procedure the use of distraction techniques should be encouraged so that the child focuses on something other than the procedure. Post-procedural support is essential to reassure the child. Rewards may be used to acknowledge bravery and to promote confidence and self-esteem.

12.3 **Nasogastric feeding**

Nasogastric feeding is usually the route of choice for enteral feeding unless long-term use is anticipated. A nasogastric tube is a polyvinyl or polyurethane tube that is passed through the nose, through the oesophagus, and into the stomach. Polyurethane tubes are more suitable for long-term use (Trigg & Mohammed, 2006). Nasogastric tubes should be changed according to the manufacturer's guidelines to prevent increased risk of bacterial contamination and erosion of the tube by gastric juices. Although nasogastric tubes are principally used for nutritional purposes they may also be used to decompress the upper gastrointestinal tract of gas and fluid, to remove gastric samples for diagnostic testing, and to alleviate nausea and vomiting or to irrigate the stomach (Stroud et al., 2003).

Nursing Alert

Nursing students should familiarize themselves with local policies and procedures regarding syringe products. It is recommended that syringes used for delivery of medications and use in enteral feeding are reverse luer, i.e. are not compatible with luer lock connections used in intravenous giving sets and connections. Additionally, many units are now moving to the use of nasogastric tubes with reverse luer connections. Use of such products will ensure that the accidental delivery of oral medications/enteral feed does not take place via the intravenous (IV) route and vice versa.

Procedure: Inserting a nasogastric tube

Preparation

To prevent the spread of infection, wash hands* with liquid soap, or an alcohol hand rub if the hands are visibly clean, and put on plastic apron. Clean the trolley prior to placement of supplies.

Ascertain whether the patient has an allergy to any adhesive material, to prevent skin irritation.

*Hand hygiene is the single most effective step in preventing the spread of infection (Department of Health and Children (DOHC), 2005).

Step-by-step guide to inserting a nasogastric tube

Step	Rationale
1 Carry out effective hand hygiene (wash hands with liquid soap, or an alcohol hand rub product if hands are visibly clean).	Hand hygiene is the single most important step in preventing the spread of infection (DOHC, 2005).
2 Put on disposable non-sterile gloves and apply apron.	To prevention cross infection.
3 Find most appropriate position for child.

Babies may be wrapped in a blanket and held in arms of the assistant (Corkin & Chambers, 2008) or lying on side with the palm of the non-dominant hand along the side of the infant's face, without hyper-extending the neck. Older child: elicit cooperation by asking him/her to slightly hyper-extend the neck, keep head still, breathe through the mouth, and swallow when instructed. | To prevent the child from pulling tube out and to maintain comfort.
Hyper-extension of an infant's neck can occlude the airway. An infant is less likely to aspirate in a side-lying position. |
| **4** Ensure nostrils are free of debris. | Infants are nose breathers, so obstruction to the other nostril may affect their patent airway. This also facilitates passage of the NG tube. |
| **5** Check tube is intact. If tube has guidewire, stretch tube and check that wire is not bent and is correctly positioned down the middle of the tube. Flush tube with approximately 10 mls of sterile water if there is a guidewire *in situ*.
Ensure that there are no contraindications to passing a nasogastric tube. | To prevent injury from guidewire.

To prevent complications and adverse outcomes. |
| **6** Measure length of tube from tip of the nose to the ear and then from ear to a point midway between xiphoid process and the umbilicus. Note or hold the marking on the tube. | To facilitate the insertion of correct tube length. |
| **7** Lubricate the end of the tube in sterile water or a water-based lubricant.
Do not use KY jelly. | To assist in the passage of tube and reduce risk of friction.
May affect pH reading. |
| **8** Ensure cap at the end of the tube is closed.
Gently put the tip of the tube into the child's nostril. Angle it slightly upwards and gently advance it along the floor of the nose into the pharynx.
Continue to feed the tube downwards. As it gets to the back of the throat, encourage an older child to have a sip of water (if not prohibited). Offer a baby a soother to help the tube go down. | Prevents leakage of stomach contents.

To ease the passage of the tube, ease discomfort, and reduce the risk of the tube passing into the trachea, as the epiglottis will cover the trachea when swallowing. |

9 Observe for signs that tube placement is in the trachea or bronchus: excessive coughing, choking, and cyanosis. If this occurs withdraw tube to the naso-pharynx and reinsert after child/infant has recovered. It may be necessary to pause in order for tube to pass through the cardiac sphincter into the stomach. Stop passing tube when the place you have marked on the tube is at the opening of the child's nostril; the tip should now be in the stomach.

Presence of the tube in the trachea or bronchus occludes the airway and is potentially hazardous.

10 Ask the person holding the child to place two fingers against the tube.

To prevent dislodgement of tube.

Check that tube is in correct position by aspirating gastric contents and testing on pH strip. Remove end cap of tube, connect a syringe to the end of the NG tube, and withdraw the plunger until fluid appears in the syringe. Only a very small amount (0.5–1 ml) of fluid is required. Disconnect the syringe and put end cap of tube in place.

To obtain gastric aspirate for testing.
To ensure tube is in correct position before proceeding to use tube.

11 Test results using colour indicator chart with pH numbers as supplied with strips.
If tube position is confirmed, remove guidewire (if present) and tape tube in place.

The National Patient Safety Agency (NPSA, 2005) recommends that feeding may take place if pH is below 5.5, as there are no known reports of pulmonary aspirate at or below this figure.
If aspirate is pH 6 or above do not feed as there is a possibility of aspirate being a bronchial secretion. Wait up to one hour and try again. The NPSA states that the most likely reason for failure to get gastric aspirate below pH 5.5 is dilution of gastric acid by enteral feed. Waiting up to an hour allows time for the stomach to empty and pH to fall.
Be aware that certain medications, such as antacids, H2 antagonists, and proton pump inhibitors, can elevate the pH level of gastric contents; therefore it is important to check if patient is on these medications.

12 Document details of pH result and proceed to post-procedural steps outlined below.

To ensure record of nursing care.

13 Procedure if aspirate is not obtained:
Insert the tube a further few centimetres or change the child's position and try again.

Tube may not be in contact with stomach contents.

14 If still unable to aspirate fluid and it is safe to do so, offer the child a drink orally and try again (Stroud *et al.*, 2003).

Absence of gastric fluid is not necessarily evidence of improper placement. The stomach may be empty, or the tube may not be in contact with stomach contents.

15 If still unable to confirm position by aspirate, an X-ray will be necessary. Contact senior colleague and conduct risk assessment.

To confirm correct position.

16 Document actions and decision, i.e. replace/reposition tube; X-ray; continue based on assessment of risk.

To ensure record of nursing care and to maintain accountability (An Bord Altranais, 2002).

Equipment

Before you begin, collect and assemble all necessary equipment. Arranging the trolley and items of equipment so that they are within easy reach helps the procedure to go smoothly and prevents undue delays. Always ensure the usability of equipment (Hankins *et al.*, 2001). If a product's integrity is compromised, it should not be used. The equipment needed includes:

- Disposable apron.
- Disposable gloves.
- Nasogastric tube (appropriate size, length, and type). Consider period of time that tube is likely to be required, whether there is a requirement for a short or long tube, and what the purpose of the tube is (e.g. some feeds and medications may necessitate a wider tube; use of the tube for aspiration of stomach contents will also require a wider tube).
- Sterile water or water-based lubricant to lubricate the nasogastric tube.
- pH indication paper (range 0–6).
- Two syringes (one to aspirate tube to confirm position and one to flush the tube):
  - 5–10 ml syringe for PVC tube.
  - 50 ml/60 ml syringe for polyurethane tube.
- A pair of clean/sterile scissors to cut tape.
- Transparent film or other suitable dressing.
- A hydrocolloid dressing may be used to provide a protective layer between the child's skin and the adhesive tape holding the tube in place. The dressing should cover two-thirds of the child's cheek between the nostril and the ear and should be three times the width of the tube itself (Hanks & McEwing, 2009).
- Tape to secure the tube (wide enough to cover tube, overlap the sides, and hold it securely in place).
- Emesis bowl.
- Soother (if the child normally uses one).

Nursing Alert

Observe for signs of vagal stimulation while passing the tube past the gag reflex area: decreased pulse, gasping, apnoea, coughing, cyanosis, gagging, and/or vomiting. If these symptoms occur withdraw the tube and wait for the child/infant's condition to stabilize before proceeding.

To minimize stress during the procedure ensure that privacy is maintained and that there is adequate lighting and ventilation. Use minimal clinical holding.

Assessment

If the child's condition allows, use a procedure room to pass the tube. This preserves the child's room as a safe environment.

Consent and communication

Locate the patient and confirm their identity. This procedure will most often require the assistance of at least two individuals. Elicit assistance where required and encourage parent/s to stay where possible, to provide a distraction.

This procedure may be distressing for the child and family. To help gain cooperation and alleviate anxiety, explain the procedure carefully using a variety of age-appropriate communication methods (NMC, 2007). A play therapist may be involved in the preparation of the child and family for this procedure.

After the procedure

Clear away equipment as per local healthcare waste disposal policies and wash hands. This promotes safety and prevents spread of infection. Inform relevant staff that the procedure has taken place. Documenting which nostril is used, the size and the length of the tube, and the date, will help in establishing if the tube has been dislodged.

Confirm tube position:

- At the time of insertion.
- Before each use.
- When the child has an episode of retching, vomiting, excessive coughing, or respiratory distress.
- Following a successful attempt to resolve a blocked tube.
- Where it appears the tube has dislodged, i.e. tube length appears visibly increased.
- Six hourly when on continuous feeds.

Nursing Alert

- If you have any concerns or doubts about the positioning of the NG tube, feeding (or other use) should not commence until the position of the tube has been checked and confirmed by a senior nurse.

- **Syringe size:** The strength of the pressure created at the tip of a syringe during aspiration is dependent on the size and type of the syringe, in addition to the amount of force used. Smaller syringes cause greater pressure on the tube and may cause it to break (Irish Nutrition & Dietetic Institute (INDI), 2007; Bowers, 2000). It is therefore important that the manufacturer's guidelines are adhered to.

- **pH indication paper:** The acidity of aspirate should be confirmed with pH indication paper rather than the blue litmus paper traditionally used. Blue litmus paper will determine acidity but not the level of acidity (Khair, 2005).

- **Confirming tube position:** Auscultation using air (via a syringe) and a stethoscope should never be used to determine the position of a nasogastric tube as sounds are similar to those heard when air is instilled into the lungs via a nasogastric tube. Therefore, it is not a reliable method to identify the position of the nasogastric tube (Metheny *et al.*, 1994).

Gastrostomy feeding

A gastrostomy is an artificial opening made in the stomach wall through which a tube is inserted for the purposes of feeding. Gastrostomy feeding is normally indicated when long-term enteral feeding is required. It is generally preferred by children because the tube is more comfortable, requires fewer changes, and is more cosmetically acceptable than a nasogastric tube (Johnson, 2007). There are three main types of gastrostomy tubes. These are percutaneous endoscopically placed gastrostomy tubes (PEG tubes), surgically placed balloon gastrostomy tubes, and the skin level 'button' devices.

The percutaneous endoscopically placed gastrostomy tube (PEG) is inserted into the stomach under endoscopic conditions and can stay *in situ* for up to two years. The surgically placed tube is used when endoscopic insertion has failed or if the patient is having a laparotomy and the tube can be placed in the stomach during the procedure.

The skin level 'button' device is a short tube that sits inside the stomach and the external part of the tube sits

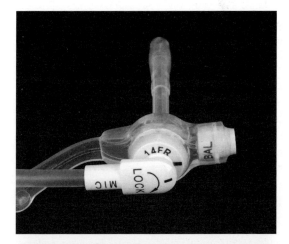

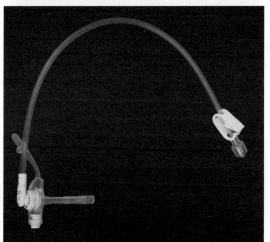

Figure 12.2 Gastrostomy tubes

flush with the skin. It is a second level gastrostomy, i.e. it is normally only inserted once a tract has been formed by a PEG or other gastrostomy tube. The major advantage of this type of device is that it has no protruding tube. An extension set is used for feeding and flushing and it is, therefore, cosmetically very acceptable. The disadvantages of this tube include the need for an established tract prior to tube insertion and the speed at which the stoma closes if the tube becomes dislodged—closure may start to occur within 6–8 hours (Johnson, 2007).

12.4 Administering continuous or bolus enteral nutrition via nasogastric tube or gastrostomy tube

Enteral feeds can be delivered via a pump or syringe driver (more appropriate for small volumes of feed or volumes delivered at a slow rate) on either a continuous or intermittent basis, or can be given by gravity or bolus feeding. Both devices guarantee a constant flow rate. The regime chosen should be individualised to suit the particular needs of the child and family. Children will generally tolerate continuous feeding better than bolus feeds and this is often chosen as the preferred method when enteral feeding is commenced (Johnson, 2007). Bolus feeds given every 3–4 hours mimic normal feeding patterns and may fit in with the family's routine or lifestyle because it provides greater flexibility. Additionally, intermittent feeding is recommended as continuous feeds result in suppression of gastric acid production and subsequent potential for bacterial growth.

Procedure: Continuous or bolus feeding via a nasogastric tube (see following page)

Preparation

Ensure the head of the bed is elevated to at least 30 to 45 degrees for gastric feeding. This reduces the risk of pulmonary aspiration and enhances gravitational flow. A small child or infant may sit on their parent's knee to promote comfort (Burns Conway, 2008).

Equipment

The equipment required to administer continuous or bolus nutrition via a nasogastric tube or gastrostomy includes:

- Disposable apron.
- Disposable gloves.
- Prescribed feed.
- Pump if continuous feeding is planned.
- Feed administration set/gravity set for bolus feed, and syringes to obtain aspirate and flush tube before and after feed.
- Water for flush. Sterile water is recommended in hospital settings. In the community it is more likely that cooled boiled water will be used.
- pH indication paper (if nasogastric tube used).
- Two syringes (5–10 ml for PVC tube/50 ml for polyurethane tube).

Consent and communication

Explain the procedure to the child and family to gain consent and cooperation, and to ease any anxiety.

After the procedure

Flushing the NG tube with water after the feed is complete ensures that the entire feed has been administered and helps to prevent blockages.

Clamp and disconnect the tubing after feeding is completed. Discard the administration set and feed containers after each feed as they are single use only.

Clear equipment and wash hands to promote safety and prevent the spread of infection. To assess the child's tolerance of feeding and detect any complications or a dislodged tube, monitor the child's condition and respiratory status, recording observations.

To decrease bacterial flora in the mouth and to prevent drying and cracking of oral mucosa, perform mouth care. This helps the patient to feel more comfortable.

Nursing Alert

The principles for administering a gastrostomy feed are the same as for a nasogastric feed except it is not necessary to check the position of the tube by gastric aspirate prior to the administration of the feed.

Step-by-step guide to continuous or bolus feeding via a nasogastric tube

Step	Rationale
1 Wash hands and put on plastic apron.	To prevent cross infection.
2 Continuous or bolus feed via feeding pump: Wipe the feeding pump with detergent and water. Switch on pump; test the alarm system on the pump.	To decontaminate the equipment. To ensure that the pump is in working order.
3 Clean preparation space with an alcohol impregnated wipe and allow to dry.	To minimize the risk of cross infection.
4 Wipe top of feed container or bottle with an alcohol impregnated wipe.	To decontaminate the container.
5 Check the prescription order sheet. It should indicate the type of formula, volume to be delivered, and rate or length of infusion of the feeds. Check the expiry date on feed.	To ensure that the correct feed is being administered and to reduce the risk of error. To ensure that the feed has not expired.
6 If child is an infant, give them a soother (non-nutritive sucking) if possible.	To facilitate non-nutritive sucking and promote a positive association between sucking and relief of hunger. It will also increase peristalsis, thus enhancing absorption of nutrients (Khair, 2003). To encourage the development of normal sucking instinct of the preterm infant and thus prevent oral aversion developing. Pinelli & Symington (2005) in their Cochrane review noted that non-nutritive sucking had a positive effect on transition from tube to bottle feeding and reduced length of stay in hospital.
7 Expose the baby to as many different touches as can be tolerated, e.g. gentle touch around mouth area, and if possible allow them to 'taste' small amounts of food or liquids (Khair, 2003).	To provide oral motor stimulation and decrease oral hypersensitivity (Khair, 2003).
8 Remove the feeding set from sterile package using aseptic non-touch technique.	To prevent contamination of feeding set.
9 Check that the seal on the lid is intact in the case of Ready to Feed formula.	To prevent contamination of the feed.
10 Shake feed.	To ensure feed is evenly dispersed within container/package.

11	Aspirate fluid from the stomach using appropriate size syringe and confirm nasogastric tube position using pH strip.	In order to prevent passage of the feed into the lungs.
	Flush tube with 5–10 ml water.	To confirm patency of the tube.
	Commence feed if aspirate is pH 5.5 or below (NPSA, 2005).	
12	Prime the feeding set tubing with prescribed feed.	Priming of the tube eliminates air. Infused air can cause discomfort.
13	Attach primed feeding administration set to feeding tube using an aseptic non-touch technique.	To prevent contamination of feed and set.
14	Set the pump to run and set rate and volume according to instructions.	To ensure the correct amount of feed is administered.
	If gravity feed, kink/pinch tubing and fill syringe with feed. Allow to flow via NG tube. Continue until feed administered.	To prevent ingestion of air thus avoiding discomfort and vomiting.
	Refer to local guidelines regarding hanging times of enteral feeds.	
	Ready to Feed formulas may be given for a whole administration session up to 24 hours (NICE, 2003).	
	Reconstituted feeds (non-sterile) should be administered over a maximum of four hours (NICE, 2003; Paediatric Group of the British Dietetic Association, 2007).	Prevents bacterial growth in set.
	The giving set should be changed on a 24-hourly basis except in the case of high risk babies, where it should be changed four hourly (Paediatric Group of the British Dietetic Association, 2007; FSAI, 2007).	
15	Label the feeding line.	To prevent confusion between feeding line and intravenous line.
16	Flush the enteral feeding tube before and after feeding or the administration of medications (NICE, 2003).	To prevent blockage of the tube by food debris and prevent damage to the tube due to the increased pressure as a result of the build-up of feed deposits.
	Fresh tap water can be used. In the case of immunosuppressed patients either cooled freshly boiled water or sterile water from a freshly opened container should be used (NICE, 2003).	
	Check the manufacturer's instructions for the amount of water to instil.	
17	Document the feeding, recording the amount taken, the type of feed administered, and duration of feed.	To record an accurate intake.

12.5 **Care of a percutaneous endoscopic gastrostomy and 'button' gastrostomy device**

Procedure: Care of a percutaneous endoscopic gastrostomy and 'button' gastrostomy device

Preparation

Wash your hands and put on gloves, to prevent cross infection. Assess the comfort and fit of the tube—if it is too loose or too tight it will need to be sized. Assess stoma for signs of redness, swelling, discharge, or leakage, and check the skin integrity around the stoma site. It is vital to maintain skin integrity and prevent complications developing.

Nursing Alert

Do not attempt to use a guidewire to unblock a nasogastric tube. This could lead to gut perforation or damage the tube.

Community perspective

As many children are discharged from hospital on enteral feeds, discharge planning should commence as early as possible if it is envisaged that this method of feeding will continue. This requires a multidisciplinary team approach and entails providing timely and appropriate education and training for the carers and sourcing of supplies (Stephens, 2005). A number of factors may influence the nature of parental roles in the home, so it is important to ascertain their readiness to take on this role. Such factors include the emotional and parenting capacity to take on the task, other factors that may inhibit capacity (financial, relationship,

Step-by-step guide to care of a percutaneous endoscopic gastrostomy and 'button' gastrostomy device

Step	Rationale
1 Clean the stoma site and tube once daily using cooled boiled water or a mild soap solution and gauze swabs. Allow to dry.	This ensures that the stoma is clean and free from infection.
2 Turn tube 360 degrees daily.	To prevent tube adhering to the child's skin (Medical Innovations Corporation, 1999).
3 Change water in the retention balloon once a week (button gastrostomy and surgically placed gastrostomy only). Refer to the manufacturer's guidelines.	Water is absorbed over time from balloon.
4 Do not insert a syringe directly into the button. Use the extension set provided.	Inserting a syringe directly into the button will damage the anti-reflux valve, causing leakage of stomach contents whenever the feeding and medication port is open.

Table 12.1 Troubleshooting

Gastrostomy tubes	
Leakage around stoma site	Proper tube fit and prompt recognition of leaking will prevent this complication. A baseline measurement of gastrostomy should be done following initial placement and weekly thereafter. This should take into account length of the tube from the abdomen (Bordewick *et al.*, 2001). Leaking can be categorized as mild (occurs only with large volume feeds), moderate (intermittent leaking of gastric contents), or severe (continuous leaking). If leaking is severe it may be necessary to replace tube with either a bigger or smaller tube or replace tube with a different type of gastrostomy.
Localised infection	Daily cleansing with soap and water should be sufficient to keep area clean and prevent infection. If infection is present, antibiotic cream may be prescribed.
Granulation tissue	This may begin to form a few weeks after tube placement. Again, ensuring proper fit may help prevent this complication. If granulation tissue becomes a problem due to bleeding or improper fit, silver nitrate may be used to remove it (Bordewick *et al.*, 2001; Grant, 1993). This is undertaken by clinician and must be prescribed.
Breaking or splitting of tube	Parents/carers are instructed to move position of clamp in order to avoid damaging the tube. Prior to discharge, parents/carers should be instructed on what action to take should this occur. Parents are issued with a prescription for a replacement connector. If the existing connector splits, it may be removed and a new one inserted into the tube. If the tube splits or becomes damaged below the connector, the clamp is moved to below the damaged area, the tube is cut just below the damaged area, and a new connector is applied.
Gastrostomy tubes and nasogastric tubes	
Blockage of tube: This can be caused by— <ul><li>inadequate flushing of the tubes</li><li>infrequent flushing of the tubes</li><li>administration of medication into the tube that has not been adequately crushed or mixed with water.</li></ul>	Flushing post-medications and feeds should prevent this complication. If tube does become blocked, flush with 10–20 ml of lukewarm water. Inject 5 ml of air using a medication syringe to attempt removal of debris from end of tube. Reattempt aspiration. Attempt push-pull technique of instilling water into the tube. Do not use high pressure to unblock the tube as pressures of less than 80 psi are sufficient to perforate the tube. Always confirm position of nasogastric tube using pH strips when a tube has been unblocked. Do not use fizzy drinks or pineapple juice as the low pH of these drinks may cause the feed to clot (INDI, 2007).

time, and other competing demands), family support, and facilities within the home. In addition the parent may simply wish to have a parenting role and not be a carer (Lewis & Noyes, 2007). On the other hand, parents may view feeding as an important parenting task and, therefore, may wish to be involved in this part of their child's care. Due to the complexity of the situation a multidisciplinary approach will best address the issues.

Parents require education prior to discharge on the following:

- Hand washing technique, because enteral feed provides an ideal environment for the growth of bacteria (Best, 2008).

- Insertion of NG tube.
- Checking position of NG tube and troubleshooting.
- Administering continuous feeds via a feeding pump and bolus feeds via a syringe or bolus feeding set.
- Caring for the tube on a daily basis.
- Administering medication correctly.
- Flushing the tube pre- and post-feeds and medications.
- Appropriate storage of feeds.
- Disposal of consumable equipment.
- Checking the water in the retention balloon (if button device in use).
- Connecting and disconnecting the feeding set to the button securely (if button device in use).
- Procedure to follow if gastrostomy is accidentally dislodged (if button device in use).

It is vital that both verbal and written information is given to the parents to assist them in meeting the needs of the child and family. An interpreter service may be required if English is not the first language of the family and written information should be translated to the appropriate language. The following information should be given to parents prior to discharge:

- Contact name and telephone number for the community children's nurse/public health nurse.
- Contact name and telephone number for community dietician.
- Written instructions/guidelines on care of the feeding pump and company contact details.
- Written troubleshooting guide.
- Written feeding regime for the child.
- Written instructions on storage, ordering, and administration of feeds (Corkin & Chambers, 2008).
- Prescription for a spare button tube and extension sets for feeding.

12.6 **Administering parenteral feeding** Ⓐ

This is *an* advanced skill. You must check whether you can assist with or undertake any aspect of this skill, in line with local policy.

Parenteral nutrition (PN) is a method of providing nutritional support (partial or complete) for patients whose gastrointestinal tract is inaccessible or non-functioning. It involves the delivery of nutrients into the circulatory system via either a central venous catheter or peripheral veins. PN may include the administration of aqueous solution, amino acids, or **lipid** infusion. PN may be indicated for a number of reasons including the following:

- Intestinal obstruction due to peritoneal sepsis or adhesions.
- Bowel fistulas.
- Inadequate intestinal length.
- Extensive body burns.
- Abdominal tumours.
- Inflammatory bowel disorders not responding to other treatments.
- High output intestinal fistulas/stomas.
- Post-operatively following major intestinal surgery, e.g. for conditions such as gastroschisis or necrotizing enterocolitis (NEC).
- Conservative management of NEC.
- Extremely low birth weight infant.
- Neonates/infants fasting longer than three days, and in older children fasting longer than seven days (European Society of Paediatric Gastroenterology, Hepatology and Nutrition & European Society of Parenteral and Enteral Nutrition, 2005). (Note: In some circumstances, it may be advisable to initiate PN earlier, e.g. preterm infants.)

Central venous access is the route of choice for PN as it allows for solutions of high osmolality and high nutritional density to be infused, and is advised in the use of long-term PN administration. Solutions are rapidly diluted resulting in minimal risk for thrombophlebitis. Peripheral access may be used for patients who require short-term PN.

Procedure: Administering parenteral feeding (see following page)

Equipment

The equipment required is as follows:

- Sterile field and gloves (one pair sterile, one pair non-sterile).
- Dressing trolley.
- Prescribed PN solution, e.g. aqueous and lipid solutions.
- PN administration sets.
- Syringes, needle free access devices, NaCl 0.9%.
- Alcohol wipes.
- Prescription sheet.
- Sharps bin.
- Non-injectable bungs.
- Parenteral nutrition (PN) bag(s).

PN is stored in a refrigerator at 2–8°C and should not be administered straight from storage. The PN bag(s) must be warmed at room temperature for 30 minutes to two hours prior to administration to the patient. The PN must not be placed in direct contact with a heated surface used to warm the bag.

To ensure that the PN is safe to administer, check the PN bag(s) for minute leaks by squeezing the bag firmly; check bag for clarity, turbidity, and particles; and check the expiry date.

Preparation

Wash and dry hands to prevent cross infection.

A two-person technique should be employed to reduce the potential risk for infection. One person will prepare the infusions under aseptic technique using a sterile field and sterile gloves. The second person will wear non-sterile gloves.

Provide a clean working area for priming and administration of PN. Clean a suitable trolley with detergent and water and allow to dry. Wipe the trolley with an alcohol wipe from the centre outwards. Employ a circular motion. Allow to dry thoroughly.

Consent and communication

Explain the procedure to the child and family to prepare them and allay anxieties. The following patient details must be checked by two nurses to make certain that the correct prescription and solution is administered to the correct child and minimize risk of error:

- Name of patient.
- Date of birth.
- Hospital number.
- Date of feeding.
- Unit number.

Check the contents of the PN and lipid bags against the parenteral nutrition prescription sheet using the patient's actual weight/working weight, to avoid the risk of over- or under-infusing fluids, nutrients, and electrolytes.

Refer to Chapter Nine for more information on care of a central line, aseptic non-touch technique, and sterile technique. Refer to Chapter Fourteen for procedure steps on blood **glucose** monitoring.

Step-by-step guide to administering parenteral feeding

This is an advanced skill. You *must* check whether you can assist with or undertake any aspect of this skill, in line with local policy.

Step	Rationale
1 Open all equipment and place on a sterile drape.	To maintain asepsis.
2 Wearing sterile gloves, prime intravenous sets with PN and lipids, taking care not to touch key parts.	To maintain asepsis.
3 Clean central line site as per local guidelines and policy.	To prevent infection.
4 A single lumen (from central line) should be reserved where possible for PN access (Birmingham Children's Hospital, NHS Trust, 2001).	To prevent infection.

5	Ensure that the fluid is run carefully through the administration set.	To expel any air bubbles that may be present in the tubing.
	Both aqueous and lipid solutions need to be protected from light.	To prevent vitamin degradation (aqueous solution) and to prevent both vitamin degradation and peroxide formation (lipid solution). It is especially important that the lipid solution is completely protected from light where infants are receiving phototherapy.
6	Attach the administration set to the line and thread through the infusion pump. A volumetric infusion pump must always be used to administer PN.	To minimize complications with rapid infusion and ensure accuracy of infusion.
7	Commence the infusion.	To begin feeding.
8	Monitoring:	To ensure that the correct infusion is being administered at the correct rate as prescribed.
	Monitor and record the infusion rate and fluid volume infused on an hourly basis.	To enable early detection and management of phlebitis and extravasation. Peripheral access must not be used where PN contains greater than 12.5% dextrose concentration.
	If a peripheral line is in use check site at 30 minute intervals for redness, swelling, oozing, or tenderness.	
	If a central line is in use, check site at hourly intervals for redness, swelling, inflammation, or oozing.	To enable early detection and management of phlebitis and extravasation.
	Check all lines hourly for leaking or kinking.	To minimize risk of infection, haemorrhage, and embolism.
	Vital signs:	To check for evidence of sepsis, i.e. poor perfusion, hypotension, lethargy, tachycardia, pyrexia, and respiratory distress.
	Monitor temperature closely, observing for pyrexia, which may be indicative of line infection. Monitor heart and respiratory rates, blood pressure, and peripheral perfusion and observe for deviations from the norm.	
9	Assess and record the child's fluid intake and output.	Early detection of fluid overload.
10	Perform urinalysis daily for glucose and ketone levels.	To detect glycosuria. If present may need to adjust glucose content of PN.
11	Blood glucose should be recorded 4–6-hourly or as condition indicates/as per doctor's instructions, and whenever glucose concentration has been increased or decreased.	To ensure blood glucose is maintained within recommended range.
12	Record weight daily/on alternate days as condition indicates or as per local guidelines.	PN and electrolytes etc. are prescribed according to weight.
		To ensure child is thriving.
13	Maintain frequent oral hygiene care (particularly in patients receiving nil orally) and inspect perineum area frequently.	To prevent oral dryness.
		Administration of PN increases potential for candidiasis due to hyperalimentation (Borzotta & Beardsley, 1999).

| **14** | **PN must *not* be disconnected for transporting patient to X-ray or to change patient's clothing**. | To assist in the detection and management of complications associated with PN administration. |
| **15** | **Refer to PN prescription sheet and patient's notes/ local instructions for frequency of laboratory instructions.** | To prevent infection. |

12.7 **Assessing dehydration**

Dehydration is a disturbance in body fluids and occurs as a result of inadequate fluid intake and/or excess losses of body fluid. It can occur for a variety of reasons, the most common cause in infants and young children being gastroenteritis, which causes vomiting and diarrhoea (Rudolf & Levane, 2006). Infants and young children are at increased risk of dehydration and electrolyte imbalance because they have a higher content of body water than adults; a higher proportion of this fluid is extracellular and extracellular fluid is more easily lost from the body than intracellular. They also have a larger surface area to volume ratio, resulting in a higher insensible loss from the skin and respiratory system, a higher metabolic rate than adults, and a reduced renal ability to concentrate urine. Therefore, prompt assessment of hydration status and treatment with rehydration therapy is crucial in preventing rapid deterioration of the child's condition. The table below outlines the steps to be followed in carrying out the assessment.

Procedure: Assessing dehydration

Step-by-step guide to assessing dehydration

Step	Rationale
1 **Wash and dry hands.**	To prevent the spread of infection.
2 **On admission obtain an accurate history from child and/or carer:** ● **Dietary history.** ● **Length of illness prior to admission.** ● **Fluid intake including type, amount, and frequency.** ● **Urine amount and frequency.** ● **Stool amount, consistency, frequency, and characteristics.** ● **Vomiting amount, type, and characteristics.**	To aid diagnosis.
3 **Observe the child's colour, general appearance, and level of consciousness.** **Check and monitor the following:** ● **Vital signs.**	Because the following are signs of dehydration: ● Altered responsiveness, e.g. irritability and lethargy. ● Tachycardia and tachypnoea (hypotension is a sign of shock). ● Sunken eyes.

Assessing dehydration

- Appearance of eyes.
- Anterior fontanelle.
- Mucous membranes.
- Peripheral pulses.
- Temperature of skin.

- Sunken fontanelle.
- Dry mucous membranes (except for mouth breather).

Pale, mottled, or cold skin is a sign of shock (NICE, 2009). Weak peripheral pulses also indicate shock.

4 Record weight on admission and daily thereafter using the same scales and at the same time of day. Fluid loss can by measured by subtracting the child's present weight from their previous weight.

As water forms a significant proportion of the child's body, weight loss is a reliable indicator of fluid deficit in the child (Kanneh, 2006). Mild dehydration is <5% loss of body weight; moderate dehydration is 5–10% body weight loss and these children have clinical signs of dehydration; and severe dehydration >10% body weight loss and these children present with shock (Lissauer & Clayden, 2007).

5 Record strict intake and output. Ask the child if he/she passed urine. Weigh all soiled nappies and request parents to keep nappies for inspection and weighing. In order to calculate output weight, dry nappy and subtract weight of dry nappy from wet one. Note 1 g = 1 ml.
Calculate the child's hourly urinary output by dividing total urine output by weight in kg, then divide by 24 hours, e.g. if an infant weighing 10 kg has a urinary output of 480 ml, then hourly output is 480/10/24 = 2 ml/kg/hr.
Note colour of urine and check specific gravity.

Decreased urinary output is a sign of dehydration.

Normal urine output is 1–2 ml/kg/hour. Babies normally have 6–8 wet nappies in 24 hours (Lambert & O'Toole, 2009).

To determine concentration of urine.

6 Record the number of soiled nappies the baby has. If stools are very loose it may be difficult to distinguish between urine and stool.

To maintain an accurate record of output.

7 Check capillary refill by applying pressure with a finger on the child's forehead or sternum for five seconds. Under normal circumstances when the pressure is released the colour returns to the area within two seconds in children and less than three seconds in neonates (RCN, 2007c).

A slow capillary refill indicates poor skin perfusion.

8 Check skin turgor by gently pinching a roll of skin on the insides of the thighs or the abdomen.

Under normal circumstances the pinched skin will return to its normal place when released. Slow return indicates dehydration.

12.8 **Administering rehydration therapy**

Rehydration therapy is normally commenced for infants and children with dehydration (Moules & Ramsay, 2008). There are two options: oral rehydration therapy using **oral rehydration salts** (ORS), which are a balanced glucose-electrolyte mixture, or intravenous fluids. The type of rehydration therapy depends on the degree of dehydration present; therefore it is important to assess the child appropriately. Oral rehydration is recommended as the first line of treatment in children with mild to moderate dehydration (Hartling *et al.*, 2006). ORS solution can be given as a supplemental drink to a child who has gastroenteritis but who is not clinically dehydrated. If a child is clinically dehydrated ORS solution should be given to replace fluid deficit as well as maintenance fluids. Intravenous fluids should be commenced if shock is suspected or confirmed, if the child shows evidence of deterioration despite oral rehydration, or if the child persistently vomits the ORS given orally or via a nasogastric tube (NICE, 2009).

Management of a child on rehydration therapy requires accurate calculation of replacement fluid volume. This is done by estimating the actual fluid loss, maintenance fluid requirements, and ongoing losses (Rudolf & Levane, 2006). Instructions for calculating replacement and maintenance fluid requirements are provided in **Box 12.4**. In addition, it is necessary in the case of gastroenteritis to determine the causative organism. The next section will deal with stool specimen collection.

Procedure: Administering oral rehydration therapy (see following page)

Preparation

Wash hands, dry thoroughly, and don gloves and gown, to reduce the risk of cross infection.

Equipment

- Oral rehydration solution.
- Fresh drinking water.

Consent and communication

Explain to the child and parents the reasons for commencing the oral rehydration therapy to allay anxiety and promote family centred care.

Box 12.4 Calculating replacement and maintenance fluid requirements

Formula:

$$\text{fluid deficit (ml)} = \text{weight} \times \text{percentage dehydration} \times 10$$

e.g. If an infant weighing 8 kg is believed on the basis of clinical examination to be 10% dehydrated, their fluid requirement is as follows:

$$\text{fluid deficit} = 8 \times 10 \times 10 = \textbf{800 ml}$$

Maintenance fluids = 100 ml/kg/day for the first 10 kg of body weight;

50 ml/kg/day for the second 10 kg of body weight;

20 ml/kg/day for each additional kg body weight.

e.g. For previous example, maintenance fluids = 100 ml × 8 kg = **800 ml**

Therefore this infant needs 800 + 800 = **1600 ml** fluid over the next 24 hours to rehydrate and then maintain normal hydration.

To calculate hourly rate in this example: 1600/24 = 66.6 ml per hour (67 ml).

Maintenance fluids cover essential urine output and insensible losses so if there are significant ongoing losses this volume may need to be increased further.

Adapted from Calculating the replacement and maintenance requirements, p 79 (Miall *et al.*, 2007, *Paediatrics at a Glance*. London: Wiley-Blackwell.)

Step-by-step guide to administering oral rehydration therapy

Step	Rationale
1 **Make up oral rehydration solution (ORS) according to the manufacturer's instructions.** **Reconstitute with cooled, boiled fresh drinking water.** **Use flavoured variety of ORS.**	To ensure the correct concentration of solution. May be more palatable to drink.
2 **Give ORS frequently in small amounts.** **ORS may be given via nasogastric tube.**	To promote fluid intake. If the child is vomiting. Enteral feeds are less likely than intravenous fluids to cause fluid/electrolyte imbalance (Hill, 2007).
3 **Increase intake as tolerated by the child.** **ORS may be supplemented with usual fluids (except fruit juices or carbonated drinks) if child refuses to take sufficient quantity of ORS solution (NICE, 2009).**	To increase oral intake. Fruit juices and carbonated drinks are high in carbohydrates, low in electrolytes, and have high osmolarity (Hockenberry & Barrera, 2007).

After the procedure

Record the intake in the fluid balance chart to ensure the child receives appropriate fluid requirements. To ensure that the child is responding to treatment, monitor and record the response to therapy by regular clinical assessment. Report any deterioration in condition to senior nursing staff and the medical team. See Essential Skills Clusters (NMC, 2007) for advice on accurately recording observations and communicating to appropriate personnel.

Many children with gastroenteritis are discharged home following initial assessment and management in the Accident and Emergency department and it is important that parents are able to continue treatment at home. Make sure that parents are advised of the correct method of preparing oral rehydration therapy before discharge from hospital.

12.9 **Collection of a stool specimen**

There are a number of indications for collecting stool samples. The most common reason in children is to identify organisms that cause gastrointestinal infections, such as rotavirus, *Giardia, E. coli, Salmonella*, or *Shigella*. Samples may also be taken for faecal occult blood. This identifies blood in the stool and thus indicates bleeding in the gastrointestinal tract. This test can be carried out on the ward using a test card, which can be obtained from the laboratory. Instructions for use are included in the packet and should be followed to ensure appropriate collection of sample. It requires samples of faeces that have been collected over a three-day period (Jasper, 2008). It is important to remember that due to the potentially contagious nature of stool specimens, strict infection control precautions should be adhered to when handling samples.

Procedure: Collecting a stool specimen

Preparation

Ensure privacy while the procedure is taking place as this may be embarrassing for the child. Consider the timing of specimen collection, as some specimens may need to be collected first thing in the morning (e.g. threadworm/pin worm) or may need to be sent fresh to the laboratory so must be collected during laboratory hours.

Equipment

The equipment required for the collection of stool specimens is as follows:

- Disposable gloves.
- A protective tray.
- A sterile container for the specimen.
- Laboratory specimen form.
- A polythene transportation bag.
- Biohazard label (if required).

Consent and communication

To elicit their help and cooperation, explain the procedure to the child and parent, and the reasons for taking the specimen. They have a right to refuse.

Step-by-step guide to collection of a stool specimen

Step	Rationale
1 Wash hands using bactericidal soap and water or alcohol hand rub before and after specimen collection.	Hand washing greatly reduces the risk of infection.
2 Wear gloves when collecting or handling specimen.	To avoid cross contamination and cross infection.
3 Assess whether specimen may be collected from a nappy/clean potty/bedpan/by placing bedpan or other suitable tray in toilet to catch specimen.	To collect specimen.
4 Where diarrhoea is present in an infant, a small piece of non-absorbent material can be placed in nappy.	To prevent sample soaking into the nappy.
5 Ask patient (if able to understand) to defecate into clinically clean bedpan.	To avoid contamination from other organisms.
6 Using a scoop (often incorporated in container) or wooden spatula, place faecal material into a container. Fill a third of specimen container if possible.	To avoid contamination. To obtain sufficient amount for examination.
7 Examine the sample for consistency, odour, or blood and record observations.	To monitor changes/trends.
8 Label and dispatch specimen promptly to laboratory with completed request form. The stool should not be allowed to dry out and if the test is not carried out immediately it should be kept in a refrigerator (Skinner, 2005).	To ensure laboratory staff receive sample in a time frame and condition appropriate to the investigation required.
9 Remove gloves and wash hands.	To prevent cross infection.
10 Document procedure in patient's clinical notes.	To record that sample has been taken and sent to laboratory.

Bowel care

There are wide variations in bowel patterns in the healthy infant, for example, a breastfed baby may pass several stools per day in the early days of breastfeeding but after a couple of months the breastfed baby may not pass stool for several days and experience no ill effects (Lissauer & Clayden, 2007). Nevertheless, constipation (which is the painful passage of hard, infrequent stool) is a common childhood problem and requires careful management. Treatment depends on severity and may range from diet alone to the use of laxatives, stool lubricants, and/or bowel stimulants. These may be administered orally or rectally as a suppository or an enema. A suppository is a medicated solid formulation that melts at body temperature and dissolves in the mucosa secretions of the rectum (Dougherty & Lister, 2008). An enema is a liquid preparation that is administered into the rectum for the purposes of evacuating the bowel or administering medication (Kyle, 2007). In addition, both these preparations may be used to empty the bowel prior to surgery or investigations, or to soothe and treat irritated mucosa (Dougherty & Lister, 2008).

The administration of a suppository or enema is an invasive procedure and is potentially uncomfortable and embarrassing for the child. Therefore, appropriate explanation and privacy is necessary. Parental presence during the procedure may help to alleviate anxiety. Refer to Chapter Seven for procedural steps on administering an enema and the insertion of suppositories. While these interventions may be used to aid normal bowel functioning, there are occasions when surgical intervention is required to ensure that waste products are excreted from the bowel, e.g. stoma formation in the case of Hirschsprung's disease.

12.10 Stoma care (colostomy/ileostomy)

A bowel stoma is a surgically created opening whereby a section of the bowel is brought to the surface of the abdomen to allow for the excretion of waste material. The majority of stoma formation in children is temporary and occurs in the neonate period during the surgical correction of congenital abnormalities such as Hirschsprung's disease and imperforate anus. In some instances a stoma may be permanent, for example, with inflammatory bowel disease, tumours, and trauma. There are two types of bowel stoma: a colostomy, where a section of the colon is brought through the abdominal wall, and an ileostomy, where a section of the ileum is used. A colostomy is usually sited in the left iliac fossa and an ileostomy in the right iliac fossa.

Although a stoma is a temporary measure for many children, it can affect the child and family physiologically, psychologically, and emotionally (Coyne, 2008). Therefore, the child and family will require appropriate preparation prior to stoma formation and ongoing support and education in managing the stoma. It is essential that carers are taught all aspects of stoma care prior to discharge into the community, therefore discharge planning should commence as early as possible after stoma formation. Referral to the community healthcare team is essential to ensure appropriate support for the child and family in the home.

There are a variety of stoma bags (pouches) available. These may be either a one- or two-piece device, and both can have a closed or an open end. A one-piece bag has an adhesive base (flange) attached, which adheres to the skin and that is removed from the skin when the bag is changed. A two-piece bag has a base (flange) that sticks to the skin and a separate pouch that attaches to the bag. The base (flange) can remain in position for several days and only the bag needs to be changed. This can help reduce skin irritation. A closed-end bag is used when stools are formed and an open-end one when stools are loose. The procedure for changing a stoma bag will now be explained.

Procedure: Changing a stoma bag

Preparation

Wash hands and apply gloves and gown, to prevent cross infection.

Equipment

Gather the equipment you need before starting the procedure, to facilitate a smooth procedure. The equipment required for this procedure is as follows:

Step-by-step guide to changing a stoma bag

Step	Rationale
1 Position a baby lying down and offer an older child the option of lying or standing.	To allow good access to stoma.
2 Use a protective material to protect patient's clothing if effluent is fluid in nature.	Avoids necessity for changing clothing.
3 Where drainable pouch is used, empty contents into measuring jug (if measuring output) before changing pouch.	For prevention of spillage and ease in handling the appliance.
4 Measure output if required and dispose of in toilet.	To maintain a record of output.
5 Remove soiled pouch carefully while supporting the skin with one hand.	To avoid trauma to the skin.
6 Dispose of used pouch in nappy sack or disposal bag.	To ensure safe disposal according to hospital policy.
7 Clean around the stoma with warm water and gauze squares. Where there is adhesive left on skin, remove first with dry gauze or adhesive remover. Do not use cotton wool.	To promote cleanliness and prevent skin breakdown. The fibres may stick to the stoma.
8 Dry the skin with dry gauze. Examine colour of stoma and assess surrounding skin. If stoma appears a darker colour, report to doctor.	The new appliance will attach more securely. A healthy stoma is red/pink. If the blood supply to the bowel is compromised the stoma will become darker in colour.
9 Cut the new pouch to fit snugly around the stoma with no peristomal skin exposed.	So that the new pouch fits well.
10 Apply new pouch. If a one-piece pouch is being used, fold the adhesive section in half. Place the pouch on the underside of the stoma first and then remove the remaining adhesive and secure in position. If a two-piece is being used, secure the base and then press the pouch firmly against base to form a tight seal.	To attach the new pouch securely.
11 If a drainable pouch is being used, ensure that the clip is secured correctly.	To prevent leakage of contents.

- Disposable gloves for hospital staff.
- Parents may opt not to wear gloves as they would not normally do so at home. However, correct hand washing technique must be taught to prevent transmission of infection.
- Bowl of warm water and mild soap if desired.
- Bag to dispose of soiled cleaning materials and pouch.
- Scissors.
- Gauze/dry wipes.
- Template pattern of the stoma size and new pouch.
- Alcohol-free adhesive remover.

Consent and communication

Before you begin, explain and discuss the procedure with the child/parents. It is vital to ensure the patient understands the procedure and gives consent.

After the procedure

Dispose of the pouch correctly. Pouches should be emptied, put in a disposal bag, and placed in clinical waste (if appropriate) or other suitable waste bin. Biodegradable pouches may be put down the toilet. Make sure you comply with your hospital waste disposal policy.

Wash hands thoroughly using bactericidal soap and water or alcohol hand rub, before documenting the procedure, noting skin and stoma condition, and how the child tolerated the procedure.

Conclusion

This chapter provides an overview of the main gastrointestinal nursing skills carried out by the children's nurse. It highlights the complexity of the care required and the student is advised to consult other chapters in the book in order to provide holistic care. Collaboration with other members of the multidisciplinary team is also part of the care plan for many of these children. As more children with complex healthcare needs are nursed in the community, the involvement of parents and parent education are paramount.

Online resource centre

You may find it helpful to work through our online resources including interactive scenarios intended to help you to develop and apply the skills in this chapter. Where material referenced below is available electronically, we're pleased to provide active web links to the source via **http://www.oxfordtextbooks.co.uk/orc/coyne/**

References

Albon, D. & Mukherji, P. (2008) *Food and Health in Early Childhood*. London: Sage.

An Bord Altranais (2002) *Recording Clinical Practice: Guidance to Nurses and Midwives*. Available at: **http://www.nursingboard.ie/**

Best, C. (2008) Enteral tube feeding and infection control: How safe is our practice? *British Journal of Nursing* **17** (16), 1036–1041.

Birmingham Children's Hospital, NHS Trust (2001) *Nutritional Care Team Protocols*. Birmingham: Birmingham Children's Hospital.

Bordewick, A., Bildner, J., & Randall, S. (2001) An effective approach for preventing and treating gastrostomy tube complications in newborns. *Neonatal Network* **20** (2), 37?40.

Borzotta, A.P. & Beardsley, K. (1999) *Candida* infections in critically ill trauma patients. *Archives in Surgery* **134** (6), 657?665.

Bowers, S. (2000) All about tubes. *Nursing* **30** (12), 41–48.

Bowling, T. (2004) Nutritional support for adults and children: A handbook for hospital practice. Oxon: Radcliff Publishing.

Burns Conway, D. (2008) Enteral nutrition: Administration. In J.K. Verger & R.M. Lebet (eds.) *AACN Procedure Manual for Pediatric Acute and Critical Care*. Missouri: Saunders Elsevier.

Chamley, C.A., Carson, P., Randall, D., & Sandwell, M. (2005) *Developmental Anatomy and Physiology: A Practical Approach*. London: Churchill Livingstone.

Corkin, D. & Chambers, J. (2008) Enteral feeding. In J. Kelsey & G. McEwing (eds.) *Clinical Skills in Child Health Practice*. London: Churchill Livingstone.

Coyne, I. (2008) Stoma care. In J. Kelsey J & G. McEwing (eds.) *Clinical Skills in Child Health Practice*. London: Churchill Livingstone.

Department of Health and Children (2005) The *Prevention of Transmission of Blood-Borne Diseases in the Health-Care Setting*. Available at: **http://www.dohc.ie/**

Dougherty, L. & Lister, S. (2008) *The Royal Marsden Hospital Manual of Clinical Nursing Procedures, 7th ed*. Oxford: Wiley-Blackwell.

European Society of Paediatric Gastroenterology, Hepatology and Nutrition & European Society of Parenteral and Enteral Nutrition (2005) Guidelines on paediatric gastroenterology and nutrition. *Journal of Pediatric Gastroenterology and Nutrition* **41**, Supplement 2.

Fergusson, D. (2008) *Clinical Assessment and Monitoring in Children*. London: Blackwell Publishing.

Food Safety Authority of Ireland (2007) *Guidance Note 22: Information relevant to the development of guidance material for the safe feeding of reconstituted powdered infant Formula*. Dublin: Food Safety Authority.

Gill, D. & O' Brien, N. (2007) *Paediatric Clinical Examination Made Easy, 5th ed*. London: Churchill Livingstone.

Grant, P.J. (1993) Percutaneous endoscopic gastrostomy: Initial placement by a single endoscopic technique and long term follow up. *Ann Surg* **217** (2), 168–174.

Hankins, J., Walsman Lonsway, R.A., Hedrick, C., & Perdue, M. (2001) *Infusion Therapy in Clinical Practice, 2nd ed*. Philadelphia: WB Saunders Company.

Hanks, C. & McEwing, G. (2009) Enteral feeding. In A. Glasper, G. McEwing, & J. Richardson (eds.) *Foundation Skills for Caring*. London: Palgrave McMillan.

Hartling, L., Bellemere, S., Wiebe, N., Russell, K., Klassen, T.P., & Craig, W. (2006) Oral versus intravenous rehydration for treating dehydration due to gastroenteritis in children. Cochrane Database of Systematic Reviews, Issue 3. Art. No.: CD004390. DOI: 10.1002/14651858.cd004390.pub2.

Hill, S. (2007) Gastroenterology. In S. Strobel, S.D. Marks, P.K. Smith, M.H. EL Habbal, & L. Spitz (eds.) *The Great Ormond Street Colour Handbook of Paediatrics and Child Health*. London: Manson Publishing.

Hockenberry, M.J. & Barrera, P. (2007) Communication and physical and developmental assessment of the child. In M.J. Hockenberry & D. Wilson (eds.) *Wong's Nursing Care of Infants and Children*. Missouri: Mosby Elsevier.

Holden, C. & MacDonald, A. (2000) *Nutrition and Child Health*. London: Bailliere Tindall in association with the RCN.

Hussain K. & Preece, M. (2006) Applied physiology: Understanding growth. *Current Paediatrics* **16**, 430–433.

Infant Feeding Survey 2005 (2008) *A commentary on infant feeding practices in the UK: A Position paper by the Scientific Advisory Committee*. Available at: **http://www.dh.gov.uk/en/Healthcare/Maternity/Maternalandinfantnutrition/DH_091337.**

Irish Nutrition & Dietetic Institute (2007) *Home Enteral Feeding Resource Pack. Nutritional Support Interest Group*. Available at: **http://www.indi.ie**

Jasper, E.V.P. (2008) Specimen collection. In J. Kelsey & G. McEwing (eds.) *Clinical Skills in Child Health Practice*. London: Churchill Livingstone.

Johnson, T. (2007) Enteral nutrition. In V. Shaw & M. Lawson (eds.) *Clinical Paediatric Dietetics*. London: Blackwell Publishing.

Kanneh, A. (2006) Caring for children with body fluid and electrolyte imbalance. In A. Glasper & J.A. Richardson (eds.) *Text Book of Children's and Young People's Nursing*. London: Churchill Livingstone Publishers.

Khair, J. (2003) Managing home enteral tube feeding for children. *British Journal of Community Nursing* **8** (3), 116–126.

Khair, J. (2005) Guidelines for testing the placing of nasogastric tubes. *Nursing Times* **101** (20), 26–27.

Kyle, G. (2007) Administering an enema. *Nursing Times* **103** (45), 26–27.

Lambert, V. & O'Toole, D. (2009) Assessing and managing hydration. In A. Glasper, G. McEwing, & J.A. Richardson (eds.) *Foundation Skills for Caring using Student-centred Learning*. London: Palgrave.

Lewis, M. & Noyes, J. (2007) Discharge management for children with complex needs. *Paediatric Nursing* **19** (4), 26–30.

Lissauer, T. & Clayden, G. (2007) *Illustrated Textbook of Paediatrics, 3rd ed*. London: Elsevier.

MacGregor, J. (2008) *Introduction to the Anatomy and Physiology of Children: A guide for students of nursing, child care and health*. London: Routledge.

Medical Innovations Corporation (1999) *The MIC-KEY G Low Profile Feeding Tube: Your guide to proper care*. Utah: Medical Innovations Corporation, Ballard Medical Products.

Metheny, N.A, Clouse, R.E., Clark, J.M, Reed, L, Wehrle, MA., & Wierema, L. (1994) pH testing of feeding tube aspirates to determine placement. *Nutrition in Clinical Practice* **9** (5), 185?190.

Miall, L., Rudolf, M., & Levane, M. (2007) *Paediatrics at a Glance, 2nd ed*. London: Blackwell Publishing.

Mitchell, M.K. (2002) *Nutrition across the Lifespan, 2nd ed*. London: Elsevier.

Moules, T. & Ramsay, J. (2008) The T*extbook of Children's and Young People's Nursing, 2nd ed*. London: Blackwell Publishing.

National Institute for *Clinical Excellence (2003) Clinical Guideline 2. Infection control: prevention of healthcare associated infection in primary and community care*. Available at: **http://www.nice.org.uk**

National Institute for Health and Clinical Excellence (2008) *Public Health Guidance 11: Maternal and child nutrition*. Available at: **http://www.nice.org.uk**

National Institute for Health and *Clinical Excellence (2009) Clinical Guideline 84: Diarrhoea and vomiting in children*. Available at: **http://www.nice.org.uk**

National Patient Safety Agency (2005) How to *Confirm the Correct Position of Nasogastric Feeding Tubes in Infants, Children and Adults*. London: NHS. Available at: **http://www.npsa.nhs.uk/advice**

Neill, S. & Knowles, H. (2004) *The Biology of Child Health: A reader in development and assessment*. Basingstoke: Palgrave Macmillan.

Nursing and Midwifery Council (2004) *The NMC Code of Professional Conduct: Standards for conduct, performance and ethics*. London: Nursing and Midwifery Council.

Nursing and Midwifery Council (2007) *Introduction of Essential Skills Clusters for Pre-registration Nursing programme, Circular07/2007*. Available at: **www.nmc-uk.org**

Paediatric Group of the British Dietetic Association (2007) *Guidelines for Making Special Feeds for Infants and Children in Hospital*. London: Food Standards Agency. Available at: **http://www.bda.uk.com**

Pinelli, J. & Symington, A.J (2005) Non-nutritive sucking for promoting physiologic stability and nutrition in preterm infants. *Cochrane Database of Systematic Reviews*. Issue 4. Art. No.:CD001071. DOI:1002/14651858.CD001071.pub2.

Royal College of Nursing (2007a) Malnutrition: What nurses working with children and young people need to know and do. An RCN position paper. Available at: **http://www.rcn.org.uk**

Royal College of Nursing (2007b) *Formula Feeds: RCN guidance for nurses caring for infants and mothers*. Available at: **http://www.rcn.org.uk**

Royal College of Nursing (2007c) Standards for assessing, measuring and monitoring vital signs in infants, children and young people. Available at: **http://www.rcn.org.uk**

Royal College of Paediatrics and Child Health (2009) UK-WHO Growth Charts: What is the difference? Available at: **http://www.growthcharts.rcpch.ac.uk**

Rudolf, M. & Levane, M. (2006) *Paediatrics and Child Health, 2nd ed*. London: Blackwell Publishing.

Skinner, S. (2005) *Understanding Clinical Investigations: A quick reference manual, 2nd ed*. London: Elsevier.

Spencer, A. & Jones, L. (2002) Understanding breast-feeding: How to offer practical help. *Current Paediatrics* **12**, 93–97.

Stephens, N. (2005) Complex care packages: Supporting seamless discharge for child and family. *Paediatric Nursing* **17** (7), 30–32.

Stroud, M., Duncan, H., & Nightingale, J. (2003) Guidelines for enteral feeding in adult hospital patients. *Gut* **52**, vii1–vii12.

Torgus, J., Bykowski, N.J., Ciagne, G., Haynes, S.G., & Cusack, J. (2006) *An Easy Guide to Breastfeeding*. Washington: US Department of Health and Human Services Office on Women's Health.

Trigg, E. & Mohammed, T. (2006) *Practices in Children's Nursing: Guidelines for community and hospital, 2nd ed*. London: Churchill Livingstone.

WHO (2003) *Global Strategy for Infant and Young Child Feeding*. Geneva: WHO.

Further reading and URLs

Dixon, M., Crawford, D., Teasdale, D., & Murphy, J. (2009) *Nursing the Highly Dependent Child or Infant: A manual of care*. Oxford: Wiley-Blackwell.

Doyle, C. (2006) Peg feeding and the child with ID. *World of Irish Nursing* **14** (4), 27–28.

Holden, C , MacDonald, A, Ward, M., *et al.* (1997) Psychological preparation for nasogastric feeding in children. *British Journal of Nursing* 6 (7), 376–385.

Miller, D. & Miller, H. (1995) A nurse's guide to tube feeding: Giving meds through the tube. RN **58**, 44–48.

National Nurses' Nutrition Group (2005) *Guidelines for Confirming Correct positioning of Nasogastric Feeding Tubes*. London: NNNG.

Taylor, S. & Goodison-McLaren, S. (1992) *Nutritional support – A team approach*. London: Wolfe Publishing.

Wong, D.L. (1999) *Nursing Care of Infants and Children, 6th ed*. St. Louis: Mosby.

13 Musculo-skeletal system

SIOBHAN McDERMOTT AND LIZ NOLAN

Skills

This chapter aims to highlight the principles of orthopaedic nursing and the skills required to perform effective musculo-skeletal care of orthopaedic injury in children.

Introduction

Musculo-skeletal injury is one of the most frequently encountered problems in children's nursing. Almost 20% of children who present with injury have sustained a fracture (Hart *et al.*, 2006). When children have fractures, they are generally brought to emergency departments. Whether the fractures are simple or complex, or they require surgical intervention or not, fractures produce a great deal of anxiety for children and their families. Children's nurses are in an ideal situation to use their nursing knowledge to provide optimal care for children with musculo-skeletal injury. The initial assessment and immediate treatment of

an injured extremity is fundamentally important in ensuring a good outcome.

Delay in recognition of neurovascular compromise can lead to a condition known as **compartment syndrome** (CS). If ignored, a limb can become seriously compromised, which could eventually lead to amputation of the limb or even the death of the patient. However, having the foundation of knowledge regarding total neurovascular function can equip the nurse with accurate assessment skills and the knowledge of the need for immediate action. **Neurovascular assessment** used correctly provides the best patient care with the best possible outcome.

Compartment syndrome is a possible complication for every patient with a fracture, sprain, or following orthopaedic surgery. Any deviation from the normal range of the neurovascular parameters should be highlighted immediately. Early identification of the symptoms will prompt immediate treatment and prevent any compromise of the limb. In addition the immature skeleton of children has unique properties that directly affect the management of fractures in children.

Learning outcomes

By the end of this chapter you will be able to:
- Explain the nursing assessment you would undertake for an infant/child presenting with musculo-skeletal injury.
- Understand the principles of neurovascular assessment and complete all the aspects involved in assessing neurovascular status.
- Understand the rationale and purpose of the musculo-skeletal nursing skills outlined such as care of the child with a cast.

Anatomy and physiology of the skeletal system

Figure 13.1 shows the skeletal system. The adult skeleton is made up of 206 bones, whereas children are born with more than 300 bones that are primarily made up of cartilage. As the child grows, normal growth and development ensures that certain parts of the skeleton fuse to form single bones, eventually resulting in the adult skeleton (Chamley *et al.*, 2005). The main function of the bones is to protect the muscles and organs of the body (see Box 13.2). In children, however, the bones are not fully formed. Indeed, the skeleton continues to grow until the age of approximately 18 to 21 years. The rate of healing in children is different, and injured growth plates can cause long-term problems. The major anatomical regions of a growing bone include: the epiphysis, growth plate (physis), metaphysis, and diaphysis. The epiphysis is the secondary ossification centre located at the end of long bones. The skeletons of children may be injured more easily than the mature skeletons of adults because the bones are more porous and the long bones are further weakened

Box 13.2 Functions of the skeleton

- It supports the body and provides a shape.
- It protects the body's vital organs, e.g. brain, heart, and renal organs.
- It provides a store for minerals, calcium, and phosphorus.
- It provides a framework for the structures of the body.
- It is essential for movement.
- It contains red bone marrow, which is responsible for producing red blood cells.

Box 13.3 Differences between children's and adults' skeletons

- Children's bones are still growing.
- Children's bones are more porous.
- Children's long bones are weakened by epiphysial plates at each end.
- Children have a lower injury rate because they are more flexible.

(Klenerman, 1994)

by the epiphyseal plates at the proximal and distal ends (see Box 13.3).

Embryology

The skeletal systems develop through a process called osteogenesis or ossification. Bone begins to form from approximately the fourth week of prenatal development

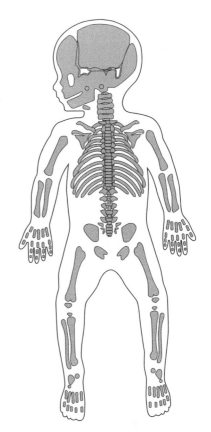

Figure 13.1 The child's skeletal system (adapted from Chamley *et al.* 2005, reproduced with kind permission of Elsevier).

by either intramembranous ossification or endochondral ossification. These processes begin with migration of mesenchymal (mesodermal) cells into the area where bone formation will occur. Most bones develop from mesenchymal cells that develop into *chondroblasts*, which condense into a hyaline cartilage precursor. The hyaline cartilage is later replaced by bone through endochondral ossification. Certain bones (facial bones and some flat bones of the skull) develop by intramembranous ossification whereby mesenchymal cells develop into *osteoblasts* that directly form bone without first passing through a cartilage stage. Whilst bone formation (ossification) begins at about the fourth week of embryonic development, ossification centres are not observed until about the eighth week. Ossification is not completed in certain bones until about 25 years of age.

Bone is continuously broken down by osteoclasts and formed by another type of cell, the osteoblasts. Osteoblasts and osteoclasts are instrumental in controlling the amount of bone tissue. Osteoblasts form bone and osteoclasts resorb bone.

Definitions

- **Osteoblasts** manufacture bone and are mesodermal in origin, arising from mesenchymal cells. They further differentiate into osteocytes.
- **Osteoclasts** resorb bone and this is an important mechanism for bone remodelling. They are derived from hematopoietic precursor cells formed by the fusion of monocytic cells at the bone sites to be resorbed.
- *Physis* is epiphyseal cartilage.
- *Epiphysis* is the end part of the long bone (not the shaft). It is a centre of ossification, separated from the shaft by layer of cartilage.
- *Metaphysis* a conical section of bone between the epiphysis and diaphysis of long bones.
- *Diaphysis* is the shaft of the bone.

Bone formation begins *in utero* as follows:

- Fourth week gestation—differentiation of connective tissue into three layers (skin, muscle, and cartilage and bone). Limb buds recognizable.
- Sixth week gestation—formation of embryonic vertebrae and digits (failure of this separation can lead to a condition called syndactylism).

- Eighth week gestation—primary ossification is evident at antenatal scan; fingers separate; human appearance; basic organs are complete.
- Twelfth week gestation—first bone (clavicle) ossifies by process of deposition of calcium; primary ossification appears in the diaphysis of most bones (Chamley *et al.*, 2005); limbs grow proportionally to form a solid framework.

Bone formation

- First stage—mesenchymal cells condense to become models for future bones.
- Second stage—rapid interstitial growth (chondrification).
- Final stage—cartilage is converted into bone by intramembranous and endochondral ossification.

Bone growth (ossification)

- Bone growth begins in the embryo at week six or seven of embryonic life and continues until 18–21 years (Chamley *et al.*, 2005).
- Intramembranous ossification—bone forms on or within loose fibrous connective tissue.
- Endochondral ossification—bone forms from within the hyaline cartilage.
- Children have a growth plate located at the epiphysis region.
- This plate is thick and elastic and is the area where growth takes place.
- It absorbs shock and protects joint surfaces from injury.
- It is the means by which limbs are able to grow and straighten.

Examples of anatomical developments

- At one year of life: centre appears at femoral head.
- At three years of life: centre appears in the patella.
- At 11–13 years of life: final height of vertebral column is reached in girls.
- At 14–16 years of life: final height of vertebral column is reached in boys.
- Puberty: ossification is complete soon after puberty.

(adapted from Chamley *et al.*, 2005)

Fractures

A fracture is a break or a crack in the continuity of a bone. A fracture occurs when the resistance of the bone against the stress being exerted yields to the stress force (Hockenberry & Wilson, 2003).

Upper extremity fractures are very common in children due to their active and adventurous nature. Children commonly fracture upper extremities during sports activities, cycling, climbing trees, or simply a fall. Nurses are often the first to assess a child when they arrive into the Accident and Emergency department. Therefore children's nurses should have a good understanding of normal growth and development and the common mechanisms of injury seen in children. The causes of fractures are as follows:

- Direct force.
- Indirect force.
- Muscular action.
- Pathological.

Common signs associated with a fracture

- A fracture is quite often very visible to the eye—check the affected against the unaffected limb to assess abnormalities.
- Fractures are generally associated with pain—assess pain using appropriate pain tools.
- The affected limb shows signs of swelling—this may be slow or fast.
- There may be discolouration of the skin—compare with the unaffected limb.
- The child may voice a tingling or numb sensation distal to the fracture site.
- The child is unable to or displays difficulty in moving the affected limb.

Common childhood fractures

Clavicle

A fracture sustained to the clavicle (collarbone) is extremely common in children.

Common mechanism of injury: Falling on an outstretched hand; fall onto the shoulder; direct trauma to the bone (Hart *et al.*, 2006).

Presenting signs: Bruising; swelling; grinding (crepitus) that is easy to palpate (Eiff & Hatch, 2003); child usually holds affected arm against the body with the unaffected hand.

Diagnosed: Anteroposterior X-ray of the clavicle.

Treatment:

- Simple sling for 2–3 weeks or until comfortable (Staheli, 2006).
- Follow-up X-ray in 4–6 weeks.
- Contact sports restricted for 2–3 weeks following clinical and radiological healing (Hart *et al.*, 2006).
- A visible and palpable bump often remains due to the excess callous formation.

Humerus

A fractured humerus is very common and is often the first suspicion upon assessment of those with consistent injuries in the 9–15 year age group (Hart *et al.*, 2006).

Common mechanism of injury: Fall or direct trauma to the proximal humerus.

Diagnosed: Physical examination reveals point of tenderness over proximal humerus; anteroposterior and lateral X-ray of the shoulder.

Treatment: Majority are non-surgical treatment, immobilized in simple sling for 3–4 weeks. Neurovascular assessment—axillary nerve must be assessed due to its close proximity to the proximal humerus.

Supracondylar fractures

These are also quite common in children, representing 60–80% of all elbow fractures (Beaty, 2003). Peak incidence in 5–7-year-olds; high complication rate.

Common mechanism of injury: Falling on an outstretched arm (hyper-extended) (Hart *et al.*, 2006).

Presenting signs: Very difficult to diagnose; extensive swelling; pain.

Diagnosed: Physical examination reveals point of tenderness over proximal humerus; anteroposterior and lateral X-ray of the shoulder.

Treatment: Type 1 (non-displaced) can be treated non-surgically in a long arm cast (Hart *et al.*, 2006). The elbow is generally held in a 90–110 degree flexion unless swelling precludes.

Type 2 and Type 3 are generally treated with closed reduction and percutaneous pinning or K-wires (Kirchner-wires). This is done in the operating room under fluoroscopic guidance by the orthopaedic surgeon.

> **Nursing Alert**
>
> Supracondylar fracture is associated with a high risk of neurovascular injury due to the location of important blood vessels and nerves surrounding the elbow. Swelling or fracture fragments can cause injury to the brachial artery as well as the radial and median nerve. Therefore children with suspected or known supracondylar fracture must receive a thorough neurovascular assessment.

Types of fractures in children

- Closed.
- Open/compound.
- Complicated.
- Greenstick.
- Impacted.
- Comminuted.
- Fissured.

Nursing care of fractures

A physical examination (see the section on assessment below) and an X-ray of the affected limb will determine the diagnosis. The main aim of treatment is to get the child back to his/her normal daily activity as quickly as possible. Once the type of fracture is diagnosed, the affected limb is very often positioned and held in place by a cast. **Plaster casts** are used to obtain complete immobilization, protection,

and correction of bony or tissue damage or deformity (Chadburn, 2006). Placing the limb in a cast or splint relieves pain and aids bone healing. It is very common for the injured limb to be placed in what is known as a backslab initially, as this allows for swelling. This type of cast maintains position but it is not a complete cast. The open area at the front of the cast allows for any subsequent swelling of the limb and prevents complications such as compartment syndrome and/or neurovascular damage. A full cast is applied once any swelling has reduced. The clinical skills involved in casts are described later in this chapter.

Sprains, strains, and contusions

Most injuries in older children and adolescents are not skeletal (fractures) but rather injuries to soft tissues, including sprains, strains, and contusions (Mandleco, 2002).

A sprain is a stretching or tearing of a ligament from the point of injury to the joint. A strain is characterized by the stretching or tearing of either a muscle or tendon from overuse, overstretching, or misuse. A contusion occurs when there is damage to soft tissue, subcutaneous structures, small vessels, and muscles, yet the integrity of the skin is not disrupted.

Nursing care

The treatment of sprains, strains, and contusions involves what is commonly known as RICE (Rest, Ice, Compress, Elevate):
- The affected limb must be **R**ested.
- An **I**cepack is placed over the affected site.
- A **C**ompression bandage is applied to the affected limb.
- The affected limb is **E**levated above the level of the heart to reduce swelling.

Moderate sprains may need to be placed in a splint or cast for 2–3 weeks in order to rest the limb and promote healing. Once the muscle has regained strength and the child's range of movement (ROM) has returned, normal activities can resume. Severe sprains may require a full cast to ensure no movement of the muscle. Rehabilitation exercises must be taught to help maintain or restore strength following a sprain and these should be tailored to suit each child. If the child requires a sling, parents or family members need to be shown how to reapply the sling. It is worth noting that the occurrence of sprains is uncommon in young children because their growth plates are weaker than the ligaments and will usually separate before a ligament will tear.

Key nursing skills

13.1 Initial assessment of musculo-skeletal injury

- Check the body for any wounds or broken skin.
- Stop any bleeding by applying pressure.
- Decrease swelling by elevating the affected limb on a pillow.
- Assess the child for any pain using appropriate tools.
- Take a history of how the injury occurred.
- Did the child continue with activities after the accident?
- When did the swelling begin? Acute swelling is more likely associated with fracture, dislocation, or ligament tear.
- Note any history of previous fractures or similar injuries.
- First aid—RICE (Rest, Ice, Compression, Elevation).
- Perform detailed neurovascular assessment.

Neurovascular assessment

The Wessex Paediatric Neurovascular Assessment Tool (WPNA) is one instrument used by nurses to assess neurovascular impairment that could lead to compartment syndrome (Wright, 2007). Assessing children with musculo-skeletal injury can be challenging for children's nurses.

Therefore it is important to use the principles of family centred care (Chapter Two) and distraction (if possible) (Chapter Five). Neurovascular assessment must include assessment of: colour of limb; temperature of limb; capillary refill; peripheral pulses; oedema; movement; sensation; and pain. It should also include appropriate documentation.

Colour

See Table 13.1.
- It is important to assess the child's general colour and skin tone, particularly as a baseline for neurovascular assessment.
- Compare affected with unaffected extremity.
- Assess respiratory status of child.
- Colour should be pink indicating normal perfusion of the limb.
- Pale/blanched/white limb may indicate arterial insufficiency.
- Dusky/blue/cyanosed/mottled limb may indicate inadequate venous return.

Temperature

See Table 13.1.
- Assess by placing dorsal or back of hand on the extremity.
- Compare with unaffected side.
- Cool indicates inadequate arterial supply.
- Warm or hot indicates venous congestion.
- Temperature is considered the least reliable sign of vascular compromise but combined with other signs is useful in neurovascular assessment.
- Observe environmental temperature—room, cool pack, ice or heat packs, recent cast application.

Table 13.1 Assessing the affected limb

	Normal	Inadequate arterial blood supply	Inadequate venous blood supply
Colour	Pink	Pale/white	Blue/cyanosed
Temperature	Warm	Cool	Hot
Capillary refill	1–2 seconds	>2 seconds	Immediate
Tissue turgor	Full	Hollow/prune-like	Distended/tense

Capillary refill

See Table 13.1.

- Helps evaluate arterial blood supply to small peripheral vessels; capillary bed furthest away from the heart.
- Evaluates peripheral perfusion and cardiac output.
- Squeeze a nail bed for 2–3 seconds until it blanches, then release and observe time for the colour to return (three seconds or less is normal).

Peripheral pulses

See Box 13.4.

- Observe blood flow through peripheral vessels.
- Palpate by applying easy pressure to pulse point using pad of index finger and middle finger.
- Graded 0–4 scale (Thompson McFarlane *et al.*, 1997):
  - ○ 0 = absent
  - ○ 1+ = diminished, weak
  - ○ 2+ = difficult to palpate
  - ○ 3+ = easily palpable
  - ○ 4+ = strong, bounding, normal.
- If pulse is difficult to palpate, an ultrasonic Doppler can be used to audibly assess the pulse (this is a hand-held instrument that audibly evaluates the blood flow through the blood vessel).
- It is important to remember that the reliability of the Doppler instrument is dependent on the skill of the person using it (Kunkler, 1999).
- Once the peripheral pulse is found it is general practice to mark the spot with an 'X' to help with locating it again.

Box 13.4 Eight major pulse points in neurovascular assessment

- Axillary
- Posterior tibial
- Brachial
- Ulnar
- Radial
- Femoral
- Dorsalis pedis
- Popliteal

Note: Check the presence and quality of the appropriate pulse. A hand-held Doppler device can be useful to document arterial patency.

- Record and report any abnormalities, as early detection is paramount.

Swelling/oedema

- Occurs as a physiological response to injury or surgery.
- Increased oedema in a confined space increases neurovascular compromise and risks compartment syndrome.
- Skin can appear swollen, taut, and stretched.
- If indentations last more than five seconds after the skin is pressed, this is known as pitting oedema.
- Grade the swelling/oedema using the 0–4 scale (Black & Matassarin-Jacobs, 1993), a widely accepted scale for measuring oedema. 0 represents no swelling and 4+ represents depression >1 cm.

Movement

Neurovascular deficit can cause muscles in affected limbs to become paralysed as a result of nerve damage (Judge, 2007). Children's nurses should be competent in assessing motor ability in children with orthopaedic injury. Both active and passive range of movement of both the affected and non-affected limbs should be carried out. In addition, children should be encouraged to participate in neurovascular assessment. The activities shown in **Figure 13.2** are recognized activities that demonstrate motor ability.

These activities can easily be made into a game, but where this is not possible due to language or developmental barriers, the movements should be carried out passively (Altizer, 2004). Parents could also be of great help here. Any reduced movement should be recorded and reported.

Sensation

All touchable/visible surfaces (including in between digits) should be checked for presence and type of sensation, and this should preferably be done with the child's eyes closed or while they are not watching (neurovascular charts often have diagrams of the nerve endings for the foot and hand):

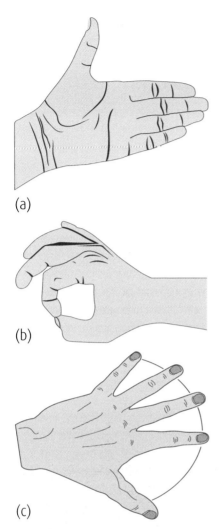

(a)

(b)

(c)

Figure 13.2 (a) L-shape using the thumb and first digit. **(b)** The thumb is brought to meet the index finger in an OK-sign. **(c)** The fingers are splayed and mild pressure is applied to the external digits to ensure the position can be maintained.

- Ask child to close eyes.
- Lightly touch extremity and ask: 'Where am I touching?'
- Ask child to describe sensations, e.g. numbness, tingling.
- Record and report any abnormalities.

Pain

The assessment of the child's pain is essential to ensure that the correct analgesia is prescribed and administered. Ineffective pain assessment will cause undue stress to a child with a musculo-skeletal injury (Clarke, 2003). Relieving pain following injury or orthopaedic surgery is a priority for the children's nurse. Further information on pain and pain management may be found in Chapter Six.

Assessing a child's pain is complex, especially in young or cognitively impaired children. While the assessment of pain in a child can be difficult, it is a vital part of paediatric practice (Bulloch & Tenenbein, 2002) as it provides an information base from which to provide effective pain management. Early studies by Twycross *et al.,* (1998), who compared nurses' assessment to children's pain scores, found that nurses consistently underestimated children's level of pain. This finding is also echoed in current literature, which finds that nurses often underestimate children's pain (Clarke, 2003). In the UK the Royal College of Nursing (Royal College of Nursing (RCN), 2007) produced guidelines to enable children's nurses to better recognize and assess pain in children.

Assessment of pain in children is dependent on the pain assessment tool used. There are a diverse range of pain assessment tools available to children's nurses. There are issues regarding their reliability, which are outlined in Chapter Six. It is important that a pain assessment tool should be clear, simple, and easy to use, and that scoring should be quick and not labour intensive. Further information on the types of pain assessment tools that may be used for children is found in Chapter Six.

Documentation

Documenting neurovascular assessment is a vital part of caring for a child with a musculo-skeletal injury. Documentation and record keeping are discussed in more detail in Chapter Five. A neurovascular chart where observations

Box 13.5 Signs and symptoms of compartment syndrome

(All signs may not be present at the same time.)
- Pain—increasing pain that is not controlled by normal levels of analgesia. Pain on passive movement.
- Tenseness—skin looks shiny and stretched.
- Muscle becomes taut and bulging.
- Change to sensation—paraesthesia.
- Muscle weakness—pressure within the muscle compartment may result in loss of movement.
- Pulse—may be present, gradually weakening, or absent.
- Absence of pulse is a late symptom.

are kept separate to vital signs is often used. Any action taken can be documented by the nurse alongside the event, for example, elevation of the limb or loosening of bandages. Documentation should take place at the time when actions are conducted (Judge, 2007). Neurovascular charts should be detailed and include the relevant observations of colour, temperature, peripheral pulses, oedema, movement, sensation, and pain. Relevant scoring including pain score, oedema grading, and peripheral pulse checks should be included.

Compartment syndrome

Action taken if compartment syndrome is suspected

- Observe—regular observations of all patients in casts.
- Listen—accept what the patient is saying.
- Lower—consider reducing elevation if you suspect CS.
- Notify medical staff immediately if you suspect CS.
- Splitting/bivalve—to relieve exacerbation of symptoms caused by the cast, the limb may need to be inspected and the circumference measured.

Once CS is diagnosed a fasciotomy (cutting of the fascia) may be undertaken to relieve the pressure.

Consideration

List the signs and symptoms of compartment syndrome and explain how this could be a potential problem if a full cast was applied to a new fracture.

Treatment of musculo-skeletal injuries and related skills

The treatment of musculo-skeletal injuries may involve manipulation (manually regaining correct position), immobilization (maintaining the correct position until bone healing occurs), and rehabilitation (regaining normal movement and function of the affected limb) (McRae, 2002).

Box 13.6 Benchmark for best practice

Child receives care from a competent and knowledgeable nurse.

(RCN, *Benchmarks for Children's Orthopaedic Nursing Care*, 2007)

13.2 **Casts**

Plaster casts are one of the gold standards for non-operative treatment of fractures. A child may require a cast as a result of trauma, e.g. a fracture or dislocation, or to correct a deformity, e.g. developmental dysplasia of the hip (DDH) or talipes equinovarus. Both children and their families are affected by prolonged casting and possible lengthy hospital stays. Preadmission preparation involving all members of the multidisciplinary team is important to support children and their families with the added burden of prolonged immobility and loss of independence. Issues such as decreased autonomy, social isolation, missed school, parental loss of earnings, and altered self-image can arise as a result of the injury (Hart *et al.*, 2006). Education and advice are key to supporting the child and family.

Nursing Alert

Parents of children with casts report less sleep, less social interaction, and more stress when their child is immobilized and dependent on them for their self-care needs (Newman, 2005).

Application of a cast can be a very stressful experience for both the child and the parent/carer, especially following a stressful trauma. The nurse needs to give clear, concise explanations of the reasons behind the application. It is important to allow for questions and answers so that the child and family understand and consent to the process. This will help gain cooperation and compliance from both the child and family. Depending on local policy, written consent or assent may be required.

Types of casts

The two most common materials used in cast application are plaster of Paris and fibreglass/resin. Plaster of Paris

Table 13.2 Types of casts

Type	Application	Uses
Arm cylinder cast	Applied from the upper arm to the wrist.	Holds the elbow muscles and tendons in place after a dislocation or surgery.
Leg cylinder cast	Applied from the upper thigh to the ankle.	Knee or lower leg fractures, knee dislocations, or after surgery on the leg or knee area.
Hip spica cast	Applied from the chest to the thighs or knees.	To hold the hip muscles and tendons in place after surgery to allow healing.
Abduction boot cast	Applied from the upper thighs to the feet. A bar is placed between both legs to keep the hips and legs immobilized.	To hold the hip muscles and tendons in place after surgery to allow healing.

has been the most common choice for many years and is relatively inexpensive. It is pliable and easy to mould, smoothing to conform almost exactly to the extremity. Plaster of Paris is the material of choice for fresh fractures, post-surgery, and where swelling or bleeding may occur. Fibreglass/resin casts are very common in children as they come in a variety of colours and are more resilient than plaster of Paris casts. This material is preferable where there is a requirement for a lighter, stronger cast with early weight bearing. This type of cast is approximately one-fifth of the weight of plaster bandage. **Table 13.2** outlines how casts should be applied for different injuries.

Procedure: Cast application

Preparation

- Analgesia should be prescribed and administered to minimize pain and also reduce the child's anxiety.
- Ensure appropriate numbers of staff are available to support the child and family during the procedure.
- Ensure the infant/child is in a position of comfort prior to commencing the procedure.
- Cast application can be messy so it is important to protect the child's clothes by placing paper sheets, an apron, or towels over them.
- Remove all jewellery from the limb to prevent disruption to circulation. This should not be replaced until the affected limb is fully recovered.

Equipment

If fibreglass is being used, allow the child to pick the colour, e.g. they may wish to pick the colour of their favourite sports team. This provides the child with an element of control and can improve compliance during the application process.

Blood loss will stain the plaster of Paris but not synthetic casts, so it is important to choose the most suitable material before application. If blood is noted on the cast, draw a line around the stain. This will allow any further oozing to be detected.

Assessment

It is important to assess the skin for abrasions/cuts before the cast is applied. Cuts and abrasions must be cleaned aseptically and covered.

Consent and communication

It is very important to use age-appropriate language and detail what the child is likely to experience throughout the procedure, e.g. the cast may feel warm when it is being applied. The cast bandages must be soaked in lukewarm water as cold water slows the setting process and hot water quickens the process. Inform the child and parent/carers that the cast will feel heavy following application. Parental involvement during the procedure will also reduce the child's anxiety.

Step-by-step guide to care of the infant/child following cast application

Step	Rationale
1 Elevate the affected limb.	To decrease any oedema of the limb underneath the cast that could restrict circulation (Bindler & Ball, 2003).
2 Position the affected limb on a pillow.	To aid drying and prevent any dents occurring.
3 Observe the cast regularly for cracking, softening, or breakdown.	May affect bone realignment and healing (Davis, 1994).
4 Mark any blood leakage that stains the cast with a marker.	So any further ooze can be easily detected.
5 Monitor the limb closely for signs of swelling and/or discolouration. This can be achieved by comparing the limb with the unaffected limb.	The most common complications associated with casts are due to circulatory and/or nerve impairment; early detection can prevent such complications (Solomon, 2005).
6 Carry out full neurovascular observations of the cast limb including the '5 Ps' (see Table 13.3).	The most common complications associated with casts are due to circulatory and/or nerve impairment; early detection can prevent such complications (Solomon, 2005).
7 It is important to handle a fresh cast with care to prevent denting or cracking, which could lead to the formation of pressure sores under the cast. Use the palm of your hands when handling rather than fingertips.	Fingertips can cause indents that could lead to pressure sores (Bindler & Ball, 2003).
8 Inspect the limb regularly for signs of infection. Check for increased heat from the limb and any unpleasant odour or exudate. Other signs include pain, staining through the cast, and pyrexia. All of these must be reported immediately and prompt treatment given.	These symptoms could indicate the presence of infection or pressure sores, which need to be treated promptly.
9 Reposition the infant/child at regular intervals.	Helps prevent complications associated with immobility. It will also help the cast to dry in a uniform fashion.
10 Particular attention must be given in relation to personal hygiene. Keeping the infant/child cool will minimize sweating, which can be very uncomfortable for a child in a cast. Frequent nappy changes for the smaller child are needed.	To keep the area as dry as possible to prevent the build-up of moisture. It is especially important to provide protection around the top of a leg cast, particularly the upper thigh in children, as the cast may become contaminated by urine and/or faeces.

11	Children in spica casts require assistance with elimination. A small bedpan can be used while the child is in this type of cast.	To avoid contamination by urine or faeces or any further complications with urinary retention. It is almost impossible for a child in a spica cast to use a toilet.
12	Infants in spica casts require frequent nappy changes. Resin casts are somewhat waterproof but the skin underneath can become irritated if moisture collects.	To avoid contamination by urine or faeces or any further complications with urinary retention.
13	Depending on where the cast is situated, the child's eating and drinking can be affected. If an upper limb is in a cast, ensure the child can manage their meals and provide assistance where necessary. Ensure a well-balanced diet.	To promote good bone healing. A diet high in fibre and fluids helps prevent constipation associated with reduced mobility.

During the procedure

- Padding over bony prominences should be applied firmly, smoothly, and evenly under the cast to avoid loosening of the cast and the incidence of pressure sores.
- It is important to regularly check the appearance of the cast and the limb for prompt detection of complications associated with the cast.
- Plaster of Paris takes approximately 24–48 hours to dry fully, so it is important not to cover the cast and to allow it to dry naturally.
- Resin or other synthetic casts dry within 30–60 minutes.
- Post-application the limb must rest on a pillow to allow it to set and also to avoid denting of the cast. If denting occurs, pressure sores may result.

Warning signs

If any of the changes in the patient's condition listed in **Table 13.3** are present, urgent action needs to be taken.

Following the procedure

Splitting and bivalving casts

If the affected limb has a large degree of swelling or if a large degree of swelling is anticipated, splitting or bivalving of the cast is undertaken. Splitting involves performing one cut down the entire length of the cast, ensuring the limb is not constricted. This is only appropriate in casts made from plaster of Paris.

Table 13.3 The 5 'Ps'

Pallor	This is due to an interruption in blood supply. It can present as pallor or an increase in the colour of the affected limb. The limb may also appear swollen and tight with the skin taking on a shiny appearance.
Paraesthesia	This is due to a tight cast impinging on nerves. The child may complain of pins and needles or numbness or just a funny sensation in the limb.
Paralysis	If a cast is very tight and this is left undetected, paralysis due to muscle damage may result.
Pain	Pain is to be expected following a fracture, but if this pain is not responding to regular analgesia, it could indicate compartment syndrome.
Pulse	It is extremely important to check the pulse of the affected limb. A weakening pulse or no pulse at all indicates circulatory damage and needs to be attended to urgently.

Bivalving involves performing two cuts down the length of the cast. Resin casts require this method because the material used does not have the same degree of flexibility as plaster of Paris casts.

Sometimes a window will be cut in the cast to aid inspection and dressing of a wound or to investigate the possibility of a pressure sore. The window must always be replaced and secured to avoid weakening of the cast.

Instructions for parents/ carers and children going home with a cast

Aim: To assist the child in partnership with the family to gain a level of mobility and activity that meets their needs (Santy *et al.*, 2005).

Nursing implications

It is essential to give clear instructions supported by written information to parents/carers prior to discharge. Simply explaining what is normal and what is not can be very helpful (guidelines for parents on recognizing symptoms of deterioration and need for referral to the GP are outlined in **Box 13.8**). The infant/child may need to be in the cast for a prolonged period of time and this can have a psychological effect on the child, especially if they are normally very independent. Educating and empowering the family in relation to such effects can help them cope and make the situation less overwhelming.

The parent/carer and child must be shown specific exercises to perform prior to discharge in order to encourage venous return to the affected area, reduce swelling, and prevent muscle wasting and stiffness. These exercises must be demonstrated and written instructions with diagrams should be given along with the written cast care instructions.

Cast care instructions must include the following:
- Keep cast exposed to air until dry.
- Keep the affected limb elevated on pillows for the first day, or as directed by the healthcare professional. The limb must be elevated on pillows when the child is resting. Upper limb casts must be elevated in a sling while the child is upright.

- Observe fingers/toes for signs of swelling and contact the healthcare provider if any is noted.
- Observe fingers/toes for discolouration (lighter or darker than comparable limb) and contact the healthcare provider if this is noted.
- Check the child's movement and sensation frequently—this can be done by getting the child to wiggle his/her fingers/toes. It is also important to change the child's position every few hours, especially if the child is in a spica cast, to avoid pressure sores. Cushions, pillows, and beanbags are useful.
- The child may experience itching. This can be relieved by placing an ice pack at the cast edges. Do not allow the child to put anything inside the cast as this may cause sores to develop and the item could get stuck down the cast.
- Avoid water as this will damage the cast and cause skin irritation under the cast. Cover the cast with plastic or cling film while attending to personal hygiene to avoid splashes.
- Cover the cast while your child is eating to prevent food spills and crumbs from entering the cast.
- Do not put powders or lotion inside the cast.
- Prevent small toys or objects from being put inside the cast.
- Encourage your child to move his/her fingers or toes to promote circulation.
- Do not use the abduction bar (hip spica cast) on the cast to lift or carry the child.
- Care guidelines for spica casts are outlined in Box 13.7.

Crutches

If the child needs crutches, they will require measuring for them and instructions on how to use them before discharge. They must be assessed firstly for suitability. Younger children less than six years or children lacking coordination may not be able to use crutches. A walking frame or wheelchair may be more appropriate. The child must be taught how to use the crutches and given the time to practise before discharge. This also applies to the child in a walking frame.

Box 13.7 Spica cast care guidelines

Parent troubleshooting guidelines developed by Clarke & McKay (2006).

How do I wash my child's body and hair?
- Wash with flannel or sponge using soap and moisturize skin.
- Wash hair over bath or basin and protect the cast from water.

Can my child be comfortable?
- Change position regularly—two-hourly, alternating back, tummy, and side.
- Use pillows to change positions.
- Encourage older children to turn themselves.
- Lift the child with the hand supported under the bottom.

How does my child go to the toilet?
- Continue with nappies if applicable.
- Use bedpan or urinal (arrangements for access to this equipment should be made for parents prior to discharge from hospital).

How can I occupy my child?
- Computer games, TV, videos, art, drawing, and other activities to prevent boredom.
- Home school/tuition can be encouraged.

Do I offer my child a normal diet?
- Yes, but smaller amounts of a nutritious, high-fibre diet with plenty of fluids.
- Use straws for drinking.
- Position the child at a 45 degree angle with the aid of pillows to assist digestion and reduce the risk of aspiration or choking.

How do I keep my child at the correct temperature?
- Light, loose clothing.
- Place room thermometer in the child's room (18 degrees is the ideal temperature).
- Check the child's temperature regularly for over- or under-heating.

Parents/carers must be given a contact number and instructed to contact or return to the hospital if they feel worried or notice anything abnormal (**see also Box 13.8**).

> **Consideration**
>
> - What are the common complications that might occur in a child in a cast?
> - What action would you undertake or instigate to resolve these?

13.3 Care of the infant/child during cast removal

Bivalving is the method used to remove a resin cast. Plaster of Paris casts are removed by using cutting shears or an

Box 13.8 When to call your general practitioner

Parents should be advised to contact their doctor if any of the following symptoms occur:
- Increase in temperature to greater than 101°F.
- Increased pain.
- Increased swelling above or below the cast.
- Any complaints of numbness or tingling.
- A drainage or foul odour from the cast.
- Cool or cold fingers or toes.

electric cast cutter. Cast saws are relatively safe to use but care must be taken and cast removal must only be performed by a member of staff experienced in this area. The saw may cut and/or burn the skin if used incorrectly and dragged along the cast rather than used in the correct in-and-out motion.

Preparation

Position the infant/child comfortably and ensure the parents are with the child if possible. They should also

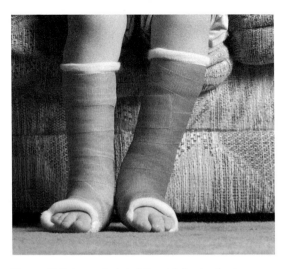

Figure 13.3 Lower limb in full cast following fracture.
© Dvane Ellison/ISTOCKPHOTO.COM

be encouraged, where appropriate, to be involved in the procedure as far as possible if they so wish. This reduces child anxiety.

Equipment

- Saw/electric cast cutter.
- Hearing protectors can also be used to reduce the infant's/child's anxiety during the procedure (Katz *et al.*, 2001).

Consent and communication

Take the time to explain the procedure to the child and family. Demonstrating the action of the saw is advisable to minimize anxiety. The electric cast cutter can be very noisy and this may cause the child to be frightened. Cast saws work by vibration; therefore they only cut hard surfaces (Katz *et al.*, 2001).

Offer explanations prior to the procedure regarding the sensations the child may feel during the procedure. The vibration from the saw can generate heat and a tingling sensation.

Procedure: Care of the infant/child during cast removal

- Mark lines down the medial and lateral sides of the cast as a guide, and avoid bivalving over bony prominences when removing a resin cast using the bivalving method. It is important to fully bivalve the cast to allow the limb to be lifted out safely.
- Stop the procedure if the child complains of heat or discomfort or becomes upset. Reassess the situation before continuing.
- Once the limb has been safely removed from the cast, inspect the skin for evidence of pressure sores or infection. The skin will be caked with dry desquamated skin. Soaking the limb in a bath usually removes this but it may take several days to remove the accumulation completely. It is important not to pull or remove any of this material with scrubbing as this may cause excoriation or skin damage.

Following the procedure

Once the cast is removed, the limb must be inspected by a doctor before weight bearing to ensure proper bone alignment. The parent/carer and the child must be advised that it may be some time before normal function resumes due to muscle and joint inactivity. A range of exercises should be demonstrated to increase the strength in the affected limb.

Internal fixation

The nature of the majority of fractures in children makes them suitable for closed management. Internal fixation is well established in the treatment of certain adult fractures; however, it is generally avoided in children. The immature skeleton is characterized by a tough periosteum, which often means that children's fractures occur with little disruption to the periosteum, heal rapidly, and are generally relatively stable. Conditions that do advocate internal fixation include Salter-Harris type III and IV, which often require internal fixation:

- Salter-Harris fractures: Fractures affecting the growth plate of a bone. Once bone growth has completed, the term 'Salter-Harris fracture' no longer applies.
  - Type III—a fracture through growth plate and epiphysis.
  - Type IV—a fracture through all three elements of the bone: the growth plate, metaphysis, and epiphysis.

External fixation

External fixation is an accepted treatment for some conditions in children, such as long bone fractures or pelvic fractures (Bernardo, 2001), correction of limb length discrepancy, and conditions such as Perthes (Caterall, 2006). Pins or wires can be attached to traction, casts, or external fixators to stabilize the fractured bone and therefore promote healing (Baird-Holmes & Brown, 2005).

Skeletal pins or wires are inserted into the bone through incisions in the skin (Baird-Holmes & Brown, 2005). The most common complication in external fixation is pin tract infection, which can result in loosening of the pin and/or necrosis of the tissue around the pin site. Pin site care requires specialized nursing care, which is initially carried out in hospital and then (following training and education) by the child or parent at home. Many parents now perform pin site care in the home using a clean technique.

13.4 **Care of pin site**

There have been huge technological advances in orthopaedic pins and wires over the last several years. Despite this, pin site infection is a common complication of external fixation (Patterson, 2005). There is much debate in the literature regarding appropriate pin site care. Studies by Davies *et al.* (2005) and W-Dahl & Toksvig-Larsen (2004) found increased infection rates with the use of normal saline as a cleaning solution compared to chlorhexidine. The frequency of pin site care has also been a source of much confusion. Baird-Holmes & Brown (2005) recommend weekly pin site care if the pin is considered problematic. However, Lee-Smith *et al.* (2001) indicate that pin site care should be carried out only if there are exudates present. The National Association of Orthopaedic Nurses (NAON) produced evidence-based recommendations for the care of pin sites (Baird-Holmes & Brown, 2005), which are shown in **Box 13.9**.

It is important for the children's nurse to be able to recognize the signs of infection and differentiate between normal healing processes and signs of infection. Signs of reaction around the pin site include change in skin colour, heat, and serous slight blood drainage at the site. Reaction at the site does not mean infection. Reaction refers to normal changes that may occur at the pin site following the insertion of the pin, which include increased warmth and serous ooze from the pin site. Colonization is present

Box 13.9 Evidence-based recommendations for the care of pin sites

- Carry out pin site care only if there are exudates present.
- If present, carry out care on a daily or weekly basis after the first 48–72 hours. This applies where the pinning is mechanically stable.
- Use chlorhexidine 2 mg/ml solution as the cleaning solution.
- There is a higher incidence of infection in areas close to soft tissue (Sims & Saleh, 2000); therefore pins located close to soft tissue are considered at greater risk of infection.
- Parents/carers should be taught pin site care before discharge from hospital. They should be provided with written instructions on care of the pin site and the signs of infection.

(Baird-Holmes, 2005)

when the skin at the pin site becomes red and warm, with increased drainage and pain. Microbes will be present in cultures. Infection is present if all the signs outlined above are present, with visible drainage of pus, pin loosening, and increased microbial growth (Lee-Smith *et al.*, 2001).

There are various grading systems to assist nurses with distinguishing pin site infection. **Table 13.4** outlines one such system, the Checketts-Otterburns grading system.

Procedure: Pin site care

Table 13.4 The Checketts-Otterburns grading system (Checketts, 2000)

Grade	Appearance	Treatment
1	Slight redness with slight discharge	Improved pin site care
2	Skin red, discharge, pain, and tenderness	Improved pin site care and oral antibiotics
3	Grade 2 with no improvement	Pins re-sited, external fixation continued
4	Severe soft tissue infection involving more than one pin	External fixation abandoned
5	Grade 4 with involvement of the bone visible on X-ray	External fixation abandoned
6	Infection occurs after the external fixation has been removed; pin track heals initially then breaks down with discharge; sequestrum formation within bone	Curettage of the pin track

Step-by-step guide to pin site care

Step	Rationale
1 Maintain a sterile procedure when carrying out pin site care while hospitalized, followed by a clean technique at home (Patterson, 2005).	Due to risk of nosocomial infection (Patterson, 2005).
2 Clean the pin site using a cleaning solution—chlorhexidine 2 mg/ml.	This has been found to decrease the rate of infection (Baird-Holmes, 2005).
3 If crusts have formed around the site, consider whether to remove or not.	Some studies suggest that the crust is a normal protective mechanism and should be left undisturbed (Baird-Holmes & Brown, 2005) while others suggest removal of the crust (W-Dahl et al., 2003). Removing the crust will allow drainage of exudate that could become a source of infection (Sims & Saleh, 2000).
4 The procedure for crust removal at the pin site is sterile saline or cooled boiled water.	To remove the crust from the site (Lee-Smith et al., 2001).
5 Pin sites should be redressed after 24 hours. Apply a dressing—absorbent non-stick dressing if there are exudates present.	To cover the pin site (Lee-Smith et al., 2001)
6 Check local policy regarding showering.	Showering is allowed in many orthopaedic centres after 5–10 days (Baird Holmes & Brown, 2005). The fixator should be dried with a clean towel afterwards (Lee-Smith et al., 2001). However, some centres recommend that the external fixator and pin site is covered with plastic during showering (W-Dahl & Toksvig-Larson, 2004: W-Dahl et al., 2003). There is little support for sterile cleaning of pin site following shower.

13.5 **Traction**

This is an advanced skill. You *must* check whether you can assist with or undertake any aspect of this skill, in line with local policy.

Traction is mainly used to provide force on bones and muscles. It occurs when a pulling force is exerted on a limb. Traction must always be opposed by counter traction or pull exerted by a fixed object. Counter traction occurs when a pulling force is exerted counter to the pull of the traction.

Types of traction

Fixed traction occurs when there is a pull between two fixed points. A Thomas splint device provides fixed traction where the extension cords are secured to the end of the splint and the counter pressure is exerted by the ring of the splint against the ischial tuberosity of the pelvis.

Balanced traction occurs when there is a pull between weights attached to skin extension cords with counter traction provided by the body weight.

Box 13.10 Principles of traction

- To regain normal length and alignment of involved bone.
- To reduce and immobilize a fractured bone.
- To lessen or eliminate muscle spasms.
- To relieve pressure on nerves, especially spinal.
- To prevent skeletal deformities or muscle contractures.

Skin traction occurs when either adhesive or non-adhesive tape is applied to the skin, holding extension cords in place and producing a traction force on the bone through the skin. It can be fixed or balanced.

Skeletal traction occurs when a strong pulling force is required and uses a metal pin inserted through the bone.

Gallows traction is sometimes used in children with developmental dysplasia of the hip (DDH). It can be used in children up to the age of three years (or four years if the child has a small, light frame). Traction tape is applied to both legs and then fixed to the overhead beam. The hips are flexed to 90 degrees and the legs are vertically extended so that the traction cords are secured to an overhead bar above the cot (fixed) or to weight and pulleys (balanced). The bottom of the cot is tilted up, the child's buttocks are raised off the bed, and the body weight allows for counter traction to occur (McRae, 2002). Gallows traction can be used for the treatment of developmental dysplasia or femoral fractures in children up to 18 months or 16 kg or below, and can also be suitable for home use if circumstances allow.

Traction using a Thomas splint is sometimes used to immobilize a child who has suffered a fractured femur. It is one of the oldest conservative methods used to treat closed femur fractures in children and is still used in some hospital settings (Houghton *et al.*, 2003).

The splint is generally applied for 10–14 days and may be followed by a period of cast application. This is done to maintain the femur length, prevent any shortening of the limb, and relieve pain or spasm. Pressure area care must be carried out, particularly observing the skin adjacent to the Thomas splint, e.g. groin area. Houghton *et al.*, (2003) recommend that skin care is observed at four-hourly intervals.

Procedure for applying skin traction

Preparation

The orthopaedic doctor's order should include:
- Type of traction.
- Amount of weight to be applied.
- Frequency of neurovascular checks if more frequent than every four hours.
- Site care of inserted pins or wires if used.
- Discontinuation of traction.

Equipment

- A skin traction pack containing foam-lined stirrups, straps, and cord.
- For balanced traction—suitable weights with holders (refer to orthopaedic team instructions).
- Traction pulley system.
- Tape.

Consent and communication

Explain the rationale for the use of traction to the child and family, the type of traction, and what is involved.

Following the procedure

Care of the child on traction

- The affected extremity must be maintained in proper alignment at all times with the ropes unobstructed and weights hanging freely.
- Cord should be checked daily for fraying and twisting.
- Check daily the overall alignment of the limb and that traction pull is in line.
- Refer to local guidelines on traction care.
- Observe the child's pressure area every two hours (RCN, 2001).
- Check skin integrity daily and inspect bandages and strapping.
- Check that sheets are clean and wrinkle free.

Step-by-step guide to applying skin traction

Step		Rationale
1	Hand washing as per local policy.	Infection control.
2	Check skin integrity of child's limbs prior to applying skin traction.	Skin traction would be contraindicated where there is evidence of skin damage, broken skin, or wounds.
3	Perform neurovascular observations including pain assessment.	To ensure the limb is not compromised prior to commencing the traction and to provide baseline observations.
4	When applying the skin traction ensure the foam-lined stirrups are positioned to allow room for the foot to dorsiflex without restriction and ensure the ankle is protected by the padded stirrup.	To prevent any compression on the peroneal nerve or pressure sores to the ankle.
5	Wrapping should be applied evenly and secured with tape.	To ensure the skin traction is securely held in place.
6	The affected leg should be supported using a pillow with the heel hanging freely over the pillow.	To prevent pressure sores.
7	The traction cord is fed through and tied with a knot at the base of the foot section. Pulleys are attached and the traction cord is fed through the pulley so that the cord runs freely over the pulley.	To ensure the correct traction force is being applied.
8	Ensure any weights that are used are hanging freely.	To ensure the correct traction force is being applied.
9	The end of bed or cot should be elevated (refer to orthopaedic team or instructions).	To provide the opposing force and ensure the child is not sliding down towards the end of the bed or cot.

- Pin site care should be carried out if skeletal traction is being used (see above section on pin site care).
- Assess the child for signs of pain using appropriate pain tools.
- Neurovascular assessment should be carried out hourly for the first 12 hours, and then at regular intervals determined by the condition of the child and local policy (Judd & Wright, 2005).

- Maintain an accurate intake and output chart.
- Encourage regular fluids through straws or non-spill cups.
- Liaise with the dietician regarding a well balanced diet to promote healing and prevent constipation (RCN, 2002).
- Offer the child a urinal or bedpan often.
- Offer a hand washing bowl after toilet facilities.

- Ensure prompt treatment of urinary tract infection if it occurs (Whaley & Wong, 1994).
- Assist with hygiene needs including washing, dressing, and hair brushing, and involve parents with this, if they so wish.
- Adapt clothing to suit the child on traction, e.g. may need Velcro along seams.
- Provide age-appropriate activities and toys to ensure social and psychological needs are met.
- Involve play therapist and school teacher as applicable.
- Encourage visiting from family and friends in accordance with local policy.

> **Nursing Alert**
>
> When skin traction is being applied check that the child has no known allergies to adhesive tape.

Rehabilitation

The priorities during rehabilitation are as follows:
- Continue to protect the limb by splinting or use of crutches, etc.
- Continue to check pain levels and offer appropriate analgesia as required.
- Introduce range of motion and muscle strengthening exercises early and as recommended by the orthopaedic team.
- Maintain exercises such as swimming for children to improve fitness.

Community perspectives

Prevention

Playground accidents can often result in fractures in children. With the number of sports related injuries such as skateboard and bicycle related injury increasing, safety is a key factor in preventing musculo-skeletal injury in children. Protection, particularly wrist guards, elbow pads, knee pads, and approved helmets, are all necessary in protecting the young child against orthopaedic injuries (Sheehan, 2003). Better education and a tighter

Box 13.11 Activities to help prevent musculo-skeletal injury in children

- Make physical activity part of a child's daily schedule.
- Encourage physical involvement in age- and size-appropriate activities such as team sports (i.e. football, basketball, dancing, swimming, tennis, and other racquet sports).
- Take the time to warm up and stretch. Research studies have shown that cold muscles are more prone to injury. Warm up with jogging on the spot or walking for three to five minutes.
- Drink plenty of water before, during, and after activities.
- It is important they take breaks if tired.
- Eat a well balanced diet, which should include sufficient calcium and vitamin D to keep bones strong.
- Be prepared for emergency situations such as dislocations, fractured wrist, or finger sprains.

supervision of children whilst skating is vital in preventing injury. Dedicated skateparks should only be used by experienced and older children. 85% of ramp injuries in skateparks occur in first or second time users (Sheehan, 2003).

Health promotion

Childhood obesity is reaching epidemic proportions. In the US 16% of children and adolescents aged 6–19 years old are considered overweight. Excess weight and inactivity can cause undue stress on children's musculo-skeletal system. The American Academy of Orthopaedic Surgeons (AAOS) stresses the importance of physical activity for children to maximize strong bone and muscle potential and combat obesity.

Community-based care

When injuries do occur it is important that the period of hospitalization is kept to a minimum for children. This can reduce the effects of hospitalization on the child (see Chapter Two). Nurses are responsible for regularly updating and maintaining their orthopaedic skills so that these children receive optimum nursing care. Procedures for the care of children with musculo-skeletal compromise such as casts, pins, and traction must be taught, demonstrated, and reinforced to children and their families so that the care can continue at home. Written instructions/information must be provided and be clear and easy to understand. In addition, parents and children must be provided with support in the community and access to relevant and up-to-date information regarding the care of their child with a musculo-skeletal injury.

> **Consideration**
>
> Having had a severe musculo-skeletal injury may be associated with a decreased risk of subsequent injury in children and adolescents. Possible explanation could be reduced exposure to risk (Keays *et al.*, 2006).

Conclusion

> **Consideration**
>
> Design a teaching plan for the family of a child with a musculo-skeletal disorder and present it to your class for discussion.

This chapter provides children's nurses with a step-by-step approach to caring for children with musculo-skeletal injury and the skills that are involved in that process. Using play and involving children in their care will encourage their participation and cooperation, which will aid their recovery. Ensuring that the child and family are informed about and involved in the care remains the responsibility of the children's nurse.

Musculo-skeletal injury can deprive children of normal development and childhood experience. Besides the physical and emotional burden that these conditions and injuries place on the patient and family, the financial burden they inflict can be enormous for the patient and healthcare system. Furthermore, complications such as compartment syndrome can be devastating for children and their families. Apart from the devastating risk to the affected limb, the length of hospital stay is also increased (Dandy & Edward, 2004). Children's nurses must be skilled in their ability to carry out neurovascular assessment and respond accordingly when a deficit is observed, so as to prevent such detrimental effects of injuries.

Online resource centre

You may find it helpful to work through our online resources including interactive scenarios intended to help you to develop and apply the skills in this chapter. Where material referenced below is available electronically, we're pleased to provide active web links to the source via **http://www.oxfordtextbooks.co.uk/orc/coyne/**

References

Altizer, L. (2004) Compartment syndrome. *Orthopaedic Nursing* 23 (6), 391–396.

Baird Holmes, S. & Brown, S.J. (2005) Skeletal pin site care: National Association of Orthopaedic Nurses Guidelines for Orthopaedic Nursing. *Orthopaedic Nursing* 24 (2), 99–107.

Beaty, J.H. (2003) Elbow fractures in children and adolescents: Instructional course. *Lectures of the American Academy of Orthopaedic Surgeons* **52**, 661–665.

Bernardo, L.M. (2001) Evidence-based practice for pin site care in injured children. *Orthopaedic Nursing* 20 (5), 29–34.

Bindler, R.C. & Ball, J. (2003) *Clinical Skills Manual for Paediatric Nursing, Caring for Children, 3rd ed.* Washington: Prentice Hall.

Black, J. & Matassarin-Jacobs, E. (eds.) (1993) *Luckmann and Sorensen's Medical-Surgical Nursing: A psychophysiologic approach, 4th ed.* Philadelphia: Saunders.

Bulloch, B. & Tenenbein, M. (2002) Assessment of clinically significant changes in acute pain in children. *Academic Emergency Medicine* **9** (3), 199–202.

Caterall, A. (2006) *Reading list: Perthes disease.* Available at: **http://www.jbjs.org.uk/misc/ RLperthesdisease.dtl**

Chadburn, L. (2006) Plaster care. In E. Trigg & T. Mohammed. *Practices in Children's Nursing: Guidelines for hospitals and community, 2nd ed.* Edinburgh: Churchill Livingstone.

Chamley, C.A., Carson, P., Randall, D., Sandwell, M. (2005) *Developmental Anatomy and Physiology of Children, 1st ed.* Edinburgh: Churchill Livingston.

Checketts, R.G. (2000) Pin tract infection and the principles of pin site care. In A. De Bastiani, A.G. Apley, & D.E. Goldberg (eds.) *Orthofix External Fixation in Trauma and Orthopaedics*. Berlin: Springer.

Clarke, S. (2003) Orthopaedic paediatric practice: An impression of pain assessment. *Journal of Orthopaedic Nursing* **7**, 132–136.

Clarke, S. & McKay, M. (2006) An audit of spica cast guidelines for parents and professionals caring for children with developmental dysplasia of the hip. *Journal of Orthopaedic Nursing* **10** (3), 128–137.

Dandy, D.J. & Edwards, D.J. (2004) *Essential Orthopaedics and Trauma, 4th ed.* Edinburgh: Churchill Livingstone.

Davies, R., Holt, N., & Nayagam, S. (2005) The care of pin sites with external fixation. *Journal of Bone and Joint Surgery* **87**, 716–719.

Davis, P.S. (1994) *Nursing the Orthopaedic Patient*. Edinburgh: Churchill Livingstone.

Eiff, P.M. & Hatch, R.L. (2003) Boning up on common pediatric fractures. *Contemporary Pediatrics* **20**, 30–42.

Hart, E.S., Grottkau, B.E., Rebello, G.N., & Albright, M.B. (2006) Broken bones: Common pediatric upper extremity fractures—Part 2. *Orthopaedic Nursing* **25** (5), 311–323.

Hockenberry, M.J. & Wilson, D. (2003) *Wong's Nursing Care of Infants and Children*. London: Mosby.

Houghton, K., Peregrina, D.G., & Herden, J. (2003) A small trial of the nursing care of patients immobilized with a Thomas splint. *Journal of Orthopaedic Nursing* **7** (4), 201–204.

Judd, J., & Wright, E. (2005) Joint and limb problems in children. In J. Kneale & P. Davies (eds.) *Orthopaedic and Trauma Nursing*. London: Churchill Livingston.

Judge, N.L. (2007) Neurovascular assessment. *Nursing Standard* **21** (45), 39–44.

Katz, K., Fogelman, R., Attias, J., Baron, E., & Soudry, M. (2001) Anxiety reaction in children during removal of their plaster cast with a saw. *Journal of Bone and Joint Surgery* **83**, 388–390.

Keays, G., Swaine, B., & Ehrmann-Feldman, D. (2006) Association between severity of musculoskeletal injury and risk of subsequent injury in children and adolescents on the basis of parental recall. *Arch Pediatr Adolesc Med* **160** (8), 812–816.

Klenerman (1994) ABC of sports medicine: Musculoskeletal injuries in child athletes. BMJ **308**, 1556–1559.

Kunkler, C.E. (1999) Neurovascular assessment. *Orthopaedic Nursing* **18**, 3.

Lee-Smith, J., Santy, J., Davis, P., Jester, R., & Kneale, J. (2001) Pin site management: Toward a consensus, part 1. *Journal of Orthopaedic Nursing* **5**, 37–42.

Mandleco, B. (2002) Paediatric Nursing: Caring for children and their families. Clifton Park, NY: Delmar Publishing.

McRae, R. & Esser, M. (2002) *Practical Fracture Management, 4th ed.* Edinburgh: Churchill Livingstone.

Newman, D. (2005) Functional status, personal health and self esteem of caregivers of children in a body cast: A pilot study. *Orthopaedic Nursing* **24**, 416–423.

Patterson, M. (2005) Multicentre pin site care study. *Orthopaedic Nursing* **24** (5), 349–359.

Royal College of Nursing (2001) *Pressure Ulcer Risk Assessment and Prevention*. London: Royal College of Nursing.

Royal College of Nursing (2002) *A Traction Manual*. London: Royal College of Nursing.

Royal College of Nursing (2007) *Benchmarks for Children's Orthopaedic Nursing*. London: Royal College of Nursing.

Santy, J., Rogers, J., Davis, P., *et al.* (2005) A competency framework for orthopaedic and trauma nursing. *Journal of Orthopaedic Nursing* **9** (2), 81–86.

Sheehan, E., Mulhall, K.J., Kearns, S., *et al.* (2003) Impact of dedicated skate parks on the severity and incidence of skateboard and rollerblade-related pediatric fractures. *Journal of Pediatric Orthopaedics* **23** (4), 440–442.

Sims, M. & Saleh, M. (2000) External fixation—the incidence of pin site infection: A prospective audit. *Journal of Orthopaedic Nursing* **4** (2), 59–63.

Solomon, L., Warwick, D., & Nayagam, S. (2005) *Apleys Concise System of Orthopaedics and Fractures, 3rd ed.* London: Hodder Arnold.

Staheli, L.T. (2006) *Practice of Paediatric Orthopaedics, 2nd ed.* Philadelphia: Lippincott Williams & Wilkins.

Thompson, J., McFarlane, G., Hirsch, J., & Tucker, S. (eds.) (1997) *Mosby's Clinical Nursing, 4th ed.* St. Louis: Mosby-Year Book Inc.

Twycross, A., Moriarity, A., & Betts, T. (1998) *Paediatric Pain Management: A multidisciplinary approach.* Oxford: Radcliffe Medical Press Ltd.

W-Dahl, A. & Toksvig-Larsen, S. (2004) Pin site care in external fixation: Sodium chloride or chlorhexidine solution as a cleaning agent. *Archives of Orthopaedic Trauma Surgery* 124 (8), 555–558.

W-Dahl, A., Toksvig-Larsen, S., & Lindstrand, A. (2003) No difference between daily and weekly pin site: A randomized study of 50 patients with external fixation. *Acta Orthopaedica Scandinavica* 74 (6), 704–708.

Whaley, L. & Wong, D. (1999) *Nursing Care of Infants and Children, 6th ed.* St Louis: Mosby.

Wright, E. (2007) Evaluating a paediatric neurovascular assessment tool. *Journal of Orthopaedic Nursing* **11** (1), 20–29.

Further reading and URLs

British Orthopaedic Association (2006) *Casting Technique Course: Compartment syndrome handout.* London: British Orthopaedic Association, Royal College of Nursing, Society of Orthopaedic and Trauma Nursing, & Association of Orthopaedic Technicians.

Broughton, N.S. (1997) *A Textbook of Paediatric Orthopaedics.* London: WB Saunders.

Glasper, E.A., McEwing, G., & Richardson, J. (2007) *Oxford Handbook of Children's and Young People's Nursing.* New York: Oxford University Press.

Prior, M.A. & Miles, S. (1999) Casting: Part 1. *Nursing Standard* **13** (28), 49–53.

http://www.rcn.org.uk/rcn
http://www.orthonurse.org/

The endocrine system

YVONNE CORCORAN

Skills

14.1 **Assessment of growth in children**
....
14.2 **Blood glucose measurement**
....
14.3 **Insulin administration in children**
....
14.4 **Dietary management of children with endocrine disorders**

Introduction

This chapter aims to explore the nursing skills required to care for the child and family with an underlying endocrine disorder both in a healthcare setting and in the community. This chapter will include an overview of the anatomy and physiology of the endocrine system, related pharmacology and microbiology, and a detailed description of the main skills involved in caring for children with an endocrine disorder and their families. Endocrine disorders in childhood are generally of a chronic nature, therefore prompt, accurate treatment and management are essential to ensure normal development into fully functioning adulthood. Disorders of the endocrine system can manifest their effects immediately or in a more gradual manner over days to months.

Endocrine disorders most commonly occur due to three main reasons: a disordered endocrine system, often as a result of a genetic abnormality; overproduction of a particular hormone; or underproduction of a particular hormone (Evans & Tippins, 2008). **Type 1 diabetes** mellitus accounts for approximately 50% of endocrine disorders in childhood with an incidence in children (0–14 years) of 13.5 per 100,000 in the UK (Raine *et al.,* 2006).

Although some general principles apply to the nursing care of children with an endocrine disorder, you will need to refer to local policy and be familiar with local protocols regarding the nursing management of these children and their families in the hospital and the community.

Learning outcomes

It is anticipated that you will be able to do the following once you have read and studied this chapter:

- Understand the anatomy and physiology of the endocrine system and how it affects many of our bodily functions.
- Understand the predominant pathological conditions related to the endocrine system.
- Understand the key nursing skills required to care for a child with an endocrine disorder and their family.

Anatomy and physiology

The endocrine system is a chemical communication system that consists of hormone producing cells, hormones, and receptors (Glasper & Richardson, 2006). This system regulates and controls the body's metabolic processes including energy production, growth, fluid and electrolyte balance, responses to stress, and sexual reproduction (Baxter *et al.,* 2004). Disorders of the endocrine system may manifest their effects either immediately or gradually over a period of time. The endocrine system consists of glands that are widely separated from one another and have no direct anatomical links (Chamley *et al.,* 2005). These glands produce and secrete hormones (chemical messengers) and are listed in **Box 14.1** below. These endocrine glands also secrete hormones directly into the bloodstream for distribution around the body, where they can alter the activity of many organs at one time. **Figure 14.1** demonstrates the location and distribution of endocrine glands in the body. **Box 14.2** further outlines the functions of the endocrine system.

Box 14.1 The endocrine glands

- Adrenal glands (2)
- Pancreatic islets
- Placenta
- Pituitary gland
- Parathyroid glands (4)
- Pineal gland
- Thyroid gland
- Ovaries (2)
- Testes (2)

The pituitary gland

The pituitary gland (hypophysis cerebri), sometimes referred to as the *master gland*, is a small oval gland situated at the base of the brain. It is divided into two parts: the anterior lobe and the posterior lobe. The release of hormones by the pituitary gland is controlled by the hypothalamus (see Chapter Ten). The anterior pituitary

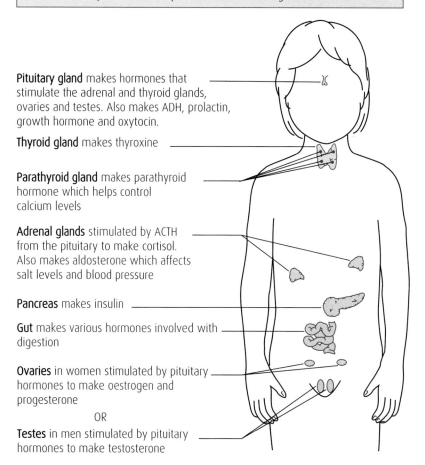

Endocrine glands make hormones. These are chemicals that travel in the blood to afftect other parts of the body. The main endocrine glands are shown here

Pituitary gland makes hormones that stimulate the adrenal and thyroid glands, ovaries and testes. Also makes ADH, prolactin, growth hormone and oxytocin.

Thyroid gland makes thyroxine

Parathyroid gland makes parathyroid hormone which helps control calcium levels

Adrenal glands stimulated by ACTH from the pituitary to make cortisol. Also makes aldosterone which affects salt levels and blood pressure

Pancreas makes insulin

Gut makes various hormones involved with digestion

Ovaries in women stimulated by pituitary hormones to make oestrogen and progesterone

OR

Testes in men stimulated by pituitary hormones to make testosterone

Figure 14.1 The location of endocrine glands in the body

Box 14.2 Functions of the endocrine system

- Regulation of the rate of metabolism in the body and effects on the rate of maturation of the tissues.
- Ion regulation in the blood (pH, sodium, potassium, and calcium).
- Regulates water balance by controlling the solute concentration in the body.
- Assists in the immune system regulation.
- Assists in the regulation of heart rate and blood pressure.
- Regulation of **blood glucose levels** and other nutrient levels in the blood.
- Controls the development and function of the reproductive system in males and females.
- Regulates uterine contractions during delivery and stimulates milk release in lactating females.

Adapted from Tate (2009).

gland consists of a collection of hormone-producing cells, which are controlled by the hypothalamus. The hormones produced by the anterior pituitary gland are:

- Human growth hormone (GH).
- Thyroid stimulating hormone (TSH).
- Prolactin.
- Adrenocorticotrophic hormone (ACTH).
- Luteinizing hormone (LH).
- Follicle stimulating hormone (FSH).

Table 14.1 further outlines these hormones, identifying their sites of action and effects.

The posterior pituitary gland does not actually produce hormones but those formed in the hypothalamus are stored there until stimulated to be released. The posterior pituitary therefore secretes two hormones: anti-diuretic hormone (ADH) and oxytocin. ADH influences the amount of fluid that the kidneys reabsorb into the circulatory system and the amount of fluid that the kidneys excrete in urine. Production of ADH is regulated by the osmolality of the circulating blood. Oxytocin causes contraction of smooth muscle cells in the uterus and initiates release of milk from the breasts in women who are breastfeeding (Tate, 2009).

The thyroid gland

The thyroid gland is highly vascular and situated just inferior to the larynx. It consists of two lobes connected by a narrow band called the isthmus. It is one of the largest endocrine glands and weighs approximately 15–20 grams. The thyroid secretes two major hormones called thyroxine (T4) and triiodothyronine (T3). Synthesis and secretion of these hormones is regulated by thyroid stimulating hormone from the anterior pituitary gland. Thyroid hormones affect nearly every tissue in the body but mostly they increase the rate of metabolism in the body. Metabolism is the amount of energy used by the

Table 14.1 Hormones of the anterior pituitary gland and their target sites

Hormone	Target site	Effects at target site
Human growth hormone	Bone, muscle, fat	Growth of tissues
Thyroid stimulating hormone	Thyroid gland	Secretion of hormones
Prolactin	Mammary glands	Milk production
Adrenocorticotrophic hormone	Adrenal cortex	Secretion of hormones
Luteinizing hormone	Testes and ovaries	Testosterone secretion/ovulation
Follicle stimulating hormone	Testes and ovaries	Sperm production/ follicle maturation

body to carry out its functions. The metabolic rate can be increased by 60–100% when blood thyroid hormone levels are increased (Tate, 2009).

In addition to secreting these hormones, the thyroid gland also produces and secretes a hormone called calcitonin. This hormone is important in maintaining calcium levels in the body.

The parathyroid glands

There are four parathyroid glands and they are situated on the posterior aspect of the thyroid gland. They secrete a hormone called parathyroid hormone, which is essential for the regulation of calcium levels in the body. While calcitonin from the thyroid is released when the calcium levels in the body are too high, parathyroid hormone is released when the levels of calcium are too low.

The adrenal glands

There are two adrenal glands and they are situated on the top of each kidney. Each adrenal gland has two layers know as the adrenal medulla (inner layer) and the adrenal cortex (outer layer). The adrenal cortex secretes hormones that are essential for life: glucocorticoids, mineralocorticoids, and sex steroids. The adrenal medulla produces the catecholamines: epinephrine and norepinephrine.

Glucocorticoids

These are steroids produced by the adrenal cortex that affect glucose metabolism and reduce the intensity of the inflammatory and immune responses in the tissues. The major glucocorticoid is called cortisol. It is a stress hormone and it is released by the body when increased energy is needed. Its release is stimulated by adrenocorticotrophic hormone (ACTH) produced in the pituitary gland during a stressful event. Cortisol causes the liver to release more sugar, causes the breakdown of fat and muscle for energy, and reduces the energy requirements of the cells in the body.

Mineralocorticoids

The effect of mineralocorticoids is directed upon the body's electrolytes or minerals and therefore has an effect on the body's water balance.

Catecholamines—epinephrine and norepinephrine

These two hormones are produced in the adrenal medulla and are responsible for the body's 'fight or flight' response in times of increased exercise, emotional excitement, injury, stress, or low blood sugar. Their release is in response to stimulation of the sympathetic neurons in the body's autonomic nervous system.

The pancreas

The pancreas is an elongated organ measuring approximately 15 cm long, which is situated posterior to the stomach and is partially covered by a loop of the first part of the small intestine. The pancreas has both an exocrine and an endocrine function; however, for the purposes of this chapter we are concerned only with its endocrine function.

The pancreatic islets

The endocrine pancreas consists of clumps of cells called pancreatic islets, approximately 500,000 to one million in number. Within the islets the alpha cells secrete glucagon while the beta cells secrete insulin. The release of insulin at times when sugar levels are high in the body, like after a meal, is designed to lower blood sugar levels. Glucagon, on the other hand, is released when sugar levels are low in an attempt to return the blood sugar levels to normal.

Endocrine conditions in children

Diabetes mellitus (DM)

Diabetes mellitus (DM) is a condition where there is a complete deficiency or an insufficient level of the hormone insulin, which results in **hyperglycaemia**. **Type 1 diabetes** mellitus accounts for approximately 50% of endocrine disorders in childhood with an incidence in children (0–14 years) of 13.5 per 100,000 in the UK (Raine *et al.,* 2006). The classic symptoms of DM include polyuria, polydipsia, and **glycosuria**. Insulin-dependent diabetes mellitus is the third most common chronic illness in childhood (Dixon, 2003).

Type 1 diabetes mellitus (T1DM) accounts for 70–90% of diabetes occurrence in children (Danne & Becker, 2007). T1DM is believed to arise as a result of auto-immune beta cell destruction resulting in insulin deficiency, and must be treated with lifelong insulin injections (Wal-lymahmed, 2006). **Type 2 diabetes** mellitus (T2DM) is characterized by insufficient production of insulin or by insulin resistance in the target cells. Both Type 1 DM and Type 2 DM can occur in children and adolescents, although T1DM is more prevalent. As children and adolescents with diabetes mellitus grow they will have special and changing needs in order that optimal glycaemic control is maintained.

Adrenal disorders

Adrenal disorders manifest themselves by either the underproduction or overproduction of the main steroids produced by the adrenal glands, which are: mineralocorticoids, glucocorticoids, and androgens. A summary of these disorders and effects is provided below; however, supplementary reading is required to develop a more in-depth knowledge of this area.

Adrenal insufficiency

Adrenal insufficiency occurs due to an inability of the adrenal glands to produce cortisol in response to stress. It can be caused by a number of diseases including Addison's disease and congenital adrenal hyperplasia (CAH). Congenital adrenal hyperplasia involves the disordered production of cortisol resulting in insufficient or excessive production of sex hormones. The most common conditions include:

- Ambiguous genitalia.
- Precocious or delayed puberty.
- Vomiting due to salt wastage.
- Excessive facial hair.
- Irregular menstrual cycle/virilization/infertility.

Addison's disease

Addison's disease is a disorder caused by disrupted functioning of the adrenal cortex. This results in decreased production of two important hormones normally released by the adrenal cortex: cortisol and aldosterone. Signs and symptoms in the early stages of the disease include fatigue, weight loss, polyuria, and increasing skin pigmentation (Raine et al., 2006).

Cushing's syndrome

Cushing's syndrome is very rare in childhood (Raine et al., 2006). The signs and symptoms include obesity, slow growth, fatigue, hirsutism, acne, and hypertension.

Congenital hypothyroidism

Congenital hypothyroidism is more common in boys than girls and is an absence or severe deficiency of thyroid hormone. If left untreated in infants it can cause permanent mental retardation and also growth failure. The incidence is approximately one in 4000 births (Raine et al., 2006).

Hyperthyroidism (Graves' disease)

This condition is characterized by excess synthesis and secretion of thyroid hormone, also known as thyrotoxicosis. It is more common in females with a peak occurrence in adolescents. It is an autoimmune disease where antibodies against the thyroid gland are produced.

Diabetes insipidus

This is a condition that occurs when the kidneys are unable to conserve water during their filtering of blood. The conservation of water is controlled by vasopressin, which is an anti-diuretic hormone (ADH).

Hypopituitarism

Hypopituitarism is a failure of the pituitary gland to secrete one or more of its hormones. This can affect any number of the body's normal functions.

Klinefelter's syndrome

This is a condition caused by chromosome aneuploidy, which is a change in the number of chromosomes. Klinefelter's syndrome-affected males have an extra X chromosome, which can reduce their fertility.

Marfan syndrome

Marfan syndrome is characterized by an abnormality of fibrillin, a connective tissue protein, leading to it being weak or elastic. This results in children being usually tall and slim with long fingers and toes and a degree of hypotonia.

Turner's syndrome

Turner's syndrome is a disorder in females. Instead of having XX chromosomes, only one X chromosome is present. Functioning female sexual characteristics are present but undeveloped.

Key nursing skills

This section will describe some of the key nursing skills required by the nurse caring for a child with an endocrine condition. The skills identified and described in this section are: assessment of growth in children; blood glucose measurement, recording, and interpretation; and insulin therapy, including administration and dietary management.

Ongoing education and support for the child and family is a key role of the children's nurse caring for a child with an endocrine disorder. Due to development of key interdisciplinary personnel such as diabetes nurse specialists, paediatric consultant endocrinologists, and dieticians, much of the child's care may be managed successfully at home with their families. As a result hospital admissions are kept to a minimum while still achieving optimal growth and development and disease management.

14.1 **Assessment of growth in children**

Accurate measurements of a child's height, weight, and growth development are vital components of the assessment of a child with an underlying endocrine condition. Accurate assessment of growth is an essential nursing skill required in order to provide ongoing care to children with an endocrine disorder and their families.

The term 'auxology' is used to describe the study of human growth and detailed measurements can provide pertinent information about a child's physical and mental development. As growth is a continuous but uneven process it is most reliably evaluated by comparing growth measurements over a period of time (Hockenberry & Wilson, 2007). Within the specialty of endocrinology the assessment of growth requires exceptional accuracy and the knowledge to perform this skill proficiently. It is a key clinical skill for nurses caring for children with endocrine disorders.

Normal human growth is divided into three phases: infancy, childhood, and pubertal growth. In infancy growth is rapid and a continuation of foetal growth but with a significant decrease in velocity. Nutrition plays the most influential part in this growth. In childhood growth is more heavily reliant on hormonal influences, particularly growth hormone (GH) and insulin-like growth factor (IGF) hormone. Normal thyroid status is also essential to maintain normal growth. In puberty growth is caused by increasing levels of androgen in boys and oestrogen in girls.

Nursing Alert

All hospitals should have local policies in place regarding the weighing of children, therefore ensure you are familiar with and adhere to the local policy where you are working.

Recording of growth assessment

Any height or weight measurement of a child must be outlined and plotted on a growth chart. Growth charts are available for different population groups and the most up-to-date charts should be used. Many charts have also been produced for different childhood diseases and disorders.

Growth charts are often sex specific and show age/time on the horizontal axis and the measurement on the vertical axis. Most charts use 'centile' spacing. There can be many variations but the most common tends to be 3rd, 5th, 10th, 25th, 50th, 75th, 90th, and 97th. Thus when a child's measurements are plotted it can be easily seen if the height and weight are proportional, and when plotted over a period of time growth velocity can be ascertained and deviations can be addressed.

Measurements should be recorded in the child's notes, with the date, in addition to on the growth chart. The measuring of a child's height and weight are important clinical observations, and are detailed in Chapter Five.

14.2 **Blood glucose measurement**

This section aims to provide you with knowledge and understanding of the skills required to carry out blood glucose measurement in a child. Blood glucose measurement is a procedure that is performed in order to establish the level of glucose in the blood. In children with some endocrine conditions, especially Type 1 diabetes mellitus, blood glucose measurement is an essential component of their care as they are very susceptible to episodes of **hypoglycaemia** and **hyperglycaemia**. Self-monitoring of blood glucose is recognized as an essential tool in the management of childhood and adolescent diabetes (International Society for Pediatric and Adolescent Diabetes (ISPAD), 2005). Self-monitoring of blood glucose levels empowers the child and their family by enhancing their understanding of how insulin, food, and exercise affect their blood glucose (Danne & Becker, 2007). Routine monitoring using a hand-held blood glucose monitor is a quick and convenient means of obtaining blood glucose values. It can be used by the nurse at the child's bedside, or the child and/or family can be instructed in how to use the equipment in the community, such as the school or the home environment. This is referred to as point-of-care testing (POCT). It facilitates holistic care and timely treatment (Royal College of Nursing (RCN), 2005), although practices may vary locally.

Considerable variations in blood glucose levels may occur depending on the time of day the sample is taken. Blood glucose levels are lowest in the morning before breakfast (Blann, 2006). Levels rise immediately after a meal and fall to fasting levels about two hours later (Skinner, 2005).

Capillary blood is used to measure glucose levels when using a blood glucose monitor, and these therefore give a whole blood measurement of glucose, while laboratory-tested blood provides plasma glucose levels. Glucose is more concentrated in plasma, so plasma levels will be higher than whole blood capillary levels (Dungan *et al.*, 2007). Some modern blood glucose monitors are capable of reporting either whole blood or plasma glucose levels (Diabetes Forecast, 2007).

Indications for performing blood glucose monitoring

The following are indications for performing blood glucose monitoring in children with an endocrine condition:

- Children receiving intravenous or subcutaneous insulin. The readings can assist the medical team to adjust insulin levels (Alexander *et al.*, 2006).
- To detect hypoglycaemia (low blood sugar) or hyperglycaemia (high blood sugar).
- To monitor patients who are taking hypoglycaemic medications.
- To eliminate diabetes mellitus as an underlying cause in those who present in an unconscious state (Skinner, 2005).

Nursing Alert

Blood glucose levels are measured in millimoles per litre (mmol/l). The normal range for a child is 3.4–5.6 mmol/l and for a neonate is 2.6–5.0 mmol/l (Skinner, 2005). The acceptable range may vary between individual children and should be determined by a doctor and recorded in the patient's notes (Jamieson *et al.*, 2002).

Staff need to be aware that certain conditions may give rise to false readings of blood glucose. In these instances a laboratory measurement using a venous blood sample is required. Results may be affected by the following:

- Dialysis treatment.
- Hyperlipidaemia.
- Severe dehydration.
- High and low haematocrit values.
- High bilirubin values.
- Peripheral circulatory failure.
- Intravenous infusions of ascorbic acid (vitamin C).
- Patients receiving intensive oxygen therapy (Medicines and Healthcare products Regulatory Agency, 2005).

Step-by-step guide to blood glucose measurement using a blood glucose meter

(measurement in mmol/l of a child's capillary blood glucose level)

Step	Rationale
1 Ensure that you are familiar with how the equipment works.	Only practitioners who are specifically trained should use the monitor.
Check manufacturer's instructions and calibrate if necessary.	To ensure accuracy.
2 Check expiry date of reagent strips and that they have been calibrated.	To ensure accuracy.
When opening a new container, record the date of opening.	Strips may need to be used within a certain time frame once opened (Jamieson *et al.*, 2002).
3 Ask patient to wash their hands, rinse thoroughly with clean water, and ensure hands are dried thoroughly.	To ensure accurate results.
Alcohol wipes should not be used to clean puncture site.	Alcohol interferes with test/reagent strips and repeated use toughens skin (Smith *et al.*, 2004).
4 If appropriate, ask patient or patient's carer to undertake or assist during the procedure.	To promote family centred care.
5 Select a suitable puncture site. The side of the finger or the side of the heel are potential sites. Avoid using the back of the heel and the fingertip.	To reduce pain and prevent damage to underlying nerves.
6 The puncture site should be alternated. The child/family can be involved in selecting the finger/site.	To reduce the risk of infection from recurrent punctures, prevent the areas becoming hard, and reduce discomfort. Involvement in site selection will help them feel empowered and that they have choice and control over the procedure.
7 Insert a lancet into the finger pricking device and select an appropriate depth thickness.	Finger prick lancets have different depth thickness settings and the appropriate setting should be chosen depending on the child's age and size.
8 Remove protective cap from lancet. Place the sterile lancet firmly against selected area and press the release button. The lancet will immediately puncture the skin.	To obtain blood sample.
Position finger in downward position.	To aid the flow of blood.

9 Gently squeeze the finger (or heel).

To produce a sufficient sample of blood to ensure accuracy of result. Sometimes, as the finger prick is so slight, blood is not immediately seen. This ensures the puncture made by the finger lancet device does not close.

Avoid massaging blood from the puncture site.

This may result in damage to the tissues and the subsequent seepage of tissue fluid will give a false result (Skinner, 2005).

10 Apply the blood to the reagent strip pad in one application only (Dougherty & Lister, 2004). Ensure that there is sufficient blood to cover the reagent/test strip.

To give an accurate result.

Do not smear or spread the blood on the strip.

May alter the result.

11 Continue as per the manufacturer's instructions.

The procedure may vary depending on the type of monitor.

12 Read and record result as soon as displayed on monitor.

To ensure accuracy.

The nurse must know the normal blood glucose range.

So that abnormalities can be recognized and treatment provided as appropriate.

13 Apply cotton wool to puncture site and apply pressure.

To prevent further bleeding and to prevent haematoma formation.

14 Dispose of lancet in sharps bin. Dispose of waste appropriately.

To reduce the risk of needle stick injury.
To prevent the spread of infection.

15 Ensure bleeding has stopped and the patient is comfortable.

To ensure patient comfort.

16 Remove and dispose of gloves and apron. Wash hands or clean with bactericidal solution.

To prevent cross infection.

17 Store the monitor and reagent/test strips according to manufacturer's instructions.

To ensure proper storage.

18 Document the blood glucose level and report any abnormal findings to relevant personnel.

To ensure accurate documentation.
So that any abnormal findings can be addressed.

Procedure: blood glucose monitoring

Preparation

Before commencing you will need to wash your hands in accordance with local hospital policy. Standard precautions should be followed strictly during the procedure, including the wearing of disposable gloves and a plastic apron.

You will also require the child to wash and dry their hands thoroughly directly prior to the procedure. Then you will select a suitable site to collect a blood sample. Recommended blood sampling sites are sides of the fingertips as the sensitivity of the fingertips is not affected (see Figure 14.2). Avoid using the thumbs and index fingers and rotate sties continually.

Nursing Alert

It is important to ensure that hands are washed as if a child has eaten something, remnants can be left on the skin and give a false result. Also, some soaps, crayons, and felt-tip pens have glycerol additives. It is also essential that hands are thoroughly dried as children can have false low results if the blood test is diluted with water on the finger.

Equipment

Gather all equipment required prior to commencing the procedure. There are a variety of blood glucose monitors available. They vary depending on size, testing speed, amount of blood needed for the test, ability to store test results in memory, and cost of meter and reagent/test strips. It is important to follow the manufacturer's instructions for storage and blood monitoring technique. Compatible test/reagent strips should be used. Monitors should be calibrated as per the manufacturer's guidelines to ensure an accurate result.

Equipment required:
- Blood glucose meter.
- Test/reagent strips.
- A spring-loaded finger pricking device and sterile lancets.

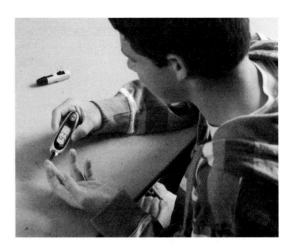

Figure 14.2 The fingertip is the recommended blood sampling site
© Mark Hatfield/istockphoto.com

- Cotton wool balls.
- Non-sterile gloves and apron.
- Sharps bin.
- Child's record sheet.
- Receptacle for waste material.

Consent and communication

Before commencing the procedure you need to explain to the child and family why the monitoring and measuring of blood glucose levels is necessary, what is involved in the procedure, the duration of the procedure, and the implications of the result (see Chapter Two for further discussion of family centred care and Chapter Five for preparation of the child for clinical observation). The appropriate use of distraction techniques, play therapy, and level of involvement of the child and family should be assessed and addressed when planning the procedure (see Chapter Two).

Following the procedure

Following the procedure you will need to ensure that the child is comfortable and that all equipment used is disposed of safely or cleaned in accordance with hospital infection control guidelines. It is important to document and record the procedure and any observations in the child's hospital notes (see Chapter Five regarding documentation). If you are uncertain regarding any issues relating to blood glucose measurement, refer to local policy or contact laboratory personnel.

Other considerations

Educating both child and family

In many cases glucose monitoring is a skill that will need to be performed when the child is at home, so instructing the child and family regarding the correct procedure to accurately measure, record, and interpret their blood glucose level is essential. The child and family will need to be competent in both the procedure and interpretation of blood glucose monitoring prior to discharge home. Support should be available in the home setting from a health visitor/public health nurse and an action plan must be in place should the child become unwell.

Blood ketone testing

The ability to test blood glucose and blood ketone levels quickly using a hand-held blood glucose monitor has greatly improved the care of children and adolescents with diabetes mellitus in the community setting (ISPAD, 2005). Both blood glucose and blood ketone levels can be measured using the same meter. The procedure for blood ketone levels is similar to that for blood glucose measurement but a blood ketone reagent strip is used in order to obtain a blood ketone measurement.

Box 14.3 Why do errors occur when measuring blood glucose?

- The margin of error in a correctly calibrated and used glucose meter is 10% (Hanas, 2007).
- An abnormal blood glucose reading may need to be verified by sending a venous sample to the laboratory.

False low reading
- Too small an amount of blood applied to the reagent strip.
- Drop of blood applied too late to the reagent strip.
- Water or saliva on the finger.

False high reading
- Unwashed hands.

14.3 **Insulin administration in children**

Background to insulin therapy in children

It is important for you as a student to develop an understanding of the knowledge and skills required to administer insulin to children with Type 1 diabetes. Normal blood glucose levels in a healthy child are maintained by the complex interaction of hormones including insulin, cortisol, and growth hormone. The result is the maintenance of the blood glucose within a normal range (see above) with little variation in times of extremes of nutrition, exercise, and physiological stress (Williams & Dunger, 2004). However, children with diabetes, either due to a resistance to insulin or a complete absence of circulating insulin, require injections of insulin in order to regulate the metabolic pathway of glucose, protein, and fat.

Insulin was first used in the early 1920s and the discovery of effective short- and long-acting insulin has revolutionized diabetes care. Human recombinant insulins are now the most commonly recommended preparations of insulin used in children (Australian Paediatric Endocrine Group, 2005). Evidence that improving glycaemic control in people with Type 1 and Type 2 diabetes can significantly reduce the risk of microvascular complications is well established (Diabetes Control and Complications Research Group, 1993; United Kingdom Prospective Diabetes Study, 1998).

The aim of insulin administration in children with Type 1 diabetes is to mimic the body's normal insulin secreting pattern, therefore alleviating the symptoms of diabetes, minimizing the risk of long-term microvascular complications, and improving the child's quality of life (Wallymahmed, 2006). There are many different forms of insulin prescribed for use in children with Type 1 diabetes. Optimal glycaemic control is essential to avoid the long- and short-term complications of Type 1 diabetes and the most suitable insulin, in terms of its particular absorption profile, is matched according to the child's needs in order obtain good glycaemic control (National Institute for Clinical Excellence (NICE), 2004).

There are five main types of insulin preparation suitable for use in children: rapid acting; short acting; intermediate acting; long acting analogue; and mixed insulin. The information below gives a brief overview of the most commonly used insulins in children, their onsets of action, their peak effects, and their durations of action.

Rapid acting insulin analogues

Rapid acting insulin is produced by modifications to the chemical structure of native insulin, which results in a shorter onset and duration of action compared to regular insulin. Insulin is usually administered between 5 and 15 minutes prior to a meal.

> **Nursing Alert**
>
> Pre-school children with Type 1 diabetes may use rapid acting insulin analogues after eating due to their unpredictable eating patterns (NICE, 2004).

Short acting insulin

Short acting insulin is used as an essential part of most daily insulin replacement regimes for children with Type 1 diabetes. It is often combined with intermediate acting insulin in a two to three daily dose regime. Peak action time for short acting insulin is approximately 30 minutes after administration.

Intermediate acting insulin

Suitable regimes for intermediate acting insulin are normally between once and three times per day (Steck *et al.,* 2007). The onset of action occurs between one and two hours following injection, and the duration of effect can be between 16 and 35 hours.

Long acting insulin analogues

Normally administered in a once daily dose in order to achieve a more constant and steady background level of insulin.

Premixed insulin

There are several premixed insulin preparations available for use in children, including combinations of rapid acting, short acting, intermediate, or long acting insulin. Premixed insulin is not generally recommended for first line use in children due to their ever changing needs in relation to their insulin regime. It can, however, be useful in situations where there are difficulties with the child or parent accurately drawing up or mixing insulin and where compliance is an issue.

Insulin administration

Total daily insulin requirements in children with Type 1 diabetes mellitus range from 0.8 units/kg/day increasing to 1–1.5 units/kg/day in adolescents. The total daily insulin requirement is normally administered in two or three daily injections. A regime of insulin administration is tailored to meet the individual requirements of the child, taking into account the child's age and lifestyle. The aim is to achieve optimal glycaemic control in order to minimize both short and long-term complications associated with diabetes.

Insulin can be delivered into the subcutaneous layer of the skin via a syringe, a specific insulin pen, or an insulin pump. Insulin can only be injected as it is destroyed by gastric juices. The choice of insulin type and regime needs to be guided by a variety of factors including the following:

- The age of the child.
- Lifestyle issues.
- Child and family preferences and management skills.
- Metabolic targets.
- Associated complications, especially hypoglycaemia (Australian Paediatric Endocrine Group, 2005).

Box 14.4 Principles of insulin storage

- Insulin can be stored at room temperature providing there are no extremes in temperature.
- Open vials should be refrigerated at 4–8°C.
- The date of opening should be recorded on the vial of insulin, and if stored in the refrigerator it will remain suitable for use for three months.
- Penfill cartridges and disposable insulin pens should be discarded after 21–28 days. Always refer to the manufacturer's instructions.
- Always check the expiry date on the vial of insulin prior to administration.

Administering subcutaneous insulin to children

When administering insulin to children, always adhere to the local hospital and national policies for the administration of medication to patients in your care. Insulin can be given via an insulin syringe or via a pen and the procedure used to perform this skill is outlined below. Depending on the age and cognitive ability of the child the administration of insulin may be the responsibility of the parent/carer, or if the child is old enough it can be done by the child under the supervision of the parent in the community setting.

Nursing Alert

Parents give insulin at home on a daily basis and they will know the most current doses.

Injection sites

Insulin should be administered into the subcutaneous layer as it is more slowly and consistently absorbed. The site of administration is also important as the rate of absorption varies depending on the anatomical location where it is administered. The suitable sites for administration in children include the abdomen, buttocks, and thighs (see Figure 14.3). Complications associated with the administration of subcutaneous injections include a condition called lipohypertrophy. This is where there is an accumulation of fat and fibrous tissue in lumps under the skin that result in poor insulin absorption. It is important to teach the child and parent the importance of site rotation to reduce these side effects.

Nursing Alert

It is important to remember that injections may be very distressing for a child.

Procedure: Insulin administration in children (see following page)

The following procedure outlines general principles when administrating insulin without using an insulin pen.

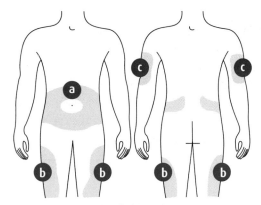

Recommended injection sites
a Either side and below the umbilicus
b Anterior thigh
c Upper and outer arms

Figure 14.3 Suitable sites for administration of insulin in children

Preparation

Check the dose prescribed for the child in accordance with the hospital drug policy. Wash and dry hands in accordance with local policy to prevent cross infection.

Equipment

Gather all equipment that you will need for this procedure, including:
- Prescription chart.
- Alcohol swabs.
- Insulin.
- Insulin syringe and needle.

Consent and communication

Explain to the parents and child that you are about to administer insulin.

Insulin pens

Insulin pens are now the most common form of device used to administer insulin. Children as young as four years old are successfully using these devices. However, when assessing a child's ability to utilize such a device it is important to remember to consider

Step-by-step guide to general insulin administration in children

Step	Rationale
1 Ensure the insulin doses have been prescribed in accordance with the hospital policy. If you have any doubt about the doses of insulin prescribed check again with the doctor who has prescribed the dose.	Double checking will ensure the correct dose is administered.
2 Check the expiry date on the vial of insulin. If the insulin has been opened, the date when the insulin was opened is recorded on the side of the label.	To check that the insulin is safe to use.
3 Select injection site taking into consideration the child's preference and the injection rotation plan.	This is important in order to reduce the complications of long-term subcutaneous injection.
4 Check the appearance of the insulin. Rapid and short acting insulin should be clear in appearance while intermediate and long acting insulin appear cloudy.	To ensure the insulin matches the label.
5 If administering intermediate or long acting insulin, gently mix the insulin in the vials by slowly rotating the vials of insulin. Do not shake the vial. Clean the tops of the insulin vials with alcohol swabs and allow to dry completely.	Insulin is unstable and can be easily damaged when shaken.
6 Withdraw the prescribed amount of insulin into the insulin syringe. Always withdraw the short acting insulin first. Once the prescribed dose of short acting insulin has been drawn up then withdraw the prescribed dose of long acting insulin into the same syringe.	To ensure the correct dose is given.
7 If an error is made when adding the long acting insulin to the short acting insulin, all must be discarded and the procedure started again from the beginning.	To ensure patient safety.
8 Remove any air bubbles by gently tapping the outside of the syringe. Ensure the prescribed dose has been drawn into the syringe.	To prevent air from entering the patient.

9	Take the insulin in the syringe and the prescription chart to the bedside. Confirm the child's identity in accordance with the hospital policy. Ensure the child's privacy during the procedure.	To ensure patient safety and dignity.
10	With one hand gently pinch about one inch of skin at the selected injection site.	Pinching ensures that you don't inject into muscle. Injecting into muscle is more painful for the child and can also affect the amount of time it takes for the insulin to act.
11	With your other hand hold the syringe like a pencil and insert into the skin at a 90° angle. Gently press the plunger in a smooth, steady action until all the insulin has been administered.	As insulin needles are short, a 90° angle is more appropriate to ensure safe delivery of insulin.
12	Remove the needle at the same angle as you inserted it and press lightly on the injection site for a few seconds.	To prevent leakage of insulin from the injection site.
13	Ensure the child is comfortable following the procedure and record administration in the child's drug prescription record.	To maintain patient's safety and comfort and to follow legal requirements.
14	Dispose of all sharps in accordance with local policy.	For safety reasons.
15	Return unused insulin to refrigerator or store in accordance with local policy.	To ensure that insulin is stored correctly.

Step-by-step guide to the administration of insulin using an insulin pen

Step		Rationale
1	Ensure the pen refill cartridge has been fitted into the pen in accordance with the manufacturer's instructions. Once the cartridge has been loaded into the pen the insulin will last for 4–6 weeks.	Always refer to manufacturer's instructions before use to ensure the pen is prepared correctly.
2	Fit a pen needle to the top of the pen. The needle is a screw top and will secure into place.	To prepare the pen.
3	Dial up a small amount of insulin and depress the push button so insulin freely flows from the needle point. Do not dial up the prescribed dose until this happens.	To ensure insulin flow.

4	Dial the prescribed amount of insulin. Always check the dose prescribed for the child in accordance with the hospital medication policy. Bring the insulin pen to the bedside and confirm the child's identity in accordance with hospital policy.	To ensure the correct dose is given to the correct patient.
	Inject the needle at a 90 degree angle. Press the push button until the insulin has been administered (the dial will return to zero).	To ensure safe delivery of insulin.
	Hold in place for ten seconds once the insulin has been administered.	Prevents leakage of insulin from the injection site.
	Remove the needle from the injection site and dispose of sharps appropriately.	For safety reasons.

individual preferences and offer both the child and family a choice when making this decision. The decision about the device used may be guided by some of the following factors: age, cognitive ability, dexterity, and family input. There are two main types of pens, preloaded (disposable) and cartridge (reloadable) pens. The accuracy and convenience of insulin pens has improved the quality of life for children with T1DM and their families (Steck *et al.*, 2007).

Procedure: Administering insulin using an insulin pen (see page 389)

14.4 **Dietary management of children with endocrine disorders**

Children with an endocrine disorder have the same basic nutritional requirements as all other children and young people. As nurses we need to be cognisant of the nutritional requirements of children and young people and provide both written and verbal information in relation to the importance of a balanced, nutritionally appropriate diet that will promote growth and development.

Information regarding the food pyramid and the provision of a balanced diet should be available both verbally and in written form to children and their parents for them to follow in the home environment. In all children with an endocrine disorder, maintaining a good, nutritionally balanced diet can be a particular challenge to both the healthcare worker and the child's family. Children and adolescents need to be encouraged to adopt a healthy eating plan in order to promote growth and development and to achieve a healthy weight (Danne & Becker, 2007). Lifestyle modifications including changes to diet have an important role in preventing and treating diabetes in children (Danne & Becker, 2007). The following sections will outline the dietary issues in relation to children with Type 1 and Type 2 diabetes.

Dietary issues related to Type 1 and Type 2 diabetes in childhood

The aims of dietary management in childhood diabetes include meeting the child's nutritional needs in order to ensure normal growth and development, contributing to overall glycaemic control in order to reduce the risk of long-term complications, and developing an eating plan individualized for the child and their family (Richmond, 2000). Education of the child and family is a key factor in order to promote good dietary management and the nurse's role is essential. Children should eat regular meals containing complex carbohydrates, reduce their intake of refined sugars, fats, and salt, and be encouraged to include high fibre foods as tolerated (Raine *et al.*, 2006).

Table 14.2 Dietary requirements of a child with diabetes

Food group	% required in diet	Food sources
Carbohydrate (unrefined)	40–50% of total dietary intake	Brown bread, pasta, potatoes
Carbohydrate (refined)	25 g as part of a healthy diet	Sweets, biscuits
Protein	15% of total dietary intake	Meat, pulses, nuts
Fat	30–35% of total dietary intake (>5 years)	Milk, dairy products, cheese
Fibre		Fruit, vegetables, pulses, wholemeal bread

An outline of the nutritional requirements of a child with diabetes, including sources, is outlined in **Table 14.2**. The incorporation of whole family involvement in similar dietary modifications can improve compliance.

Dietary approach

The two main approaches to dietary management in a child with diabetes can be described as either a qualitative or quantitative approach. Prior to selecting an approach for the child, a detailed history of the child's normal eating pattern including the child's lifestyle and insulin regime should be recorded by the nurse.

A qualitative approach adopts a healthy eating plan that includes the requirements of a diet high in fibre, low in salt, and with at least 40% of the child's daily intake from carbohydrates. The importance of eating regular meals, normally three meals and three snacks daily, underpins this approach. Education and support for the child and family are essential to the success of this approach. This can be done by developing a therapeutic relationship with both child and family (see Chapter Two) in order to provide support. Education can be provided to both child and family using a variety of means, including verbal explanation, leaflets, and DVDs. Support groups and national associations can also be helpful to the family in this regard.

A quantitative approach involves using a measured amount of carbohydrate as an exchange system, where 10 g of carbohydrate is equivalent to one exchange and the contents of meals are based on the number of 'exchanges' required (Raine *et al.*, 2006). A formula of 120 g of carbohydrate plus 10 g for every year of age is often used (Richmond, 2000). The total amount of carbohydrate required is calculated and this is then given to the child in multiples of 10 g portions throughout the day. Both the child and the family will need to understand how to assess the amount of carbohydrate in each food and the concept of how to exchange foods of similar value as required.

A combination of both approaches can be successful depending on the child and family's preferences and lifestyle. Dietary issues need to be followed up on an outpatient basis and support and advice will need to be ongoing to avoid complications. The age of the child will have an impact on the dietary approach adopted and should always be considered when selecting a dietary management approach.

Conclusion

In this chapter we have provided you with a practical approach to developing both the knowledge base and nursing skills required to care for a child with an endocrine disorder and their family. In most cases, following the initial diagnosis and stabilization of the underlying endocrine disorder, the care of these children and their families is maintained at primary care level with the ongoing support and advice of a paediatric endocrinologist and specialized interdisciplinary team including nurses, dieticians, and child psychologists. Although most endocrine disorders in childhood are of a chronic nature, good management of the conditions can result in the development of the child into a normally functioning adult who is not compromised by any physical or mental restraints (Raine *et al.,* 2006). The promotion of holistic care underpinned by a philosophy of family centred care is essential in the nursing care of children with an endocrine disorder. The skills described in this chapter should always be practised in conjunction with local policies and guidelines in your healthcare facility. The information in this chapter can be used in conjunction with the recommended reading in order to develop your skills and knowledge further.

Online resource centre

You may find it helpful to work through our online resources including interactive scenarios intended to help you to develop and apply the skills in this chapter. Where material referenced below is available electronically, we're pleased to provide active web links to the source via **http://www.oxfordtextbooks. co.uk/orc/coyne/**

References

Alexander, M., Fawcett, J.N., & Runciman, P.J. (2006) *Nursing Practice Hospital and Home: The adult, 3rd ed*. London: Churchill Livingstone.

Australian Paediatric Endocrine Group (2005) *Clinical Practice Guideline: Type 1 diabetes and adolescents*. Australia: National Health and Medical Research Council, Australian Government Publication.

Baxter, J.D., Ribeiro, R.C.J., & Webb, P. (2004) Introduction to endocrinology. In F.G. Greenspan & D.G. Gardner. *Basic and Clinical Endocrinology, 7th ed*. USA: McGraw Hill Publishing.

Blann, A. (2006) *Routine Blood Tests Explained: A guide for nurses and allied health professionals*. Keswick: M & K Update Ltd.

Chamley, C.A., Carson, P., Randall, D., & Sandwell, M. (2005) *Developmental Anatomy and Physiology of Children: A practical approach*. Oxford: Churchill Livingstone.

Danne, T. & Becker, D (2007) Paediatric diabetes: Achieving practical, effective insulin therapy in type 1 and type 2 diabetes. *Acta Paediatrica* **96**, 1560–1570.

Diabetes Control and Complications Research Group (1993) The effect of intensive treatment of diabetes on the development and progression of long term complications of insulin dependent diabetes. *New England Journal of Medicine* **329**, 977–986.

Diabetes Forecast (2007) Blood glucose monitoring and data management systems. *Diabetes Forecast* **60** (1) Suppl., RG36–51.

Dixon, L. (2003) A normal lifestyle? Challenges facing children with diabetes and their families. *Paediatric Nursing* **15** (8), 35.

Dougherty, L. & Lister, S. (2004) *The Royal Marsden Hospital Manual of Clinical Nursing Procedures, 6th ed*. Oxford: Blackwell Publishing.

Dungan, K., Chapman, J., Braithwaite, S.S., & Buse, J. (2007) Glucose measurement: Confounding issues in setting targets for inpatient management. *Diabetes Care* **30** (2), 403–409.

Evans, C. & Tippins, E. (2008) *Foundations of Nursing: An integrated approach*. UK: McGraw Hill Publishing.

Glasper, A. & Richardson, J. (2006) *A Textbook of Children's and Young People's Nursing*. UK: Churchill Livingstone.

Hanas, R. (2007) *Type 1 Diabetes in Children, Adolescents and Young Adults, 3rd ed*. London: Class Publishing.

Hockenberry, M.J. & Wilson, D. (2007) *Wong's Nursing Care of Infants and Children*. USA: Mosby.

International Society for Pediatric and Adolescent Diabetes (2005) *Consensus Guidelines for the Management of Type 1 Diabetes in Children and Adolescents*. ISPAD medical forum.

Jamieson, E.M., McCall, J.M., & White, L.A. (2002) *Clinical Nursing Practices, 4th ed*. London: Churchill Livingston.

Medicines and Healthcare products Regulatory Agency (2005) *Point of Care Testing: Blood glucose meters. Advice for healthcare professionals*. Available at: **http://www.mhra.gov.uk**

National Institute for Clinical Excellence (2004) *Type 1 Diabetes (Childhood): Diagnosis and management of Type 1 diabetes in primary and secondary care*. London: NICE.

Raine, J.E., Donaldson, M.D., Gregory, J.W., Savage, M.O., & Hintz, R.L. (2006) *Practical Endocrinology and Diabetes in Children*. Oxford: Blackwell Publishing.

Richmond, H. (2000) Childhood diabetes: Dietary aspects. *Nursing Standard* **14** (50), 48–52.

Royal College of Nursing (2005) *Competencies: An education and training competency framework for capillary blood sampling and venepuncture in children and young people*. London: RCN.

Skinner, S. (2005) *Understanding Clinical Investigations: A quick reference manual*. London: Balliere Tindall.

Smith, S.F., Durell, D.F., & Martin, B.C. (2004) *Clinical Nursing Skills: Basic to advanced skills, 6th ed*. New Jersey: Pearson Prentice Hill.

Steck, A.K., Klingensmith G.J., & Fiallo-Scharer, R. (2007) Recent advances in insulin treatment for children. *Paediatric Diabetes* **8** (6), 49–56.

Tate (2009) *Hole's Essentials of Human Anatomy and Physiology, 10th ed*. New York: McGraw Hill.

United Kingdom Prospective Diabetes Study Group (1998) Intensive blood-glucose control with sulphonylureas or insulin compared with conventional treatment and risk of complications in patients with type 2 diabetes (UKPDS 33). *Lancet* **352** (9131), 837–853.

Wallymahmed, M. (2006) Insulin therapy in the management of Type 1 and Type 2 diabetes. *Nursing Standard* **21** (6), 50–56.

Williams, R.M. & Dunger, D.B. (2004) Insulin treatment in children and adolescents. *Acta Paediatric* **93**, 440–446.

Further reading and URLs

Aslander-van Vliet, E., Smart, C., & Waldron, S. (2007) Nutritional management in childhood and adolescent diabetes. ISPAD clinical practice consensus guidelines 2006–2007. *Paediatric Diabetes* **8**, 323–339.

Australian Paediatric Endocrine Group (2005) *Clinical Practice Guideline: Type 1 diabetes and adolescents*. Australia: National Health and Medical Research Council, Australian Government Publication.

Department of Health (2001) Standard principles for preventing hospital acquired infection. *Journal of Hospital Infection* **47** (suppl), 21–37.

Diabetes Control and Complications Research Group (1993) The effect of intensive treatment of diabetes on the development and progression of long term complications of insulin dependent diabetes. *New England Journal of Medicine* **329**, 977–986.

Food and Drug Administration (2005) *Diabetes Information: Glucose Meters and Diabetes Management*. Available at: **http://www.fda.gov/diabetes/glucose**

Greenspan, F.S. & Gardner, D.G. (2004) *Basic and Clinical Endocrinology, 7th ed*. USA: McGraw Hill Publishing.

Hall, D. & Elliman, D. (2003) *Health for all Children, 4th ed*. New York: Oxford University Press.

Hanas, R. (2007) *Type 1 Diabetes in Children, Adolescents and Young Adults, 3rd ed*. London: Class Publishing.

Mohammed, T.A. & Trigg, E. (2006) *Practices in Children's Nursing: Guidelines for Hospital and Community*. UK: Churchill Livingstone.

Nursing and Midwifery Council (2002) *Code of Professional Conduct*. London: NMC.

Patel, L., Dixon, M., & David, T.J. (2003) Growth and growth charts in cystic fibrosis. *Journal of the Royal Society of Medicine* **96** (Suppl. 43), 35–41.

Pickup, J. & Williams, G. (2004) *A Textbook of Diabetes, 3rd ed*. Oxford: Blackwell Science.

Royal College of Nursing (2006) *Malnutrition in Children and Young People: What nurses working with children need to know and do. An RCN position statement*. Available at: **http://www.rcn.org.uk**

15 Integumentary system

JACINTA KELLY AND JOAN SIMONS

Skills

15.1 **Care of pressure sores**

Introduction

The skin is an organ that serves many functions in maintaining homeostasis in the body (Bryant, 2000). A wide range of diseases manifest in changes in the skin and its appendages, and because the skin is visible and its disorders are often disfiguring, skin disorders can cause emotional and psychological stress for children and their families (Ball & Bindler, 2007). Skin diseases affect 20–33% of the population at any one time, seriously interfering with activities in 10% (Byrant, 2000). Epidemiological evidence suggests that many cases of skin disease do not reach the general practitioner (GP) or even the local pharmacist; nevertheless, each year about 15% of the population consult their GPs about skin complaints (Bryant, 2000). Skin disorders are among the most common health problems in children (Butcher & White, 2005). The infant and child are possibly more vulnerable to the effects of skin disorders and breakdown due to their underdeveloped integumentary system. Understanding the normal condition of the skin can help in the identification of abnormal signs and prompt treatment of skin disorders (Butcher & White, 2005). This chapter will focus on the integumentary system of the child, with reference to the normal structure of the skin together with common alterations and injuries to the skin of the child and the skills required for their nursing management.

Learning outcomes

At the end of this chapter you should be able to do the following:
- Understand the normal child skin anatomy and physiology.
- Understand the fundamentals of a skin assessment in a child.
- Develop an awareness of the management of common skin alterations.
- Understand the nature and treatment of a child with a skin injury.

Anatomy and physiology

The skin of an infant or child is normally fundamentally the same as that of an adult, although the blood and nerve supplies are immature and the **dermis** thinner, with less collagen and fewer elastic fibres. This means that the skin is fragile and can be more easily damaged through physical and mechanical trauma (Table 15.1) (Turnball, 2007). The skin of a newborn is found to have **lanugo**, which is a very fine, soft, and unpigmented coat of hairs covering its body until it is shed about 14 days after birth. Infants have less developed hypodermal fat and as a result are at risk for hypothermia. The sweat

Table 15.1 Variants in children's skin at different ages

Age group	Expected variant
Infant	Smooth skin Lack of terminal hair Lanugo Less hypodermal fat Decreased sweat gland activity
Child	Some bruising
Adolescent	Sweat gland and sebaceous gland activity Terminal axillary and pubic hair development

glands do not begin to function until one month of age and are not fully functional until adolescence (Morton *et al.*, 2005).

The structure of the skin

The skin or integumentary system is one of the most complex and largest organ systems of the body. It has two main components: the cutaneous membrane and the **accessory structures**. The cutaneous membrane consists of **epidermis** or superficial epithelium and the dermis, an underlying connective tissue. The accessory structures include the hair, nails, and sebaceous (eccrine) and sweat (apocrine) glands (Smeltzer & Bare, 2008). Beneath these layers is the subcutaneous or **hypodermis** layer, which is composed largely of adipose tissue and separates the integument from the deep fascia around other organs such as muscle and bones (**Figure 15.1**).

The epidermis

The outermost layer of the skin is the epidermis, which is a thin cellular layer with no blood vessels. Blood vessels in the dermis provide nutrients for the epidermis (Holloway & Jones, 2005). The epidermal layer is composed of stratified squamous epithelium, keratinocytes, melanocytes, Langerhans cells, and Granstein cells (Russell, 1998). The epidermis has a maximum of five *strata* or layers—stratum basale, stratum spinosum, stratum granulosum, stratum lucidum, and stratum corneum—and has many essential functions (**Box 15.1**).

Nursing Alert

Infants have fewer melanocytes than adults, which increases photosensitivity, and therefore nurses need to advise families to protect infants from strong sunlight with sunshades and appropriate clothing.

The dermis

The **dermis** is a thick layer of strong connective tissue containing blood vessels, nerves, glands, and hair follicles

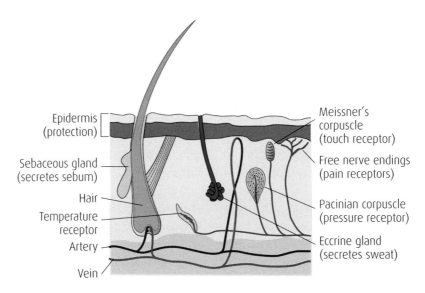

Epidermis (protection)
Sebaceous gland (secretes sebum)
Hair
Temperature receptor
Artery
Vein
Meissner's corpuscle (touch receptor)
Free nerve endings (pain receptors)
Pacinian corpuscle (pressure receptor)
Eccrine gland (secretes sweat)

Figure 15.1 The structure of the skin

Box 15.1 Epidermal layers and functions

Stratum basale

The innermost epidermal layer is the stratum basale, which contains melanocytes or pigment cells that produce melanin. Together with carotene, which exists in the subcutaneous layer, and haemoglobulin, which circulates in red blood cells, melanin determines the child's skin colour. The amount of melanin is genetically determined and increased by sunlight (Massey, 2006). Merkel cells are also found on the stratum basale, which act as sensory receptors.

Stratum spinosum

The stratum spinosum contains Langerhans cells, which participate in the immune response by stimulating a defence against micro-organisms and superficial cancer cells. The cells in this layer are living cells and are constantly replacing the basal layers above (Lloyd-Jones, 2007).

Stratum granulosum

The epidermal layer above the stratum spinosum is the stratum granulosum and contains keratinocytes, which at this point are non-viable, irregularly shaped granular cells. This hard layer is most prominent on the soles of the feet and palms of the hands (Tongle, 1999).

Stratum lucidum

The stratum lucidum covers the stratum granulosum and contains flattened, densely packed cells. It is only found at points in the body that are exposed to friction such as the fingertips, palms, and soles (Holloway & Jones, 2005).

Stratum corneum

The epidermal layer nearest the surface is the stratum corneum or horny layer, containing flattened layers of keratinized cells that are constantly worn away and replaced every 15 to 30 days. They act as a barrier to bacteria, chemicals, and water (Russell, 1998).

Basement membrane zone

The basement membrane zone (BMZ) is also known as the dermo-epidermal junction and is a cellular layer that separates the epidermis from the dermis. This semi-permeable membrane regulates the transfer of proteins and other materials across the BMZ from the dermis to the epidermis (Tongle, 1999).

(Bianchi & Cameron, 2008). These structures are held in position by a matrix of collagen and elastin that is used in temperature regulation and excretion of excess body heat, and acts as a cushion against physical and mechanical damage (Russell, 1998). A lymphatic system network is found in the dermis flowing alongside the vascular structure. Lymphatic vessels act as a filter and overflow channel, transporting extra fluid back to the venous system (Tongle, 1999). There are several types of nerve fibres present in the skin and either together or alone they convey touch, pain, temperature, pressure, and itch from all over the body. Hair follicles originate from the dermis, alongside sebaceous glands, which lubricate the surface, maintain the skin surface, and maintain the skin's acid mantle at around pH 5.5 (Holloway & Jones, 2005). The main cells in the dermis are macrophages and fibroblasts, which aid wound healing (Tongle, 1999).

The papillary and reticular layers

The dermis is divided into two main layers, the papillary layer (found immediately below the BMZ) and the reticular layer (which connects with the epidermis via concrete ridges called dermal papillae) (Tongle, 1999). In the dermal papillae are capillary loops that supply the epidermis with nutrients and oxygen. The papillary layer also contains Meissner's corpuscles, which act as nerve endings responsible for touch (Russell, 1998). The reticular layer is below the papillary dermis and contains thicker collagen fibres. This layer contains Pacinian corpuscles or nerve endings, which are sensitive to pressure (Russell, 1998).

The hypodermis layer

The **hypodermis** lies beneath the dermis and is the innermost layer of the skin. It is made up of adipose tissue, which provides a cushion between the skin layers, muscles, and bones. It promotes skin mobility, moulds body contours, and insulates the body. The subcutaneous tissues and the amount of body fat deposited are important factors in body temperature regulation (Smeltzer & Bare, 2008). The superficial region of the subcutaneous layer contains large arteries and blood vessels (Lloyd-Jones, 2007).

The surface area of the skin of an average adult is 1.8 m² (Russell, 1998), whereas the ratio of skin surface to body volume is greater in infants and small children, contributing to the risk of greater absorption through the skin (Ball & Bindler, 2007).

Developmental issues

At birth the infant's skin is thin with little underlying subcutaneous fat, and because of this the newborn loses heat more rapidly, has greater difficulty regulating body temperature, and becomes more chilled than an older infant. Older infants and small children have extensive 'baby fat' that provides extra insulation and helps reduce heat loss. Subcutaneous fat also serves as a substantial energy reserve and as a shock absorber for the rough-and-tumble of early years (Martini, 2006).

Nursing Alert

Topical medications should also be avoided in infants less than six months as their increased rate of absorption could cause toxicity.

Accessory structures

The accessory structures of the skin include hair and hair follicles, sebaceous and sweat glands, and nails, and are considered appendages of the skin (Martini, 2006).

Hair

Hair first appears after roughly three months of embryonic development and these hairs are collectively known as lanugo. They are extremely fine and unpigmented and are shed before birth and replaced by vellus hairs (located over much of the body surface) and terminal hairs (located on the head, eyebrows, and eyelashes) (Martini, 2006). Hair projects above the surface of the skin almost everywhere except the sides and soles of the feet, the palms of the hands, the sides of the fingers and toes, the lips, and portions of the genitalia (Smeltzer & Bare, 2008). Although located in the dermis, hair follicles project through the epidermis to the integumentary surface (Martini, 2006).

Nails

Nails are plates of tightly packed, hard, non-living, keratinized cells of the epidermis. Each nail consists of a nail body, a free edge, and a nail root (Tortora & Derrickson, 2006). The nail body is the portion of the nail that is visible, the free edge is the part that extends past the end of the fingers and toes, and the nail root is the portion that is not visible (see Figure 15.2). Most of the nail body is pink because of the underlying blood capillaries. The whitish semi-lunar area near the nail root is called the lunula due to the thickened stratum basale in this area. The nails protect the distal end of the fingers and toes (Massey, 2006), help us grasp and manipulate small objects, and allow us to scratch various parts of the body (Tortora & Derrickson, 2006).

Capillary refill test

Because the nail bed is so vascular, it is generally an excellent location to assess the adequacy of the patient's peripheral circulation and is a useful indicator of fluid status in adults (Morton et al., 2005). This quick test is performed on the nail beds and monitors tissue perfusion and dehydration. Pressure is applied to the nail bed until it turns white and is then removed; a pink colour should return in less than two seconds after blanching. Blanch times that are greater than two seconds may indicate dehydration, shock, or hypothermia; however, in children this is most accurate when obtained by pressing on the forearm.

Sebaceous glands

The eccrine glands are widely distributed and open directly onto the skin surface. These glands are responsible for sweat production and have a role in maintaining the

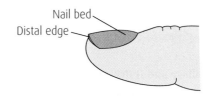

Figure 15.2 Anatomy of the nail

body temperature. Because babies are small the reduced skin surface area in relation to body mass means that glands are closer together and function irregularly; as a result infants have a reduced ability to sweat, and can become prone to overheating (Turnball, 2007). The apocrine glands are found chiefly in the axillary and genital regions, usually open into hair follicles, and are stimulated by emotional stress (Massey, 2006). These glands do not function fully until the child reaches puberty (Turnball, 2007).

> **Nursing Alert**
>
> Nurses need to advise parents that eccrine glands do not reach mature function until age two or three years, making infants and young toddlers less able to regulate their body temperature.

Functions of the skin

The five main functions of the skin consist of body temperature regulation, protection, sensation, excretion, and absorption, production, and synthesis of vitamin D (**see Table 15.2**) (Tortora & Derrickson, 2006). Skin also provides a function of identification and communication.

Thermoregulation

An important function of the skin is to protect the body from cold and heat, achieved through the complex vascular system within the skin. In warm periods the vessels dilate, the skin becomes reddened, and beads of sweat form on the surface. Secretion and evaporation of sweat from the surface of the skin help to cool the skin (Tongle, 1999). In cold periods the blood vessels constrict, preventing heat from escaping.

Protection

The skin, when intact, acts as a waterproof barrier and protects against bacteria and viruses as well as physical trauma (Lloyd-Jones, 2007). The epidermis (composed of hard, keratinized cells) together with the various barrier lipids synthesized in the stratum corneum form the basis for the protective function of the skin and prevent entry of toxins, microbes, and insect bites (Smeltzer & Bare, 2008). Hair on the head protects the scalp from ultraviolet radiation, helps to cushion light blows to the head, and insulates the skull (Tortora & Derrickson, 2006). Hairs guarding the entrance to nostrils and external ear canals help prevent the entry of foreign particles and insects, and eyelashes perform a similar function for the surface of the eye (Martini, 2006). A root hair plexus of sensory nerves surrounds the base of each hair follicle and provides an early warning sensory mechanism that may prevent injury (Martini, 2006).

Sensation

Nerve receptors in the skin are sensitive to pain, pressure, touch, itch, and vibration, as well as hot and cold (Lloyd-Jones, 2007).

Excretion

The stratum corneum has the capacity to absorb water, thereby preventing water and electrolyte loss from the

Table 15.2 Functions of the skin

Function	Skin layer
Protection	Horny layer, melanocytes, Langerhans cells, nails
Temperature regulation	Blood vessels, eccrine sweat glands
Insulation	Subcutaneous fat
Sensation	Specialized nerve endings
Lubrication/waterproofing	Sebaceous glands
Calorie reserve	Subcutaneous fat
Vitamin D synthesis	Keratinocytes
Body odour	Apocrine sweat glands
Psychosocial/display	Skin, lips, hair, and nails

body and retaining moisture in the subcutaneous tissues (Smeltzer & Bare, 2008).

Vitamin production

Skin exposed to ultraviolet light can convert substances necessary for synthesizing vitamin D (cholecalciferol). Vitamin D is essential for preventing osteoporosis and rickets, a disease that causes bone deformities and results from deficiency of vitamin D, calcium, and phosphorous (Smeltzer & Bare, 2008).

Identification and communication

The skin serves the purpose of identification of one another through a unique combination of facial characteristics, hair and skin colour, and even fingerprint. In addition, through paling, blushing, and other expressions regulated by the autonomic nervous system, the skin serves as a communication system.

Skin assessment

Assessment of the skin encompasses a detailed history of the child's skin condition (including duration, occurrence, and any variations), a general assessment (including state of mind of the child, physical abilities, present medication, cultural needs, and physiological status), and a specific physical examination of the child's skin and hair (Lawton, 2001). Assessment of the skin involves the entire skin area, including the mucous membranes, scalp, hair, and nails, using techniques of measurements, palpation, and inspection (Smeltzer & Bare, 2008). The child's privacy should be considered throughout the skin assessment process.

Palpation

Nurses should make a point of palpating or touching patients where appropriate and with permission in order to gain important information about the skin texture and temperature (Lawton, 2001). Assess the skin for moisture or dryness, and check the face, hands, axilla, and skin folds and assess for signs of diaphoresis or dehydration. Symmetrically feel each part of the body, compare upper areas with lower areas, and assess for hypothermia and hyperthermia. Assess the temperature of the skin with the backs of the fingers against an area of the patient's skin. Skin turgor, possible oedema, and elasticity are assessed by palpation. Skin turgor measurement, whilst part of the initial assessment of children with suspected dehydration, is only moderately reliable and other clinical signs such as behavioural changes, tachycardia, and decreased urinary output should be sought to confirm this diagnosis.

> **Nursing Alert**
>
> Good hand hygiene before and after examining the child is preferable to wearing gloves as the latter can make the child feel stigmatized and unapproachable.

Skin turgor test

The skin turgor of a child may be tested quickly and non-invasively on the skin of the forearm or sternum. Skin mobility and turgor is assessed by lifting a fold of skin and observing the ease with which the skins lifts up (mobility) and the speed with which it returns into place (turgor). Decreased mobility would be evident in oedema, while decreased turgor would be observed in dehydration.

Pitting oedema test

Pitting oedema on the skin is the accumulation of fluid in the intercellular spaces. It can be diagnosed through an equally unobtrusive test. To check for oedema, imprint your thumbs firmly against the ankle malleolus or tibia. If the pressure leaves a dent in the skin, pitting oedema is present.

Inspection

Good lighting in the examination environment is particularly important when inspecting the child's skin, especially one who is dark-skinned, as alteration may occur in synthetic lighting (Lawton, 2001). A penlight may be used to highlight lesions. The room should be warm and comfortable so as to encourage the child to cooperate during the examination. A selection of suitable toys and books are useful to distract the child if necessary when examining them (Turnball, 2007) (see also Chapter Five for detail on other distraction techniques).

Skin colour

Erythema is a redness of the skin resulting from congestion of capillaries caused by an increase in temperature, inflammation, or infection. Ecchymosis or bruising are diffuse areas that are usually black and blue and result from injuries, whereas petechiae—small pinpoint haemorrhages—can denote some type of blood disorder. Practitioners should observe the skin for any other changes, for example, jaundice may be present in the sclera as well as in the lips, hard palate, under the surface of the tongue, and most obviously the skin. The skin is observed for variations of colour such as cyanosis (blue tinge) or pallor (loss of rosy glow). Cyanosis is easily observed in the extremities, nail beds, lips, and mucous membranes. In dark-skinned people, the skin assumes a greyish cast. Central cyanosis is best observed in the lips, oral mucosa, and the tongue, and most reliably through the capillary refill test.

Skin lesions

It is important to inspect for any rashes or primary lesions and to note colour, elevation, pattern or shapes, size, location, and distribution on the body, together with any exudates or pruritus (itching). A metric ruler is used to measure the size of the lesions so that any further extension can be compared with this baseline measurement (Smeltzer & Bare, 2008). When examining a rash, the skin is stretched gently to decrease the reddish tone and make the rash more visible, with the aid of a pen torch pointed laterally across the skin. The differences in the skin texture are examined by running the tips of the fingers lightly over the skin (Smeltzer & Bare, 2008).

Hair and nails

Inspect the hair for texture (whether coarse or elastic), quality (whether shiny or dull), and distribution. The scalp is also inspected for ticks and lice. Hair type is related to race and this needs to be considered as, for example, Afro-Caribbean hair can be easily damaged by heat and chemicals (Manning, 2007). Inspect the shape and contour of the nails, whether curved or flat, and check that the edges are smooth, rounded, and clean. Nail consistency should be smooth, regular, not brittle or splitting and should be adequately thick and firm. Normal colour of the nail is translucent where its pink colour is provided by the nail bed.

Common childhood skin alterations

Alterations in skin are classified according to non-infectious and infectious skin conditions, and skin injuries. As there is a vast array of skin alterations in childhood only the common alterations will be discussed here.

15.1 **Care of pressure sores**

Skin breakdown in children can result in pain, infection, disfigurement, altered body image, and mortality. Pressure sores can result in increased length of hospital stay and increased cost (Baharestani & Ratliff, 2007). Cho et al. (2003) found that pressure sores led on average to a 1.84 day increase in length of stay in hospital. Pressure sores can develop at any point on the body but particular pressure points for children include the bony prominences, the sacrum, heels, and the occiput (Baldwin, 2002).

Prevalence

McLane et al. (2004) found the incidence of pressure ulcers in 1000 children to be 4%. Two thirds of the pressure sores were hospital-induced, indicating that there is a need for nurses to be diligent in assessing risk and preventing pressure sores.

Nursing Alert

Immobile children should be identified as being at significant risk of developing pressure sores.

Developmental issues

In infancy the head is proportionately larger compared to the body than in an adult, putting the occiput and ears at greater risk than the sacrum when lying down. In time, as the child grows, the proportions become more adult-like so that the areas of greatest risk include the sacrum, heels, and elbows (Murdoch, 2002).

Nursing Alert

Nurses need to be aware of the need to assess pressure sore risk differently in young children from in older children, due to the difference in weight distribution across the body as children grow.

Intrinsic and extrinsic causes of pressure sores

Factors that cause pressure sores can be divided into two main groups: extrinsic causes and intrinsic causes, as shown in **Table 15.3** (Moules & Ramsay, 2008). As well as extrinsic and intrinsic causes, friction and shear both contribute to pressure sores (Hockenberry & Wilson, 2007).

Friction

Friction occurs when the surface of the skin rubs against another surface such as sheets on a bed. The skin may have the appearance of an abrasion. The damage is usually limited to the epidermal or upper layers and most often occurs over the elbows or heels. By itself friction does not cause pressure sores, but when it acts with gravity it causes shear injury.

Table 15.3 Extrinsic and intrinsic causes of pressure sores

Extrinsic causes	Intrinsic causes
Weight	Nutrition
Temperature	Neurological factors
Moisture	Age
Mobility	

Shear

Shear is the result of the force of gravity pushing down on the body and friction of the body against a surface such as the bed or chair.

Nursing Alert

Nurses need to avoid/eliminate the possibility of a child encountering friction or shearing when moving children.

Special considerations

Some children are more at risk of developing pressure sores, such as those nursed in intensive care, neonates, children undergoing prolonged surgical procedures, and those with a spinal injury. Children in intensive care are particularly at risk and should have their positions changed regularly; if this is not possible, pressure prevention devices should be used (Dyer & Embling, 2006).

Nursing Alert

The immobile child should have their position monitored carefully to minimize extended periods of pressure on vulnerable areas of the body.

Assessment of pressure sores

Whilst risk assessment should be performed immediately on admission to hospital, this assessment may take time to fully complete if information is not readily available. Assessment should also be ongoing and frequency of reassessment should be dependent on changes in the patient's condition (European Pressure Ulcer Advisory Panel (EPUAP), 1998).

Risk assessment tools

The best method to assess the risk of a child developing a pressure sore is through the use of a validated risk assessment tool (Keast et al., 2008). Waterlow (1997) and the Royal College of Nursing (2001; 2005) recommend a full assessment of pressure risk. Although there are a range of well-established and validated adult tools, there are few tools specifically developed for children. Two examples of paediatric tools are the Braden Q tool and Glamorgan Scale.

The Braden Q tool

The Braden Q is an adaptation of an adult tool that was developed for pressure sore risk identification in children aged 21 days to eight years (Curley & Quigley, 2003). This scale contains the original six subscales for use with adults and an additional subscale of tissue oxygenation and perfusion. The original subscales were also modified to make them developmentally appropriate for children. The purpose of the scale was to match the unique developmental needs of infants and children.

The minimal score for each subscale is one (more risk) and the maximum score is four (less risk). Potential total scores range from 7–28. The lower the score, the higher the potential risk of developing a pressure sore. Acutely ill children with a Braden Q score of 16 can be considered at risk of a grade II pressure sore.

Nursing Alert

It is important to remember that the use of a risk assessment tool should only be as an *aide memoire*, and should not replace clinical judgement (National Institute for Clinical Excellence, 2001).

The Glamorgan Scale

This tool was developed specifically for children. There are many adult pressure sore risk assessment scales (Salzberg, 1999), and many scales that have been

Box 15.2 The Braden Q risk assessment tool subscales

Intensity and duration of pressure
- Mobility
- Activity
- Sensory

Tolerance of the skin and supporting structures
- Moisture
- Friction and shear
- Nutrition
- Tissue perfusion and oxygenation

adapted for use with children (Quigley & Curley, 1996; Garvin, 1997; Samiengo, 2003), but few that have been developed specifically for children. Most pressure ulcer risk assessment scales give similar weightings to each subscale, such as nutrition, continence, or mobility. Pressure sores are caused by prolonged pressure on the skin, shearing, or friction when the skin rubs against a surface. In order to prevent pressure sores in children, these are the factors nurses need to monitor and take preventive action to avoid. This scale has been developed using a review of the literature, feedback from clinical experts, and data from 60 hospitalized children with pressure sores and 265 children with no pressure sores (Willock *et al.*, 2007; Willock *et al.*, 2008) (see Table 15.4).

Nursing Alert

To be effective, risk assessment scales must identify those at risk, their level of risk, and the factors that are contributing to that risk. It is important not to think of pressure ulcer risk as a single score but to consider each element of the risk in order to alleviate or reduce the overall risk.

Classification of pressure sores

Nurses can be assisted in the recognition of pressure sores through the use of a standardized classification system. Once a pressure sore has been classified, a plan of care can be developed. The European Pressure Ulcer Advisory Panel (1998) have devised a classification system that is recommended by the National Institute for Health and Clinical Excellence (NICE, 2005) in the UK and is in line with the American National Pressure Ulcer Advisory Panel (2007) (Table 15.5).

Nursing Alert

The identification of the grade or degree of a pressure sore is the first step in planning care to promote healing of the pressure sore.

Table 15.4 Glamorgan Paediatric Pressure Ulcer Risk Assessment Scale

Child cannot move without great difficulty or deterioration in condition/general anaesthetic.

Unable to change his/her position without assistance/cannot control body movement.

Some mobility, but reduced for age.

Normal mobility for age.

Equipment/objects/hard surface pressing or rubbing on skin.

Significant anaemia (Hb <9 g/dl).

Persistent pyrexia (temperature >38°C for more than four hours).

Poor peripheral perfusion (cold extremities/capillary refill >2 seconds/cool, mottled skin).

Inadequate nutrition (discuss with dietician if in doubt).

Low serum albumin level (<35 g/l).

Weight less than 10th centile.

Incontinence (inappropriate for age).

Risk Score	Category	Suggested action
10+	At risk	Inspect skin at least twice a day. Relieve pressure by helping child to move at least every two hours. Use an age- and weight-appropriate pressure redistribution surface for sitting on/sleeping on.
15+	High risk	Inspect skin with each positioning. Reposition child/equipment devices at least every two hours. Relieve pressure before any redness develops. Use an age- and weight-appropriate pressure redistribution surface for sitting on/sleeping on.
20+	Very high risk	Inspect skin at least hourly. Move or turn if possible, before skin becomes red. Ensure equipment/objects are not pressing on the skin. Consider using specialized pressure-relieving equipment.

Table 15.5 Pressure sore classification

Grade	Description of pressure sore
Grade 1	Non-blanchable erythema of intact skin. Discolouration of the skin, warmth, oedema, induration, or hardness may also be used as indicators, particularly on individuals with darker skin.
Grade 2	Partial thickness skin loss involving epidermis and/or dermis. The ulcer is superficial and may present as an abrasion or blister.
Grade 3	Full thickness skin loss involving damage or necrosis of subcutaneous tissue, which may extend down to but not through underlying fascia.
Grade 4	Extensive destruction and tissue necrosis or damage to muscle, bone, or supporting structures, with or without full thickness skin loss.

Procedure: Care of pressure sores

It is not enough just to treat the pressure sore, it is necessary to also treat the cause of the pressure sore (Sibbald *et al.*, 2004). Once a pressure sore has developed the likelihood of healing will depend on the ability of the care team to address both intrinsic and extrinsic factors affecting the skin (NICE, 2005).

Pressure-relieving devices

Children who have a pressure sore or are considered to be at risk of a pressure sore should be nursed on a pressure-relieving device, which works by conforming to the shape of the child's body and distributing the weight of the body over a large surface area, rather than allowing increased pressure on one bony prominence such as the occiput or sacrum. In infants the areas of greatest risk when lying down are the occiput and ears. In older children the areas

of greatest risk are the sacrum, heels, and elbows. It is important to be particularly vigilant when nursing a child requiring equipment, as every device can potentially cause pressure on a child's skin. Traction equipment or infusion, feeding, oxygen, or urinary or wound drainage tubing should be placed so that they are not causing pressure. Bean bags rather than angled bed rests can be used to reduce friction and shearing forces on a child's skin. When making beds, care should be taken to ensure tight bottom sheets to prevent pressure from creases. Crumbs and small toys are also risks for small children who are immobile (Moules & Ramsay, 2008). Low risk children can be nursed on a standard mattress. For children at medium risk of developing a pressure sore, use a pressure relieving mattress or overlay. Silicone gel or foam pads may also be used. High risk children, e.g. children having lengthy surgical procedures, should be nursed with the appropriate pressure-relieving aids on the theatre table. There are a number of support surfaces that can be used

Step-by-step guide to care of a child with a pressure sore

Step	Rationale
1 **Use pressure-relieving devices.**	Conform to the shape of the child's body and distribute the weight of the body over a large surface area, rather than allowing increased pressure on one bony prominence.
2 **Management of moisture and incontinence: gently clean the skin and change linen without delay with warm water and mild cleansing agent.**	To avoid moisture and incontinence contributing to skin breakdown.
3 **Assess the child's pain using an age-appropriate, validated pain tool, and provide analgesics if required, reassessing their effectiveness.**	In order to manage the child's pain.
4 **Reduction of infection: vigilance in hand washing and wound cleansing along with protection from contamination.**	Promotes wound healing in pressure sores.
5 **Debridement.**	Required in large extensive pressure sores to prevent infection from necrotic tissue.
6 **Education of child and family.**	Working in partnership with the child and family increases the likelihood of preventing pressure sore formation.

Table 15.6 Static and dynamic support systems for use in prevention and treatment of pressure sores

Static support systems	Dynamic support systems
Standard mattresses	Alternating air: large air cushions alternately over-inflate and under-inflate in sequence
Foam overlays	Low air loss: air-filled cells circulating air across the skin to reduce moisture and help maintain a constant skin interface pressure
Foam mattresses	Turning/rotation: assists patient position changes
Static flotation mattresses involving air cells or gel overlays	Air fluidized: patient is 'floating' on silicone beads

to assist in the prevention or relief of pressure sores. Support surfaces can be categorized as static or dynamic (Keast *et al.*, 2008), as in **Table 15.6**.

The most recent developments in the treatment and prevention of pressure sores suggest the use of computerized pressure mapping devices to evaluate a surface. A thin, pressure-sensitive mat is placed between the patient and the surface. Interface pressure is then translated into an image on the computer. This system can also be used as a biofeedback mechanism (Keast *et al.*, 2008).

Wound management

Pressure sore wound care involves the debridement of non-viable tissue, assessment and management of colonization, and management of exudate through appropriate dressing selection. Nurses need to prevent infection and promote wound healing. For grade 2 and 3 pressure sores (**Table 15.5**), dressings that are moist may be used to keep the wound clean but moist. Nursing assessment should be carried out if the skin or underlying tissue dies,

Step-by-step guide to wound management in pressure sores

Step	Rationale
1 Assessment of the pressure sore.	To determine the extent of tissue damage and to determine care required.
2 Assessment of colonization and exudate and appropriate dressing selection.	To prevent infection and promote wound healing.
3 For pressure sores involving partial or full thickness skin loss (i.e. grade 2 and 3), dressings that are moist may be used.	To keep the wound clean but moist.
4 Determine the need for debridement.	To reduce the risk of infection from dead tissue and promote healing.
5 For severe extensive pressure sores (i.e. grade 4), debridement is likely to be needed. Any dead or necrotic tissue will need to be removed with forceps or scissors.	To prevent infection.

to determine the need for debridement to reduce risk of infection and promote healing. For grade 4 pressure sores (**Table 15.5**), debridement is likely to be needed and some may need further surgery. Any dead or necrotic tissue around the area of the pressure sore will need to be removed with forceps or scissors to prevent infection. Minimal mechanical force should be used when cleansing or irrigating the ulcer. Showering may be used to clean the wound or irrigation can be useful for cleaning a cavity ulcer. Antiseptics should not routinely be used to clean wounds but may be considered when infection needs to be controlled (after clinical assessment). Ideally antiseptics should only be used for a limited period of time until the wound is clean and surrounding inflammation reduced (EPUAP, 1998). There are a number of appropriate dressings available that provide an optimum wound healing environment for treatment of pressure sores in children, e.g. hydrocolloids, hydrogels, foams, films, alginates, soft silicones, and gauze (NICE, 2005; Harris *et al.*, 2003). It is necessary to determine the condition of the wound and establish treatment objectives before selecting a dressing, e.g. grade of pressure sore, wound bed, infection, level of exudate, pain, surrounding skin, position, and patient's preference. Regular observation will demonstrate the progress of healing and whether there is a need to change treatment objectives.

Management of moisture and incontinence

When a child soils the area of the pressure sore, skin should be cleansed gently at the time of soiling with a mild, pH-balanced, non-sensitizing cleansing agent. Warm water is recommended to minimize drying and irritation.

Nursing Alert

Wet skin is fragile and more susceptible to friction injuries (Keast *et al.*, 2008).

The use of cotton sheets is recommended to promote evaporation, skin aeration, and faster drying of skin that is moist from perspiration. There are a number of chemical factors that can lead to skin damage. Faecal incontinence, especially when mixed with urine, and wound drainage around gastrostomy tubes can erode

the epidermis. Moisture barriers, gentle cleansing as soon after exposure as possible, and skin barriers can be used to prevent damage caused by chemical factors (Hockenberry & Wilson, 2007).

Management of pain

There is a need to assess the impact of pain on mobility and the possibility of increasing the risk of pressure sore development. Pressure sores can cause a child significant pain and discomfort. Pain control measures may involve analgesics, therapeutic positioning, support surfaces, and covering the pressure ulcer with appropriate wound dressings (Registered Nurses Association of Ontario, 2005). (Please also see Chapter Six for more information on pain assessment and management.)

Reduction of infection

Pressure ulcers in children can become infected, most frequently by *Staphylococcus aureus*. In severe cases this can lead to osteomyelitis (Bar-on *et al.*, 2003). To reduce the risk of infection and enhance wound healing, nurses must be vigilant in hand washing as well as wound cleansing. It is important to consider antimicrobial therapy in the presence of systemic and/or local signs of infection (NICE, 2005). When there are clinical signs of infection that do not respond to treatment, X-rays should be taken to exclude osteomyelitis and joint infection. Where appropriate, systemic antibiotic therapy should be commenced for children with bacteraemia, sepsis, advancing cellulitis, or osteomyelitis. Pressure sores should be protected from external sources of contamination (e.g. faeces) (Howard & Sippel, 2005).

Debridement

Deeper pressure sores involving extensive tissue damage will require surgical debridement and closure. In large pressure sores, which can have a negative impact on a child's body image, surgical closure is a viable option to reduce disfigurement. According to adult guidelines (Bergstrom *et al.*, 1994), when a stable **eschar** (dead tissue) is overlying the **calcaneal** region without signs of infection, pressure should be relieved and the eschar left undisturbed to serve as its own biologic covering.

Education of child and family

Nurses and families should be educated in risk assessment and the use of equipment, and carry out pressure area care using evidence-based practice. Children and their families should be informed of the risks of developing pressure sores. Individual care plans can provide information on personal risk factors for pressure sore development, sites of the body at greatest risk, how to inspect the body for damage and recognize changes in the skin, and how to care for the skin including methods of pressure relief or reduction (Dyer & Embling, 2006). By children's nurses working in partnership with parents, the likelihood of preventing pressure sore formation will be increased.

Special considerations

Within children's nursing there are special considerations that need to be noted when caring for vulnerable groups. In relation to pressure sores, neonates of less than 32 weeks gestation are more vulnerable to pressure sores because of the immaturity of their skin. It is recommended that water, air, and gel mattresses and sheepskin and gel pads placed at the joints, behind the ears, and behind the occiput should be used for pressure sore prevention (Lund, 1999). Nursing care should also include regular assessment of the risk of these small babies developing pressure sores.

Skin infections

Most children will have a skin infection at some time and for that reason skin infections are a common reason for consultation in primary care and dermatology practice (Sladden & Johnston, 2004). Skin infections in childhood include bacterial, fungal, parasitic, and viral infections as well as viral exanthems or rashes. Bacterial skin infections affect children with compromised immune systems—those with debilitating illnesses, immune deficiency disorders, or those receiving immunosuppressive drug therapy (Potts & Mandleco, 2007).

Bacterial—impetigo

Impetigo is a very contagious bacterial infection of the epidermal layer of the skin with a prevalence of occurrence in children in late summer (Millard, 2008). Impetigo is caused by *Staphylococcal* or *Streptococcal* organisms and its diagnosis is either primary (where there is direct invasion of the skin) or secondary (when infection is secondary to some underlying skin disease such as eczema, insect bites, or scabies, or trauma that disrupts the skin barrier (Millard, 2008)). Two major forms exist: (1) impetigo contagiosa, which is the most common and is characterized by 'honey-coloured' crusted lesions; and (2) bullous impetigo, characterized by fragile bullae where lesions of both forms most often appear on the face around the mouth and nares (Potts & Mandleco, 2007).

Family can help prevent the spread of infection by always using a clean washcloth and towel each time the child is washed, and not sharing towels, clothing, or other toiletries with other family members. Hands should be washed thoroughly after touching the skin lesions and children should not attend school when lesions are weeping (Millard, 2008). Mild infection may be treated by improved hygiene and using an antibacterial soap, along with a prescription antibacterial cream. For severe cases, oral flucloxicillin is the drug of choice (Millard, 2008).

> **Nursing Alert**
>
> If impetigo is left untreated, it can spread to other areas of the body and cause boils, abscesses, and even toxic shock.

Bacterial—cellulitis

Cellulitis is a non-contagious bacterial skin infection involving the dermis and subcutaneous tissue and is characterized by a painful and tender area of erythema that may spread through the surrounding tissue (Nazarko, 2009). Systemic symptoms can be evident with fever, chills, and malaise, together with lymphangitis (red streaks leading from the affected area) and lymphadenopathy (lymph node swelling) being common (Potts & Mandleco, 2007).

Streptococcus pyrogenus and *Staphylococcus aureus* are the most common offending organisms and therefore immediate administration of antibiotics such as cephalosporins or erythromycin is essential (Nazarko, 2009). The child with limited cellulitis may be managed in the community if family members are instructed on how to provide antipyretic, antibiotic, and anti-inflammatory agents, in addition to comfort measures such as hot and cold compresses, elevation of the extremity, and close observation for response to treatment (Potts & Mandleco, 2007).

> **Nursing Alert**
>
> Children with facial cellulitis are at risk of meningitis.

Fungal—candidiasis

Candidiasis is a fungal infection of the skin or mucosa membrane commonly called a yeast infection or thrush, and is most common in infants, obese children, adolescents, the chronically ill or immunocompromised, or children receiving antibiotic or steroid treatment (Burns *et al.*, 2009). *Candida albicans*, a commensal fungus of the mouth and gastrointestinal tract, is the most common causative organism of fungal infection. Although systemic infections are reported, the majority of *Candida* infections are superficial, occurring as oropharyngeal candidiasis and as candidial nappy **dermatitis** (Potts & Mandleco, 2007). Candidiasis presents on the mouth as white plaques on an erythematous base that adhere to mucous membranes, or it can present on the corners of the mouth—fissured and inflamed (angular cellulitis). In intertriginous areas such as the neck, axillae, or groin, bright erythema in flexural folds occur, while in the nappy area candidiasis appears as moist, beefy-red macules and papules with sharply-marked borders and satellite lesions (Burns *et al.*, 2009). Topical antifungal agents such as nystatin, miconazole, and ketoconozaole applied to the skin are used in the management of candidiasis, as well as topical steroid cream if inflammation is present and oral antibiotics if secondary bacterial infection occurs (Lansdell-Smith, 2001). Family must be educated to keep the affected areas dry and cool, and frequent nappy changes or leaving the nappy open to air are necessary. Rubber pants must be avoided and mild soap and water should be used for cleansing, avoiding nappy wipes and rinsing well (Burns *et al.*, 2009).

Fungal—tinea infections

Fungal infections caused by the dermaphytes are grouped under tinea and supplemented by a word describing the site of infection, such as pedis (foot), capitis (head), corporis (body), or cruris (groin) (Lansdell-Smith, 2001). Tinea pedis and tinea cruris most commonly occur in adolescence. Tinea pedis (athlete's foot) is often acquired from contaminated showers or locker room floors and presents as scaly, red, and pruritic lesions between the toes. It may be treated with azole creams. Tinea cruris (jock itch) affects the groin area as scaly, red-brown eruptions with defined borders, and often causes intense pruritis. It is managed with clotrimazole creams and by keeping the affected area dry (Potts & Mandleco, 2007). Tinea corporis (body ringworm) and tinea capitis (scalp ringworm) are most common in children. Tinea corporis presents as ring-shaped lesions and is usually contracted from animals such as kittens and puppies (Lansdell-Smith, 2001). Tinea corporis usually responds well to topical agents such as miconazole and clotrimazole creams applied twice daily for two to three weeks. If still persisting, such as is possible in an immunocompromised host, an oral agent such as itraconazole is indicated (Burns *et al.*, 2009). Tinea capitis occurs most frequently in children in crowded living conditions and lower socioeconomic groups, but can occur in schools and day care centres (Potts & Mandleco, 2007). It presents mainly as moist, boggy scalp scaling with or without alopecia (hair loss). Oral administration of griseofulvin for a minimum of eight weeks remains the gold standard of treatment (Fuller *et al.*, 2003). Family are advised to thoroughly clean all objects that have come into contact with the infected child's hair, such as combs, brushes, and hats, to prevent possible spread (Lansdell-Smith, 2001).

Viral—*Molluscum contagiosum*

Viral infections are responsible for many childhood communicable diseases, which can be benign or cause serious complications (Potts & Mandleco, 2007). *Molluscum contagiosum* is a benign, self-limiting viral infection of the skin caused by a poxvirus. It generally affects children over the age of one who swim or bathe together, or who are immunosuppressed. The lesions appear as multiple dome-shaped, pearly, flesh-coloured papules with a central depression, which usually appear on the trunk and flexural areas (Sladden & Johnston, 2004). Parents may wish their GP to treat these lesions with curettage or cryotherapy due to the stigma the condition attracts and also the potential for scarring, but are advised that the condition is benign and typically resolves spontaneously without the use of painful treatments (Sladden & Johnston, 2004).

Viral—warts

Cutaneous viral warts are benign epithelial proliferations caused by the human papilloma virus, which consists of four basic types: *Verruca vulgaris*, *Verruca plana*, *Verruca plantaris*, and *Condyloma acumination* (Watkins, 2005). Their transmission is largely skin-to-skin contact and auto-inoculation (self-infection) (Burns *et al.*, 2009). Many children and caregivers will want warts removed for cosmetic reasons and due to the associated embarrassment they often experience, whereas plantar warts are usually removed because of pain and difficulty walking (Potts & Mandleco, 2007). The first line treatment of the verrucae include application of topical agents once or twice daily, such as salicylic acid solutions to the affected area only, together with the application of petroleum jelly to protect the non-affected area. Cryotherapy or 'freezing' of the wart is considered a second line therapy for verrucae (Potts & Mandleco, 2007).

Viral—*Herpes simplex*

In the active state, *Herpes simplex* virus (HSV) causes contagious infections of the skin and mucous membrane ranging from mild to life-threatening (Burns *et al.*, 2009). There are two types of HSV, HSV1 and HSV2, and both may be passed on by direct contact or through infected items such as towels, and may even be transmitted by an individual with no active lesions (Watkins, 2003). A primary infection with HSV1 often occurs in childhood and may be associated with fever, malaise, sore throat, and decreased fluid intake. With recurrent infection, tingling, parasthesia, and itching of the involved site is common (Burns *et al.*, 2009). HSV1 is the most common type and is usually related to cold sores in and around the mouth, while HSV2 is usually sexually transmitted and more likely to present in the genital areas (Watkins, 2003).

> **Nursing Alert**
>
> Genital lesions in children may indicate the possibility of sexual abuse.

Diagnosis of HSV1 can be made based on appearance but viral cultures can aid diagnosis through swabbing of the lesion (Watkins, 2003). Mild, uncomplicated primary infections require supportive measures such as hygiene, analgesia, and hydration, while more severe cases of primary or recurrent infection may require administration of oral acyclovir (Potts & Mandleco, 2007). Families are educated to ensure that children with active lesions do not pick at lesions and transmit HSV to unaffected areas of the body. Family can also be advised that triggers for recurrence include psychological stress, trauma, fever, exposure to UV light, menses, and extreme weather, and that acyclovir cream applied in the prodromal phase may relieve symptoms (Watkins, 2003).

Skin infestations

Parasites are organisms that depend on their human host for survival. Infestations from pediculosis and scabies are amongst the most common contagious diseases affecting children. They can reach epidemic proportions and be very discomforting for children and family (Potts & Mandleco, 2007).

Parasitic—lice

Children are most affected by head lice because they often put their heads together at school during study and play (Cook, 2002). Head lice (*Pediculus humanus capitis*) are tiny insects either grey or brown in colour and no larger than the head of a pin, which live on the hair and feed from the human scalp by sucking blood from the skin. When the lice lay their eggs (nits) they glue them to the strands of hair so that they cannot be easily removed (Cook, 2002). Lice can be dislodged by combs, towels, and by mere air movement, facilitating their transmission, with the most significant mode of transmission of head lice being head-to-head contact (Sharma *et al.*, 2007). The main detection of head lice is itching, although mild fever, malaise, and lymphadenopathy may also be present (Potts & Mandleco, 2007). The most common areas affected in head louse infestation include the scalp, back of the neck, and post-auricular areas (behind the ears) (Mandell, 2005). The most effective way to detect lice is the wet combing method using a special lice detector available from pharmacies, as the teeth of an ordinary comb are too wide to detect lice (Cook, 2002). Excoriations may be present at the site of infestation. If this is the case, secondary infection (impetigo) should be excluded. Bite reactions manifest as pruritic papules and/ or wheals, depending on the length of time since the last blood meal. Healed bites may reappear when new bites occur in other areas. Untreated head lice infestations can last for months (Sharma *et al.*, 2007).

Treatment of *Pediculosis capitis*, both lice and eggs in one application, is with anti-lice lotions such as Malathion, Phenothrin, or Permithrin (Cook, 2002). Gloves do not necessarily have to be worn during inspection and application but careful hand washing should be carried out. However, pediculicide resistance has become an increasing issue worldwide due to poor technique, non-compliance, and re-infestations (Potts & Mandleco, 2007). Therefore, parents should be advised once they have eradicated the lice that empty egg cases remaining stuck on the hair need to be removed with conditioner and a fine comb, and that careful examination of all family members should be encouraged (Cook, 2002). Contaminated combs and brushes should be immersed in boiling water and floors and furniture should be vacuumed thoroughly. Parents should be encouraged to notify schools or day care centres where the affected child attended so that other affected children may be identified and treated (Potts & Mandleco, 2007).

Non-infectious diseases

Non-infectious diseases are often inflammatory skin disorders that react to intrinsic or extrinsic factors. They may occur in children of any age, are chronic in nature and challenging to manage, and most importantly can impact on the child's quality of life and self-esteem (Potts & Mandleco, 2007). Common non-infectious disorders of childhood, including acne, eczema, and psoriasis, will be discussed.

Acne

Acne vulgaris is an inflammatory disorder of the pilosebaceous unit in which excess sebum, keratinous debris, and bacteria accumulate, producing microcomedones

(blackheads) (Burns *et al.*, 2009). It is thought that hormonal influences of androgens are the initial trigger in puberty, and it may also have a hereditary component and be associated with the use of drugs such as steroids, lithium, iodides, and some antiepileptic medications (Watkins, 2008). Superficial blockage of the sebaceous duct leads to the development of greasy skin on the face and upper trunk (mild acne); this may progress to papule and pustule formation (moderate acne) and deeper blockage leads to the development of painful nodules and cysts (severe acne). In addition normal skin becomes colonized by micro-organisms (Watkins, 2003). Mild acne treatments include topical preparations such as benzoyl peroxide or salicylic acid, alone or in conjunction with an antimicrobial. The area should be first washed with soap or an antiseptic cream and then the cream or gel should be applied once or twice a day. Moderate acne may be treated with oral antibiotics such as oxytetracycline or erythromycin for at least three months, in addition to the topical treatments. Severe and persistent acne can be treated with dramatic results using oral isotretonoin, which acts by reducing sebum production. However, it has some undesirable side effects such as teratogenic effects (causing harm to the foetus) and depression (Watkins, 2008). Other approaches include phototherapy, but this brings with it the risks associated with sun damage of the skin (Watkins, 2008).

Atopic dermatitis (AD)

Characterized by remissions and exacerbations atopic dermatitis (AD) or eczema is a common inflammatory skin disorder that develops in early childhood usually before three months of age (Burns *et al.*, 2009). AD is often associated with asthma and hay fever and its incidence appears to be increasing in the West (British Association of Dermatologists, 2005). The cause of atopic eczema is unknown, although it is believed that genetic, environmental, immunological and biochemical factors all play a part (Lawton, 2009). It manifests itself as persistent pruritis and scratching mainly at night-time where is it believed the 'itch' causes the 'rash'. During infancy the lesions appear on the face, scalp and **extensor** surfaces of the extremities. However, by two years of age the lesions appear on the **flexural** surfaces such as antecubital and popliteal fossae, wrists, ankles and neck (Potts & Mandleco, 2007). AD occurs as: *acute lesions* characterized by extremely

pruritic erthymateous papules, which may occur with excoriation; erosion and serous exudate and crusting; *subacute
lesions* where the papules are excoriated with fine scaling
with mild **lichenification** or thickening of the skin, and as
chronic lesions where marked lichenification is evident (Potts
& Mandleco, 2007). There is no cure for AD and therefore the
treatment strategy is based on interrupting the itch-scratch
cycle, correcting skin dryness with moisturizing, eliminating
offending agents i.e. irritants and allergic triggers and treating secondary bacterial or viral infections (Burns *et al.*, 2009).

Families can be advised about non-pharmacological
approaches to interrupting the itch-scratch cycle, such as
keeping the child's nails short in order to avoid trauma to
the skin from scratching, using distractions (as the child may
not understand that they should not scratch), and promoting cool environmental temperatures (Potts & Mandleco,
2007). Hydration is a key element in the treatment of AD,
and therefore daily bathing in lukewarm water using a mild
soap, followed by patting dry and application of an occlusive
product such as a cream or ointment to seal in moisture,
can be helpful. Moisturizing emollients should be applied
freely throughout the day (Burns *et al.*, 2009). Open wet
compresses are used if lesions are weeping, oozing, or
there are signs of inflammation. Topical corticosteroids comprise the main pharmacological treatment of acute lesions,
where a thin layer of 1% cream is applied to affected areas
three to four times a day. In addition, immunomodulators
such as tacrolimus 0.03% ointment can be used, but only
in severe AD cases in children two years of age and older
(Lawton, 2009). Diphenhydramine hydrochloride (Benad-
ryl) for children older than two years is useful for its anti-
histamine and sedative properties, especially to prevent
itching at night in order to facilitate a good night's sleep
(British Association of Dermatologists, 2005). Systemic antibiotic therapy such as cephalosporins is essential if secondary infection with *Staphylococcus aureus* or *Streptococcus
pyogenes* is evident, as otherwise a severe illness, eczema
herpeticum, could develop. However, topical application
(with the exception of mupirocin) is contraindicated (Burns
et al., 2009).

Nursing Alert

Exposure to identified irritants and triggers such as dust
mites, pets or animal dander, pollens, soaps, food allergies, textiles, or emotional stressors should be avoided.

Nappy (diaper) dermatitis

Any child wearing nappies is at risk of developing nappy
dermatitis and for this reason dermatitis or 'nappy rash'
is the most common irritant contact dermatitis of childhood (Potts & Mandleco, 2007). 'Classical' nappy rash or
ammoniacal dermatitis is caused by prolonged exposure
of the 'nappy' area to urine and faeces and is found on
those areas that are most often in contact with these
waste products (Herreboudt & Sigalov, 1997). It is a frequent cause of fretful, crying babies and often a source
of exasperation and guilt to parents who find their child
inconsolable (Alison, 2000). On physical examination,
erythema, oedema, and vesiculation are observable
in the acute phase, whereas scale, lichenification, and
increased or decreased pigmentation are noted in chronic
conditions (Potts & Mandleco, 2007). Families should be
educated that the following reduce the severity and frequency of nappy rash: frequent nappy changes; cleansing the area well but not vigorously with water and mild
soap; avoiding wipes; using a greasy lubricant if skin is
dry, using a protective ointment such as petroleum at the
first sign of irritation; and avoiding rubber or plastic pants
(Alison, 2000).

Treatment of nappy (diaper) rash is with sitz baths in
warm water for 10–15 minutes four times a day, exposing
the nappy area to air by leaving the nappy off three or
four times daily, Burrow's solution soaks or compresses
four times daily if the skin is weepy, calcium decylenate
powder to decrease friction and moisture, and hydrocor-
tisone 0.5% or 1% applied thinly three times a day for a
maximum of five days. Fungal (Candidal) infections are
common and require topical and oral antifungal treatment.
(Burns *et al.*, 2009). Secondary infections with bacteria,
viruses, or fungi can occur and need to be treated without
delay.

Psoriasis

Psoriasis is a complex chronic inflammatory skin disease
thought to be influenced by genetic and environmental factors, where trigger factors include infection, local
trauma, stress, and certain drugs (Burns *et al.*, 2009).
There are many types of psoriasis (**Box 15.3**) which affect
2–3% of the population and are associated with exacerbations and remissions (Page, 2007).

Box 15.3 Types of psoriasis

- **Chronic plaque psoriasis:** Well-demarcated, pink plaques with dry, silvery-white scale, seen in 90% of patients. The elbows, knees (extensor surfaces), lower back, and scalp are most affected. If the scales are picked off, there is likely to be pin-point bleeding (Auspitz's sign).
- **Guttate psoriasis:** Small, round, red spots appear suddenly on the trunk and become scaly. Lesions are small, extensive, and superficial, and are described as looking like raindrops. Usually seen in children and adolescents. Trigger: tonsillitis or a streptococcal sore throat. Often clears in 2–3 months and tends to be self-limiting. Some individuals have recurrent attacks of guttate psoriasis and occasionally lesions coalesce to become plaque psoriasis.
- **Scalp psoriasis:** One of the commonest sites for psoriasis. Scalp may be dry and flaky or red and inflamed with well-defined plaques. Areas affected: behind the ears and just below the hairline. Scaling is thick and may form hard lumps on the head, which can lead to temporary hair thinning and loss. Hair loss will almost always resolve spontaneously after the psoriasis clears.
- **Flexural psoriasis:** Most common in women and obese patients. Affects submammary, axillary, and anodental folds. Not scaly but the glistening red plaques are clearly demarcated. There is often cracking in the depths of folds.
- **Pustular psoriasis:** Palmoplantar psoriasis is a localized, painful condition affecting the palms and soles. The white or (emergency referral) yellow pustules are 3–10 mm in diameter and lie on top of inflamed red skin. The pustules can heal to (if generalized) leave brown marks. Palmoplantar psoriasis is often the most resistant to treatment. More common in females and associated with smoking.

- Generalized pustular psoriasis can be a complication of longstanding psoriases, or due to the withdrawal of corticosteroid therapy, hypoglycaemia, infections, and local irritants. It often follows an unstable phase and is usually seen in middle age. The top layer of skin may come away in sheets and the patient can become acutely ill.
- **Erythrodermic psoriasis:** The whole body becomes red with patches of scaling. The scaling (emergency referral) is different from that seen in chronic plaque, as it is fairly superficial. Oedema of the limbs develops, and cardiac failure and impaired liver and kidney function can also result from vasodilation. Triggers include: severe sunburn; withdrawal of systemic steroids; irritation of the skin from coal tar and dithranol; and internal infections.
- **Psoriatic arthropathy:** Arthritis occurs in up to 7% of psoriasis patients, most often in finger and toe joints. Other patterns may involve the sacroiliac joints and spine, or a single large joint. Blood tests for rheumatoid arthritis will be negative, but arthropathy may be present for years before any skin signs appear. The prognosis in psoriatic arthropathy appears to be better than in rheumatoid arthritis and there is generally less pain and disability.
- **Napkin psoriasis:** Develops in the nappy area of an infant to cause a bright red, weeping rash or more typical psoriasis plaques.
- **Nail psoriasis:** Psoriasis affects the matrix or nail bed in up to 50% of patients. Thimble pitting is the commonest change, followed by onycholysis (separation of the distal edge of the nail from the nail bed). Treatment is often difficult.

In psoriatic skin the epidermal cycle is accelerated and cell turnover time, which should be 28 days, is reduced to four days, resulting in a failure of cells to mature appropriately (Ryan, 2008). Plaque psoriasis is the most common type and is characterized by the development of single or multiple well-defined red plaques with silver scales, which can appear anywhere on the skin, but most often on the elbows and knees (Ryan, 2008). Psoriasis can be painful and itchy but also unsightly. As a result the patient's body image can be significantly affected with potential psychological debilitation (Lawton, 2000). For this reason, sensitivity and tactfulness must be exercised with patients with psoriasis. Psoriasis treatment can

be categorized broadly as topical for mild to moderate disease, phototherapy for moderate to severe disease, and systemic treatments for very severe disease (Ryan, 2008). Mineral or olive oil and warm towels can be used to soak and remove thick plaques and topical treatments such as emollient creams, Eucerin and Aquaphor, can be applied liberally for their soothing, hydrating, and moisturizing effects (Lawton, 2000).

Topical corticosteroids should be applied accurately with the use of fingertip unit (**Figure 15.3**) and are reserved for areas such as the face, flexural areas, and genitalia (Page, 2007). Tar can be used but is quite smelly and messy; keratolytic shampoos (e.g. Nizoril)

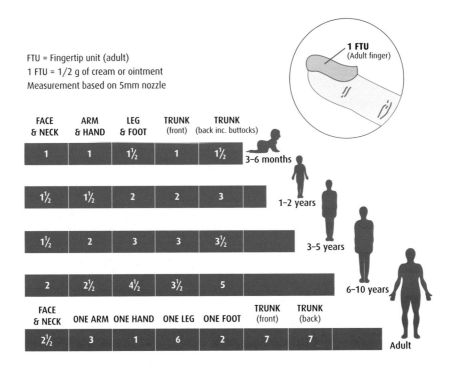

FTU = Fingertip unit (adult)
1 FTU = 1/2 g of cream or ointment
Measurement based on 5mm nozzle

1 FTU (Adult finger)

FACE & NECK	ARM & HAND	LEG & FOOT	TRUNK (front)	TRUNK (back inc. buttocks)	
1	1	1½	1	1½	3–6 months
1½	1½	2	2	3	1–2 years
1½	2	3	3	3½	3–5 years
2	2½	4½	3½	5	6–10 years

FACE & NECK	ONE ARM	ONE HAND	ONE LEG	ONE FOOT	TRUNK (front)	TRUNK (back)	
2½	3	1	6	2	7	7	Adult

Figure 15.3 The fingertip unit method

can be used on the scalp. Antralin ointment or vitamin D derivatives such as Calcipotril can be effective for plaques resistant to steroid treatment, but family must be cautioned that Antralin causes staining and extensive use of Calcipotril ointment can lead to hypercalcaemia (Lawton, 2000).

Sun exposure and UVB in moderate amounts is believed to alleviate lesions alone or with other treatments, but sunburn should be avoided (Page, 2007). For severe psoriatic disease systemic treatment is administered in the form of cyclosporine, methotrexate, and retinoid, and psoralens may also be considered as well as immunotherapy (Burns *et al.*, 2009). Patients and family need to be motivated and educated to become involved in self-care and self-management so as to minimize not only the unpleasant symptoms of psoriasis but also complications that can ensue, from the less serious *Candida* infection in the nappy area to the more serious erythrodermic and pustular psoriasis causing fever, malaise, electrolyte and temperature instability, and leukocytosis (Moules & Ramsay, 2008). Preventative measures to avert complications include moisturizing of skin, avoidance of stressors such as skin injury, itching, bites, oral

steroids, NSAIDs, and stress, as well as keeping fingernails short and gentle brushing of the hair if the scalp is affected (Burns *et al.*, 2009). When dealing with psoriasis sufferers sensitivity and tactfulness is paramount due to the psychological impact of the disease. Support groups can be beneficial for patients and families to overcome the psychosocial impact of the disease.

Skin injury

Because children are less able to protect themselves, injury to the skin of the child resulting from bites, stings, and burns are the most common causes of injury in children and can have serious sequelae (Potts & Mandleco, 2007).

Bites and stings

Insect bite and sting injuries are extremely varied but essentially there are insects that either sting (venomous) or bite (non-venomous) (**Table 15.7**). An insect that bites is non-venomous as the insect is piercing the skin to feed on

Table 15.7 Causes of insect stings or bites

Causes of insect bites	Causes of insect stings
Midges	Bees
Gnats	Wasps
Mosquitoes	Hornets
Horseflies	Ants
Fleas	
Ticks	
Bedbugs	

Box 15.4 Measures to avoid insect stings and bites

- Avoid perfume and bright-coloured clothing to reduce the risk of bee stings.
- Control odours at picnics, garbage areas, etc. that can attract insects.
- Destroy or relocate hives or nests close to your home.
- Don't leave pools of stagnating water as these attract mosquitoes.
- Electrical insect repelling devices and lit coils may be effective.
- Cover all parts of the body with clothing, hats, socks, and gloves if going into areas where there is a high likelihood of getting bitten or stung.
- Maintain good personal and household hygiene.
- De-flea cats, dogs, and other household pets regularly.
- Use insect repellents, which are readily available from pharmacies or supermarkets. Those containing DEET (diethyltoluamide) are the most effective.
- Permethrin can be applied to clothing to give protection for two weeks, through two washings. It can also be applied directly to exposed skin, keeping the insects away for a few days.
- Thiamine (vitamin B1) can be used as a systemic insect repellent (the skin has a characteristic smell).

its victim's blood and the insect's saliva frequently causes a localized allergic reaction characterized by pruritic papule (Stevens, 2008). An insect sting causes a stinging sensation or pain with redness and swelling of the area, which occurs when the insect injects venom into its victim as a defence mechanism. Both stings and bites can become infected with the risk of cellulitis and the risk of anaphylaxis occurring in sensitive children (Stevens, 2008).

In some parts of the world, insect bites can be even more problematic as the insects are carriers or vectors of diseases such as malaria, lyme disease, rickettsial disease, and Dengue fever. Parents should be made aware of simple measures that can prevent insect stings and bites (**Box 15.4**). In the event of an insect bite, such as a tick bite, the tick can be removed with tweezers and resting and elevating (if a limb) and using cold compresses are effective in reducing inflammation. A topical steroid cream and oral antihistamines can combat the itch and topical anaesthetics may also provide relief, as can the application of calamine lotion (Stevens, 2008). In the case of tick bites, oral antibiotics are indicated (Stevens, 2008).

In sting injuries it is more common to observe a systemic allergic response such as generalized pruritis and hives, nausea, shortness of breath, and wheezing resulting from airway swelling (anaphylaxis), which can progress to shock and become life-threatening (Potts & Mandleco, 2007). The stinger should be removed by using the firm edge of a knife or credit card placed against the skin and dragged across to remove the stinger (DermNet NZ, 2009) and in addition to the comfort measures applicable to insect bites, subcutaneous epinephrine should be administered (Stevens, 2008). Many children who have had such an experience will be given an emergency epinephrine kit (e.g. Epipen) which is available for self-administration in the event of reoccurrence.

Dog bites

The most common victims of dog bites are children, and the face is the most frequent target in dog bites (Bermant, 2009). Dog bites in children often require emergency department (ED) treatment for wound repair, rabies evaluation, and infection prevention (Bernardo *et al.*, 2000). Injuries should be cleansed with sterile saline under irrigation and repair of the wounds may require simple closure, removal of injured tissue, and reconstructive surgery. Underlying nerve and bone injuries may need repair and sometimes completely severed tissue can be replaced as a graft or reattached with microsurgical repair of tiny blood vessels (Bermant, 2009). Dog bites to the hand, foot, and face, puncture wounds, wounds requiring surgical debridement, wounds involving joints, tendons, or ligaments, suspected fractures, and children who are at high risk of infection (such as those who are diabetic, cirrhotic, or immunosuppressed) require a seven day course of antibiotics (co-amoxiclav) to prevent and treat wound infection (Clinical Knowledge Summaries, 2007). Immediate rabies prophylaxis is necessary for individuals bitten by domestic animals suspected of being rabid (Potts & Mandleco, 2007). Appropriate tetanus therapy should also be administered to children who have not been immunized within the last ten years (Presutti, 2001).

Almost one half of all reported cases of dog bites involve an animal owned by the victim's family or neighbours. Several dog breeds have been identified in fatal dog bite attacks, namely pit bull breeds, malamutes, chows, Rottweilers, huskies, and German shepherds (Presutti, 2001). To prevent dog bites to children, parents need to be advised that dogs with a history of aggression are unsuitable for households with children and they need to teach basic safety tips to children and review them regularly (**see Box 15.5**).

Burn injury

Burns are the fifth leading cause of death in children in the European Union (Eurosafe, 2009). There are about

Box 15.5 Dog bite prevention measures

- Do not approach an unfamiliar dog.
- Do not run from a dog or scream.
- Remain motionless (e.g. 'be still like a tree') when approached by an unfamiliar dog.
- If knocked over by a dog, roll into a ball and lie still (e.g. 'be still like a log').
- Do not play with a dog unless supervised by an adult.
- Immediately report stray dogs or dogs displaying unusual behaviour to an adult.
- Avoid direct eye contact with a dog.
- Do not disturb a dog that is sleeping, eating, or caring for puppies.
- Do not pet a dog without allowing it to see and sniff you first.
- If bitten, immediately report the bite to an adult.

250,000 burn injuries each year in Britain seen in NHS hospitals, many of which are preventable, and some 16,000 are admitted to hospital, many to non-specialist units. The majority of burns in children are scald injuries in children under two years of age (British Burns Association (BBA), 2009). Some 16% of burn injuries are due to child abuse and therefore physical findings inconsistent with the reported findings, unclear history, a delay in seeking treatment, or conflicting stories about how the injury occurred should alert the health professional to the possibility of an inflicted injury (Burns *et al.*, 2009).

There are four major sources of burns, namely thermal (flame, scald, contact, flash), electrical (low/high voltage and flash), chemical (acids/alkalis), and radiation (UVA/UVB). The severity of the burn is classified according to the depth of the burn, percentage of total body surface area (TBSA) involved, location of the burn, and association with other injuries (Potts & Mandleco, 2007). There are three types of burn depth: superficial, partial-thickness (superficial and deep), and full-thickness. Superficial or epidermal burns are typified by sunburn, which affects only the epidermis with erythema and seldom blistering. They are treated with analgesia and fluid hydration and heal within a week (Papini, 2004). Parents are advised to encourage the use of sunscreen and shades and to avoid the midday sun and long periods in the sun, in order to reduce the risk of reoccurrence and the long-term risk of skin cancer (Burns *et al.*, 2009).

Partial thickness burns involve the epidermis and the dermis. Superficial partial thickness burns are red, painful, mottled, and blistered and heal in 10–21 days with no scarring, whereas deep partial thickness burns are very painful, appear pale yellow, and are weepy. They take about three weeks to heal and may result in scarring (Papini, 2004). Full thickness burns are major thermal injuries where the dermis and appendages (tendons, muscles, and bones) are destroyed and the skin appears whitish or leathery. They result from prolonged exposure to hot liquids or fire or electrical burn injuries, require excision and skin grafts, and are associated with permanent scarring (Potts & Mandleco, 2007).

First aid measures should include removing the child from the source of the burn; if clothing is alight the 'drop and roll' procedure is followed and where electricity is involved the source should be turned off before giving help (Benson *et al.*, 2006). The burn should be cooled with lukewarm water for at least 20 minutes (longer for chemical burns); ice or very cold water should be avoided. Polyvinyl or 'cling film' can be used as a dressing to allow wound assessment and wound protection. In assessing a burn further and planning resuscitation, careful examination of all body surfaces is necessary and a useful assessment method in the acute setting is Wallace's 'rule of nines', or using the patient's palmar surface of the hand, which approximates 1% of the total body surface area (Fowler, 1998). However, in children, whose proportions are different to those of adults, the Lund and Browder chart (**Figure 15.4**) is used for a more accurate assessment (Malic *et al.*, 2006).

Nursing Alert

Simple erythema should not be included in the Lund and Browder TBSA calculation.

Once the type, depth, and extent of burn injury is known, together with associated injuries, age, and pre-existing conditions, the burn injury can be determined as minor, moderate, or major (Potts & Mandleco, 2007). Children with burns meeting the British Burns Association (BBA) referral criteria must be admitted to a specialist burn injury unit (**see Box 15.6**). Children with simple, minor, or moderate burn injury should have debris removed from the wound with mild soap and water before paraffin gauze dressings are applied; hydrocolloid dressings are useful on hands or other small areas. Large friable blisters should be 'de-roofed' prior to treatment (pierce and remove the blister top using a sterile technique), although small blisters may be left intact. Antibiotics are not required for a child who has minor burns but the

Box 15.6 Criteria for referral to Burn Unit

- Associated airway injury.
- Partial thickness burns greater than 5% TBSA in a child.
- Partial or full thickness burns to face, perineum, external genitalia, feet, and hands, and over joints.
- Circumferential injury.
- Chemical and electrical burns.
- Non-accidental injury.
- Comorbidity.
- Non-healed injury three weeks after injury.

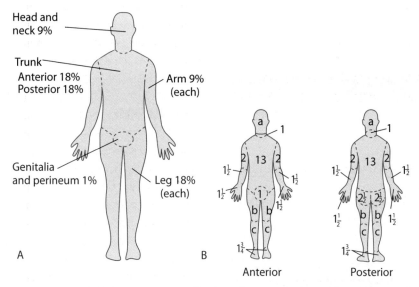

Relative percentage of body surface area (% BSA) affected by growth

	Age				
Body Part	0 yr	1 yr	5 yr	10 yr	15 yr
a = 1/2 of head	9 1/2	8 1/2	6 1/2	5 1/2	4 1/2
b = 1/2 of 1 thigh	2 3/4	3 1/4	4	4 1/4	4 1/2
c = 1/2 of 1 lower leg	2 1/2	2 1/2	2 3/4	3	3 1/4

Figure 15.4 Lund and Browder TBSA calculation, with permission from Elsevier

tetanus status of the child should be established (Benson *et al.*, 2006).

Major burn injuries are essentially managed according to the following protocol: **A** = Airway and spine control; **B** = Breathing and ventilation; **C** = Circulation and haemorrhage control; **D** = Disability; **E** = Exposure and environmental control; **F** = Fluid resuscitation (British Burns Association, 2000). Airway and respiratory complications can be anticipated if the burn occurred in an enclosed space or if loss of consciousness is evident and therefore oxygen should be administered if hypoxia is apparent. Chest expansion should be observed as full thickness burns affecting the trunk may obstruct breathing due to constricting eschar and may require an incision into restricting eschar (escharotomy) to restore peripheral blood circulation and to release the chest restriction (Potts & Mandleco, 2007). Arterial blood gases or non-invasive electronic CO-oximetry meters (e.g. Masimo RAD57) may reveal the presence of carbon monoxide poisoning or smoke inhalation. A child who has upper body or facial injury or soot in the nose or mouth is at risk of airway obstruction from oedema and will need to be evaluated by an anaesthetist for endotracheal intubation (Benson *et al.*, 2006). Children with major burn injuries are at risk of hypothermia and therefore temperature needs to be monitored and warming measures instigated.

Nursing Alert

Pulse oximetry is an unreliable respiratory assessment tool in the presence of inhalation injury.

Fluid resuscitation is of major importance in seriously burned children, initially to prevent hypovolaemic shock and subsequently to maintain stability (Potts & Mandleco, 2007). The BBA (2000) recommends the use of the Parkland Formula, but also recognizes that intravenous fluids should be guided by patient response, such as adequate urinary output (1–2ml/kg/hr) measured via a urinary catheter of, stable vital signs and oriented mental status. Fluid resuscitation is calculated from time of injury as opposed to time of presentation. To calculate the fluid requirements 3–4mls Hartmann's solution/kg body weight/% total body surface area, plus maintenance fluid 4% glucose in 0.25% N Saline (Benson *et al*, 2006).

For the first 24 hours half of this fluid is given in the first eight hours and half over the subsequent 16 hours of 3–4 ml Hartmann's solution/kg body weight/% TBSA, plus maintenance fluid 4% glucose in 0.25% N Saline (Benson *et al.*, 2006). Pain is managed with the administration of intravenous morphine sulphate in the acute phase and this should be administered regularly, and particularly before painful procedures. Major wounds need to be soaked, cleansed, and debrided daily, either manually with forceps or mechanically with hydrotherapy, followed by the application of topical antimicrobial agents such as silver sulfadiazine and dressings (Fowler, 1998). Excision of the burned skin may also be necessary, and reconstruction with split skin grafts taken from the patient in single or multiple stages, which may be combined with cadaveric skin grafts if the patient has insufficient donor skin (Benson *et al.*, 2006). Nutritional support is essential for recovery as the burned child will require 2–3 times the normal amount of calories in order to heal (Potts & Mandleco, 2007). Physiotherapy and occupational therapy are necessary to prevent complications, to preserve and restore function with exercise and splints, and to minimize scarring with the aid of pressure garments (Fowler, 1998). Psychological support of the child is paramount to facilitate a successful recovery and this can be enhanced by involving family members in care and the provision of burn camps for the child (Potts & Mandleco, 2007).

Conclusion

The integumentary system is a vitally important organ of the body that is responsible for many physical and social functions, and therefore when the integrity of the skin is compromised both physiological and psychosocial consequences can ensue. Infectious and non-infectious diseases of the skin together with skin injuries are very varied and many chronic skin conditions are very challenging and potentially life-threatening; however, it has to be said that many conditions are preventable, especially pressure ulcers, bites and stings, and many burn injuries and skin cancers.

Online resource centre

You may find it helpful to work through our online resources including interactive scenarios intended to help you to develop and apply the skills in this chapter. Where material referenced below is available electronically, we're pleased to provide active web links to the source via 🌐 **http://www.oxfordtextbooks.co.uk/ orc/coyne/**

References

Alison, F. (2000) Nappy rash: An overview. *Practice Nursing* **1** (17), 17–19.

Baharestani, M.M. & Ratliff, C.R. (2007) Pressure ulcers in neonates and children: An NPUAP White Paper. *Advances in Skin & Wound Care* **20** (4), 208–220.

Baldwin, K.M. (2002) Incidence and prevalence of pressure ulcers in children. *Advances in Skin and Wound Care* **15** (3), 121–124.

Ball, J. & Bindler, R. (2007) *Paediatric Nursing—Caring for Children.* Upper Saddle River, New Jersey: Prentice Hall.

Bar-on, E., Weigl, D., Parvari, R., Katz, K., Weitz, R., & Steinberg, T. (2003) Congenital insensitivity to pain. *The Journal of Bone and Joint Surgery* **84** (2), 252–257.

Benson, A., Dickson, W.A., & Boyce, D. (2006) ABC of wound healing: Burns. *British Journal of Medicine* **332**, 649–652.

Bergstrom, H., Bennet, M.A., Carlton, C.E., *et al.* (1994) *Treatment of Pressure Ulcers: Clinical Practice Guideline No. 15.* Rockville MD: AHCPR Publication.

Bermant, M. (2009) *Dog bite prevention.* American Board of Plastic Surgery. Available at: **http://www. plasticsurgery4u.com/procedure_folder/dog_ bite.html**

Bernardo, L.M., Gardner, M.J., O'Connor, J., & Amon, N. (2000) Dog bites in children treated in a paediatric Emergency Department. *Journal of the Society of Paediatric Nurses* **1** (6), 2000.

Bianchi, J. & Cameron, J. (2008) Management of skin conditions in the older population. *British Journal of Community Nursing* **13** (3) Suppl. S26–S32.

Bryant, R. (2000) *Acute and Chronic Wounds: Nursing management.* London: Mosby.

Burns, C.E., Dunn, A.M., Brady, M., Starr, N.B., & Blosser, C.G. (2009) *Paediatric Primary Care, 4th ed.* New York: Saunders Elsevier.

Butcher, M. & White, R. (2005) The structure and function of the skin. In R. White (ed.) *Skin Care in Wound Management Assessment and Treatment.* Aberdeen: Wounds UK.

Cho, S.H, Ketefian, F., & Barkauskas, V.H. (2003) The effects of nurse staffing on adverse events, morbidity, mortality and medical costs. *Nursing Research* **52**, 71–79.

Clinical Knowledge Summaries (2007) *Bites—Human and animal.* Available at: **http://www.cks.nhs. uk./bites_human_and animal/view_whole_ guidance**

Cook, E. (2002) How to detect and control head lice. *Practice Nursing* **13** (6), 257–258.

Curley, M.A. & Quigley, S.M. (2003) Pressure ulcers in pediatric intensive care. Incidence and associated factors. *Pediatric Critical Care Medicine* **4**, 284–290.

DermNet NZ (2009) *Insect bites and stings.* Available at: **http://dermnetznz.org/arthropods/bites/html**

Dyer, L. & Embling, B. (2006) Pressure area care. In E. Trigg & T.A. Mohammed. *Practices in Children's Nursing.* Edinburgh: Churchill Livingstone.

European Pressure Ulcer Advisory Panel (1998) *Pressure Ulcer Treatment Guidelines.* Oxford: European Pressure Ulcer Advisory Panel.

Fowler, A. (1998) Nursing management of minor burn injury. *Nursing Standard* **12** (49), 47–52.

Garvin, G. (1997) Wound and skin care for the PICU. *Critical Care Nursing Quarterly* **20** (1), 62–71.

Harris, A., Coker, K.L., Smith, C.G., Uitvlugt, N., & Doctor, B. (2003) Case report of a pressure ulcer in an infant receiving extracorporeal life support: The use of a novel mattress surface for pressure reduction. *Advances in Neonatal Care* **3**, 220–229.

Herreboudt, A. & Sigalov, J. (1997) Nappy rash at a glance: From top to bottom. *British Journal of Midwifery* **5** (7), 42–46.

Hockenberry, M. & Wilson, D. (2007) *Wong's Nursing Care of Infants and Children, 8th ed.* Saint Louis (USA): Mosby Elsevier.

Holloway, S. & Jones, V. (2005) The importance of skin care and assessment. *British Journal of Nursing* **14** (22), 1172–1176.

Howard, A. & Sippel, V. (2005) Coding for decubitus ulcer. *For the Record* **17** (1), 47.

Keast, D.H., Parslow, N., Houghton, P.E., Norton, L., & Fraser, L. (2008) Best practice recommendations for the prevention and treatment of pressure ulcers: Update 2006. *Advances in Skin Wound Care* **20**, 447–460.

Lansdell-Smith, J. (2001) Diagnosis and management of fungal skin infections. *British Journal of Community Nursing* **6** (4), 186–192.

Lawton, S. (2000) Psoriasis. *Nursing & Residential Care* **2** (5), 220–225.

Lawton, S. (2001) Assessing the patient with a skin condition. *Journal of Tissue Viability* **11** (3), 113–115.

Lawton, S. (2009) Dermatology in schools: Understanding skin conditions. *British Journal of School Nursing* **4** (1), 11–14.

Lloyd-Jones, M. (2007) Tissue viability part 1: The effects of ageing on the skin. *British Journal of Healthcare Assistants* **1** (1), 22–24.

Lund, C. (1999) Prevention and management of infant skin breakdown. *Nursing Clinics of North America* **34**, 907–920.

Malic, C.C., Karoo, R.O., Austin, O., & Phipps, A. (2007) Resuscitation burn card—a useful tool for burn injury assessment, *Burns* **33** (2), 195–199.

Mandell, G. (2005) Pediculosis. In: G. Mandell (ed.) *Principles and Practices of Infectious Diseases, 6th ed*. Edinburgh: Churchill Livingston.

Manning, J. (2007) The assessment of dark skin and dermatological disorders. *Nursing Times* **100** (22), 48.

Martini, F.H. (2006) *Fundamentals of Anatomy and Physiology, 7th ed*. San Francisco: Pearson Education.

Massey, D. (2006) The value and role of skin and nail assessment in the critically ill. *Nursing in Critical Care* **11** (2), 80–85.

McLane, K.M., Bookout, K., McCord, S., McCain, J., & Jefferson, J.S. (2004) The 2003 national pediatric pressure ulcer and skin breakdown prevalence survey: A multisite study. *Journal of Wound Ostomy & Continence Nursing* **31** (4), 168–178.

Millard, T. (2008) Impetigo: Recognition and management. *Practice Nursing* **19** (9), 432–434.

Morton, P.G., Fontaine, D.K., Hudak, C.M., & Gallo, B.M. (2005) *Critical Care Nursing: A holistic approach, 8th ed*. Philadelphia: Lippincott, Williams & Wilkins.

Moules, T. & Ramsay, J. (2008) *The Textbook of Children's and Young People's Nursing, 2nd ed*. Oxford: Blackwell Publishing.

Murdoch, V. (2002) Pressure care in the paediatric intensive care unit. *Nursing Standard* **17** (6), 71–76.

National Institute for Clinical Excellence (2001) *Pressure Ulcer Risk Assessment and Prevention*. London: NICE.

National Institute for Health and Clinical Excellence (2005) *The Prevention and Treatment of Pressure Ulcers*. London: NICE.

National Pressure Ulcer Advisory Panel (2007) *Updated Staging System*. Washington: NPUAP.

Nazarko, L. (2009) Providing outpatient antibiotic therapy for cellulitis in primary care. *British Journal of Community Nursing* **13** (11) 520–524.

Page, B. (2007) Psoriasis management in primary care. *Practice Nursing* **18** (10), 497–500.

Papini, R. (2004) Management of burn injuries of various depths. *British Journal of Medicine* **329**, 158–160.

Potts, N. & Mandleco, N.L. (2007) *Paediatric Nursing: Caring for children and their families, 2nd ed*. London: Thomson Delmar Learning.

Presutti, R.J. (2001) Prevention and treatment of dog bites. *American Family Physician* **63**, 1567–1572.

Quigley, S.M. & Curley, M.A.Q. (1996) Skin integrity in the paediatric population: Preventing and managing pressure ulcers. *Journal of the Society of Pediatric Nurses* **1** (1), 7–18.

Registered Nurses Association of Ontario (2005) *Nursing Best Practice Guideline: Risk Assessment and Prevention of Pressure Ulcers*. Toronto: RNAO.

Royal College of Nursing (2001) *Risk Assessment and the Prevention of Pressure Ulcers*. London: RCN Publishing.

Royal College of Nursing (2005) *The management of pressure ulcers in primary and secondary care. A clinical practice guideline*. London: RCN Publishing.

Russell, L. (1998) Physiology of the skin and prevention of pressure sores. *British Journal of Nursing* **7** (18), 1084–1100.

Ryan, S. (2008) Psoriasis characteristics, psychosocial effects and treatment options. *British Journal of Nursing* **17** (5), 284–290.

Salzberg, C.A. (1999) Predicting pressure ulcers during initial hospitalization for acute spinal cord injury.

Wounds: A Compendium of Clinical Research and Practice **11** (2), 45–57.

Samiengo, I.A. (2003) A sore spot in paediatrics: Risk factors for pressure ulcers. *Paediatric Nursing.* **29** (4), 278–282.

Sharma, D., Kaliaperumal, C., & Choudhari, K.A. (2007) An overview of headlice in neurosurgical patients. *British Journal of Nursing* **16** (16), 982–989.

Sibbald, R.C., Williamson, D., Orsted, H.L., *et al.* (2004) Preparing the wound bed. Debridement, bacterial balance and moisture balance. *Ostomy/Wound Management* **46** (11), 14–35.

Sladden, M.J. & Johnston, G. (2004) Common skin infections in children. *British Medical Journal* **329**, 95–99.

Smeltzer, S. & Bare, B. (2008) *Brunner & Suddarth's Medical Surgical Nursing, 11th ed.* Philadelphia: Lippincott, Williams & Wilkins.

Stevens, D. (2008) Insect bites and stings. *Practice Nursing* **19** (8), 411–413.

Tongle, H. (1999) The structure and function of the skin. *Nursing & Residential Care* **1** (1), 48–55.

Tortora, G.J. & Derrickson, B. (2006) *Introduction to the Human Body: The essentials of anatomy and physiology.* Philadelphia: Wiley.

Turnball, R. (2007) Skin assessment in children: A methodical approach. *Nursing Times* **96** (41), 33.

Waterlow, J.A. (1997) Pressure sore risk assessment in children. *Paediatric Nursing* **9** (6), 21–24.

Watkins, J. (2003) Dermatology clinic: Herpes simplex. *Practice Nursing* **14** (7), 327–330.

Watkins, J. (2005) Tinea corporis. *Practice Nursing* **16** (5), 230–234.

Watkins, J. (2008) Acne vulgaris and its management. *British Journal of School Nursing* **3** (1), 20–24.

Willock, J., Anthony, D., & Baharestani, M.M. (2007) A risk assessment scale for pressure ulcers in children. *Nursingtimes.net* **103** (14), 32–33.

Willock, J., Anthony, D., & Richardson, J. (2008) Inter-rater reliability of the Glamorgan Paediatric Pressure Ulcer Risk Assessment Scale. *Paediatric Nursing* **20** (7), 14–19.

Further reading and URLs

Bliss, M. (2000) Pressure sores: Demographic perspectives. *Journal of Tissue Viability* **10** (3), 106–114.

British Association of Dermatologists patient information. Available from: **http://www.bad.org.uk/site/796/default.aspx**

British Burn Association. *Emergency Management of Severe Burns Course Manual, UK version.* Wythenshawe Hospital, Manchester, 1996.

Chamley, C.A., Carson, P., Randall, D., & Sandwell, M. (2005) *Developmental Anatomy and Physiology of Children.* Edinburgh: Elsevier.

Emmet, A., Uchida, T., & Wagner, R. (2008) *Dermatology Online Journal.* Available at: **http://dermatology.cdlib.org/141/commentary/sunburn/wagner.html**

Eurosafe: European Association for Injury Prevention and Safety Promotion. Available at: **http://www.paulinchen.de/fileadmin/content/Renate_Krohn/Downloads/2009-03-23_burns_and_scalds.pdf**

Fisher, P. & Holmes, P. (2000) Sunburn. *Practice Nursing* **10** (12), 31–35.

Fuller, L.C., Child, F.J., Midgley, G., & Higgins, E.M. (2003) Diagnosis and management of scalp ringworm. *British Medical Journal* **326**, 539–541.

Guy, H. (2007) Best Practice: Pressure ulcer risk assessment and grading. *Nursing Times* **103** (15), 38–40.

James, S.R. & Ashwill, J.W. (2007) *Nursing Care of Children—Principles and practice.* St. Louis, Missouri: Saunders Elsevier.

Jeans, P., Rand, W., & Blake, F. (1946) *Essentials of Pediatrics.* Philadelphia: J.B. Lippincott Company.

Nazarko, L. (2007) Scabies: An overview of the condition. *British Journal of Healthcare Assistants* **1** (9), 401–404.

Nicholson, M. (2004) Not simple at all: Herpes simplex virus. *Practice Nursing* **15** (10), 480–486.

Rawlins, J., Khan, A., Shenton, A., & Sharpe, D. (2007) Etiology and outcome analysis of 208 children with burns attending at Emergency Department. *Pediatric Emergency Care* **23** (5), 289–293.

Sheridan, R., Petras, L., Lydon, M., & Salvo, P. (1997) Once-daily wound cleansing and dressing change: Efficacy and cost. *Journal of Burn Care & Rehabilitation* **18** (2), 139–140.

Thompson, J. (1995) Atopic eczema and skin infections. *Practice Nursing* **7** (3), 11–13.

Watkins, J. (2004) Viral warts. *Practice Nursing* **15** (9), 452–456.

Willock, J. & Maylor, M. (2004) Pressure ulcers in infants and children. *Nursing Standard* **24** (18), 56–62.

Wilson, D. & Hockenberry, M.J. (2008) *Wong's Clinical Manual of Paediatric Nursing 7th ed.* St Louis, Missouri: Mosby Elsevier.

Young, A. & Chambers, T. (2005) Standards for care of critically-ill children with burns. *The Lancet* **365**, 1911–1913.

http://www.nice.org.uk/guidance/B
http://www.epuap.org

http://www.npuap.org
http://www.woundsresearch.com/archives.cfm
http://www.headlice.org
http://www.psoriasis.org
http://www.skincancer.org
http://nationaleczema.org
http://www.DermNET NZ.org
http://www.britishburnassociation.co.uk/
http://www.euroburn.org/news.php

16 Reproductive system

SAM CHENERY-MORRIS AND AILEEN LYNCH

Skills

16.1 **Preparing the child for pelvic examination** 🅐

....

16.2 **Preparing the child for a swab procedure** 🅐

....

16.3 **Care of dressings on genitalia postoperatively** 🅐

Introduction

This chapter describes a number of clinical procedures related to the reproductive system that commonly occur in children. After completing this chapter you will have a working knowledge of the reproductive system and will have accomplished the following learning objectives.

Learning outcomes

After reading this chapter you should be able to:
• Describe the anatomy of the female reproductive system including the external genitalia, the ovaries, the accessory reproductive structures, and the mammary glands.
• Describe the ovarian and menstrual cycles and the hormones that regulate them.
• Describe the anatomy of the male reproductive system including the external genitalia, the testes, the internal ducts, and the glands.

• Discuss the procedures involved in preparing the child for pelvic examination, demonstrating an awareness of the cultural, ethical, and legal implications of this examination.
• Explain and prepare the child for a swab procedure.
• Undertake the post-operative care of dressings on genitalia.

Prior knowledge

Before embarking on this chapter it would be helpful to read through Chapter Two and Chapter Four, to provide you with relevant background skills required in this context. Informed consent and child protection are quite important related issues, and are covered in great detail in Chapter Four. The initial part of this chapter describes the anatomy and physiology of the reproductive system as a background towards understanding the relevant nursing care. This discussion is not intended to replace detailed study of anatomy and physiology, and for further and more detailed instruction on the topic you ought to consult a key text such as Martini & Nath (2008).

Anatomy and physiology of the reproductive system

Female reproductive system

The female reproductive system is regulated in a cyclical manner by hormones. The onset of the first menstrual cycle

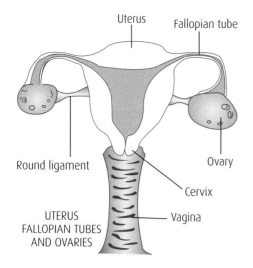

Figure 16.1 The female reproductive system
© EMIS and PiP 2009, as directed on http://www.patient.co.uk

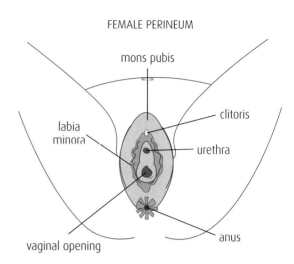

Figure 16.2 External genitalia of the female
© EMIS and PiP 2009, as directed on http://www.patient.co.uk

(**menarche**) occurs at **puberty**, and the female has the capacity to become pregnant up until the **menopause**, when the menstrual cycle ceases. The essential sex organs of the female reproductive system are the ovaries, which release one ovum (egg) each month. The fallopian tubes, uterus, vagina, and the mammary glands (breasts) make up the female accessory reproductive structures. The anatomy of the female reproductive system is illustrated in **Figure 16.1**.

External genitalia

Apart from the vulva and breasts (discussed further below), all of the female reproductive structures are located internally (Martini & Nath, 2008). The vulva comprises the external female genitalia, which surround the opening to the vagina, and this is illustrated in **Figure 16.2**. The mons pubis is a fat-covered region over the pubic bone, which is covered by hair after puberty. The clitoris is an erectile structure similar to the penis in males. The elongated folds of the labia majora contain hair follicles, sweat glands, and sebaceous glands. Its inner surface contains the labia minora, which (unlike the mons pubis and the labia majora) remain hair-free even after puberty. The area between the labia minora is called the vestibule and contains the openings to the vagina and urethra. There are glands called Bartholin's glands (or greater vestibular glands) on each side of the vaginal opening that secrete a mucus-like lubricating fluid into the vestibule. The perineum is the area between the vaginal opening and the anus,

and sometimes it is surgically cut (episiotomy) in order to assist childbirth (Martini & Nath, 2008).

Essential sex organs

Ovaries

The paired ovaries are the essential organs of reproduction in the female. Mature egg cells (ova) are developed in and released from the ovaries. The ovaries have both exocrine (ova producing) and endocrine (hormone producing) functions. Within the ovaries are ovarian follicles, which are fluid-filled sacs containing the oocytes (immature eggs). When a baby girl is born she has the full complement of ovarian follicles (about two million) and when the menstrual cycle is initiated she has about 250,000 follicles remaining. One ovum is released each month under hormonal regulation (discussed further later in the chapter). The ovaries also produce and release the female sex hormones, oestrogen and progesterone, thus fulfilling their endocrine function. Oestrogen is also responsible for development of the **secondary sex characteristics** after puberty: development of the external genitals, uterus, and breasts; hair growth in the pubic area and axillae (armpits); and broadening of the female pelvis in preparation for childbearing.

Accessory reproductive structures

In the female the purpose of the accessory reproductive structures, which extend from the ovaries to the exterior, is to transport the ova and aid in **fertilization** and in pregnancy. They comprise the fallopian tubes (or oviducts or uterine tubes), uterus, and vagina. The fallopian tubes arise from the uterus and end in funnel-shaped fimbriae that receive the released ovum from the adjacent ovary. The ovum remains in the distal end of the fallopian tube for a few days and degenerates if it is not fertilized by a sperm. If the ovum is fertilized, it remains in the fallopian tubes while it divides and becomes a **blastocyst**. Peristaltic movements and the movement of cilia lining the tubes then thrusts the blastocyst towards the uterus where it is implanted and further develops.

The uterus is a muscular, thick-walled organ and has three functions: **menstruation**, pregnancy, and labour (Martini & Nath, 2008). It is composed of three layers (**see Figure 16.1**): the outer perimetrium, the muscular myometrium, and the inner **endometrium**. The endometrium undergoes major changes during each menstrual cycle (discussed later in the chapter). If fertilization does not occur, the endometrium is shed via the vagina (menstruation or 'having a period') and is slowly replaced again over the next month to be prepared for the next possible fertilized ovum.

Menstruation begins at puberty at about the age of 12 years and ceases at the menopause (around age 50). Menarche, the first menstrual period, can start as early as eight years old (though this is rare) and it is thought that the timing of menarche is influenced by both genetic and environmental factors, including nutritional status. Improved nutrition, the attainment of larger body mass (Frisch, 1987), and the increased incidence of childhood obesity are factors that have been linked with the earlier onset of menarche (Kaplowitz, 2008). Other potential contributing factors include exposure to environmental contaminants, which may mimic oestrogens and thus modulate the timing of menarche (Euling *et al.*, 2008).

If fertilization does occur, the fertilized ovum is implanted in the endometrium and develops into a foetus during pregnancy. At the time of delivery the uterus undergoes powerful rhythmic contractions during labour. The anatomy of the uterus is composed of the upper region, the body, and the narrow lower region is the **cervix**. The fundus is where the fallopian tubes enter the uterus (**Figure 16.1**). The cervix is a cylindrical structure containing openings at each end: the internal and external os (**Figure 16.1**). The vagina (or birth canal) is a tubular organ that extends from the external os of the cervix to the exterior and its function is to receive the male sperm during intercourse.

The glands

The mammary glands or breasts and the Bartholin's glands (mentioned above) are the key glands of the female reproductive system (Martini & Nath, 2008). The breasts secrete milk, which provides nourishment to the newborn. Though primitive breasts are present in men and children, it is only in females that they become fully developed after puberty. Milk-secreting alveolar glands become activated under the influence of prolactin, which is released by the pituitary gland after birth. These glands are located in lobules that combine to form 15–25 lobes. Lactiferous ducts converge at the protruding nipple (**Figure 16.3**).

Oxytocin stimulates the ejection of milk in response to the suckling of the infant. During pregnancy and at the time of childbirth colostrum is secreted, so milk is produced about three days after birth.

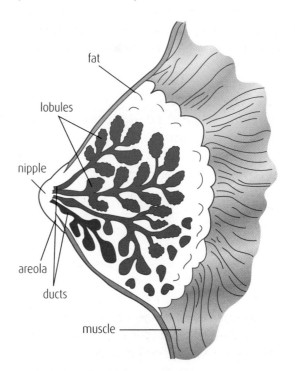

CROSS SECTION THROUGH THE BREAST

Figure 16.3 The female breast

Female reproductive cycle

There are two cycles that occur in the female post-puberty. One occurs in the endometrial lining of the uterus, the menstrual cycle, and the second occurs in the ovaries, the **ovarian cycle** (Martini & Nath, 2008). There are distinct phases to each cycle that at first glance seem complicated. Analogous to the role of a referee regulating two teams in a football match over a defined time frame, hormones tightly regulate the two cycles in the course of a month. The aim is that both the menstrual and ovarian cycles are in phase, so that once the released ovum is fertilized, the endometrial lining is ready for implantation. The female reproductive cycle during the childbearing years varies from 21 to 40 days, but the average length is 28 days. **Figure 16.4** illustrates the concurrent events in the ovaries and endometrium over a 28 day cycle.

Ovarian and menstrual cycles

Day one of the menstrual cycle is marked by the onset of menstruation (menstrual phase) when the endometrium is shed. This lasts for four or five days. Gonadotropin-releasing hormone is released by the hypothalamus and stimulates the release of follicle stimulating hormone (FSH) from the anterior pituitary. As the name indicates, the role of this hormone is to stimulate the development of primary follicles in the ovary.

One of these will become the mature Graffian follicle containing the ovum, and this is the follicular phase. The maturing follicles release oestrogen, which triggers the repair of the endometrium (proliferative phase). Oestrogen levels peak about 32 hours before **ovulation**. These high levels switch off FSH production and trigger the release of luteinizing hormone (LH) from the anterior pituitary. LH levels surge prior to ovulation, signalling the release of the ovum from the Graffian follicle, which occurs around day 14. Kits aimed at detecting increased LH levels in urine have been manufactured commercially to predict ovulation, thereby indicating a female's most fertile period, which lasts only a few days.

Following ovulation and under the influence of LH, the ruptured Graffian follicle is transformed into the corpus luteum, which releases large levels of progesterone in addition to oestrogen. In the ovary, this phase is called the luteal phase. The rising level of progesterone further thickens the endometrium and promotes vascularization (secretory phase) to facilitate implantation of the fertilized ovum.

If unfertilized, the ovum disintegrates and is reabsorbed. In the ovary, the corpus luteum degenerates to become the corpus albicans, which results in falling levels of oestrogen and progesterone. This dearth of hormonal stimulation signals to the endometrium to shed, and thus initiates menstruation and the next menstrual cycle.

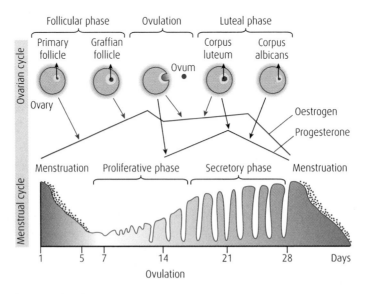

Figure 16.4 Ovarian and menstrual cycles

MALE REPRODUCTIVE SYSTEM

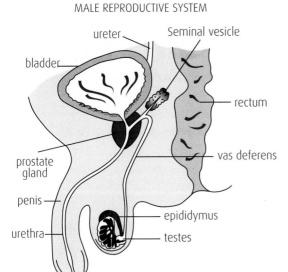

Figure 16.5 The male reproductive system
© EMIS and PiP 2009 as directed on http://www.patient.co.uk

If after sexual intercourse the ovum is fertilized, the corpus luteum continues to produce oestrogen and progesterone, which assists with implantation in the endometrium. Within eight to ten days after fertilization, the **embryo** and placenta produce human chorionic gonadotropin, which is the basis of the home pregnancy kit signifying early pregnancy.

Male reproductive system

The male reproductive system produces, stores, and transports sperm outside the body. In the male, the testes are the essential sex organs or gonads and are the organs that produce sperm and the male sex hormone, testosterone (Martini & Nath, 2008). Sperm production and maturation takes about 72 days and once puberty occurs, this is a continual process. The accessory reproductive structures comprising glands and ducts help in the maturation, nutrition, and transportation of the sperm through the male reproductive system and into the female's body for fertilization. The anatomy of the male reproductive system is illustrated in **Figure 16.5**.

External genitalia

The penis and scrotum comprise the external structures of the male reproductive system. The penis delivers sperm

into the female reproductive system, and urine to the exterior. It is covered by a loose layer of skin and the tissue at the end forms the glans penis. In uncircumcised males the glans penis is covered by a fold of loose skin, the foreskin or prepuce. The penis contains spongy erectile tissue and a large vascular supply so that during sexual arousal, the arteries dilate and fill the spongy tissue with blood, resulting in an erection. The scrotum is a loose sack of skin and contains the testes, which are suspended by the spermatic cords. This arrangement ensures that the temperature in the testes is about 3°C cooler than normal body temperature, which is optimal for sperm development.

Essential sex organs

Testes

The pair of testes develops within the abdomen but about two months before birth (or sometimes just before or just after birth), they descend into the scrotum. Occasionally one or both testes fail to descend and remain in the abdomen or in the inguinal canal, so surgery may be required to reposition them. Within each testis are lobules comprising the seminiferous tubules lined by epithelial cells, which develop into sperm following cell division. This is called **spermatogenesis** and is driven by FSH released by the anterior pituitary gland. The seminiferous tubules are supported by loose connective tissue containing interstitial Leydig and Sertoli cells.

At puberty, LH activates the Leydig cells to secrete testosterone, which is responsible for the secondary sex characteristics: facial hair, hair growth in the pubic area and axilliae, deepening of the voice, larger bone structure, and increased muscle mass. The Sertoli cells have a role in releasing the mature sperm into the tubules. Therefore analogous to the ovaries in the female, the testes also have exocrine (sperm producing) and endocrine (testosterone producing) functions and these duties are performed by different cell populations in the testes (Martini & Nath, 2008).

Accessory reproductive structures

Ducts

The duct system functions as the sperm transport system and include the epididymis, deferent duct (vas deferens), ejaculatory duct, and urethra. The seminiferous tubules of the testes open into the epididymis, which comprises a tightly coiled tube attached to the back of the testes. The sperm reside in the epididymis for up to two weeks while they mature. The deferent duct begins at the epididymis and exits the scrotum to enter the abdominal region of the body. After passing over the bladder, the deferent duct combines with the duct of the seminal vesicle forming the ejaculatory duct. This duct passes through the prostate and joins the urethra, which is a tube running from the bladder to the end of the penis. Because the urethra is shared by the urinary and reproductive systems, muscular sphincters automatically regulate the transport of semen when urine is flowing and vice versa.

The glands

Three glands—the seminal vesicles, the prostate gland, and the bulbourethral glands (**Figure 16.5**)—produce secretions that when combined with sperm form seminal fluid or semen. The seminal vesicles are located behind the bladder and produce a viscous alkaline secretion that makes up about 60% of the seminal fluid. This secretion contains fructose and nutrients to provide the sperm with energy. The prostate gland is located below the bladder and produces a thin, milky-white, alkaline fluid that helps maintain the mobility of the sperm and comprises 30% of the seminal fluid. The bulbourethral glands or Cowper's glands are located below the prostate gland. These glands secrete thick, clear, alkaline mucus that acts as a lubricant during sexual intercourse and makes up 5% of the seminal fluid. The alkaline secretions neutralize the acidity of the urethra caused by any residual traces of urine, and the acidic environment of the female reproductive tract (Martini & Nath, 2008).

Semen and sperm

Not only does the seminal fluid provide the sperm with essential nutrients, but it also dilutes them and provides a medium through which the sperm can move. Sperm contain three parts: a head region, which contains the DNA and is encapsulated by the **acrosome**; a midpiece that contains the mitochondria necessary to generate ATP to propel the tail; and the tail itself (Martini & Nath, 2008).

Semen contains an antibiotic, seminalplasmin, which can destroy certain bacteria. Two to five millilitres of semen is normally ejaculated, which contains somewhere between 50 to 150 million sperm per millilitre, though only one is required to fertilize the ovum.

Now that the anatomy and physiology have been described, the remaining sections of this chapter will describe the clinical skills most frequently practised in the context of the reproductive system. In particular, the external genitalia will be discussed again in the following sections describing the preparation of a child for pelvic examination, swab procedure, and post-operative care of dressings on genitalia.

16.1 **Preparing the child for pelvic examination** 🅐

This is an advanced skill. You *must* check whether you can assist with or undertake any aspect of this skill, in line with local policy.

Definition

A pelvic examination is a clinical procedure in which a healthcare practitioner examines some or all of the male or female reproductive organs (described earlier in the sections on external genitalia). The pelvic area is a sensitive and private area of the body for any child, and pelvic examinations can cause discomfort or pain. The role of the nurse is to communicate with compassion (Nursing and Midwifery Council (NMC), 2006) and prepare the child for this examination, but an understanding of the anatomy and physiology and of the procedure is also important. Further reading of Chapter Two will help with your understanding of communicating with children and family centred care.

Studies have indicated that children and young adults are often not well prepared for procedures and that their participation in the decision making processes is limited (Runeson *et al.*, 2007). More information and preparation time for the child and their family is therefore needed prior to the procedure. This information needs to be tailored to the child's understanding, which can vary according to age and experience, hence the importance of good communication skills (NMC, 2006), clear explanations, and adequate time to consent to and ask questions about the examination.

In the female, the pelvic examination looks at the reproductive organs (**see Figures 16.1** and **16.2**), the bladder, and the rectum; refer back to the anatomy section above. The examination involves four stages: an abdominal palpation, observation of the external genitalia, insertion of a **speculum** to look inside the vagina, and lastly **digital examination** of the vagina.

In the male the examination involves inspection of the external genitalia including the penis (**Figure 16.5**), looking for abnormalities such as **hypospadias** (a congenital abnormality of the urethral opening; see the Glossary for further information). It may also involve palpating the testes to ascertain if they have descended, which means that the testes have moved down from the abdomen, where they grew and developed in the foetus, to the scrotum. Look at the anatomy and physiology section above to remind yourself about the male reproductive system.

Pelvic examinations are used for a variety of reasons: to screen for infections or abnormalities, to diagnose infections, and to treat reproductive and sexual health problems (see the further reading section for more resources on **sexually transmitted infections**, adolescent consent to sexual intercourse, and sexual health). They are intimate examinations. Nurses need to be sensitive to the individual's needs and maintain the dignity of the child or young person; to care with compassion (NMC, 2006).

Nurses also need to be aware of childhood sexual awareness development (Rollins *et al.*, 2005) and to tailor their care appropriately to each child. All of this care and preparation has to be delivered in partnership with the family. This involves full consultation with the family, including explaining procedures and clarifying any questions. This is essential to ensure the child feels in control of this intimate examination and helps reduce their anxiety about the procedure. Consider how the child might feel in this situation and be sensitive to their needs. A full discussion of family centred care is provided in Chapter Two.

Context

The skill of preparing a child for a pelvic examination takes time to develop. It is dependent upon establishing a good rapport with the child or young person, and

their family if this is appropriate—some adolescents will require preparation and examination without their parents' knowledge.

The psychological preparation of a three-month-old baby with a congenital abnormality will be entirely different from that of a six-year-old with a need for surgery. The skill with the three-month-old baby is in preparing the parents and ensuring the room is warm enough for the baby to be undressed and examined in. The six-year-old will need more knowledge of what is going to happen to them, and the nurse will also need to reassure the parents and empower them to assist in their child's care.

Empowering parents is an important nursing skill. A trusting, caring relationship with parents allows partnership working and sharing of information and perceptions (Coleman, 2002). However, a sexually active sixteen-year-old adolescent will need an entirely different approach. Undertake this skill in a safe, legal, and ethical manner with awareness that the adolescent is capable of autonomy. The nurse will need to be able to empower and inform the adolescent so they can make informed decisions for themselves, with appropriate support and knowledge. There may also be an opportunity for health promotion, a topic that you will be familiar with from reading Chapter Four.

Many problems can present to healthcare professionals working with children that require a pelvic examination. It is important to always establish the underlying physical need to examine the genitalia. Observations of vital signs and other clinical observations (as outlined in Chapter Five) may also be required, depending on the child's condition. As the child's nurse you should understand the clinical need for the pelvic examination, so will be best placed to assess the child's need for other clinical observations. You also have an important role in preparation of and providing explanations to the child and their parents. The underlying condition may require either medical or surgical treatment, or both.

Males may present with infections, **undescended testes**, **retractile testes**, hypospadias, and some types of tumour (Prem, 2006). In female children the need for pelvic examination may be related to **menstrual problems** in puberty, infections, or even the removal of a foreign body. Revise the anatomy and physiology section above and **Figure 16.4** to familiarize yourself with the female reproductive cycles.

Sexually active adolescents may need to have a pelvic examination (Daley & Cromwell, 2002) to screen for sexually transmitted infections in both sexes. In females it may be required to fit an **internal contraceptive device** (Faculty of Sexual and Reproductive Healthcare (FSRH), 2007) if the benefits of long-term contraception outweigh the risks. In males the adolescent may become aroused and embarrassed during the examination (Grundy-Bowers & Davis, 2006). It is essential that the nurse does not become embarrassed too. The nurse must reassure the young person that arousal is perfectly normal.

A pelvic examination is not normally used in child protection cases (this is where there is suspected child abuse) as the child will need to be examined again by police staff. A pelvic examination may subject the child to even greater emotional or psychological distress, and children's nursing aims, where possible, not to cause trauma (Taylor, 2006). The examination of young people in cases of suspected child abuse is usually undertaken by specifically trained forensic personnel (medically trained staff involved in criminal cases, as child abuse is a crime). If you are asked to prepare a child for a pelvic examination in child protection cases, it is important that you ensure you act as the advocate for the child: say no, refer to a more senior member of staff, and document the rationale. For more information on child protection look at the further reading resources at the end of this chapter, in particular the *Every Child Matters* and Childline websites. In addition, the examination of prepubescent young people should always be performed by trained paediatricians.

Alternative interventions

In many cases a swab of the area, abdominal palpation, and abdominal ultrasound may be performed to reduce the need for a pelvic examination. A swab, palpation, and ultrasound are less invasive to the young person and may reveal as much or more than an observation of the genitals would.

Communication skills relating to family centred care

Families, children, and young people need information prior to situations about which they may have little or no understanding. Informing children and their families prior to clinical examinations is important (Lawes *et al.*, 2008). The preparation of the child and family is the role of the nurse. Revisit Chapter Two for more detail on communication skills.

Ensure that consent is sought prior to the pelvic examination and that the rights of the child are respected. Verbal consent is adequate for this examination as long as the nurse has ensured that the meaning of consent is understood. There is a tension between respecting the rights of the child or young person and family centred care. Read Chapter Four to familiarize yourself with issues of consent and preparation of a child for procedures.

Communication skills are utilized to ensure the family understands the need for the examination, using language appropriate to their social, cultural, and developmental capability. Communication is also vital to help the child cope with the examination and is an essential skill (NMC, 2006). Staff and parental behaviour and coping styles have been shown to have an impact in reducing the child's distress (Lawes *et al.*, 2008). As the child's nurse you can support and educate the parents to use distraction techniques, such as reading a book, watching a video, or talking prior to the examination. Educating parents also empowers them to be involved in their child's care, if they so wish. During the examination using breathing techniques, such as blowing bubbles, can be effective in reducing stress. The role of the parent or carer also needs to be explained before the examination, especially if the child is to sit on their lap, so the parent knows what is expected of them. Chapters Two and Five provide more information on these techniques.

Multicultural aspects

Any intimate examination needs to be considered within the cultural and religious beliefs of the family. This may include considering the sex of the practitioner undertaking the clinical skill, as religious beliefs may prohibit this being undertaken by someone of the opposite sex (NMC, 2008). Female genital mutilation is still practised in some African cultures (Taylor, 2007) and nurses need to be aware of this practice. In the UK this practice is illegal.

Procedure: Preparing the child for pelvic examination

Preparation

Proper preparation is vital. The NMC (2006) stipulate this as a skill: organization of aspects of care.

Preparing the child/young person

Preparation of the child and their family is paramount. Use of play (Jun-Tai, 2008) can help comfort and reassure children during an unfamiliar or frightening procedure such as a pelvic examination. The use of play can help prepare a child and their family for the procedure (look back at Chapter Two to read more about the use of play). Ensure valid consent has been obtained before any procedure and double check that the environment has been prepared with the necessary equipment (see below).

The young person needs to empty their bladder prior to the procedure. They can wear their own clothes but remove their lower garments at the last minute. The young person is then covered in a small sheet for privacy.

Positioning of the child or young person is important in minimizing pain and trauma (Thomas *et al.*, 2002). More than one appointment may be needed to gain sufficient trust and confidence. The recommended position for young girls is supine, lying on their back, (Thomas *et al.*, 2002). The young person can be on their carer's lap, with a frog-legged position. The examination may require the young person to turn into the left lateral to view the perineum.

In pre-pubertal boys, the recommendation is that the examination can also be carried out on the carer's lap (Thomas *et al.*, 2002). The external genitalia can be inspected and the foreskin, if present, should be gently retracted to view the urethral meatus and frenulum. The scrotum should be gently palpated to assess the presence and descent of both testes. The examination may be completed in the left lateral position to view the perineum. Revisit the anatomy and physiology section above if these terms are still new to you, to help you visualize the anatomy.

Post-pubertal females can be screened according to local protocols for female adults if tolerant of speculum examination. Remember, in some pubertal females it may be impossible to pass a speculum.

Equipment/environment

Before the examination ensure all the equipment is gathered and in working order. All preparation of the environment and equipment should be completed before the child and their parent or chaperone enters the examination room. This is important as it helps to reduce their anxiety and time spent waiting for the examination. Prior preparation also minimizes the time the child or young person is exposed.

The examination should take place in a closed room that cannot be accessed while the examination is in progress. Toilet facilities should be available to the young person; they may need to go to the toilet both before and after the examination. If an examination table is used it should be placed facing away from the door. This will help the young person feel more secure. The examination table may be omitted depending on the child or young person's age and wishes. A carer's lap may be used instead, to comfort and hold the child. A chair may therefore be needed for the carer or parent. A flexible light source is used for the inspection of the genitalia; ensure the light is in working order prior to the child or young person entering the examination room.

In females, vaginal specula (plural of speculum) may be required in various sizes to allow for the correct speculum to be chosen for the young person. These are either reusable or disposable. Warm running water will be needed to warm the speculum and to cleanse the vaginal area prior to and following the examination. Water will also be required for hand washing, both for the practitioner performing the examination and the child if they assist with the examination to point out the problem. Lubricating jelly is also required for ease of insertion of the speculum and the practitioner's fingers during the digital examination.

Methods of documentation

Following any procedure, all the events need to be recorded (NMC, 2007) and all records should contain accurate documentation of what happened. If the young

Step-by-step guide to preparing the child for pelvic examination

This is an advanced skill. You *must* check whether you can assist with or undertake any aspect of this skill, in line with local policy.

Step	Rationale
1 Keep young person covered as much as possible.	To ensure young person is treated with dignity and respect.
2 Show compassion for young person.	To deliver care that meets the physical and emotional needs of the young person.
3 Communicate appropriately with the child or young person.	To encourage young person and reduce their anxiety.
4 Help the young person relax with breathing or distraction techniques.	To reduce the child or young person's anxiety.
5 As the nurse responsible for the child's welfare, question another practitioner if their practice is not evidence based.	To safeguard the young person.
6 Stop examination if appropriate.	The children's nurse must recognize and respond to the emotional discomfort of the young person.

person found the examination particularly difficult, document this, to protect them from further harm. It is also worth documenting what distraction techniques or breathing exercises were helpful to the child, so they may be utilized again (more information on this can be found in Chapter Five).

After the procedure: Observations/results and next action

After the procedure it is important to encourage the young person to redress, assisting them if appropriate. Thank the young person for their cooperation, reassure them that they did very well, and give positive feedback. If the young person is female and has had a speculum examination, inform them that there may be some slight bleeding following the examination.

Nursing Alert

Nurses need to be sensitive to children's and young people's previous experiences, which may involve sexual abuse, when preparing a young person to be examined intimately. Nurses working with children and young people have an obligation to safeguard children from harm. Presumptive indicators of sexual abuse include direct disclosure from the child or young person, genital or rectal trauma, and a sexually transmitted infection in a prepubescent child. Abnormal behaviour may also raise staff suspicion. Physical indicators include recurrent or persistent vaginal discharge. See the Department for Education and Skills (2006) publication *What to do if You're Worried a Child is being Abused* for the next steps to take.

The community setting

Sexual healthcare and preparation for a pelvic examination may be the role of the nurse in the community, in a GP practice, in a family planning clinic, or even in the school as a school nurse. All care is the same as previously documented, even though the setting has changed.

16.2 **Preparing the child for a swab procedure** Ⓐ

This is an advanced skill. You *must* check whether you can assist with or undertake any aspect of this skill, in line with local policy.

Definition

A swab is a cotton wool-tipped stick (similar to a cotton bud but longer) used to obtain a specimen. Specimens are samples of tissue, body fluids, secretions, or excretions. Nurses often have the responsibility of collecting, labelling, and sending specimens to the laboratory for further analysis. The collection of a swab specimen is a clinical skill, supported by the NMC (2006) essential skills clusters, which include infection prevention and control. The validity of a swab result is dependent upon good infection control procedures and swab technique.

In nursing children, the key skill is in preparing the child and family for the procedure, i.e. communication (NMC, 2006). A swab of the reproductive system is usually taken to identify an infection, or for screening purposes in sexually active adolescents. A swab of the reproductive system may be a non-invasive procedure, such as a swab of a wound. It may also be invasive, such as inside the vagina for screening purposes. Swab procedures are only to be used when there is a clinical need for the investigation to be carried out (Perry, 2007).

The Health Protection Agency (2007) shows that rates of sexually transmitted infections in young people are still rising. According to the World Health Organization (2008), the most common cause of sexually transmitted infection is a bacterium called *Chlamydia trachomatis*, commonly just called *Chlamydia*. Rates of *Chlamydia* are also rising in the United States (Chiaradonna, 2008) and the UK (Bradley-Stevenson, 2007).

Context

It is important to consider that vaginal infections can be adequately diagnosed without a speculum, by use of a swab (Blake *et al.*, 2000). Even if an adolescent is sexually active, a speculum examination is a more invasive swab procedure than might be necessary. Check the clinical need for the swab procedure and consider not performing a speculum examination to undertake the swab procedure.

The UK's National Chlamydia Screening Programme (2007) recommends that young people perform their own swab procedure. This is supported by other international research as a valid technique for *Chlamydia* screening (Langille *et al.*, 2008).

Alternative interventions

As a swab should only be undertaken when clinically indicated, there are not usually any alternative interventions. Clinical indications of an infection include pyrexia (raised temperature), tachycardia (a rapid heart rate), redness (erythema), swelling, increased pain, and offensive discharge. In the case of screening for sexually transmitted infections, a urine test is sometimes sufficient but a swab is usually more accurate. For screening purposes the swab may be undertaken by the individual themselves, thus reducing their embarrassment and increasing the uptake of the screening process.

Procedure: Preparing the child for a swab

Preparation

A private room, with the appropriate nursing and supportive adults, is suitable for the collection of the swab for the comfort, safety, and dignity of the child or young person. Swabs taken for microbiology need to be taken before treatment starts. This means that if an infection is suspected in a postoperative wound, the wound should be swabbed prior to antibiotics being prescribed and administered. This is to ensure the correct antibiotics are prescribed for the microbe growing in the wound.

Equipment

All essential equipment should be prepared prior to the child or young person entering the treatment room.

Step-by-step guide to the swab procedure

This is an advanced skill. You *must* check whether you can assist with or undertake any aspect of this skill, in line with local policy.

Step	Rationale
1 Ensure the child is comfortable.	Avoids unnecessary discomfort for the child.
2 Maintain the dignity of the child or young person, minimizing the exposure of the child.	To ensure young person is treated with dignity and respect.
3 Reassure the child or young person.	To deliver care that meets the physical and emotional needs of the young person.
4 Use distraction techniques suitable for the age and development of the individual.	Avoids unnecessary discomfort for the child.
5 If the lesion is dry, dampen a bacteriology swab with sterile saline. If the lesion is crusted, soak it with sterile saline before sampling.	To ensure appropriate specimen collection techniques are used and that the practitioner is performing evidence-based care.
6 Sweep the swab across the entire lesion in a zig-zag, turning the swab as you go (Hickin, 2008).	To obtain the specimen.
7 Question another practitioner if their practice is not evidence based.	To act as the child's advocate.
8 Stop the procedure if necessary.	To respond to the child's emotional needs.

The room should have hand washing facilities and sterile equipment including protective clothing, gloves, specimen container, request forms, and specimen bags. A working light source is essential to visualize accurately the infected area or area for screening.

Consent and communication

Consent prior to any specimen collection is paramount; see Chapter Four for more about issues of consent prior to procedures. Ensure you as the nurse understand the clinical need for the procedure and the relevant anatomy and physiology. Remember that adolescents can consent for themselves.

It is important to reduce any anxiety that the child and their parents may have. A swab of an infected or postoperative wound may be painful; this has to be considered prior to the specimen collection. Information is delivered verbally or in a written pamphlet (or both) so that the child and family understand why the swab procedure is necessary and how it will be undertaken. If as the child's nurse you do not know why the swab is being taken, you will not be able to inform the child and family, so it is imperative you understand the clinical need for the investigation. Consent is only valid if the reasons for the procedure are explained in full; without full information the child and their family are unable to participate in the decision making process (Runeson *et al.*, 2002).

Step-by-step guide to labelling the specimen form

This is an advanced skill. You *must* check whether you can assist with or undertake any aspect of this skill, in line with local policy.

Step	Rationale
1. Label with patient name and date of birth.	To identify the patient accurately (there may be two patients with the same name).
2. Label with hospital number and ward.	To identify the patient and determine which ward the results need to go back to.
3. Label with date and time of specimen collection.	To ensure the specimen is fresh.
4. Label with specimen type, for example, low vaginal swab, urethral swab.	To determine what is normal flora and what is abnormal growth.
5. Include diagnosis, signs and symptoms, or screening purpose. Example: Possible infection due to discharge.	To aid in testing and diagnosis.
6. Include relevant history. Example: Recurrent previous infections.	To aid in testing and diagnosis.
7. Include current drug treatments. This is especially important if already on antibiotics.	To aid in testing and diagnosis.
8. Include contact details of requesting practitioner.	For laboratory staff to contact if needed.
9. Include whether the specimen is a known biohazard.	So the laboratory knows whether further precautions are needed with the specimen.

Chapter Two and Chapter Four provide more information on communicating with children and their families and preparing for procedures. Simple distraction techniques may assist the child prior to the swab procedure, such as talking about non-hospital events (for example football or school), which may take the child's mind off the procedure. Blowing bubbles and using breathing as a distraction technique during the swab procedure may also alleviate some of the anxiety and pain associated with a painful or frightening event. Preparation prior to the procedure is important in reducing the child's anxiety and preparing the parent for their part in the procedure.

Methods of documentation

The collection and sending of the specimen should be recorded in the patient's clinical notes. The specimen form should be fully completed by the practitioner undertaking the specimen collection.

Specific observations to undertake following the skill

If the young female has had a speculum examination to obtain the swab, there may be some bleeding following the procedure. This needs to be communicated to the individual; it is usually self-limiting (it stops without treatment) but ensure that the young person has the contact number of the ward or department to use if she is concerned or needs further reassurance.

Remember that children that are nursed in the hospital or community reflect a multicultural community and cognisance needs to be taken of this and their particular needs. As with the previous section, any intimate examination needs to be considered within the context of the cultural and religious beliefs of the family. This may include considering the sex of the practitioner undertaking the clinical skill, as religious beliefs may prohibit this being undertaken by someone of the opposite sex (NMC, 2008).

Postoperative swab procedures may be taken in the community in the child's own home. Signs of infection frequently appear four days postoperatively when the child would already have been discharged from hospital.

Sexual health screening

Sexual health screening may be carried out in a variety of care settings, including GP practices, Genito-Urinary Medicine clinics, family planning clinics, and school health check-up clinics. All practitioners working in these areas need to have the knowledge and skills to deal with adolescents who request sexual health screening.

Aftercare

Encourage or assist the child to redress as appropriate. Reassure the child or young person and their family. Thank the child for their cooperation.

Next steps

The specimen needs to be transported to the laboratory following collection. Ensure the correctly labelled specimen is placed in the appropriate location for transportation. As a swab is only taken if there is a clinical need, the results need to be given to the young person and

their family. Ensure the communication of swab results is transparent, i.e. that the family knows how they will receive the results and when to expect them.

> **Nursing Alert**
>
> It is recommended that routine cultures of the pharyngeal, rectal, and vaginal areas be taken in all cases of suspected child sexual abuse, regardless of clinical findings. The presence of two infections, namely *Neisseria gonorrhoea* and *Chlamydia trachomatis*, remain the only conclusive markers for sexual abuse. Children do not contract these infections without having been exposed to sexual abuse.

Perhaps one of the most controversial areas of consent is when a young person requests sexual health treatment. The tests of Gillick competence and Fraser guidelines have been used as the benchmark (Grundy-Bowers & Davis, 2006). The law states that a child under the age of 16 can consent to their own treatment without their parents' knowledge or permission. If the young person is considered to be competent then the practitioner can go ahead and provide the treatment requested. In order to provide clarity on this issue for the practitioner, the Department of Health (2004a) has published guidelines for practitioners.

The increasing prevalence of sexually transmitted infections is not just a problem in terms of how much money it costs to treat such infections, but in the sequelae (the events that can occur following the infection, such as reduced fertility). Sexual health has long-term implications for health and fertility. Therefore there is a growing need for sexual health screening needs to be addressed by all health practitioners within children's services. There is also a national *Chlamydia* screening programme in the UK (Department of Health, 2004b).

The community setting

In the community setting adolescents are encouraged to make positive decisions about their sexual health and to undertake screening procedures (such as *Chlamydia* screening) if they have had sexual intercourse. The school nurse or family planning practitioner may provide information to the adolescent who is able to make informed decisions about their own care.

There are many environments outside of the hospital setting where swab procedures may be required. The transfer of children to their home environment as soon as possible postoperatively means there are more nurses working within the community. Any sign of a postoperative infection may require a swab procedure.

In adolescents there are several community initiatives requiring swab procedures, including *Chlamydia* screening.

16.3 **Care of dressings on genitalia postoperatively**

This is an advanced skill. You *must* check whether you can assist with or undertake any aspect of this skill, in line with local policy.

Definition

The most frequent operations on the genitalia are on males and can be divided into problems that are congenital (born with) and those that are acquired (develop) (Steinbrecher & Malone, 2008). The congenital abnormalities include **cryptorchidism** (undescended testes (one in twenty births; Great Ormond Street Hospital, 2004)), **hydrocele**, and hypospadias (two to eight cases per 1000 with the incidence rising; Pierik *et al.*, 2002). Acquired problems requiring surgery include **torsion**, **hernias**, tumours, and **phimosis** (tightness of the foreskin). Any surgery is traumatic for children and parents, but surgery on the genitals seems to have further consequences, including future fertility, psychological damage, and future sexual function.

Children tend to heal quicker postoperatively than adults but the need for careful selection of dressings and for the participation of children and their families in the care of dressings postoperatively is paramount. Children are naturally inquisitive, therefore any dressing is a source of interest to them and their safety must be maintained in relation to the appropriateness of the dressing used. Care of dressings and removal of dressings on the genitalia are a source of anxiety for parents and children alike. Wound management and dressings are frightening procedures for children and a lot of psychological support and preparation will be required.

All wounds are associated with pain, and this pain has to be assessed and managed by the child's nurse. The principles of wound management in children are to alleviate pain, minimize emotional distress, and minimize

scarring. The ethos of family centred care is that children are transferred to their home environment as soon as possible following surgery. Parents are often involved in caring for their children whilst their postoperative dressings are still intact, especially with a child still in nappies.

Infection control principles also apply (see Chapter Five); however, it is important to apply these principles with reference to child and family centred care. The purpose of a sterile postoperative dressing is to reduce the potential for bacterial contamination, a serious postoperative complication in children. Merei (2004) questions the need for paediatric patients to have dressings at all on clean surgical wounds. This research suggested there was no significant difference in acquiring wound infections in dressed or non-dressed surgical wounds in children. Considering how distressing wound care can be for some children and their parents, this area of care needs further research to clarify what constitutes best practice. Consult with local policies and guidelines when considering the best approaches to use in your situation.

Context

The child's nurse should have a working knowledge of the anatomy and physiology of the affected area and understand the process of healing prior to undertaking the care of a dressing.

The child and their family must be psychologically prepared for the procedure prior to the dressing. The presence of a wound places a child or young person at increased risk of infection due to the breach of the skin, the body's natural defence mechanism. Wound infection can delay healing and compromise the child. Preventing infection by wound management is vital for the rapid recovery of the child or young person. Review the section on wound assessment and management in Chapter Six.

Alternative interventions

The use of dressings and deciding which dressing constitutes best practice is a sphere of nursing that is continually evolving. The rationale for dressing use postoperatively is to apply a dressing that prevents swelling, provides support for the healing tissues, and reduces pain and discomfort. It is acknowledged that dressing removal is often a traumatic and painful experience for the child and their parents. The clinical need for a dressing and the most appropriate dressing following a particular surgical procedure is constantly changing as new evidence-based research emerges.

Common standard postoperative practice for hypospadias repair (this example is used because it is one of the most common genital anomalies in boys) is that there is still no one best practice example of which dressing to use postoperatively. Some authors (McLorie *et al.*, 2001; Van der Werff, 2002) advocate no dressing. These authors suggest there is no significant difference in surgical outcome with no dressing when compared to a standard dressing. Hence these authors suggest a no dressing policy is best practice as it minimizes the difficulty of dressing care and removal. Other authors advocate one dressing over another (Van Savage *et al.*, 2000).

Consider standard practice in your area and use up-to-date research to challenge any practice that is not best evidence based. During your nursing career the area of wound management and what constitutes best practice will need to be constantly renewed and reviewed.

Communication skills relating to family centred care

The psychological and emotional impact of a wound on a child cannot be underestimated. Wound healing is a complex process, which fortunately requires little nursing intervention as intervention is a source of stress for many children and their families. But wound management and dressing removal do require nursing intervention. Information and participation in painful or anxiety-provoking procedures, including dressing changes, assists in the psychological preparation of the child and their parents. As stated in the previous sections, other factors that reduce the stress of the child during the procedure include nurses' ability to maintain a competent attitude and parental coping styles. Parents are often unsure of how to help their child to cope during the procedure. By explaining the procedure to the child and parent/s, the nurse can reduce parental and child distress. If the parent is included (if appropriate) they can be encouraged to distract the child during the procedure, resulting in a greater reduction in the pain and anxiety felt by the child (Lawes *et al.*, 2008).

Procedure: Care of dressings on genitalia postoperatively

Preparation

As in the previous sections the equipment and environment should be prepared in advance out of sight of the child; this minimizes their waiting times and reduces their anxiety. Reducing the time the child waits in the treatment room minimizes further distress in the child and parent/s. If all equipment is prepared prior to the child's arrival the procedure can commence as soon as the child is ready and be completed as expediently as possible. For some children seeing the equipment prepared increases their anxiety levels. That is not to say that the child should not look at what equipment is to be used. Indeed if appropriate, show the child the new dressing. This will help them understand what is involved and how the dressing will be applied to their body.

Before dressing changes and removal, especially following surgery, the child is offered analgesia. Depending on the type of dressing various practices are used to reduce the anxiety. It is common practice for hypospadias repair, for example, for the child with a dressing to soak in the bath prior to dressing removal, to soak and loosen the dressing. You will find more information about pain assessment and management and wound care in Chapter Six.

The environment is prepared. Windows should be closed, to prevent the child from getting cold and to reduce the contamination risks. Dressings should not take place in a hospital environment when bed making and routine cleaning are being carried out, as these activities generate dust. The surrounding environment should be as clean as possible. All equipment, such as the dressing trolley, should be cleansed prior to and following use.

Ensure the correct number of people are present, to maintain a safe environment for the child, emotionally and physically. Is there someone capable of distracting the child, blowing bubbles, reading a book, or talking, which are all effective methods of distraction? It is beneficial to have someone available to encourage the child; the parent is not always able to encourage the child during the procedure, as they may be anxious.

Step-by-step guide to the postoperative dressing procedure

This is an advanced skill. You *must* check whether you can assist with or undertake any aspect of this skill, in line with local policy.

Step	Rationale
1 Position child comfortably.	To maximize comfort and dignity.
2 Use distraction techniques.	To reduce stress.
3 Deliver care that is interpreted as kind, warm, sensitive, and compassionate.	To provide care that meets the child's emotional needs and anticipates their anxiety.
4 Decontaminate hands.	Demonstrates effective hand hygiene and the appropriate use of standard infection control precautions.
5 Loosen existing dressing and dispose of appropriately.	This dressing is contaminated and must be disposed of according to infection control policies.
6 Cleanse hands again to open dressing pack.	To take effective measures to prevent and control infection, in accordance with local and national policy.
7 Add any cleansing solutions and new dressing to sterile field.	Ensures these dressings remain sterile.
8 Decontaminate hands.	Demonstrates effective hand hygiene and applies appropriate use of infection control policies.
9 Apply sterile gloves.	Adheres to local infection control policies.
10 Cleanse wound if required using a warmed solution.	Cleansing fluids should be warmed to body temperature to promote wound healing.
11 Assess wound for signs of infection or reaction to previous dressing.	To safely perform basic wound care.
12 Apply new dressing.	To safely perform basic wound care.
13 Dispose of clinical waste.	To dispose of waste in accordance with local policies.

Relevant protective clothing should be worn, an apron and sterile gloves. Hands should be decontaminated prior to and following dressing procedures.

Equipment

Appropriate sterile equipment is used and you must ensure that the outer packaging is clean and dry and not damaged. Check the expiry date of the sterile package. Resources include a sterile dressing pack, a warm solution for cleaning the wound, and a new sterile dressing, if required. The room should also be conducive to maintaining the child's privacy, and warm enough, as they will be exposed while the dressing is taking place.

Consent and communication

Through careful questioning, assessment, and observation check that the family and child have been thoroughly prepared for the procedure. Do they appear to understand what procedure is going to take place? Have they consented to the dressing care? Ensure that the meaning of consent to the treatment and care is understood. If you consider that preparation has not been complete, pause the proceedings to fully assess their information needs, address the gaps in their knowledge appropriately, and gain further consent.

Methods of documentation

As with every nursing intervention, all care provided should be documented by the relevant practitioner (NMC, 2007). Remind yourself about the principles of good record keeping by consulting Chapter Five.

Specific observations to undertake following the skill

Although the nurse will probably have given the child pre-dressing analgesia, the child must also be assessed for pain following the procedure. Adequate pain management is essential in caring for children postoperatively.

Aftercare

Children should wear loose clothing following genital surgery for comfort. Postoperative complications include

infection and bleeding; always assess the wound for signs of infection, which include redness, swelling, increasing pain, and discharge. Still be alert to alternative signs of infection including an elevated temperature and tachycardia.

The child's nurse is required to assist in providing accurate information to children and their parents on the management of a wound, so as to prevent and control infection and to promote healing.

Other factors to consider

The commonest male surgical procedure is circumcision (Malone & Steinbrecher, 2008) because routine infant circumcision is practised in many countries for religious and cultural reasons. There are calls for a ban on female genital mutilation (World Health Organization, 2008) for legal, ethical, cultural, and medical reasons, and the campaign has recently been extended to include male circumcision for non-medical reasons (Anonymous, 2008). Those in favour of male circumcision give lowering urinary tract infections and sexually transmitted infections as the benefits of male circumcision. Those against male circumcision say it causes pain and long-term sexual and psychological trauma. As a nurse, lifelong learning and keeping up to date with evolving campaigns and strategies to protect children are all essential aspects of your career. This area of child health and protection will no doubt be discussed and debated for many years to come. What we consider to be acceptable practice today may change in the future.

Nursing Alert

Postoperative dressings are associated with anxiety and pain. Offer analgesia to the child prior to the dressing procedure to reduce their pain. Prepare the child and their family appropriately to reduce their anxiety.

The community setting

Gormley *et al.,* (2007) have studied home dressing removal following hypospadias repair. Their findings demonstrate positive results; with community support the child can be discharged home sooner, which minimizes the impact on their families. All areas of nursing are branching out into the community. Home dressing removal of hypospadias repair and many other postoperative dressings may become commonplace in the community over the next few years, as research informs and enhances what constitutes best practice.

Conclusion

The skills necessary for preparation for pelvic examinations, swab procedures, and postoperative dressings on the genitals require knowledge of anatomy and physiology and child development, in conjunction with family centred care.

Nurses working with children and their families should remain mindful that some procedures could cause distress. Through partnership working and education, nurses can support the child and family to understand the need for the clinical examination or procedure and enable them to make decisions about their own care.

Thorough preparation is vital, both of the child and their accompanying parents. Distraction techniques are a valuable tool for the nurse during any clinical procedure.

Online resource centre

You may find it helpful to work through our online resources including interactive scenarios intended to help you to develop and apply the skills in this chapter. Where material referenced below is available electronically, we're pleased to provide active web links to the source via 🌐 **http://www.oxfordtextbooks.co.uk/ orc/coyne/**

References

Anonymous (2008) Campaigners call for male circumcision ban. *Nursing Standard* **23** (1), 8.

Blake, D., Duggan, A., Quinn, T., Zenilman, J., & Joffe, A. (2000) Evaluation of vaginal infections in adolescent women: Can it be done without a speculum? *Pediatrics* **105** (1 Pt 1): 156–157.

Bradley-Stevenson, C. (2007) Adolescent sexual health. *Paediatrics and Child Health* **17** (12), 474–479.

Chiaradonna, C. (2008) The Chlamydia cascade: Enhanced STD prevention strategies for adolescents. *Journal of Pediatric Adolescent Gynecology* **21** (5), 233–241.

Coleman, V. (2002) Empowerment: Rhetoric, reality and skills. In L. Smith, V. Coleman, & M. Bradshaw (eds.) *Family Centred-Care: Concept, theory and practice*. Basingstoke: Palgrave.

Daley, A. & Cromwell, P. (2002) How to perform a pelvic exam for the sexually active adolescent. *Nurse Practitioner* **27** (9), 28–43.

Department for Education and Skills (2006) *What to do if You're Worried a Child is being Abused*. Nottingham: DfES publications.

Department of Health (2004a) *Best Practice Guidance for Doctors and Other Health Professionals on the Provision of Advice and Treatment to Young People under 16 on Contraception, Sexual and Reproductive Health*. London: Department of Health.

Department of Health (2004b) *The National Chlamydia Screening Programme in England. Programme overview, core requirements and data collection*, 2nd ed. London: Department of Health.

Euling, S.Y., Selevan, S.G., Pescovitz, O.H., & Skakkebaek, N.E. (2008) Role of environmental factors in the timing of puberty. *Pediatrics* **121** (Suppl. 3), S167–S171.

Faculty of Sexual and Reproductive Healthcare (2007) *Intrauterine Contraception: Clinical Effectiveness Unit, Faculty of Sexual and Reproductive Healthcare Clinical Guidance*. London: Faculty of Sexual and Reproductive Healthcare.

Frisch, R.E. (1987) Body fat, menarche, fitness and fertility. *Human Reproduction* **2** (6), 521–533.

Gormley, A., Fishwick, J., & Withall, B. (2007) Home dressing removal following hypospadias repair. *Journal of Child Health Care* **11** (2), 158–162.

Great Ormond Street Hospital (2004). Available at: **http://www.ich.ucl.ac.uk/gosh_families/ information_sheets/undescended_testicles/ undescended_testicles_families_booklet.pdf** (last accessed July 2008).

Grundy-Bowers, M. & Davies, J. (2006) *Advanced Clinical Skills for GU Nurses*. West Sussex: Wiley.

Health Protection Agency (2007) *Sexually Transmitted Infections, Epidemiological Data*. Available at: **http://www.hpa.org.uk/web/HPAwebFile/ HPAweb_C/1215589014474**

Hickin, L. (2008) Managing skin and nail infections. *Practice Nurse* **35** (10), 19–21.

Jun-Tai, N. (2008) Play in hospital. *Paediatrics and Child Health* **18** (5), 233–237.

Kaplowitz, P.B. (2008) Link between body fat and the timing of puberty. *Pediatrics* **121** (Suppl. 3), S208–S217.

Langille, B., Proudfoot, K., Rigby, J., Aquino-Russell, C., Strang, R., & Forward, K. (2008) A pilot project for Chlamydia screening in adolescent females using self-testing: Characteristics of participants and non-participants. *Canadian Journal of Public Health* **99** (2), 117–120.

Lawes, C., Sawyer, L., Amos, S., Kandiah, M., Pearce, L., & Symonds, J. (2008) Impact of an education programme for staff working with children undergoing painful procedures. *Paedictric Nursing* **20** (2), 33–37.

Malone, P. & Steinbrecher, H. (2008) Medical aspects of male circumcision. *British Medical Journal* **335** (7631), 1206.

Martini, F.H. & Nath, J.L (2008) The reproductive system. In F.H. Martini & J.L. Nath (eds.) *The Fundamentals of Anatomy and Physiology, 8th ed*. London: Pearson Benjamin Cummings.

McLorie, G., Joyner, B., & Herz, D. (2001) A prospective randomised clinical trial to evaluate methods of postoperative care of hypospadias. *The Journal of Urology* **165**, 1669–1672.

Merei, J. (2004) Pediatric clean surgical wounds: Is dressing necessary? *Journal of Pediatric Surgery* **39** (12), 1871–1873.

National Chlamydia Screening Programme (2007) *Maintaining momentum*. London: Health Protection agency. Available at: **http://www.chlamydiascreening.nhs.uk/ps/assets/pdfs/AnnualReport0607.pdf**

Nursing and Midwifery Council (2006) *Advance Information Regarding Essential Skills Clusters for Pre-registration Nursing Programmes. NMC Circular 35/2006*. London: NMC.

Nursing and Midwifery Council (2007) *Record Keeping*. London: NMC.

Nursing and Midwifery Council (2008) *Chaperoning*. London: NMC.

Perry, C. (2007) *Infection Prevention and Control*. Oxford, UK: Blackwell Publishing.

Pierik, F., Burdorf, A., Nijman, J., de Muinck Keizer-Schrama, S., Juttmann, R., & Weber, R. (2002) A high hypospadias rate in The Netherlands. *Human Reproduction* **17** (4), 1112–1115.

Prem, A. (2006) Common paediatric problems. *British Medical Journal* **333**, 486–489.

Rollins, J.A., Bolig, R., & Mahan, C.C. (2005) *Meeting Children's Psychosocial Needs Across the Health-Care Continuum*. Austin, TX: Pro-Ed, Inc.

Runeson, I., Hallstrom, I., Elander, G., & Hermeren, G. (2002) Children's needs during hospitalisation: An observational study of hospitalised boys. *International Journal of Nursing Practice* **8**, 158–166.

Runeson, I., Mårtenson, E., & Enskär, K. (2007) Children's knowledge and degree of participation in decision making when undergoing a clinical diagnostic procedure. *Pediatric Nursing* **33** (6), 505–511.

Steinbrecher, H. & Malone, P. (2008) Testicular problems in children. *Paediatrics and Child Health* **18** (6), 264–267.

Taylor, M. (2006) Mapping the literature of pediatric nursing. *Journal of the Medical Library Association* **94** (2 Suppl.), E128–E136.

Taylor, V. (2007) Female genital mutilation: Cultural practice or child abuse? *Paediatric Nursing* **15** (1), 31–33.

Thomas, A., Forster, A., Robinson, K., & Rogstad, A. (2002) For the Clinical Effectiveness Group (Association of Genitourinary Medicine and the Medical Society for the Study of Venereal Diseases): National guideline for the management of suspected sexually transmitted infections in children and young people. *Sexually Transmitted Infections* **78**, 324–331.

Van der Werff, J. (2002) Re: A prospective randomised clinical trial to evaluate methods of postoperative care of hypospadias. *Journal of Urology* **167** (4), 1803–1804.

Van Savage, J., Palanca, L., & Slaughenoupt, B. (2000) A prospective randomised trial of dressing versus no dressing for hypospadias repair. *Journal of Urology* **164**, 981–983.

World Health Organization (2008) *Initiative for Vaccine Research: Sexually transmitted diseases*. Available at: **http://www.who.int/vaccine_research/diseases/soa_std/en/index.html** (last accessed October 2008).

Further reading and URLs

European Society for Paediatric Urology (2006) *Guidelines on Paediatric Urology*. World Health Organization. Available from: **http://who.int/ mediacentre/factsheets/fs241/en/index.html**

European Society for Paediatric Urology (2008) *Female Genital Mutilation Fact Sheet*. World Health Organization. Available from: **http://who.int/ mediacentre/factsheets/fs241/en/index.html**

Lloyd, M., Law, G., Heard, A., & Kroese, B. (2008) When a child says 'no': Experiences of nurses working with children having invasive procedures. *Paediatric Nursing* **20** (4), 29–35.

National Screening Committee policy (2006a) *Cryptorchidism Screening*. UK: National Screening Committee.

National Screening Committee policy (2006b) *Chlamydia infection screening*. UK: National Screening Committee.

Nursing and Midwifery Council (2008) *The Code*. London: NMC.

Paul, R. & Johnson V. (2008) Childhood circumcision. *Surgery (Oxford)* **26** (7), 314–316.

Royal College of Nursing (2004) *Sexual Health Competencies: An integrated career and competency framework for sexual and reproductive health nursing*. London: RCN.

Royal College of Nursing (2006) *Chaperoning: The role of the nurse and the rights of the patient*. London: RCN.

Royal College of Nursing (2006) *Vaginal and Pelvic Examination*. London: RCN.

Brook Advisory Centre. Consent to sexual relationships: **http://www.brook.org.uk/content/M5_1_ consent.asp**

Brook Advisory Centre. Sexually transmitted infections: **http://www.brook.org.uk/content/M8_3_STIs. asp**

Childline. Being sexually abused: **http://www. childline.org.uk/Info/AbuseSafety/Pages/ Sexual.aspx**

Department for Education and Skills (2006) What to do if you're worried a child is being abused. DfES Publications: **http://www.everychildmatters. gov.uk/_files/34C39F24E7EF47FBA9139FA01 C7B0370.pdf**

Family Planning Association (2009) Teenagers: Sexual health and behaviour: **http://www.fpa.org.uk/ Information/Factsheets/Teenagers**

Family Planning Association (2009) Under 16s: Consent and confidentiality in sexual health services: **http://www.fpa.org.uk/Information/ Factsheets/consent**

http://www.brook.org.uk/content/

http://www.childline.org.uk/Pages/default. aspx

http://www.everychildmatters.gov.uk

http://www.fpa.org.uk/Homepage

http://www.gosh.nhs.uk/gosh_families/infor- mation_sheets/hypospadias/hypospadias_ families.html

http://www.gosh.nhs.uk/gosh_families/ information_sheets/operation/operation_dis- charge.html

http://www.gosh.nhs.uk/gosh_families/infor- mation_sheets/pain_day_surgery/pain_day_ surgery_families.html

http://www.gosh.nhs.uk/gosh_families/ information_sheets/undescended_testicles/ undescended_testicles_families.html

Glossary

Abdominal palpation Involves inspecting and feeling the abdomen.

Absorption response The way a drug enters the body and reaches the bloodstream.

Abuse and neglect Forms of maltreatment of a child. Somebody may abuse or neglect a child by inflicting harm, or by failing to act to prevent harm. Children may be abused in a family or in an institutional or community setting; by those known to them or, more rarely, by a stranger.

Accessory structures Accessory structures of the skin include hair, nails and glands.

Accommodation Changing or altering our existing schemas or ideas as a result of new information or new experiences.

Acrosome A cover on the sperm head containing enzymes that degrade the covering of the ovum to allow sperm entry.

Acute pain Pain that follows injury or surgery and starts to diminish with pain relief and as healing takes place.

Agonist A drug that occupies and activates a receptor, thereby producing a cellular response.

Analgesia A drug with specific action for the relief of pain.

Antagonist A drug that occupies a receptor but that does not activate the receptor.

Anterior fontanelle A diamond-shaped 'soft spot' that is located between the two parietal bones and the frontal bones of newborns.

Anticonvulsant therapy Treatment involving medication that stops or prevents convulsions.

Antiseptic A substance that inhibits the growth of bacteria.

Aphasia An inability to produce and/or understand language.

Apnoea The temporary cessation of breathing due to infection, disease or inhalation of a foreign body.

Apraxia Loss of the ability to carry out learned purposeful movements.

Arrhythmia An abnormality of electrical conduction through the heart.

Assimilation The process of taking in new information into our previously existing schemas.

Asthma Condition causing inflammation of the airways in response to an allergen. This causes the muscles around the airway walls to tighten, the lining to swell, and the production of mucus.

Attachment An emotional bond between a child and another person.

Attachment figures Any person with whom a child has an emotional bond.

Auscultation The process of listening, usually with a stethoscope, to sounds such as gas or liquid within the body.

Bioavailability The percentage of the drug dose that is absorbed into the systemic circulation after administration.

Blastocyst A hollow ball of cells at the stage of early embryonic development.

Blood brain barrier (BBB) The blood brain barrier refers to the rate-limiting factor in determining permeation of therapeutic drugs into the brain, as unlike most body capillaries that contain pores, the brain's capillaries are tightly joined together and covered on the outside by a fatty barrier called the glial sheath.

Blood glucose level The level of glucose in the blood measured in mmol/L.

Body language The non-verbal actions of one's body such as facial gestures, positioning, or demeanour.

Body mass index (BMI) An index for estimating an individual's weight in relation to their height. Used to detect obesity.

Body surface area (BSA) A measure of the overall size of a person calculated from height and weight. Body surface area is expressed as meters squared or m².

Bradypnoea Slowing of the respiratory rate.

Buccally Buccal relates to the cheek or mouth area. Buccally refers to administering medication in the cheek where it is absorbed into the oral mucosa.

Calcaneal Relates to the calcaneus or heel bone, which is the largest of the tarsal bones of the foot.

Cannulation The process of inserting a cannula into a body cavity or vein. During insertion of the cannula a trocar fills the lumen of the small tube in order to stiffen it. This is removed once the cannula is *in situ* and the small tube is left in place.

Capillary refill time Rate at which blood returns to the capillary bed following digital compression.

Carbohydrate Compounds made up of different types of sugars.

Centile chart Growth charts that are sex specific and show age/time on a horizontal axis and the measurement on a vertical axis.

Cerebral oedema Swelling due to an accumulation of fluid within the brain.

Cerumen Commonly referred to as ear wax. This is produced in the ear canal, is usually honey coloured, and darkens in colour as it is exposed to air.

Cervix The neck-like end portion of the uterus leading to the vagina.

Charrière The measurement used to express the diameter of a catheter.

Child Anyone who has not yet reached his or her 18th birthday.

Child development Refers to the biological and psychological changes that occur in human beings between birth and the end of adolescence, as the individual progresses from dependency to increasing autonomy.

Child protection (or child safeguarding) Process of protecting individual children identified as either suffering, or at risk of suffering, significant harm because of abuse or neglect.

Child Protection Conference
A formal inter-agency meeting, following an enquiry under Section 47 of the Children Act (UK), which decides whether the child is at continuing risk of significant harm and whether the child is to be subject to a child protection plan.

Chronic pain Pain that persists beyond the time span when normal healing would have taken place; it can last for several months or years.

Cilia Tiny, hair-like projections on the cell surface that move in a wave-like manner.

CMV (cytomegalovirus) A virus that is a member of the herpes virus family. Many people contract this virus with no adverse effects. However, it can cause serious complications in a child if their immune system is not working properly; for example, a child with leukaemia receiving chemotherapy.

Cognitive development Development of the ability to think and reason in a child.

Cognitive immaturity Usually refers to young children whose thought processes have not developed yet.

Cognitive psychology The study of human internal mental processes.

Compartment syndrome A painful condition that results from increased pressure (swelling) in a fascial compartment containing muscle. This pressure and swelling can block the blood flow to the muscle leading to necrosis of muscle and nerve if left untreated.

Computed tomography (CT) A diagnostic procedure used for examining soft tissue.

Congenital abnormalities When a baby is born with some sporadic structural abnormality that is not hereditary or related specifically to the birth process.

Core assessment An in-depth assessment that addresses the central or most important aspects of the needs of the child and the capacity of his or her parents or caregivers to respond appropriately to these needs within the wider family and community context.

Cranium The part of the skull that directly covers the brain.

Critical period A period of time during development when the human is especially responsive to and learns from a specific type of stimulation.

Cryptorchidism The absence of one or both testes from the scrotum.

Cyanosis A bluish discolouration of the skin and mucous membranes, resulting from an inadequate amount of oxygen in the blood.

Cystic fibrosis A hereditary disease affecting the cells of the exocrine glands, resulting in the production of thick mucus. This obstructs the intestinal glands, pancreas and bronchi. Respiratory infections, which can be severe, are a common complication.

Depolarization Loss of difference in charge between the inside and the outside of a cell. In the cardiac cycle this occurs just before contraction of atria or ventricles.

Dermatitis Inflammation of the skin caused by contact with an irritant substance such as urine.

Dermis A thick layer of connective tissue containing blood vessels, nerves, glands and hair follicles.

Digital examination Refers to the professional use of gloved finger/s to examine an internal structure; for example, the rectum.

Distribution Where a drug goes in the body after it has been absorbed following administration.

Domain This term is synonymous with a metaphorical field, e.g. 'the domain of child development'; the specific expert knowledge within a particular field.

Drug formulation This is the physical state in which the drug is present, which can be liquid or solid.

Drug tolerance A state of decreasing responsiveness to a toxic effect of a chemical resulting from prior exposure to that chemical or to a structurally related chemical.

Dyspnoea Laboured or difficult breathing due to obstruction to the flow of air in and out of the lungs.

Electroencephalography (EEG) The recording of electric currents arising in the brain.

Electromyogram (EMG) A recording of the electrical activity of a muscle.

Elimination The route by which a substance, or its metabolites, leave the body after administration.

Embryo The first two months of human development after conception.

Encephalitis Inflammation of the central nervous system.

Endometrium The inner lining of the uterus.

Enteral feeding An artificial means of providing nutrients via a tube in the gastrointestinal tract.

Epidermis The outermost layer of the skin consisting of five layers and four principal types of cells.

Epidermolysis bullosa A rare genetic disorder whereby the sufferer develops large fluid-filled sacs and blistering on their skin, from any slight friction to their skin.

Epilepsy A condition in which there are recurrent seizures.

Equilibration The mechanism by which the balance between assimilation and accommodation is achieved.

Eschar Non-viable burn tissue resulting from full-thickness burn injury.

Ethology The study of animal behaviour.

External fixation A method of immobilizing bones to allow a fracture to heal. External fixation is accomplished by placing pins or screws through the bone on both sides of the fracture.

Extravasation The leakage of vesicant (fluid that if it escapes from a vein causes tissue damage), intravenous fluids or medicines into surrounding tissue. Damage can occur to the tissues, tendons, nerves and joints for weeks and months following the insult and in the worst cases reconstructive surgery or amputation may be required.

Exudate Fluid or cells that have moved out of the blood vessels during the inflammatory phase.

Febrile convulsion A seizure that occurs in association with a raised body temperature.

Fertilization Fusion of the nuclei of the male's sperm and female's egg (ovum).

Fibroblasts Connective tissue cells necessary for wound healing.

First-pass metabolism The metabolism of a drug in the liver before it enters the systemic circulation after administration. Consequently, the amount of drug that reaches the site of action after the first-pass effect is reduced.

Fore-milk Milk produced during the early stage of the breast feed. Contains more milk sugars and more protein than the hind milk that follows it.

Frankfurt plane An imaginary line from the centre of the ear hole to the lower border of the eye socket that is used to ensure correct positioning when measuring height.

Genetic epistemology The study of the development of knowledge or how we come to know what we know (intelligence).

Genogram Diagram showing relationships between related family members.

Gestation The period during which a fertilized egg cell develops into a body that is ready to be delivered.

Glucose A simple carbohydrate.

Glycosuria The detection of the abnormal presence of glucose in the urine.

Haematuria The detection of the abnormal presence of blood in the urine.

Haemolysis Destruction of the walls of red blood cells releasing haemoglobin.

Half life (t$_{\frac{1}{2}}$) The time necessary for the plasma drug concentration or the amount of drug in the body to decrease by half following administration.

Head injury Any trauma or injury to the head.

Healthcare-associated infection (HCAI) Any infection that occurs as a result of contact with healthcare-associated activities that are carried out in the acute hospital service, nursing home, patient's own home, or in general practice.

Hernia Soft tissue swelling where one tissue has protruded into another body space.

Hidden harm This is a term used with reference to the impact of parental substance misuse on children and young people.

Homeostasis Attempt to regulate distress by maintaining a stable psychological constant.

Human evolutionary biology The origin of human species.

Hyaline Very fragile membranes.

Hydrocele Accumulation of fluid around the testes.

Hyperglycaemia Abnormally raised blood glucose level.

Hyperplastic Flexible structures, 'bendy'.

Hypodermis The innermost layer of the skin. It provides a cushion between the skin layers, muscles and bones and promotes skin mobility, moulds body contours, and insulates the body.

Hypoglycaemia A lower than normal blood glucose level.

Hypospadias Congenital abnormality of the urethral opening in males; instead of opening at the tip of the penis it opens on the underside of the urethral shaft, in varying degrees.

Hypothermia A dangerously low body temperature.

Hypoxemia Denotes a lack of oxygen in arterial blood.

Hypoxia A deficiency of oxygen to the tissues of the body.

IDDM Insulin dependent diabetes mellitus.

Infiltration The inadvertent administration of an IV drug, or portion of a drug, into the tissues surrounding a vein rather than into the intravascular space of the vein, for which it was intended.

Information-limiting strategy Using actions to limit the amount of information directed at oneself.

Internal contraceptive device A contraceptive device that is inserted into the uterus of a woman's body by a health professional.

Internal working model Mental representation of oneself.

Intracranial pressure (ICP) Refers to pressure within the brain (cranium). This pressure is maintained through the production and absorption of cerebral spinal fluid.

Intracranial pressure (ICP) monitoring This involves the insertion of a fibre optic sensor into part of the brain. The sensor is attached to a machine that monitors the pressure levels.

Intra-thecal Inserting a substance between the meninges of the brain and spinal cord by means of an injection.

Intravenous (IV) Refers to substances that may be injected directly into a vein.

Ketones Fat is broken down into fatty acids when the cells are starved due to a lack of glucose. These fatty acids convert to ketones in the liver.

Ketosis Increased presence of ketones in the blood.

Korotkoff sounds Audible sounds related to the heart beat that are heard when undertaking manual blood pressure measurement.

Lanugo A very fine, soft and unpigmented coat of hairs covering the newborn's body until it is shed about 14 days after birth.

Laryngeal spasm (or laryngospasm) The involuntary closure of the larynx, obstructing the flow of air to the lungs.

Last offices The final nursing care that is given to patients when they die.

Leicester height metre A portable instrument for the accurate measurement of children's height, recommended by the Child Growth Foundation (UK).

Leucocytes White blood cells found in the blood.

Ligand A substance that is capable of binding specifically and reversibly with a binder.

Lipid A fatty substance present in the body.

Local anaesthetic Pain-relieving medication, which blocks the nerves and numbs the area surrounding the pain.

Lumbar puncture A diagnostic test used to remove and examine cerebral spinal fluid.

Magnetic resonance imaging (MRI) An advanced scanning technique that provides unique information about the chemical makeup of tissues.

Multi-Agency Public Protection Arrangements (MAPPA) The name given to the assessment and management of the most serious sexual and violent offenders in England and Wales.

Multi-Agency Risk Assessment Conferences (MARAC) The name given to multi-agency meetings, which focus on the victims of domestic violence where there is a high or very high risk (UK).

Mechanical ventilation Mechanical support provided to a patient who is unable to breathe normally for themselves. Devices maintain airflow in and out of the lungs either completely or partially (with patient assistance).

Menarche A girl's first menstrual period/onset of menstruation.

Meningitis Inflammation of the meninges (the protective membranes surrounding the brain and spinal cord).

Meningoencephalitis Inflammation of the meninges and the brain.

Menopause The physiological end of menstrual cycles.

Menstrual problems Problems of duration, frequency, or flow of the menstrual cycle.

Menstruation/menstrual period The monthly discharge of blood from the uterus from puberty to menopause.

Metabolism/ biotransformation Refers to how a substance is changed by the body.

Micro-organism A minute animal or vegetable, particularly a virus, a bacterium, or a protozoon.

Micturition The actual physical act of passing urine out of the body.

Milestones The changes in specific physical and mental abilities (such as walking and understanding language) that mark the end of one developmental period and the beginning of another.

mmHg An abbreviation of measurement, to indicate millimetres of mercury (pressure).

Modular feeds A feed that is formulated from separate ingredients. It allows adjustment of protein, carbohydrates, and fats to meet the needs of individual patients.

Morphology Rules governing the formation of meaningful words from sounds.

Nature versus nurture The importance of an individual's innate qualities, genetic makeup, and biology (nature), versus personal experiences ('nurture') in determining or causing individual differences in physical and behavioural traits.

Necrosis The death of some or all of the cells in an organ or tissue. Caused by disease or injury.

Nerve conduction velocity (NCV) A test that measures the speed and intensity of electrical signals travelling along the nerves.

Neurovascular assessment Evaluation of the neurological and vascular integrity of a limb.

Non-accidental injury (NAI) An injury that occurs as a result of deliberate action. It is suspected when the rationale for an injury is inconsistent with the explanation given or when there is reasonable suspicion that the injury was inflicted.

Normal flora Micro-organisms such as bacteria that normally live on body tissues and have a beneficial effect.

NSAIDs Non-steroidal anti-inflammatory drugs, a group of non-narcotic pain relieving medicines that also reduce fever.

Opioid A group of substances called narcotics that contain strong pain relief and cause side effects such as drowsiness.

Oral aversion Occurs in infants who have constant negative oral stimulation and who do not commence oral feeds.

Oral rehydration salt A balanced glucose-electrolyte mixture, which when mixed with water is used to treat dehydration.

OTC (over the counter) Refers to medication that may be purchased in a pharmacy where a prescription is not normally required to purchase these products. One example of an OTC medication is paracetamol.

Ovarian cycle The monthly cycle of follicle development, ovulation, and corpus luteum formation in the ovary.

Ovulation The release of an ovum (egg) from the ovary.

Papilloedema Swelling of the optic disc.

Partial agonist Produces less than a maximal response even when it occupies all of the receptors.

Pathogenic micro-organisms Disease-causing micro-organisms.

Patient group direction (PGD) Legal framework (within the UK) that allows certain healthcare professionals to supply and administer specific medications to patients that meet exact criteria outlined within the PGD. For further information see **http://www.npc.co.uk/** for National Prescribing Centre guidelines on PGDs.

Personal protective equipment (PPE) Items, equipment, and clothing that can be used by a person during work activities to protect their health and safety.

Pharmacokinetics The process by which drugs are absorbed, distributed, metabolized, and excreted from the body.

Phimosis Where the foreskin is not retractable over the head of the penis.

Phlebitis Inflammation of a vein that can be classified according to its cause: chemical caused by solutions irritating the lining; mechanical caused by physical trauma including the cannula moving in the vein; and caused by infection. When the inflammation is caused by blood clots accumulating in the vein it is referred to as thrombophlebitis.

Phonology Refers to the basic units of sound or phonemes that are used in a language and the rules for combining these sounds.

Physical dependence An adaptive physiological state that manifests itself by intense physical disturbance when the administration of a drug is suspended.

Plaster cast An orthopaedic casting tape used to encase a fracture in the required shape to allow a broken bone to heal naturally and protect damaged muscle.

Pragmatics Principles that underlie the effective and appropriate use of language in social contexts.

Prescription only medications (POMs) Drugs and other preparations that require a prescription in order to acquire them.

Psychoanalysis The study of human psychological functioning.

Psychological dependence Refers to a strong compulsion or desire to experience the effects of a drug because it produces pleasure or reduces psychic discomfort.

Puberty The time reproductive organs become functional.

Pyrexia A rise in body temperature to any point between 37 and 40 degrees centigrade.

Ready-to-use feeds Feeds that are prepared by the manufacturer and only require attaching to the administration set or feeding tube.

Reagent strips Chemical analysis strips.

Receptor The reactive site of a cell or tissue that can be occupied by a drug and result in a pharmacological response.

Renal calculi Kidney stones.

Retinopathy Damage to the retina of the eye, caused by a lack of oxygen in neonates.

Retractile testes Where the testes do not stay in the scrotum.

Safeguarding and promoting the welfare of children The process of protecting children from abuse or neglect, preventing impairment of their health and development, and ensuring they are growing up in circumstances consistent with the provision of safe and effective care, which is undertaken so as to enable children to have optimum life chances and enter adulthood successfully.

Schema The mental and physical actions involved in understanding and knowing. Schemas are categories of knowledge that help us to interpret and understand the world.

Secondary sex characteristics External anatomical characteristics that develop under the influence of sex hormones.

Section 17 Section of the Children Act 1989 that imposes a duty on Children's Services Social Care to safeguard and promote the welfare of children in their area who are in need (UK).

Section 47 Enquiry Section 47 of the Children Act requires every Children's Services Social Care department to make enquiries about children thought to be at risk, enabling them to decide whether they need to take further action to safeguard and promote the child's welfare (UK).

Seizures Malfunctions of the brain's electrical system.

Self-determination Being able to have some say in what you want or do.

Semantics Refers to the meanings expressed in words and sentences.

Semi-Fowler's position Semi-upright position. Head and shoulders elevated.

Sensitive period A period of time in development when a particular type of stimulation is particularly important or effective.

Separation anxiety A child's fear of separation from their parents or other caregiver.

Sexually transmitted infection Refers to a group of infections that are given and received through sexual contact.

Significant harm Harm to a child who meets the criteria for an application to court under Section 31 of the Children Act 1989. Harm means ill treatment, or impairment of physical or mental health, or physical, intellectual, emotional, social, or behavioural development.

Social agency Means being able to act on behalf of yourself or in your own self-interest.

Social development/ psychosocial development The process by which a child learns to interact with others, involving aspects of social and psychological behaviour.

Speculum A metal or plastic instrument used for looking inside the vagina.

Spermatogenesis Production of sperm cells in the male, which involves meiosis.

Status epilecticus A continuous seizure that lasts for more than 30 minutes or a series of seizures in which the patient does not regain consciousness.

Strategy for Anti-microbial Resistance in Ireland (SARI) Health Service Executive's national strategy for the prevention and control of antibiotic resistance in the Republic of Ireland.

Subarachnoid haemorrhage A haemorrhage (bleed) into the subarachnoid space of the brain.

Surfactant A complex mixture produced by type 2 pneumocytes, which determine the surface tension in the lungs. It is detectable from 25 weeks gestation, but is not sufficient for alveolar stability. The most common breathing problem in neonates is surfactant deficient lung disease. Exogenous (external) surfactant is given to all premature neonates requiring artificial respiratory support.

Syntax Study of the principles and rules for constructing sentences. The term syntax is also used to refer directly to the rules and principles that govern the sentence structure of any individual language. Syntax is the way in which words are combined.

Theorists Individuals who develop theories.

Theory An organized set of principles that is designed to explain and predict something, for example development. A theory makes generalizations about observations and consists of an interrelated, coherent set of ideas and models.

Torsion A twist in the testes, needing surgery.

Type 1 diabetes Insulin dependent diabetes that is caused by a failure of the pancreas to produce insulin.

Type 2 diabetes Non-insulin dependent diabetes caused by an increased resistance to insulin that is produced in the pancreas.

Unconsciousness A state of unawareness and inability to perceive. It may occur as a result of shock, severe trauma, or serious illness.

Undescended testes The absence of one or both testes from the scrotum, also known as cryptorchidism.

Universal precautions Precautions to be observed when handling any body fluids including wearing a disposable plastic apron and wearing disposable gloves.

Urinalysis Testing of urine specimens.

Urine sample A small amount of urine that is obtained and sent to the laboratory for examination.

Venepuncture The insertion of a needle into a vein in order to obtain a sample of the circulating blood volume. May be performed by a wide variety of staff including phlebotomists, nurses, and medical staff. The needle is removed once the specimen is obtained.

Wilm's tumour Cancer of the kidney.

Working weight Weight at which medications/diet/ nutrition is prescribed. May not be the actual weight.

Xiphisternum Also referred to as the xiphoid process, it is the lowest segment of the sternum. It consists of cartilage during infancy and childhood. During CPR if the hands are not correctly positioned it is possible to fracture the xiphisternum, which may cause damage to other internal organs.

Index